D1766062

Emergency abdominal surgery

surgery

med on or

Emergency abdominal surgery

in infancy, childhood and adult life

Third edition

Edited by

Peter F. Jones, MChir, FRCSEng, FRCSEd

Honorary Consulting Surgeon, Royal Aberdeen Children's Hospital and Aberdeen
Royal Infirmary; Emeritus Clinical Professor of Surgery, University of Aberdeen

Zygmunt H. Krukowski, PhD, FRCSEd

Consultant Surgeon, Aberdeen Royal Infirmary; Clinical Reader in Surgery,
University of Aberdeen

George G. Youngson, PhD, FRCSEd

Consultant Paediatric Surgeon, Royal Aberdeen Children's Hospital; Clinical Senior
Lecturer in Paediatric Surgery, University of Aberdeen

CHAPMAN & HALL MEDICAL
London · Weinheim · New York · Tokyo · Melbourne · Madras

Published by
**Chapman & Hall, an imprint of Lippincott–Raven Publishers Inc.,
2–6 Boundary Row, London SE1 8HN, UK**

Lippincott–Raven Publishers Inc., 227 East Washington Square, Philadelphia, PA 19106–3780, USA

First edition 1974, second edition 1987, published by Blackwell Scientific

Third edition 1998

© 1998 Chapman & Hall

Typeset in 10/12 Times by Genesis Typesetting, Laser Quay, Rochester, Kent

Printed in Great Britain by St Edmundsbury Press, Bury St Edmunds, Suffolk

ISBN 0 412 81950 3

A catalogue record for this book is available from the British Library

Library of Congress Catalog Card Number:98–71425

♾ Printed on acid-free text paper, manufactured in accordance with ANSI/NISO Z39.48–1992 (Permanence of Paper).

To the General Surgeons of the Future, in recognition of their hard-won skills and judgement, their concern for their patients, and their continued commitment to emergency care.

Contents

Contributors

Frederick H. Bagley, MD, FACS
Assistant Clinical Professor of Surgery, University of Vermont, Rutland, Vermont, USA

Lynne W. Baker, MSc, FRCS, Hon Fellow AAST
Professor Emeritus of Surgery, University of Natal, Durban, South Africa.

Peter W. Brunt, MD, FRCP, FRCPEd
Consultant Physician/ Gastroenterologist, Aberdeen Royal Infirmary; Clinical Professor of Medicine, University of Aberdeen, UK

Jetmund Engeset, ChM, FRCSEd
Consultant Vascular Surgeon, Aberdeen Royal Infirmary; Clinical Senior Lecturer, University of Aberdeen, UK

L. Peter Fielding, MB, BS, FRCSEng, FACS
Director, Surgical Service Line, Chairman, Department of Surgery, York Hospital, York; Professor of Clinical Surgery, Pennsylvania State University College of Medicine, PA, USA

Marion H. Hall, MD, FRCOG
Consultant in Obstetrics and Gynaecology, Aberdeen Royal Hospitals NHS Trust; Clinical Reader in Obstetrics and Gynaecology, University of Aberdeen, UK

Kevin Jennings FRCP, FESC
Consultant Cardiologist, Aberdeen Royal Infirmary; Clinical Senior Lecturer in Medicine, University of Aberdeen, UK

Peter F. Jones MChir, FRCSEng, FRCSEd
Honorary Consulting Surgeon, Royal Aberdeen Children's Hospital and Aberdeen Royal Infirmary; Emeritus Clinical Professor of Surgery, University of Aberdeen, UK

Ronald A. Keenan ChM, FRCSEd
Consultant Surgeon, Aberdeen Royal Infirmary; Clinical Senior Lecturer in Surgery, University of Aberdeen, UK

Derek J. King, FRCPEd, FRCPath
Consultant Haematologist, Royal Aberdeen Children's Hospital; Clinical Senior Lecturer
in Medicine, University of Aberdeen, UK

N. Mathew Koruth ChM, FRCS
Consultant Surgeon, Aberdeen Royal Infirmary; Clinical Senior Lecturer in Surgery,
University of Aberdeen, UK

Zygmunt H. Krukowski PhD, FRCSEd
Consultant Surgeon, Aberdeen Royal Infirmary; Clinical Reader in Surgery, University of
Aberdeen, UK

Joe Legge MD, FRCP, FRCPEd
Consultant Physician, Aberdeen Royal Infirmary; Clinical Senior Lecturer in Thoracic
Medicine, University of Aberdeen, UK

John R. C. Logie PhD, FRCSEd, FRCSEng, FRCSGlas
Consultant Surgeon, Raigmore Hospital, Inverness; Clinical Senior Lecturer in Surgery,
University of Aberdeen, UK

Alasdair Munro ChM, FRCSEd
Consultant Surgeon, Raigmore Hospital, Inverness; Clinical Senior Lecturer in Surgery,
University of Aberdeen, UK

David W. Noble BMedBiol FRCA
Consultant in Anaesthesia and Intensive Care, Aberdeen Royal Infirmary; Clinical Senior
Lecturer in Anaesthesia, University of Aberdeen, UK

Donald W. M. Pearson BSc, FRCPGlas, FRCPEd
Consultant Physician, Diabetic Clinic, Aberdeen Royal Hospitals NHS Trust; Clinical
Senior Lecturer in Medicine, University of Aberdeen, UK

Robert J. C. Steele, MD, FRCS
Professor of Surgical Oncology, University of Dundee, UK

Sandie R. Thomson, ChM, FRCS Ed, FRCSEng
Associate Professor and Reader in Surgery, University of Natal, Durban, South Africa

George G. Youngson, PhD, FRCSEd
Consultant Paediatric Surgeon, Royal Aberdeen Children's Hospital; Clinical Senior
Lecturer in Surgery, University of Aberdeen, UK

Preface

Emergency abdominal surgery cannot be learned from the pages of a book. So practical a subject must be studied at the bedside, and experienced in the operating theatre, where the accuracy of diagnosis and the details of operative technique are practised, at first under the guidance of a senior colleague. Training is increasingly concentrated and lessons must be learned from each patient seen. These experiences mean much more if each one is seen against a background of the whole field, and the first aim of this book is to give such a background. Each chapter can be read straight through as a review of the subject and its literature, and has been written with the practical requirements of the surgical trainee in mind.

A second aim has been to provide a handbook for consultation on a specific problem, with detailed advice on management and technique.

The first edition was written in the early 1970s when the registrar and senior registrar on duty in a busy district hospital might expect to see a number of emergency admissions, some requiring an urgent operation while others would be placed under observation. An evening operating list might start at about 7.00 pm and finish in the early hours. A newly arrived acute appendix might need to be slipped into theatre at 7.00 am before the normal day's work began again at 8.00 am.

The technical challenges of these spells of duty were considerable, at a beginner's level for the newly appointed registrar and at quite an advanced level for the senior registrar or resident still building experience in major abdominal surgery. Then it was appropriate for the dedication to be made to – 'The Night Watch – my registrar colleagues over the years, in recognition of their hard-won skills and judgement, their concern for their patients, and their continued dedication to emergency care'.

One of the consequences of this training was that registrars were taught to perform the least extensive procedure that would enable the patient to survive. This minimalist approach was a survivor from the first 40 years of the century, when anaesthesia was in a relatively primitive state, often administered by a house surgeon, little was known about fluid and electrolyte balance, and antibiotics were at an early stage of development. However, by the 1970s there had been great progress in the specialty of anaesthesia and in the conduct of pre- and postoperative care, and the first edition had to reflect these developments by recording the work of pioneers who had demonstrated during the 1950s and 1960s the possibility of using major definitive surgery in the immediate treatment of gastrointestinal perforation, obstruction and haemorrhage, and the leaking abdominal aortic aneurysm.

This development heralded an important change in the organization of emergency work, because these operations required an experienced surgeon and anaesthetist for their safe and expeditious performance. They demonstrated to senior registrars and residents the contribution that definitive treatment could make to emergency surgery.

When the second edition was written in 1984–1986 this change was well under way and the trainees, now consultants, were regularly demonstrating the advantage to the patient of having their problems dealt with in one stage.

This change was perhaps most marked in vascular and colorectal surgery. It had soon become clear that the demands of the elderly patient with a ruptured abdominal aortic aneurysm could only be met with generally favourable results by an experienced vascular team. At the same time general surgeons who had developed an interest in colorectal surgery were demonstrating the advantages of selective immediate resection, followed in some cases by immediate anastomosis, in the neoplastic and inflammatory emergencies of the large bowel. These demonstrations revealed the quality of work that could be offered when interested surgeons become involved in emergency abdominal surgery. This experience has a particular relevance now, coming at precisely the time when the hours of duty of surgical trainees have statutory limits and the length of higher training is reduced to 5 years. Just as the number of patients attending with an acute appendix or a perforated peptic ulcer has been falling, the exposure of the individual trainee to this work has diminished quite noticeably. The chance for the trainee to share, in turn, in the work of units each with a particular interest in gastroduodenal, colorectal, paediatric, vascular or cardiothoracic surgery is more restricted, and advanced training offers a more intensive study of new specialized aspects of surgery.

This book has had to adapt to this change, and the range of our contributors reflects the fact that one surgeon can no longer cover adequately all aspects of emergency abdominal surgery. The newly appointed registrar will still find an introduction to this important aspect of their work. The specialist registrar or resident who needs to revise an unfamiliar subject will find a detailed account, written by an expert. Consultant posts are now filled by surgeons who have gained most of their experience in one or two specialized fields, yet, when on emergency call in a district hospital, they remain general surgeons who are responsible for the full range of emergency work; until the time comes when several surgeons with different interests share a spell on call, we hope that this book will prove to be a useful work of reference. As in previous editions, it is our hope that the surgeon who works alone, when faced with an unfamiliar problem, may find some practical suggestions from an experienced specialist.

We are very grateful for the time and effort of our contributors, and for their tolerance of editorial suggestions and amendments. We are most appreciative of the secretarial skills of Pauline Bennett. Once again it is a pleasure to thank Dr Paul Lawrence and the staff of Aberdeen University Medical School Library for providing so willing and effective a service. New illustrations are again the work of Nigel Lukins of the University Department of Medical Illustration, and we thank him warmly for his patience and skill in the interpretation of our sketches. Our wives are already far too experienced in coping with additional demands on our time, but this does not lessen our deep appreciation of their tolerance and encouragement.

Peter F. Jones
Zygmunt H. Krukowski
George G. Youngson
Aberdeen, February 1998

1

Introduction

1.1 INTRODUCTION

For the abdominal surgeon it is a familiar experience to sit, ready scrubbed and gowned, in a corner of the quiet theatre, with the clock pointing to midnight. The scrub nurse is arranging her trolley and from the anaesthetic room comes the sound of the induction of anaesthesia. In a few minutes the patient will be wheeled in and another emergency laparotomy will commence. This is the culmination of a process which began a few hours previously with the surgeon meeting with and examining the patient, reaching a diagnosis, and making a plan of action.

The waiting surgeon, mulling over the features of the case, experiences a distinctive mixture of excitement and curiosity, of challenge and of responsibility. It is the nature of emergency surgery that however clear the diagnosis may appear to be, one can never be certain of what will be found, or of the correctness of one's decisions, or of one's ability to cope with the unexpected. At the start of training these apprehensions are extremely acute as one approaches even the simpler procedures. They do not disappear with increasing experience because, although the surgeon is better able to cope with the unexpected, that wider experience teaches that the acute abdomen is a field in which one never ceases to learn, to be surprised, and to have one's resources fully extended. Therein, of course, lies its fascination, however late the hour at which it has to be practised.

This introduction appears in the second edition of this book and it still expresses some of the enduring features of emergency work. However, surgical training is continuously undergoing change – the period of formal training is shorter, hours on call are fewer and it is generally recognized that it is better for patients and for staff if most emergency surgery takes place during the 'daytime' hours. It is necessary, therefore, to take every opportunity to participate actively in this field. Emergency admissions to general surgical wards contribute nearly half the workload and, whatever the special interests of the surgeons of the unit, these patients require knowledgeable care.

Emergency abdominal surgery remains one of the few areas of medical practice in which the essential ingredients in reaching a diagnosis and deciding on a plan of action are provided by the patient's history and by the signs that are elicited at the bedside. Special investigations play a relatively small part in this process. Sound clinical judgment is one of the most important elements in a surgeon's equipment, and the thoughtful acquisition of a body of

Emergency Abdominal Surgery. Edited by Peter F. Jones, Zygmunt H. Krukowski and George G. Youngson. Published in 1998 by Chapman & Hall, London. ISBN 0 412 81950 3.

experience in emergency work, with discussion and teaching at the bedside and in the operating theatre, is one of the best ways of developing this skill. To be the first to see an emergency, to form conclusions, to have them tested in theatre and exercise newly acquired skills in the treatment of this particular patient is to experience, in a very personal manner, both the satisfaction and challenges that make surgery a subject of continuing deep interest. Emergency abdominal surgery covers a wide field and it is important to acquire as wide an experience as possible. Surgical training currently encourages the development of an interest in one or two sub-specialties, but patients who arrive as emergencies have not been subject to any selection process and the surgeon must be ready to offer a high standard of care over a wide field. At times the urgency and time constraints of the emergency situation mean that important decisions have to be taken speedily and recovery depends on skilful surgery practised in difficult circumstances. Surgeons in training need to immerse themselves in this subject and take every available opportunity to gain and widen experience.

1.1.1   HISTORY

It is in the nature of emergency admissions for them to occur at odd and often unsocial hours when everyone is busy, but, because bedside assessment is so important, it is necessary to take time over it. It helps to shake hands, exchange names and then sit down and perhaps feel the pulse; the patient will then sense that the busy surgeon will not immediately dart away and is ready to listen. One must remember that the patient is likely to be frightened, uncomfortable and worried about outcome, work and, more often than not, the care of the family at home. It requires patience and understanding to obtain a clear history, but it will contain vital information and it is wise to allow time for it to emerge. It can help to start the conversation with some generalities and this may show that the surgeon is prepared to spend time with the patient and is sufficiently attentive and interested. It is not unusual, however, for the urgency of the illness or the degree of pain to be such that only essential points can be obtained. Sometimes there are language difficulties and, in children, parents may have to interpret. Useful insights can come from relatives and from the referring doctor's letter.

One needs to learn as much detail as possible about the characteristics of acute abdominal pain. The site is very helpful – intestinal colic is referred to the midline, ureteric colic is lateralized in one flank and groin. If the moment of onset can be clearly remembered, it must have been sudden, such as occurs when a peptic ulcer perforates. Shift of pain and areas of referred pain can be significant, including pain referred *via* the phrenic nerve to the supraclavicular region and down an intercostal nerve to the abdomen. Severity can be judged by the behaviour of the patient and by comparison with other pains. The character of the pain needs analysis – the intermittent nature of intestinal colic is different from the steady pain of the parietal peritoneal reaction to perforated appendicitis. Factors that aggravate pain can be helpful – for example, the pain of peritonitis is made worse by movement and coughing.

Current medication and any allergies must be recorded. The past medical history can be very relevant and the notes of previous admissions, if available, should be scrutinized. It is the responsibility of the surgeon to strive to establish the fitness of the patient before the acute event, e.g. the patient with a ruptured abdominal aortic aneurysm or the respiratory patient who becomes ventilator-dependent postoperatively. Sometimes a question about family history or social circumstances can prompt valuable information.

The ethnic origin of a patient can have an important bearing on perioperative care, e.g. the sickle-cell status of an Afro-Caribbean patient, in whom hypoxia may herald a crisis (p. 540)

1.1.2 THE EXAMINATION

It is a mistake to think that the examination starts only after the history has been taken. It begins from the time that the surgeon reaches the foot of the bed and forms an immediate impression of the patient. The pallor of internal haemorrhage, the tense, ill, unmoving patient with peritonitis, the restless patient with colic all give an important and immediate message.

It may or may not be right to proceed to examine in an orderly manner from head to toe; it is certainly necessary not to concentrate so much on abdominal examination that other systems are overlooked – as becomes very clear when the differential diagnosis is considered. It is useful to sit and count the pulse and quietly observe the respiration rate, which is sometimes significant. This gives a pause in which the patient can relax and the course of the examination can be explained. The blood pressure must be taken at a convenient moment.

When the time comes to examine the abdomen, it is essential to have the patient lying flat, with the head on one pillow. The whole abdomen should be exposed and if, out of a reasonable consideration for the patient's feelings, the genitalia are kept covered, then these must be uncovered later and the hernial orifices and scrotum examined. It is wise first to sit and look at the abdomen, preferably with light shining across it. This sometimes reveals visible peristalsis or a localized swelling and it always shows the degree of respiratory movement of the abdominal wall. Occasionally bruising (perhaps from a seat belt in blunt abdominal trauma) can be seen, or the ecchymosis in the flank or round the umbilicus that denotes retroperitoneal haemorrhage in acute pancreatitis.

It is desirable to have warm hands when palpating the abdomen and to palpate gently, and therefore informatively, when sitting or kneeling at the bedside. It is wise to start where it is unlikely there will be tenderness and to progress slowly towards areas likely to be sore, gaining impressions of tenderness and of tone of the abdominal muscles. The gentle approach is vital and any sudden pressure on a tender area will generate voluntary generalized guarding (p. 41). It is much easier to be gentle if the forearm and the hand are kept in a straight line, and careful 'dipping' into the abdomen is produced by flexing the straight fingers at the metocarpo-phalangeal joints (Figure 1.1).

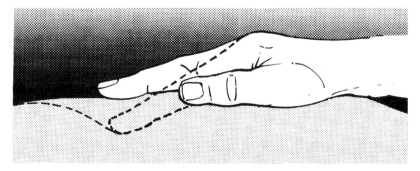

Figure 1.1 Abdominal palpation. The forearm and hand are kept straight and horizontal. Pressure is exerted by gentle flexing of the straight fingers at the metacarpophalangeal joints.

It helps to move the hand around in a circular manner, the skin moving with the hand over the subcutaneous tissues. Throughout, it is better to watch the patient's face rather than the abdomen. Great care must be exercised over eliciting the signs of rebound tenderness (p. 42). Auscultation can provide essential information in intestinal obstruction but to pronounce on the 'absence' or 'presence' of bowel sounds may require auscultation to continue over several minutes.

Details of abdominal examination are considered in the section on abdominal pain in childhood (p. 91), acute appendicitis (p. 41), intestinal obstruction (p. 188) and abdominal trauma (p. 423). Rectal and vaginal examination are essential in some circumstances and are described on p. 44, and in Chapters 12 and 13.

The emergency surgeon must be able to read plain X-rays of the chest and abdomen, and know when an emergency contrast examination, or a scan, can provide vital information. The interpretation of emergency blood counts and biochemical tests must be familiar ground.

1.1.3   THE DIAGNOSTIC PROCESS

In hospital practice most patients are referred by their family doctor, but these doctors see comparatively few patients with an acute abdomen. Fry (1983) calculated that, in his practice of 7500 patients, the three partners saw, as individuals in the course of a year, only two patients with acute appendicitis and one with intestinal obstruction. Surgeons with a much wider experience often find diagnosis difficult, so at a brief interview in the home it is particularly difficult for family doctors to do much more than decide on the need for admission. The letter that accompanies these patients often contains vital information but the provisional diagnosis is what it says – provisional.

The surgeon, therefore, needs to approach the patient with an open mind and allow patients to tell their own story. We have found a structured record form (Figure 1.2) very useful.

It acts as a prompt, because it is easy to forget to ask a vital question. It makes for accurate observation to write down exactly the signs that are observed. Then it is a valuable exercise always to write down a differential diagnosis, a provisional diagnosis and a proposed line of action, and later to check these against the final diagnosis and outcome.

There has been much debate over the last 20 years over the merits of computer-aided diagnosis, but there is general agreement that a major factor in the improvement in diagnostic accuracy that was attributed to computer analysis was due to the attention given to accurate completion of the forms. The thought given to writing down the differential diagnosis, the steady growth in experience as the final result in each patient was compared with this first impression, and regular reviews of results at unit meetings, means that everyone is involved in maintaining a high standard of emergency work.

The majority of abdominal surgical emergencies that require an operation cause either: peritoneal irritation due to inflammation or rupture of an organ or vessel; obstruction of a hollow organ; or haemorrhage into the alimentary tract. Another significant group are those who do not require operation, e.g. many patients with a ureteric calculus or acute pancreatitis, or those who, at the time of discharge, prove to be one of the considerable number of patients with non-specific abdominal pain (NSAP), which settles without treatment and is described on pp. 49–52.

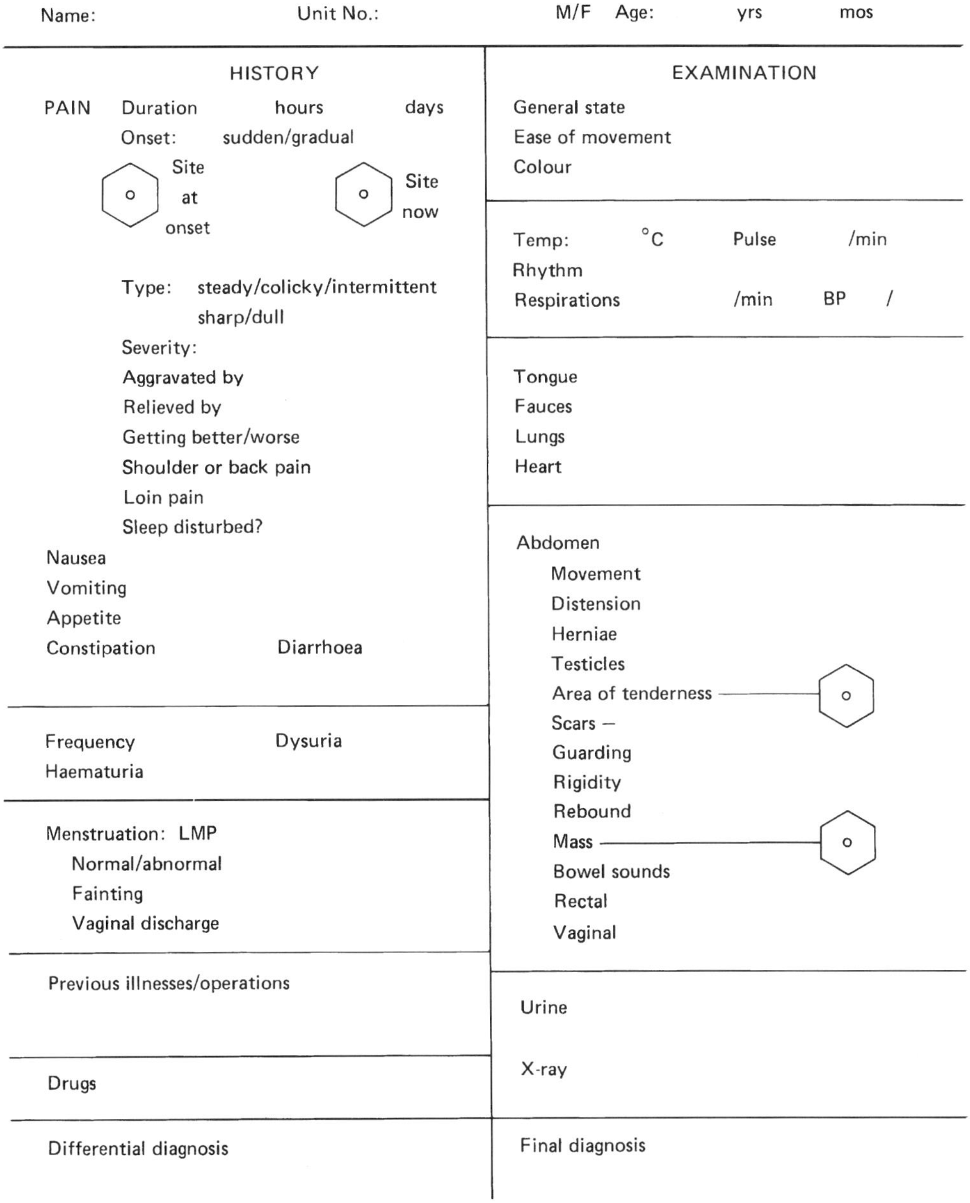

Name: Unit No.:   M/F   Age: yrs   mos

HISTORY	EXAMINATION
PAIN Duration hours days	General state
Onset: sudden/gradual	Ease of movement
Site at onset Site now	Colour
Type: steady/colicky/intermittent	Temp: °C Pulse /min
sharp/dull	Rhythm
Severity:	Respirations /min BP /
Aggravated by	Tongue
Relieved by	Fauces
Getting better/worse	Lungs
Shoulder or back pain	Heart
Loin pain	
Sleep disturbed?	Abdomen
Nausea	Movement
Vomiting	Distension
Appetite	Herniae
Constipation Diarrhoea	Testicles
	Area of tenderness
	Scars —
Frequency Dysuria	Guarding
Haematuria	Rigidity
	Rebound
Menstruation: LMP	Mass
Normal/abnormal	Bowel sounds
Fainting	Rectal
Vaginal discharge	Vaginal
Previous illnesses/operations	Urine
Drugs	X-ray
Differential diagnosis	Final diagnosis

Figure 1.2 Record sheet for the patient with acute abdominal pain.

Tables 1.1–1.3 show the relative frequency of common emergencies in the adult and paediatric age groups.

This is useful because the range of surgical diseases in children is comparatively restricted but the incidence varies greatly among adults below, as opposed to those above, 50 years of age. The tables also show the substantial number of patients who present with NSAP and is

Table 1.1 Acute abdominal pain at various ages

Adult*	%	Children†	%
Acute appendicitis	28	Acute appendicitis	24
NSAP	34	NSAP	52
Acute cholecystitis	10	Medical conditions	18
Small bowel obstruction	4	Constipation	11 (60%)
Gynaecological	4	Urinary tract infection	3 (16%)
Acute pancreatitis	3	Gastroenteritis	2 (10%)
Renal colic	3	Ovulation pain	2 (10%)
Perforated peptic ulcer	3	Other surgical conditions	5
Malignancy	2	Intussusception	
Diverticulitis	2	Splenic/liver injury	
Dyspepsia	1	Adhesive obstruction	
Liver abscess	1		
Miscellaneous	6		

* Data from de Dombal, 1988
† Data from Driver and Youngson, 1995

Table 1.2 Acute lower abdominal pain in women (Data from de Dombal, 1991)

	Proportion (%) within each age range				Overall frequency (%)
	< 20 years	20–30 years	30–40 years	> 40 years	
Acute appendicitis	50	20	15	15	22
NSAP	57	26	11	6	48
Salpingitis	34	44	18	4	14
Urinary tract infection	37	32	9	22	12
Ovarian cyst	18	38	14	30	4
Ectopic pregnancy	4	54	38	4	1
Incomplete abortion	13	47	33	7	1

Table 1.3 Spectrum of disease in patients above and below 50 years of age (Reproduced from Telfer *et al.*, 1988)

6317 patients under 50 years		2406 patients over 50 years	
NSAP	39.5	Cholecystitis	20.9
Appendicitis	32.0	NSAP	15.7
Cholecystitis	6.3	Appendicitis	15.2
Small bowel obstruction	2.5	Small bowel obstruction	12.3
Pancreatitis	1.6	Pancreatitis	7.3
Diverticulitis	<0.1	Diverticulitis	5.5
Cancer	<0.1	Cancer	4.1
Hernia	<0.1	Hernia	3.1
Vascular	<0.1	Vascular	2.3
Other	17.7	Other	13.6

a reminder that diagnosis is by no means always clear at the time of admission and that a period of close observation is often a correct first line of action.

1.1.4 MAKING A PLAN OF ACTION

Provisional diagnosis and decision on a line of action in fact go hand in hand, are often dictated by the urgency of the situation and take one of four general directions.

(a) Immediate surgery

It is unusual and generally undesirable for a patient to be 'rushed to theatre'. Uncontrolled haemorrhage is the main indication. In acute rupture of a tubal pregnancy (p. 497) and in acute rupture of an abdominal aortic aneurysm (p. 518) it is vital not to waste time in attempts at resuscitation but to take the patient directly to theatre – surgical arrest of haemorrhage is an essential element of resuscitation. In these young women and elderly men the whole picture is highly suggestive of the diagnosis and immediately leads to action.

(b) Patients who need a period of preoperative preparation

Anyone who has vomited repeatedly, who has been bleeding over a period of time or who has serious sepsis must be prepared for surgery. In a child with a perforated appendix and peritonitis, some hours spent in giving intravenous fluid, including colloid and parenteral antibiotics, converts a potentially unstable situation into a safe and controlled operation (p. 84). At this age appendicitis is much the most likely diagnosis; later in life there are more numerous possible causes of general peritonitis, but the decisions in management in these patients are largely made on the basis of the existence of peritonitis and its correct staged treatment, rather than the precise cause.

In patients with an acute small-bowel obstruction, the cause may be apparent (e.g. a strangulated external hernia) or probable (e.g. the scar of a previous laparotomy, making adhesions the likely cause). The priorities lie in spending some time on rehydration before the laparotomy (p. 190). In patients who continue to bleed from the alimentary tract there is a balance to be struck between preoperative resuscitation and operation to stop the bleeding (p. 350). Some patients with a medical condition, e.g. diabetes mellitus, may need a period of careful preparation before it is safe to operate (p. 537).

In these situations, the initial clinical assessment is concerned mainly with identifying the major threat, be it peritonitis or bowel obstruction, preparing the patient and then discovering and treating the actual cause when it is revealed at laparotomy.

(c) Patients who need a period of rest, hydration and analgesia before operation

Many patients come into this category, including the majority with acute appendicitis. Some will have had an uncomfortable ambulance journey and all will benefit from early relief of pain and a period of rest in a warm bed.

Analgesia
For many years it has been traditional teaching that a patient with acute abdominal pain should not receive an analgesic until a diagnosis has been made, but this teaching of Zachary

Cope, dating from 1921, has had an unduly long life. He was then rightly concerned that family doctors would often give a patient with an acute abdomen up to 30 mg of morphine: this certainly gave relief but then, hours later when the doctor returned, the situation had deteriorated and when Cope arrived he found a gravely ill patient. In fact, if opiates are used wisely, they can provide early relief of pain without obscuring signs or delaying decisions.

In 100 patients admitted with acute abdominal pain in Coventry, Attard *et al.* (1992) randomly administered at the time of admission either a saline injection or up to 20 mg papaveretum (12.5 mg morphine), depending on age and weight. Over 90% of the treated group received useful relief of pain. The question is whether the analgesia so modifies abdominal signs that a misleading impression is received. In the event, when the surgical registrar examined the treated patients an hour or so later, the decisions made then proved on later review to have been correct. When we made a similar trial in 1980 we found the greater comfort of the treated group made it easier to detect and localize true areas of tenderness and guarding in the abdomen.

Rehydration
Anyone who has felt ill and nauseated for 24 hours will have had little to drink and may have vomited. These losses should be replaced with an intravenous infusion of 0.45% saline and 5% dextrose.

If there has been vomiting a size 18 FG Anderson sump-effect nasogastric tube must be passed and the stomach emptied before the patient goes to theatre. Anaesthetizing the anterior nasopharynx with lignocaine gel makes the experience of passing a nasogastric tube more acceptable to all patients and possible in a number in whom it would otherwise prove impossible. Care must be taken in patients with ischaemic heart disease because its effect on blood pressure and heart rate may provoke myocardial ischaemia. Prophylactic sublingual glyceryl trinitrate may be helpful (Kristensen *et al.*, 1991).

(d) Patients who need observation

Many patients do not immediately require an operation. The clinical picture of acute pancreatitis (p. 382) and acute cholecystitis (p. 402) are fairly typical and will suggest the need for investigation to confirm the diagnosis and a spell of observation while the correct line of treatment is chosen. A considerable number of patients are admitted with a provisional diagnosis of acute appendicitis but, as Tables 1.1–1.3 show, a large proportion steadily improve, with a retrospective label of non-specific acute abdominal pain (NSAP). This syndrome is discussed in Chapter 2 (p. 49) and the important point to remember is that a number of careful surveys have shown that, when the symptoms and signs leave doubt about the presence of acute appendicitis, it is quite safe to 'wait and see' – the urine is examined and a white cell count and C-reactive protein are estimated and the situation reviewed in 3–4 hours. In some of these patients it will become clear there are more definite signs of appendicitis; in others there will be steady improvement.

Each patient needs to be considered as an individual and the correct course worked out, remembering to discuss with the patient each step on the way. Oliver Wendell Holmes wrote about surgeons when he was Professor of Anatomy at Harvard in 1860, 7 years before Lister's first paper on antisepsis – 'Some men grow more and more thoughtful and compassionate in the midst of their cruel experience. They become less nervous but more sympathetic. They have a truer sensibility for others' pain, the more they study pain and disease in light of science.'

1.1.5 PREPARATION FOR SURGERY

There are few patients who need to be 'rushed to theatre'. Most benefit from a period of rest and analgesia. In a minority who are gravely ill, skilful preparation has to be coordinated with the need for early operation to arrest haemorrhage or remove the source of major sepsis.

Haemorrhagic shock

It is not difficult to recognize hypovolaemic shock in a patient bleeding from an external wound, but in most abdominal emergencies the bleeding is internal and the fact that there has been serious loss, and that it is continuing, has to be deduced from the signs.

The adult weighing 70 kg has a blood volume of about 5 litres, and in a healthy person the loss of 500 ml – as in a blood donation – is readily accommodated through peripheral vasoconstriction. When the loss continues beyond this point, vasoconstriction begins to have harmful effects. Outwardly the patient is pale, there is a frost of sweat on the brow, the dependent hand is cold, with no venous filling, there is some cyanosis of the nail beds and the capillary return is poor, with refill time after skin compression exceeding 5 seconds. These are vital warning signs because, though the pulse may be quickened, the blood pressure may be held at the misleading level of 100 mmHg. In spite of this, cardiac and renal perfusion will already have fallen and any further loss can be followed by a sudden and serious collapse of the blood pressure. Administration of a general anaesthetic in these circumstances is particularly hazardous.

Recognition of these signs of vasoconstriction must lead immediately to rapid replacement of blood volume to restore circulation. Under these circumstances the imperative is volume replacement and the various merits of differing solutions are largely academic for the first litre. In practice, a crystalloid solution (not 5% dextrose) is always to hand and a rapid transfusion of 200 ml of 0.9% saline or Hartmann's solution should produce a response; if bleeding has stopped, infusion of 1 litre should produce noticeable improvement. Pending the arrival of cross-matched blood, an albumin solution can be given. On balance, the synthetic plasma substitutes such as dextran, gelatin and starch solutions all carry some risk of anaphylaxis or derangement of clotting when given to excess (more than a litre in 24 hours), but they may still be useful (and are certainly inexpensive) when albumin or blood is unavailable.

The response of the skin circulation and blood pressure give indications of progress, but renal function is of major concern and a urinary catheter should, in the adult, yield at least 30 ml in the hour. To achieve this the aim is to restore blood volume: use of diuretics and dopamine in a patient who is not fully volume-resuscitated is not appropriate (Cuthbertson and Noble, 1997).

Oxygen should be administered through a tight-fitting face mask at 15 l/min (though care, and a lower inspired oxygen concentration, is needed to maintain the hypoxic drive in patients with chronic lung disease).

Accurate measurement of fluid intake and output is vital. This must be emphasized because review of fluid balance charts shows how often the prescription of suitable volumes and types of intravenous fluids can go awry. There is also a limit to how much blood should be given in serious haemorrhage and this is considered on p. 424. In older patients it can be difficult to judge these matters sufficiently accurately by clinical assessment alone and measurement of central venous pressure (CVP) should be available as soon as possible. In these acutely ill patients it is wise to avoid subclavian vein puncture, with its risks of pneumothorax, and to use the internal jugular vein. The use of a hand-held ultrasound probe, if available, reduces the morbidity of this cannulation (Denys *et al.*, 1993). It is always unwise to attempt to cannulate a collapsed central vein, and if the external jugular veins do not fill with a head-down tilt it is inevitable that the internal vein will also be relatively collapsed. The imperative under these circumstances is further rapid transfusion guided by pulse and blood pressure until venous filling improves and permits safe cannulation. A CVP of 6–12 cmH$_2$O is normal and it should not rise above 14–15 cm. It provides a good indication, in an otherwise healthy person, of the restoration of blood volume in haemorrhagic shock. The CVP is especially useful in the young, as a guide to how much fluid to give, and in the elderly, in whom it is important to avoid overtransfusion.

The timing of the decision to operate can be particularly difficult in internal haemorrhage, with the exception of patients with prolific bleeding, as in ruptured aneurysm, in whom resuscitation and operative arrest of bleeding go hand in hand. In bleeding from, for instance, a peptic ulcer, careful and repeated clinical observation with endoscopy are needed to decide whether bleeding has stopped or whether it continues and operative haemostasis must not be delayed (Chapter 8).

Septic shock

The patient with septic shock has considerable occult sequestration of extracellular fluid. In 204 children who died of acute appendicitis in England and Wales in 1963–1967, the commonest identifiable cause of death was failure to correct hypovolaemia secondary to the fluid lost in the peritoneal exudate and obstructed bowel of paralytic ileus (Pledger and Buchan, 1969). This needs repair with physiological saline, with some plasma to replace colloid, along with vigorous antibiotic treatment (p. 140). The lesson of audit of preoperative resuscitation (McIlroy *et al.*, 1994) of these patients is that the priority should be operation to remove the source of peritoneal contamination, as soon as reasonable correction of the hypovolaemia has been obtained. This is a particularly important principle in the treatment of elderly patients: they have often been ill for some days and their ECF deficit can amount to 4–6 litres. The CVP can be particularly helpful in this situation in striking a balance between adequate restoration of blood volume and the need to proceed to laparotomy.

Dehydration

This situation develops over some days, particularly in small-bowel obstruction, and it should be corrected more gently than in acute haemorrhage or sepsis. If examination shows loss of skin turgor and sunken eyes, and there is severe thirst, this indicates a need for some 3 litres of physiological saline over 24 hours, in addition to normal maintenance infusion volumes. Once the blood pressure and urine flow show a return to normality, potassium will need to be added at the rate of 10 mmol/litre physiological saline. Particular care needs to be exercised in the rehydration of older patients, with a twice-daily check on the biochemical and haematological parameters, and measurement of CVP may well be required.

In distal small-bowel obstruction there is a considerable volume of extracellular fluid sequestrated in the distended bowel: this is difficult to estimate, so a continuing clinical and biochemical watch on the patient is essential.

When dehydration develops slowly the circulating blood volume is preserved at the expense of the extracellular fluid compartment, so rehydration must proceed cautiously: half-strength saline solution (0.45% saline and 4% dextrose) is a useful solution.

General preparation

In all patients proceeding to operation there are several elements that must not be forgotten:

Informed consent
The recommendation for operative surgery needs to be discussed with the patient. It is preferable that this is offered by the operating surgeon, who is best equipped to provide information and to answer the patient's questions, before written consent is given. Inability on the part of the patient to sign the appropriate form requires either authorization from a legal guardian or confirmation by a witness that verbal consent has been given by an otherwise competent patient.

Assessment of general health
Preparation for emergency surgery requires prompt assessment of fitness for anaesthesia; a chest X-ray and an electrocardiogram will be required in the older (>65 years) patient. Concomitant disease requires evaluation and is considered in Chapter 15. The coexistence of significant heart disease and diabetes mellitus can have a considerable bearing on preoperative preparation. However, the extent of preoperative investigation is dictated by the urgency of intervention, as indeed is the time available for resuscitation, with some situations requiring resuscitation coincident with operation.

The haematological and biochemical status must be defined as a baseline on which to judge further change rather than indicating a need for specific action on the measured level. This is particularly the case in anaemia, which might be chronic in origin and not require corrective transfusion. The haemoglobin level has implications for oxygen carriage if further operative loss is anticipated and intraoperative transfusion is necessary.

The medication history
This points to certain requirements, e.g. serum potassium measurement in patients on diuretic therapy. Patients taking anticoagulants need coagulation studies (p. 542) to be performed and non-steroidal anti-inflammatory drugs that inhibit platelet aggregation, compromising haemostasis, need to be discontinued.

Drug withdrawal may be a considerable problem for patients presenting with an acute abdomen. If the illness has developed over a number of days the patient may already have been without his/her regular drug intake. Postoperative 'ileus' compounds these difficulties. Drugs may include prescription drugs as well as recreational drugs such as alcohol.

Some drugs are better discontinued in the perioperative period. They include: long-acting oral sulphonylurea hypoglycaemics; biguanides such as metformin; monoamine oxidase inhibitors (MAOI); and tricyclic antidepressants, which may predispose to anticholinergic syndromes as well as tachyarrhythmias. Drug interactions should be anticipated. For example administration of pethidine (meperidine) to a patient taking a non-selective MAOI could precipitate a fatal hyperpyrexic crisis. Anticoagulation or antiplatelet therapy may increase the hazards of certain procedures such as central venous line insertion and, in particular, regional anaesthesia.

Septicaemia

While treatment of sepsis must often precede bacteriological confirmation, appropriate samples should be taken before initiating therapy whenever practical. Often antibiotics will have been commenced before the patient reaches the surgeon but appropriate blood, sputum, urine or other relevant fluid culture should be performed.

Sepsis from an enteric source requires antibiotics directed at *Escherichia coli*, *Bacteroides* spp. and *Enterococcus*. Aminoglycosides, third-generation penicillins, or third-generation cephalosporins when combined with metronidazole and ampicillin, provide effective cover and should be given as soon as the diagnosis is made (Chapter 4). In contrast, prophylactic antibiotics are given as a single dose following induction of anaesthesia (Schein *et al.*, 1994).

Prevention of venous thromboembolism

Patients presenting as emergencies should be offered the same protection against pulmonary embolism as the elective surgical patient (Torngren and Engstrom, 1991). Prophylactic measures comprise elastic hose, preoperative subcutaneous heparin (5000 IU subcutaneously b.d. stimulates antithrombin III, which inhibits activation of factor X without prolonging bleeding time) and peroperative pneumatic compression. Some patients undergoing emergency laparotomy for gastrointestinal conditions may already have been hospitalized in medical wards for another condition for a significant time period. This group, especially if suffering from a gastrointestinal malignancy, are at an increased risk from venous thromboembolism.

1.1.6 PERIOPERATIVE PLANNING

The anaesthetist should be contacted early and can play an important role in the preparation and resuscitation of the patient. This emphasizes the essential interdependence of surgeons and anaesthetists, which can make a vital difference to patient care and to a good working atmosphere. Ideally the appropriate assessment, resuscitation and planning should be well in hand by the time the anaesthetist arrives, such that the management is a collaborative and not a confrontational event.

It is also of the first importance that the team in the emergency theatre should know as early as possible that a patient is being resuscitated. There is often a fairly short period during which the maximum benefit of resuscitation has been achieved, consistent with the earliest possible relief that will come from operative arrest of bleeding or clearance of sepsis. Everyone concerned needs good notice to make the best use of this opportunity.

Thought also needs to be given by both surgeon and anaesthetist to the early recovery period and the arrangements that may need to be made with the intensive therapy unit (ITU) or high-dependency unit (HDU; Table 1.4).

If, at the end of the operation, the patient needs the facilities of the ITU it is vital that the surgeon makes a full contribution to the work of the team in the unit. No-one but the surgeon

Table 1.4 Indications for intensive care and high-dependency care

Intensive care is appropriate for:	High-dependency care is appropriate for:
• Patients requiring or likely to require advanced respiratory support alone • Patients requiring support of two or more organ systems • Patients with chronic impairment of one or more organ systems sufficient to restrict daily activities (co-morbidity) and who require support for an acute reversible failure of another organ system	• Patients requiring support for a single failing organ system, but excluding those needing advanced respiratory support • Patients who can benefit from more detailed observation or monitoring than can safely be provided on a general ward • Patients no longer needing intensive care, but who are not yet well enough to be returned to a general ward • Postoperative patients who need close monitoring for longer than a few hours

fully understands the details of the operation, the points that caused anxiety and the aspects that may cause later problems and that require close, at least twice-daily, supervision. The monitoring apparatus of the unit plays an important role, but there is no substitute for the clinical assessment of the patient by the surgeon. This in no way diminishes the skills that the intensive therapy specialist brings: these skills and the insights of the surgeon are complementary.

In many of these patients the treatment of peritoneal sepsis (Chapter 4) and the supervision of the recovery of intestinal function (Chapter 6) will raise a number of problems that require joint assessment. In this situation there is a particular risk of development of complications, so continuing close observation is needed until – and beyond – the time of leaving the unit.

For the majority of patients, who do not require urgent entry to the theatre, planned emergency theatre use has great advantages. Previous studies into the increased morbidity and mortality associated with emergency surgery (Seagroatt and Goldacre, 1994) have pointed to the benefits to patient care when surgery performed in the early hours of the morning is avoided. The availability of senior operating staff is better during the day and thus the opportunity for training in emergency techniques is enhanced. Such a policy requires the availability of a dedicated daytime emergency operating theatre (Campling *et al.*, 1993). All surgeons should endorse this policy.

The timing of surgery is often influenced by extraneous factors other than the patient's condition. It is just as harmful to compromise on preparatory care in order to secure expeditious access to an available operating theatre as it is to delay intervention unnecessarily. The patient is ready for theatre when all preparatory procedures are complete. As already indicated, the main exceptions to this are those circumstances where the effectiveness of resuscitation is dependent on an operative manoeuvre to arrest bleeding, such as cross-clamping an aorta in a case of ruptured abdominal aortic aneurysm.

Proper preparation also includes clear communication with the anaesthetist who will be responsible for the case as well as lucid communication with theatre staff as to the detail of the intended procedure so that the correct and appropriate instrumentation may be prepared.

Plans for the early recovery period should also be laid out at this point and the need for a place in a high-dependency unit or even intensive care unit made clear to the appropriate staff. In exceptional circumstances, and multiple injury is one such example, transfer into an intensive therapy facility is commended for preoperative assessment, physiological parameter measurement and preparation for surgery.

REFERENCES

Attard, R. .A., Corlett, M. J., Kidner, N. J. *et al.* (1992) Safety of early pain relief for acute abdominal pain. *BMJ*, **305**, 554–556.

Campling, E. .A., Devlin, H. B., Hoile, R. W. *et al.* (1993) *The Report of the National Confidential Enquiry into Peri-operative Deaths 1991–1992*, National Confidential Enquiry, London.

Cuthbertson, B. and Noble, D. (1997) Dopamine in oliguria. *BMJ*, **314**, 690–691.

De Dombal, F. T. (1988) The OMGE Acute Abdominal Pain Survey. *Scand. J. Gastroenterol.*, **33**(Suppl. 144), 35–42.

De Dombal, F. T. (1991) *Diagnosis of Acute Abdominal Pain*, 2nd edn, Churchill Livingstone, Edinburgh.

Denys, B. G., Uretsky B. F. and Reddy P. S. (1993) Ultrasound-assisted cannulation of the internal jugular vein. *Circulation*, **87**, 1557–1562.

Driver, C. P. and Youngson, G. G. (1995) Acute abdominal pain in children: a 25-year comparison. *Health Bull.*, **53**, 167–172.

Fry, J. (1983) The 'acute abdomen', in *Common Diseases: Their Nature, Incidence, and Care*, 3rd edn, MTP Press, Lancaster, pp. 261–266.

Kristensen, M. S., Gellett, S., Bach, A. B. *et al.* (1991) Hemodynamics and arterial oxygen saturation during preoperative emptying of the stomach. *Acta Anaesthesiol. Scand.*, **35**, 342–344.

McIlroy, B., Miller, A., Copeland, G. P. *et al.* (1994) Audit of emergency preoperative resuscitation. *Br. J. Surg.*, **81**, 200–202.

Pledger, H. G. and Buchan R. (1969) Deaths in children with acute appendicitis. *BMJ*, **iv**, 466–468.

Schein, M., Assalia, A. and Bachus, H. (1994) Minimal antibiotic therapy after emergency abdominal surgery: a prospective study. *Br. J. Surg.*, **81**, 989–991.

Seagroatt, V. and Goldacre, M. (1994) Measures of early postoperative mortality: beyond hospital fatality rates. *BMJ*, **309**, 361–365.

Telfer, S., Fenyo, G., Holt, P. R. *et al.* (1988) Acute abdominal pain in patients over 50 years of age. *Scand. J. Gastroenterol.*, **23** (Suppl. 144), 47–50.

Torngren, S. and Engstrom, L. (1991) Deep venous thrombosis after emergency gastrointestinal operations: a pilot study. *Eur. J. Surg.*, **157**, 389–391.

1.2   POSTOPERATIVE CARE

1.2.1   PATHOPHYSIOLOGY OF CRITICAL ILLNESS

The essence of postoperative care is to assist the repair of the body by providing a stable physiological milieu in which the multisystem sequelae arising from both the disease process and the therapeutic intervention can be accommodated. Healing and restoration of normal organ function is thus facilitated. The initial delivery of therapy may not immediately result in a beneficial patient response and, particularly after trauma, therapy may coincide with the next phase of critical illness known as the systemic inflammatory response syndrome (SIRS; Consensus Conference, American College of Chest Physicians and Critical Care Society, 1992). The precise contribution of the differing elements involved in this response remains ill-defined but the role of cytokines such as tumour necrosis factor, interleukin-1 and interleukin-6, along with the effects of free radicals such as the highly toxic oxygen radical superoxide (O_2^-), which is released following reperfusion of ischaemic tissue, in the SIRS process is increasingly evident (Schlag *et al.*, 1991). It is the resulting insult to cellular metabolism and the integrity of the basement membrane and cell envelope that produces organ malfunction (Davies and Hagen, 1997). A better understanding of these processes should help the clinician to maintain homeostasis and restore normal organ function in the postoperative period. The ability to manipulate organ function, both individually and in combination, provides the challenge for high-quality postoperative management.

1.2.2 SEVERITY SCORING

The more severely ill the patient the more complex recovery is likely to be and prediction of the likely outcome can be made on the basis of a several variables, including age, past illness, current illness, response to treatment and social issues. A number of severity scoring systems have been evolved, including the Acute Physiology and Chronic Health Evaluation (APACHE) score, the Simplified Acute Physiological Score (SAPS), the Mortality Prediction Model (MPM) and the Paediatric Risk of Mortality (Prism) score (Pollack *et al.*, 1996). These systems have now been refined and are now second- or third-generation. The APACHE II scoring system is the most widely applicable to surgical illness (Lemeshow and Le Gall,1994). This severity of disease classification, devised by Knaus *et al.* in 1985, measures 12 variables (acute physiology score) and an evaluation of premorbid health. When this is applied in the first 24 hours following surgery, an estimate of likely outcome can be made. However, for the present, these scoring systems do not supplant, although they might complement, clinical judgement.

1.2.3 MULTIDISCIPLINARY CARE

When surgical patients require the facilities of an intensive therapy unit, it is essential that the surgeon continues to be active in postoperative management to complement and supplement the expertise of the intensivist and hence ensure optimal postoperative care. Conflict in responsibility must be avoided and good communication will ensure a clear delineation of areas of responsibility at the outset.

1.2.4 MONITORING

Wherever the postoperative patient is cared for, the basis of effective management is a good supply of informative feedback; and monitoring equipment must be used to provide much of the data. Once again this starts with clinical examination, and an overdependency on monitor-based information must not develop since malfunction of an electronic device should not in itself compromise patient recovery. Early identification of complications in the first 24 hours enables pre-emptive steps to be taken, so forestalling a cascade of subsequent difficulties in recovery. Therefore an especially close watch in the early postoperative phase is particularly important because of the predictive value of events in this time period (Gammil and Fanning, 1991).

Temperature, pulse rate, respiratory rate and blood pressure are measured on an hourly basis, if not more frequently in an unstable patient. The general condition dictates the need for the intensity of monitoring but measurement of adequate oxygenation and documentation of an adequate fluid balance are universal requirements, with urine output often being used as an indicator of tissue perfusion and hence cardiac output. Judgement on the significance of urine volumes must recognize the potential influence of antidiuretic hormone and the urine output must also be interpreted in the light of heart rate, blood pressure, peripheral venous filling and peripheral temperature. An overly aggressive attitude towards prescription of crystalloid solutions in the postoperative period will tip a fragile patient with brittle cardiovascular performance into heart failure. A restricted regime should be considered in such patients, sufficient to provide maintenance of cardiac output and a moderate urine output (0.5 ml/kg/h), remembering that, although acute renal failure often manifests as oliguria, oliguria itself can be a physiological response and in itself is a poor predictor of acute renal failure (Sweny, 1991).

Concern over the adequacy of perfusion should prompt a fluid challenge with plasma (400 ml) and the failure of a prompt response indicates the need for venous pressure measurement; any initial concern over urine output or an anticipation of such problems constitutes an indication for a urinary catheter. In distinction to fluid administration in children, fluid losses in adults are usually summated over a 24-hour period and replaced similarly over the ensuing 24 hours with the appropriate solution (usually 0.9% NaCl with KCl 10 mmol/500 ml).

1.2.5   RECOVERY AND CONVALESCENCE

The desire to utilize valuable resources has resulted in earlier discharge policies than in previous years but the process of recovery has changed little over this time interval: indeed, the advances in care and support technology perhaps result increasingly in survival of frail and elderly patients. Good nursing care is the essence of convalescence and if a surgical unit, because of disparate demands to accommodate more patients, is expected to discharge these patients more rapidly, it remains a clinical duty to ensure that the patient's recovery to health will not be compromised by the failure to provide proper convalescence. Increasing pressure to discharge patients early, based on economic grounds, must recognize professional opinion. The surgeon remains the patient's best advocate in this regard.

When discharge is arranged, due notice must be given to carers so they can make necessary arrangements for care, and clear communication must be established with those in the community who will be responsible for continuing care, particularly when there is an active component such as wound care, mobilization or changes to medication. This communication must be prompt for reasons of both courtesy and efficiency.

REFERENCES

Consensus Conference, American College of Chest Physicians and Critical Care Society (1992) Definitions for sepsis and organ failure and guidelines for the use of innovation therapies in sepsis. *Crit. Care Med.*, **20**, 864–874.

Davies, M. G. and Hagen P. O. (1997) Systemic inflammatory response syndrome. *Br. J. Surg.*, **84**, 920–935.

Gammil, M. and Fanning, A. (1991) The first 24 hours after surgery. A study of complications after 2,153 consecutive operations. *Anaesthesia*, **46**, 712–715.

Knaus W. A., Draper E. A., Wagner D. P. *et al.* (1985) APACHE II: a severity of disease classification system. *Crit. Care Med.*, **13**, 818–829.

Lemeshow, S. and Le Gall, J. (1994) Modelling the severity of illness of ICU patients. A systems update. *J.A.M.A.*, **272**, 1049–1055.

Pollack, M. M., Patel, K. M. and Rittimann, U. E. (1996) PRISM III: an updated pediatric risk of mortality score. *Crit. Care Med.*, **24**, 743–752.

Schlag, G., Redl, H. and Hallstrom, S. (1991) The cell in shock: the origin of multiple organ failure. *Resuscitation*, **21**, 137–180.

Sweny, P. (1991) Is post-operative oliguria avoidable? *Br. J. Anaesth.*, **67**, 137–145.

1.3 PAIN CONTROL AND ANAESTHETIC CONSIDERATIONS

1.3.1 PAIN RELIEF

Once the diagnosis is clear and the decisions in management have been made, consideration must be given to pain control. As has been already indicated (p. 8), there is no need for any patient with peritonitis to be denied analgesia while awaiting laparotomy. Care must be taken with the severely hypotensive patient, where afterload reduction created by intravenous administration of opiates may create a precipitous change in haemodynamics. In shock states, there may be erratic absorption of opiates if given by the intramuscular route, and the preferable option is to resuscitate the patient and then titrate small boluses of morphine (2 mg) until suitable analgesia is obtained.

The patient suffering from abdominal trauma will benefit from analgesia, particularly in the early phase of care when the necessary movement during radiological investigation and transfer will produce pain. The choice of analgesic is important in hypovolaemic shock and non-steroidal analgesics that will interfere with platelet adhesiveness, e.g. diclofenac or indomethacin, should be avoided,

Adequate pain management is required not only for humanitarian reasons but also because outcome is better if pain is well managed. Techniques must be tailored to the needs of the patient and full use made of the expertise of the pain team, if available.

Patients' needs for analgesic drugs vary significantly. Often a single drug type is used for pain control but increasingly a multimodal approach is being used to attempt to modulate pain pathways at different points.

Opioid analgesics remain the mainstay of pain management after abdominal surgery, provided by either the intravenous or the epidural route. Pethidine may lower smooth muscle tone more than morphine but these potential benefits following bowel anastomosis are unproven and in many units morphine remains the favoured analgesic. The longer duration of action of morphine when given by the intramuscular route may partially account for its continued popularity.

Local anaesthetics, most commonly the longer-acting bupivacaine, can be used for infiltration analgesia, through nerve blocks, e.g. intercostal or ilioinguinal/iliohypogastric blocks, or in epidural blocks alone, or in combinations with adjuvants.

Non-steroidal anti-inflammatory analgesics (NSAIDs) may be of benefit alone for minor to moderate pain. Often they are effective in combination with opioid and can be opioid-sparing. This may be beneficial when otherwise high doses of opioid could produce clinical problems of respiratory depression and/or somnolence. However, they can impair haemostasis by their effects on platelet function, may precipitate bronchospasm in aspirin-sensitive individuals and, particularly in compromised individuals, may precipitate acute renal insufficiency. Intravenous, intramuscular, rectal and buccal routes are available for different NSAIDs.

Routes of administration

Following major abdominal surgery opioid drugs are the mainstay of effective analgesia and for many years the intramuscular route has dominated. This route will provide effective pain relief provided there is a ward protocol for its use. The disadvantages of the i.m. route include painful injections, erratic absorption, and the time lag between onset of pain and pain relief. Other routes of administration include oral, intravenous, buccal, inhalation, transdermal, topical and spinal or epidural routes. Intravenous routes and epidural/spinal administration have recently gained popularity. Morphine is a very effective and rapid method of dealing with acute pain when given intravenously in small boluses of 1–2 mg, repeated several minutes apart, until the adequate analgesia is achieved. The patient must be in an environment where there is someone to administer these boluses and monitor their effect if the technique is to be applied safely. Continuous intravenous infusions have also recently gained popularity with the more widespread availability of infusion pumps.

Patient-controlled analgesia (PCA) has become routine for major surgery. Most PCA pumps allow for adjustments for bolus dose and a period of time after the bolus dose following which, in the interests of safety, the patient cannot successfully receive a further dose ('lockout'). A background continuous infusion is another option but has been shown to be of no benefit and indeed may increase adverse effects. As with ordinary infusion pumps, these pumps should be located at or below patient level as leaks in syringes have been associated with siphoning of the contents into patients if the syringe is above the patient.

Epidural analgesia provides the most effective analgesia for major abdominal surgery. Local anaesthetics, most commonly bupivacaine, and/or opioids such as fentanyl, morphine or diamorphine are employed. They may be inserted at operation and continued postoperatively in carefully selected cases of patients suffering with an acute abdomen, but other simpler techniques listed above will be indicated in the majority of patients.

1.3.2   ANAESTHETIC CONSIDERATIONS

Mortality and morbidity are much higher following emergency surgery than in elective procedures. Inadequate preoperative assessment, uncorrected hypovolaemia, pulmonary aspiration, inadequate monitoring, problems with tracheal intubation, inadequate supervision of the patient in the postoperative period and postoperative ventilatory failure may individually or collectively contribute to this mortality. The recommendations that have followed from mortality studies have advised careful attention to preoperative assessment, full resuscitation before operation with CVP measurement where appropriate, greater use of monitoring equipment and better recovery facilities (Derrington and Smith, 1987).

Common problems of significance to the anaesthetist include hypovolaemia, vomiting risk, hypokalaemia, atrial fibrillation, cardiorespiratory compromise and response to sepsis as well as inadvertent drug withdrawal.

It must be stressed again that in many patients with abdominal pathology, who are hypovolaemic, the sympathetic stress response compensates until hypovolaemia becomes extreme, and then sudden decompensation occurs. Nearly all intravenous and inhalational anaesthetics cause myocardial depression, vasodilation and baroreceptor reflex inhibition, so compensated hypovolaemia may be rapidly converted into decompensation on induction of anaesthesia. Resuscitation must be sufficient to prevent this complication, unless resuscitation and surgery must proceed simultaneously, as in a ruptured abdominal aortic aneurysm.

Many abdominal conditions, pain, alcohol intoxication and opioid administration increase residual gastric volume and preoperative nasogastric tube drainage of the stomach must not be forgotten.

Hypokalaemia is common in patients presenting with acute abdomen. Medication such as diuretics, corticosteroids and β_2-adrenoreceptor agonists contribute and hypokalaemia may be exacerbated by vomiting. The adverse effects of hypokalaemia include predisposition to cardiac arrhythmias, metabolic alkalosis with compensatory hypoventilation, muscle weakness and postoperative ileus. A judgement has to be made on the relative need to correct the potassium deficit and the urgency of the surgery. Correction of hypokalaemia is by intravenous infusion of potassium chloride, which should not exceed 40 mmol/h and should be administered with ECG monitoring.

Sepsis may compromise cardiovascular function, with vasodilation and myocardial depression superimposed on relative hypovolaemia. Adequate monitoring of the circulation by means of central venous and/or pulmonary artery flotation catheter, together with appropriate fluid and inotropic or vasopressor therapy, may be required to maintain adequate tissue perfusion. Such patients should be admitted to an intensive care environment before operation if at all possible.

1.3.3 INTRAOPERATIVE CARE

The role of the anaesthetist in the operating room, quite apart from the maintenance of appropriate surgical anaesthesia, is to monitor and support vital physiological functions and to attempt to prevent or treat maladaptive responses. The patient will effectively receive intensive care during the operative period.

The measures necessary to maintain cardiorespiratory function vary from minimal to full-scale intensive resuscitation and support, depending on circumstance. Minimal cardio-respiratory monitoring in adult patients would include ECG, pulse oximetry, capnography and non-invasive blood pressure recording. Severe acute pathology or coexisting disease might necessitate more invasive monitoring such as direct arterial pressure measurement (which will also allow frequent measurement of blood gases and acid–base status), a record of central venous pressure and left heart filling pressures (pulmonary artery flotation catheter). More recently the importance of maintaining normothermia on outcome has been highlighted (Sessler, 1997).

1.3.4 POSTOPERATIVE CARE

The period spent in the recovery area provides a vital opportunity for observation of the patient before return to an appropriate environment, as well as allowing adequate and safe initial management of oxygenation, postoperative pain and maintenance of circulating blood volume. For high-risk patients, thought must be given as early as possible to their transfer to intensive care (Department of Health, 1996).

Avoidance of hypoxaemia following anaesthesia is by provision of supplemental oxygen administered by face-mask. Nasal spectacles are often better tolerated if oxygen flow rates are no more than 2 l/min. For patients at special risk of postoperative respiratory failure, controlled oxygen therapy by Venturi mask is best. Pulse oximetry has been a great advance in detection and management of hypoxaemia; however oximetry cannot provide information on adequacy of ventilation or acid–base status and arterial blood gases are required for this purpose.

These observations are a reminder of the major contribution that the anaesthetist can make to the care of the patient with an abdominal emergency.

REFERENCES

Department of Health (1996) *Guidelines on Admission to and Discharge from Intensive Care and High Dependency Units*, NHS Executive, London.

Derrington, M. C. and Smith, G. (1987) A review of studies of anaesthetic risk, morbidity and mortality. *Br. J. Anaesth.*, **59**, 815–833.

Sessler, D. I. (1997) Mild perioperative hypothermia. *N. Engl. J. Med.*, **336**, 1730–1737.

1.4 TECHNIQUE

1.4.1 MIDLINE INCISION AND CLOSURE

In adult surgery a midline incision is routinely used for emergency laparotomy, with the exception of specific diagnoses, e.g. gridiron incision for appendicectomy (p. 60) or preperitoneal approach to the strangulated femoral hernia (p. 216). A midline incision is preferred because it can be made rapidly, with minimal tissue trauma. Protection of the abdominal parietes from contamination with intestinal or infected peritoneal content is simple and reduces the wound infection rate (Krukowski and Matheson, 1988). Our preference is to use wound towels supplemented by a plastic ring wound protector and to apply the discipline of a 'red danger towel' technique. Although the value of these mechanical manoeuvres is perceived by some to be unproven by rigorous scientific study, there is no doubt that sound surgical technique and attention to detail are rewarded by a low complication rate. These findings have been validated through continuing prospective audit (Table 1.5).

Table 1.5 Prospective audit of abdominal wound infection

	1977–1986*			1991–1996		
	No.	WI	%	No.	WI	%
Clean/contaminated	1199	25	2.1	939	16	1.7
Contaminated	606	18	3.0	301	6	2.0
Dirty	401	32	8.0	178	10	5.6
Total	2206	75	3.4	1418	32	2.3

* Data from Krukowski and Matheson, 1988

Closure of the midline incision by the continuous tension-free 'mass suture' technique (Jenkins, 1976) depends on distributing the distracting forces on the abdominal wall between large tissue bites. A suture:wound length ratio of at least 4:1 should be employed. This technique, used correctly, has abolished wound dehiscence and evisceration without recourse to 'tension sutures'. It is not necessary to include the peritoneum in the 'mass' closure, which incorporates only the linea alba and adjacent rectus muscle and sheath. Below the umbilicus and the linea semilunaris the well developed linea alba becomes deficient and the rectus muscle can pout between the large sutures. A small bite of the edge of the sheath between each of the large bites provides more anatomical alignment and prevents muscle protrusion. A long-lasting synthetic monofilament suture (polydioxanone) on a large needle is used, although if this is not available a monofilament (polypropylene or nylon) is perfectly acceptable although associated with a higher risk of late wound pain and sinus formation (Krukowski *et al.*, 1987).

After midline closure only skin need be approximated. If there is concern about a large subcutaneous cavity in the obese, this is better accommodated by insertion of a suction drain than a 'fat stitch'. The skin is closed with a continuous subcuticular absorbable suture, unless the procedure is classed as 'dirty', in which case interrupted skin sutures (monofilament polyamide) or skin staples may be preferred. The combination of careful technique to minimize wound contamination and antibiotic lavage of the subcutaneous space before closure of the skin permits routine primary wound closure even after operations classed as 'dirty'. Many centres apparently enduring a higher wound infection rates may not share our confidence in tetracycline lavage and recommend delayed primary closure of the wound in 'contaminated' and 'dirty' procedures. We have not found this necessary in our continuing prospective audit of wound infection, which includes follow-up at 6 weeks (Krukowski and Matheson, 1988; Table 1.5).

1.4.2 INTESTINAL ANASTOMOSIS

1.4.2.1 Introduction

Primary healing is the objective of surgical repair in most instances. Intestinal anastomoses heal by primary intention if the divided ends of the well-perfused bowel are accurately apposed without tension. Even when alignment is suboptimal, as is inevitable in inverting anastomoses, rapid healing by secondary intention usually occurs. Systemic factors (e.g. old age, debility, anaemia and jaundice) exert a negative influence on anastomotic healing but their contribution is small, except in circumstances of extreme derangement. The single most important local factor is a good blood supply to the divided bowel ends. This depends on two key issues: accurate dissection of the supplying vessels (Figure 1.3) and perioperative fluid management.

The influence of the latter on anastomotic perfusion is vital because splanchnic blood flow is reduced disproportionately in response to a fall in cardiac output. Some pathological states, particularly sepsis and obstruction, result in increased blood flow to the bowel but are associated with a higher leak rate than in uncomplicated resections; the associated cardiovascular instability, hypoxaemia, bacterial contamination and tissue friability often negate any benefit. When local and systemic factors combine to make the risk of anastomotic failure high, the wisdom of performing an anastomosis should be questioned.

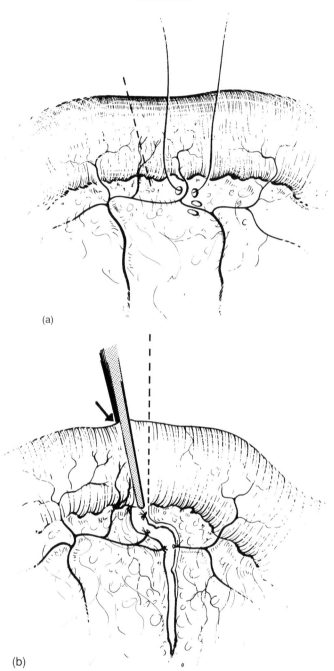

(a)

(b)

Figure 1.3 **(a)** Ligation of mesenteric vessels. The proposed site for division of the bowel is shown as a dotted line. Division of the vessels close to the bowel protects the blood supply to the end of the bowel that is to be retained. **(b)** The mesentery has been divided and the Schumaker clamp applied at an angle of 80° to the axis of the retained bowel. The bowel will be divided against the clamp (arrow).

Which anastomotic technique?

All anastomotic techniques compromise healing because they interfere with local blood flow, cause tissue disorganization and incorporate foreign material. With the plethora of techniques described for intestinal anastomoses it is important for a surgeon to choose a method in which he/she should aim to become proficient. Such a method should be based on sound theoretical concepts and supported by prospectively audited outcomes. Furthermore it behoves every surgeon to make a sustained effort to document accurately his/her own performance in this key area. Translation of clinical activity into numerical terms and application of the same process to anastomotic leaks is a revealing process, which provides an objective focus often at variance with clinical impression. After a clinical anastomotic leak the next 50 consecutive anastomoses, no matter how difficult and under what unfavourable circumstances they may be constructed, must remain intact to achieve a satisfactory standard. An overall leak rate of 1–2% should be the aim of all gastrointestinal surgeons and while this can be achieved in low-risk areas it is a continuing challenge when emergency surgery and high-risk areas such as the oesophagus and rectum are included.

Mucosal inversion and serosal apposition are traditional objectives in intestinal anastomoses but conventional two-layer techniques effect excessive inversion, with an inner layer of con-

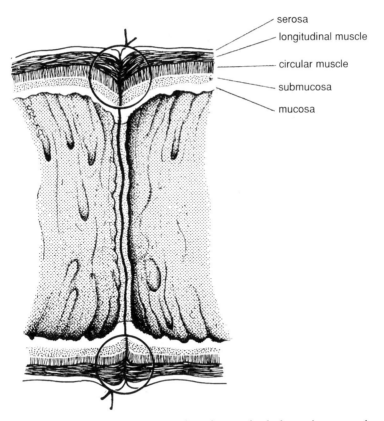

serosa
longitudinal muscle
circular muscle
submucosa
mucosa

Figure 1.4 Idealized end-to-end anastomosis using a single-layer interrupted serosubmucosal suture technique.

tinuous absorbable sutures incorporating all layers of the bowel and an outer layer of interrupted seromuscular structures. The apparent sense of security instilled by this method is hard to justify and there are theoretical and practical arguments in favour of a single-layer technique.

Experimental single-layer anastomoses are superior to two-layer anastomoses because healing is faster as a result of more accurate alignment of muscle and mucosa, less tissue strangulation and luminal reduction and more rapid angiographic healing. Matheson's interrupted single-layer technique, which he termed 'serosubmucosal' to stress the importance of the submucosal layer (Figure 1.4), first recognized by Halsted in 1887, is a simple, reliable and reproducible technique.

It has been consistently shown to be associated with the lowest reported leak rates in a variety of situations and by a number of authors. The technique as originally described (Matheson and Irving, 1976) uses interrupted braided nylon sutures and this remains the foundation (Irwin *et al.*, 1990; Carty *et al.*, 1991; Pye and Steele, 1996) particularly in areas of limited access or when the risk of failure is increased. In low risk situations with good access and tissue perfusion in which distension of the anastomosis is unlikely to be a problem, a continuous serosubmucosal suture with a synthetic absorbable monofilament suture is equally effective (Max *et al.*, 1991; Steele, 1993).

By their nature, stapled anastomoses cannot achieve primary healing. Non-alignment of corresponding layers of the bowel is inevitable and healing by secondary intention obligatory. This is not an issue when perfusion is good but becomes increasingly relevant as perfusion declines. This probably accounts for the higher incidence of anastomotic strictures reported after stapled oesophageal and rectal anastomoses.

1.4.2.2   Sutured anastomosis

Open end-to-end anastomosis

A universally applicable technique for open end-to-end anastomosis in accessible sites in the gastrointestinal tract is shown in Figure 1.5.

An appositional anastomosis requires minimal 'cleaning' of the bowel, and clamps are unnecessary on the bowel used in the anastomosis. Adequacy of blood supply at the divided ends can be observed directly, and haemostasis secured by accurate, fine diathermy. The interrupted technique permits anastomosis of bowel varying in diameter by up to 30% without an antimesenteric slit; the elasticity of the tissue accommodates well when the sutures are placed proportionately. When there is a large discrepancy in diameter, e.g. between the ileum and transverse colon following right hemicolectomy, the solution is to make an antimesenteric (Cheatle) slit (p. 275). The individual sutures are conveniently supplied in proprietary 'control release' packs of eight sutures. Braided nylon (3/0, 2 metric) is preferred for its balance of handling, knotting and relative inertness in tissue, though particular attention to secure knotting is essential.

Limited access

When access is limited and rotation of the bowel is not possible, e.g. low anterior resection or gastroduodenal anastomosis, it is easier to insert the posterior row of sutures from the anterior aspect and tie the knots on the mucosal aspect (Figure 1.6).

It is usual to insert the posterior row of sutures with the bowel ends widely separated. Once all the sutures are in place they are placed under gentle tension and the proximal bowel is slid along the sutures to appose the bowel ends.

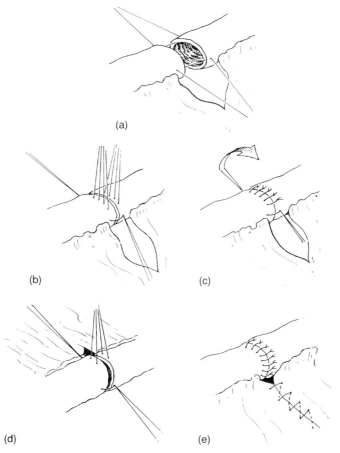

(a)

(b)   (c)

(d)   (e)

Figure 1.5 End-to-end anastomosis in accessible sites. **(a)** The first sutures are inserted into the mesenteric and antimesenteric borders, entering about 5–6 mm from the cut edge and exiting in the submucosal plane. The suture enters the opposing bowel in the same plane. The suture is tied. The second stitch is inserted in a similar fashion diametrically opposite and tied. These sutures are held in artery forceps. **(b)** The anterior row of sutures is placed sequentially using a midpoint marking suture for all but the smallest calibre bowel. The individual sutures should be no less than 5 mm apart; it is important to avoid inserting too many sutures, which can impair perfusion. **(c)** The anterior sutures are tied and cut. The stay suture on the mesenteric aspect is passed through the mesenteric defect, and the anastomosis is rotated through 180°. **(d)** The posterior row of sutures is inserted, tied and cut. **(e)** The stay sutures are cut and the mesenteric defect is closed including peritoneum only to avoid pricking a vessel.

Colorectal anastomoses

Colorectal anastomoses are easier if the posterior row of sutures is inserted with the proximal colon at some distance from the rectal stump. A series of artery forceps or, preferably, a spring-loaded device holds the sutures securely in sequence (Figure 1.7).

A double-curved Stratte needle holder is useful for insertion of sutures into the rectal stump low in the pelvis. This method is also suitable for oesophagojejunal anastomoses,

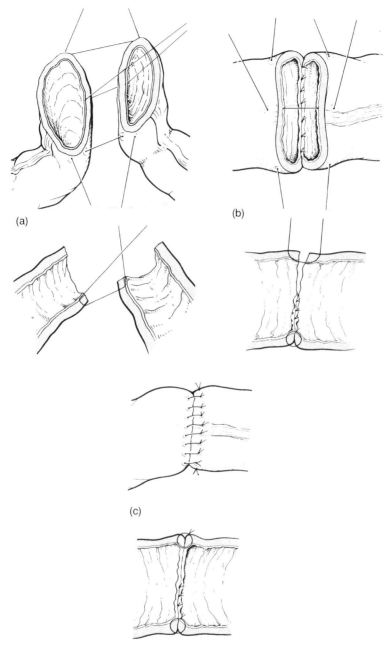

Figure 1.6 End-to-end anastomosis in inaccessible sites. (**a**) Horizontal stay sutures are inserted in diametrically opposite points of the proximal and distal bowel. A midpoint marking suture is inserted in the centre of the posterior layer with the ends of bowel held apart. The posterior row of sutures is inserted, the bowel ends are slid together and the knots are tied and cut. (**b**) The anterior row of sutures is then placed, again beginning with a midpoint marking suture. (**c**) The corner stay sutures are tied, followed by the anterior row of sutures. All the sutures are cut and the anastomosis is complete.

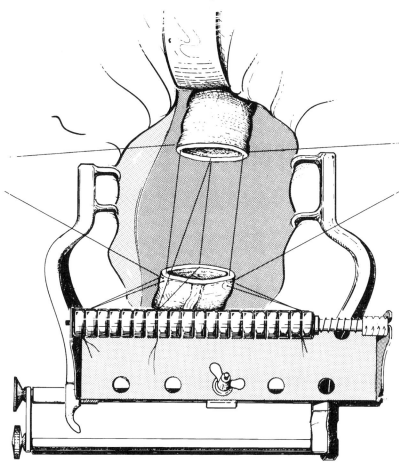

Figure 1.7 Inaccessible colorectal sutured anastomosis using a suture holding clamp resting on a Balfour self-retaining retractor.

except that some prefer full-thickness sutures for the oesophagus, in which the strength of the mucosa compensates for the absence of a strong submucosa.

Gastroenteric anastomoses

Gastroenteric anastomoses are privileged in so far as the profuse blood supply tolerates variations in technical detail that would be disastrous in low colorectal anastomoses. Conventionally, an inner layer of sutures is required to ensure haemostasis, but single-layer gastroduodenal or gastrojejunal anastomoses are straightforward. If gastric resection is followed by routine reconstitution of a new lesser curve, both end-to-end gastroduodenal or end-to-side gastrojejunal anastomoses can be made without recourse to long suture lines or 'valves' (Figure 1.8).

The new lesser curve is fashioned with a two-layer technique with an inner all-coats suture for haemostasis followed by a deep seromuscular layer. The profusion of the blood supply in

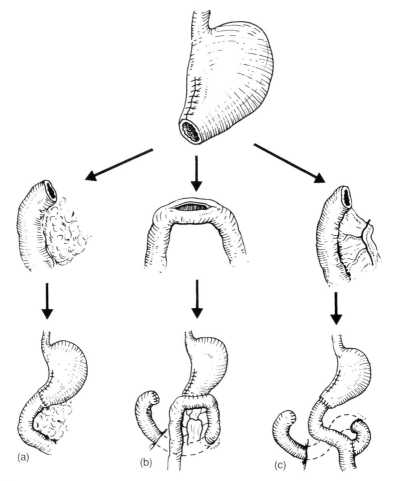

Figure 1.8 Reconstruction after partial gastrectomy. The new lesser curve is reconstituted with two layers of continuous 3/0 polydioxanone. **(a)** Gastroduodenal (Billroth I). **(b)** Gastrojejunal (Polya/Billroth II). **(c)** Gastrojejunal with a Roux-en-Y loop.

the gastric wall makes this the only site in the GI tract where a two-layer technique is used routinely. In contrast, at the open gastroenteric anastomosis actively bleeding vessels can be seen and controlled by diathermy or suture and a single-layer interrupted technique is used.

Pyloroplasty

Although the Heinecke–Mickulicz method is widely regarded as the standard method of pyloroplasty it is our experience that the modified Finney pyloroplasty is superior. It permits tension-free closure of even a long pyloroduodenotomy, such as may result from suture of a bleeding duodenal ulcer (p. 359), and if the initial incision if fashioned with a slight convex curve upwards towards the superior aspect of the pylorus the subsequent closure is even easier (Figure 1.9).

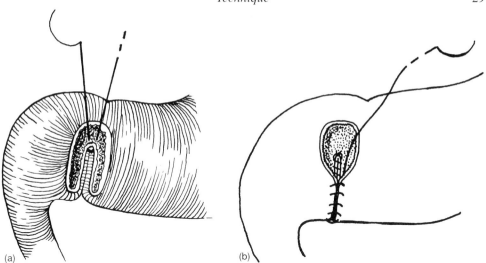

Figure 1.9 Modified Finney pyloroplasty. **(a)** A stay suture is inserted above the midpoint of the pyloromyotomy and retracted superiorly. The posterior suture is inserted from the mucosal aspect of the midpoint of the inferior edge of the incision, passing back into the lumen, and tied with the knot on the mucosal aspect. The tail of the suture is also held superiorly, converting the longitudinal pyloromyotomy into an inverted U shape. The suture is inserted as a continuous all-coats stitch from the mucosal aspect, which draws the apices of the gastric and duodenal limits of the incision together. **(b)** The stitch is locked on the serosal aspect of inferior point of the suture line and the tail of the stitch on the luminal aspect is cut. The posterior suture line is pushed back into the lumen and the closure is completed as a serosubmucosal suture to the apex of the pyloroplasty.

Closure of the duodenum, jejunum or rectum

These are the commonest situations in which the end of an open viscus requires closure. When the tissue is healthy this is readily achieved by an open continuous single-layer serosubmucosal method with 3/0 polydioxanone (Figure 1.10). The closed method is occasionally preferred for the duodenum when it has been transected between clamps (Figure 1.11).

In this circumstance the Schoemaker clamp is oversewn with 3/0 polydioxanone, the clamp is slipped out and, after tightening the suture, this is locked on the serosal aspect. The same suture inverts the first suture line. The open technique, particularly in emergency colonic surgery, has the considerable advantage of permitting direct assessment of the arterial perfusion of the open bowel.

1.4.2.3 Stapled anastomoses

Stapling in emergency abdominal surgery

Staplers have a certain appeal for their ease of use, improvement in performance when compared with suboptimal suturing techniques, and attraction to the technophile, which, in the editors' opinion, does not justify their routine use in emergency surgery. Stapling is

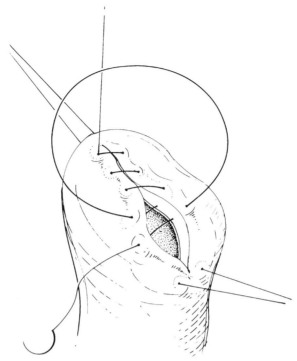

Figure 1.10 Open closure of duodenum, jejunum or rectum. A continuous serosubmucosal 3/0 monofilament absorbable suture provides a secure closure in most situations when an open end of gut requires closure. In the rectum access is improved by placing two non-absorbable (polypropylene or polyamide) stay sutures at the corners, which are subsequently tied and cut with 4–5 cm long tails to facilitate subsequent identification of the rectal stump at reoperation.

expensive, occasionally very expensive when used in a profligate manner, and may require supplementary suturing either for haemostasis or completion of a stapled procedure. There is no convincing evidence to support their universal use and we include a description of standard stapling techniques for completeness rather than recommendation.

Randomized trials show no significant difference in anastomotic failure rate between stapled and sutured anastomoses (West of Scotland and Highland Anastomosis Study Group, 1991), although stapling was quicker but considerably more expensive. Most surgeons have individual views on anastomotic technique and, despite a preference for suturing anastomoses, stapling instruments are convenient for sites in the gastrointestinal tract where access is a problem. These can include low colorectal, oesophagojejunal or oesophagogastric anastomoses.

Relative indications are when multiple anastomoses are required at the end of a lengthy procedure and marked discrepancy in the diameter of the two ends of the bowel when the functional end-to-end anastomosis is appropriate. Staplers facilitate construction of colonic or small-bowel pouches and, although this is rarely necessary during emergency procedures, the move towards more daytime and definitive emergency surgery makes it conceivable that this will increase. The only situation in which stapling is paramount is in the patient who

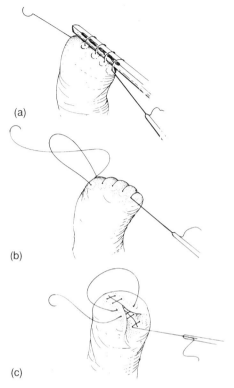

(a)

(b)

(c)

Figure 1.11 Closed suture of the duodenal stump. **(a)** An over-and-over suture of 3/0 monofilament absorbable material is inserted at the inferior margin of the duodenum below the Schoemaker clamp and tied. This is continued as an over-and-over suture over the clamp which is then slipped out. **(b)** The monofilament nature of the suture allows this to be easily tightened from the superior aspect before locking the suture. **(c)** The suture then returns as a continuous seromuscular suture inverting the first suture line.

requires oesophageal transection for uncontrollable bleeding from oesophageal varices, when the circular stapler is ideal.

Stapling instruments

Linear staplers (Figure 1.12(a)). These instruments generally come in three sizes, 30 mm, 55–60 mm and 90 mm, and are used for closure of viscera with a double row of staggered staples.

Linear cutters (Figure 1.12(b)). This is one of the most useful devices and comprises two limbs, which are inserted through the open ends of bowel or through small punctures in the sides of adjacent loops to form a fork, which is closed before forming the two rows of three lines of staples. A knife blade passes between the two rows, dividing the tissue to make a common lumen. The instruments come in sizes ranging from 30 mm (for laparoscopic use) to 90 mm. They are used for side-to-side anastomoses, functional end-to-end anastomoses and fashioning small or large bowel pouches.

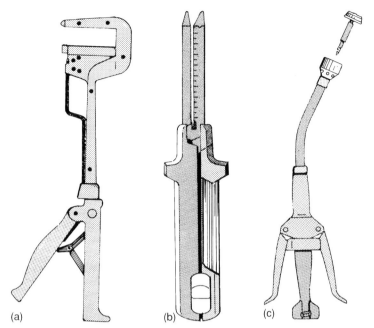

(a) (b) (c)

Figure 1.12 Stapling instruments. (**a**) Linear stapler. (**b**) Linear cutter/stapler. (**c**) Circular stapler. (Not to scale.)

Circular staplers (Figure 1.12(c)). These consist of handle, cartridge and anvil connected by a central shaft. The anvil and cartridge approximate or separate as the wing nut at the end of the handle is rotated. The cartridge contains a circular double row of staples and an inner circular knife. When the instrument is fired the staples are bent against the anvil and the circular knife cuts a window inside the double row of staples to produce an end-to-end anastomosis.

Stapling technique

The standard stapling techniques are illustrated in Figures 1.13 and 1.14. The technique of end-to-end colorectal anastomosis is well covered in standard texts on operative surgery and we would not recommend those unfamiliar with the technique to make their first attempts during an emergency operation.

Pitfalls of stapling

Good results with stapling require as much care as with suturing. Staples may not produce haemostasis and a common problem in stapled anastomoses, particularly in the upper gastrointestinal tract, is bleeding. Bleeding on the outer aspect of the anastomosis is under-run with a 3/0 monofilament suture and must not be diathermied for fear of electroconduction along the staples producing tissue damage and later leakage. The inner aspect of the anastomosis must also be inspected and any bleeding secured. A stapled gastrojejunostomy is the most likely to bleed intraluminally. If this does not stop spontaneously the stomach should be emptied with a large-bore orogastric tube and the bleeding point injected endoscopically with 1:10000 adrenaline solution.

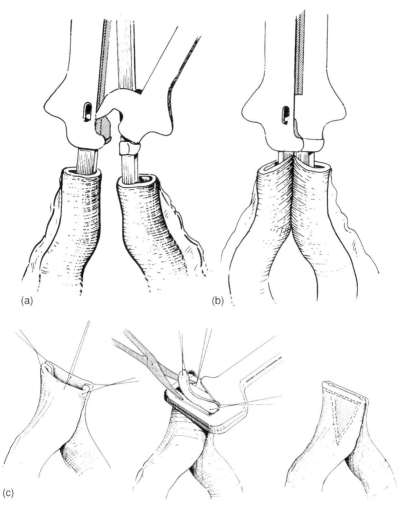

Figure 1.13 Functional end-to-end stapled anastomosis. **(a)** The bowel ends are approximated with the antimesenteric borders adjacent. **(b)** One limb of the linear cutter is inserted into each lumen and positioned symmetrically along the full length of the stapler. The instrument is closed, fired and withdrawn. **(c)** Stay sutures are inserted at the end of each staple line and midway between. The stay sutures are placed under tension and a linear stapler is used to close the open end of bowel completing the anastomosis. Scissors are used to trim off the redundant bowel beyond the suture line.

A further potential problem arises when multiple converging and overlapping staple lines are used to construct an anastomosis. The blood supply to the bowel at intersecting staple lines may be impaired and lead to later anastomotic leakage.

Particular care is required in emergency abdominal surgery when the gut is obstructed with hypertrophy of the muscularis, and in inflamed and oedematous bowel. When staples are used care must be taken to ensure that staples do not cut out. If this occurs the staple line must

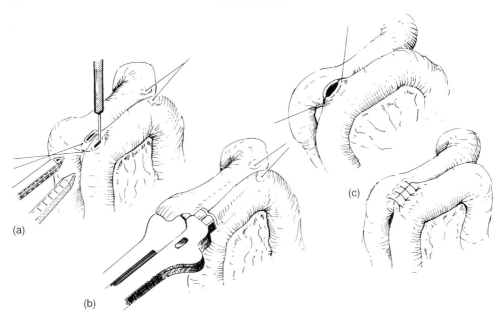

Figure 1.14 Side-to-side stapled anastomosis. **(a)** The two loops to be anastomosed are held in parallel with stay sutures and small enterotomies are made with cutting diathermy at one end of the anastomosis. **(b)** One limb of the linear stapler is inserted into each lumen and aligned evenly to use the full length of the instrument. The stapler is closed, fired and withdrawn. **(c)** The enterotomies are closed with serosubmucosal sutures.

be oversewn. The variable thickness of the gut wall is accommodated to a certain extent by different sizes of staple and the ability to control the degree of compression of tissue. Nevertheless the possibility that the staple line is too loose, encouraging leakage, or too tight, promoting ischaemia, exists.

Finally there is debate as to whether staple lines should be oversewn. Although some surgeons do this routinely it is probably only necessary to oversew when closing the duodenum after gastrectomy; we have experience of leakage of bile through otherwise intact staple lines.

The healing abilities of the gut and peritoneal structures are such that most techniques afford reasonable clinical results under favourable circumstances. However, the chosen technique must perform equally well under suboptimal conditions such as prevail in emergency surgery. The single-layer technique that we advocate and illustrate in Figure 1.5 consistently produces excellent clinical results both in elective and in emergency situations. Adoption of a standard method that is suitable (with minor modifications) for all situations in the gut allows the surgeon to develop familiarity, sensitivity and selectivity in fashioning anastomoses.

REFERENCES

Carty, N. J., Keating, J., Campbell, J. *et al.* (1991) Prospective audit of an extramucosal technique for intestinal anastomosis. *Br. J. Surg.*, **78**, 1439–1441.

Irwin, S. T., Krukowski, Z. H. and Matheson, N. A. (1990) Single layer anastomosis in the upper gastro-intestinal tract. *Br. J. Surg.*, **77**, 643–644.

Jenkins, T. P. N. (1976) The burst abdominal wound: a mechanical approach. *Br. J. Surg.*, **63**, 873–876.

Krukowski, Z. H., Cusick, E. L. C., Engeset, J. *et al.* (1987) Polydioxanone or polypropylene for closure of midline abdominal incisions: a prospective comparative trial. *Br. J. Surg.*, **74**, 828–830.

Krukowski, Z. H. and Matheson, N. A. (1988) Infection after abdominal surgery: a ten year computerised audit. *Br. J. Surg.*, **75**, 857–861.

Krukowski, Z. H. and Matheson, N. A. (1994) Hand sewn techniques for gastric anastomoses, in *Rob and Smith's Operative Surgery. Surgery of the Upper Gastrointestinal Tract*, 5th edn, (ed. G. G. Jamieson), Chapman & Hall, London, pp. 88–107.

Matheson, N. A. and Irving, A. D. (1976) Single layer anastomosis in the gastrointestinal tract. *Surg. Gynecol. Obstet.*, **143**, 619–624.

Matheson, N. A., McIntosh, C. A. and Krukowski, Z. H. (1985) Continuing experience with single layer appositional anastomosis in the large bowel. *Br. J. Surg. Suppl.*, S104–S106.

Max, E., Sweeney, W. B., Bailey, H. R. *et al.* (1991) Results of 1000 single layer continuous polypropylene intestinal anastomoses. *Am. J. Surg.*, **162**, 461–467.

Pye, G. and Steele, R. J. C. (1996) Anastomoses involving the colon and rectum: an eight year experience. *J. R. Coll. Surg. Edin.*, **41**, 95–96.

Steele, R. J. (1993) Continuous single-layer serosubmucosal anastomosis in the upper gastrointestinal tract. *Br. J. Surg.*, **80**, 1416–1417

West of Scotland and Highland Anastomosis Study Group (1991) Suturing or stapling in gastrointestinal surgery: a prospective randomized study. *Br. J. Surg.*, **78**, 337–341.

2

Acute appendicitis

Emergency abdominal surgery came into being in the last years of the 19th century, when acute appendicitis was first recognized as a potentially fatal disease that could be successfully treated by a surgical operation. It has remained the most common surgical emergency, and has long been one of the young surgeon's first testing grounds, where some of the skills of bedside examination, surgical diagnosis, operative treatment and postoperative care are progressively, and sometimes memorably, acquired. Its study enables most aspects of the care of patients with acute abdominal disease to be reviewed.

2.1 HISTORY

The second half of the 19th century saw surgery develop from what the young Joseph Lister called, in 1853, 'this bloody and butcherly department of the healing art' into a specialty that had a respectable scientific basis and was conducted in a recognizably modern manner. The combination of the arrival of anaesthesia in the late 1840s, and Lister's own pioneering work in the late 1860s, enabled the abdomen to be opened, for the first time, in a reasonably safe and civilized manner.

Perityphlitis was a condition regularly reported during the 19th century, although a few pioneers suspected that these cases originated in the appendix. Hancock in 1848 in London recognized that an inflammatory mass medial to the iliac spine was probably of appendicular origin, and he successfully drained an abscess and removed a faecolith. Willard Parker of New York reported in 1867 that the appendix caeci could become gangrenous and perforate, forming an abscess: he reported four successful drainage operations and 'for twenty years the Parker operation dominated the treatment of right iliac abscess' in North America (Smith, 1986). In England Lawson Tait, following in the footsteps of Spencer Wells, had greatly extended the scope of gynaecological surgery. In 1880 Tait operated on a girl of 17 with an inflammatory mass in the right lower abdomen: he drained a large abscess and removed a gangrenous appendix lying within it (Shepherd, 1956).

The term 'acute appendicitis' was coined by Reginald Fitz, who was Professor of Pathology at Harvard. He read his classic paper to the Association of American Physicians in June 1886: the title was 'Perforating inflammation of the vermiform appendix: with special

Emergency Abdominal Surgery. Edited by Peter F. Jones, Zygmunt H. Krukowski and George G. Youngson. Published in 1998 by Chapman & Hall, London. ISBN 0 412 81950 3.

reference to early diagnosis and treatment'. He analysed the clinical history and post-mortem findings in 257 patients and said:

> If, after 24 hours from the onset of the severe pain, peritonitis is evidently spreading and the condition of the patient is grave, the question should be entertained of an immediate operation for exposing the appendix and determining its condition with reference to its removal . . .. The vital importance of the early recognition of perforated appendicitis is unmistakable. Its diagnosis in most cases is comparatively easy. Its eventual treatment by laparotomy is generally indispensable.

Such clear-cut advice to surgeons from a professor of pathology only emphasizes that good surgery is based on a close study of morbid anatomy. The following year, 1887, T. G. Morton in Philadelphia was the first to make a preoperative diagnosis of appendicitis, followed by successful urgent appendicectomy. Charles McBurney in New York published his classic paper in 1889, based on his experience of 11 patients. He seems to have performed his first appendicectomy for unruptured acute appendicitis on 23 May 1888, and at a meeting of the New York Surgical Society that day it was recognized how much safer it would be to operate 'at a time when the process was still limited to the appendix' (Smith, 1986).

Perhaps because these early communications on the nature and treatment of appendicitis had appeared in the North American journals, progress in Great Britain was slower. Frederick Treves, who was a pioneer of the early operative treatment of intestinal obstruction, favoured waiting until an abscess formed before operating. In 1896 Moynihan in Leeds gave strong support to early appendicectomy and, in Aberdeen, Riddell in 1900 said 'no case of acute perforative appendicitis if left to nature recovers, but with operation the patient has a chance'. In 1902, when Treves drained the appendicular abscess of King Edward VII 2 days before he was due to be crowned, the hospital mortality of appendicitis was 26%. By 1912 this figure had fallen to 4%, probably as a result of speedier diagnosis and treatment (Lett, 1914). In Edinburgh in 1924 mortality still stood at 4.9% but by 1948, in the same wards, overall mortality was 1.1% (Gilmour and Lowdon, 1952). This improvement was largely due to progress in the treatment of peritonitis, with intravenous fluids and the arrival of the sulphonamides and antibiotics. Further developments in anaesthesia and in patient care have brought mortality rates to their present very low levels of about 1 in 650 (Registrar General for Scotland, 1996).

Since the middle of this century the incidence of acute appendicitis in Western countries has fallen steadily. The number of patients discharged from hospital in England and Wales with a diagnosis of appendicitis was 113 000 in 1966, 80 000 in 1976 and 51,200 in 1985 (Hospital In-Patient Enquiry, 1989). In Scotland the number of appendicectomies showed a similar trend, from 8332 in 1977 to 4597 in 1993 (Scottish Health Statistics, 1994). In the United States a national survey found that the overall incidence of primary appendicectomy fell by 22% between 1970 and 1984 (Addiss et al., 1990).

However this fall has not been seen among patients with perforated appendicitis. In Jonkoping, Sweden the incidence per 100 000 of the population for non-perforated appendicitis showed a steady fall from 152 in 1970–1974 to 111 in 1985–1989, but perforated appendicitis remained steady throughout at 21 per 100 000 (Andersson *et al.*, 1994), and it remains a dangerous condition. It is most often seen at the extremes of age, and in patients aged 80 and over the mortality rate is about 5% (Luckmann, 1989). In this connection we need to remember the words of Mason Brown (1956): 'We cannot entirely overcome the handicap which late diagnosis entails, and many of the very ill patients who survive do so by a narrow margin.'

2.2 PATHOLOGY

The serious risk presented by acute appendicitis which has progressed to perforation was made very clear by Fitz (1886). He found that in 60% of perforated appendices there was evidence of obstruction, and Wilkie in 1914 drew particular attention to the pathological and clinical differences between 'obstructive' and 'non-obstructive' appendicitis. In cats on a meat diet he demonstrated that the acutely obstructed appendix is a form of closed-loop intestinal obstruction (p. 185). Within it he found rapid proliferation of bacteria, formation of faeculent pus and the onset of gangrene, and this went on to perforation and a grave form of peritonitis. Wilkie was impressed with the rapidity of these changes and the importance of recognizing the clinical picture (p. 55).

However, the development of gangrene and perforation is not confined to appendices obstructed by a faecolith, a band or a fibrous stricture dating from a previous episode of inflammation. Shaw (1965) studied faecoliths and found them to be synonymous with calculi, in so far as they were both laminated and generally radio-opaque. In 63 patients with a gangrenous or perforated appendix, 31 contained a calculus and 32 did not, but Shaw found that when inflammation develops it is more severe and more likely to progress to perforation in the presence of a calculus.

What causes an appendix to become acutely inflamed remains uncertain. It seems likely that it is due to swelling of the lymphoid tissue in the submucosa which is responding to viral or bacterial infection. If there is a calculus present the inflammation progresses more rapidly. If the obstruction is incomplete then a phlegmonous appendicitis is more likely to develop. Inflammation spreads through the wall to the serosa, which is covered in fibrin and pus, but the appendix is not likely to perforate. When gangrene does develop it is probably related to secondary thrombosis in the appendicular artery, which supplies the distal appendix through end-arteries (Lindgren and Aho, 1969).

In most large series (Lewis *et al.*, 1975; Pieper *et al.*, 1982) some 20% of all patients have a perforated appendix. Below the age of 5 and above the age of 60 some two-thirds of patients have perforated (pp. 92 and p. 75).

2.3 AETIOLOGY

The reasons for the relatively sudden appearance of acute appendicitis in the last 30 years of the 19th century, its remarkable frequency in the first half of the 20th century and its steady decline since then are still not clear.

For a time the observations of Burkitt (1971) on the rarity of appendicitis among the tribes of sub-Saharan Africa seemed to be strong evidence in favour of the protective effect of a high-fibre diet. This coincided with the historical fact that appendicitis became common at the same time as the adoption of mechanical milling of flour led to the general consumption of white bread. This theory, however, is not consistent with the fact that the incidence of appendicitis in the UK remained unchanged throughout the Second World War, in spite of the universal consumption of a high-fibre, low-sugar diet (Barker, 1985). In Lund, Sweden, the incidence of appendicitis was halved between the 1940s and the 1970s, although the fibre content of the diet was slightly reduced (Arnbjornsson *et al.*, 1982).

Another possible explanation for the emergence of acute appendicitis as a common disease is that it coincided with the progressive introduction into Western countries, from the 1870s, of a pure water supply and municipal drainage of sewage. Children living in primitive hygienic conditions develop a relative immunity to all but virulent enteric infections, so as hygiene was improved this protection was removed. Consequently, when contaminated food was eaten, invasion of the mucosa by unfamiliar organisms led to a brisk reaction in the submucosal lymphoid tissue of the gut, including the appendix, and this could produce a measure of obstruction of the lumen, which would favour the development of appendicitis. Over the last 40 years food and domestic hygiene has improved so much that enteric infections have been fewer, and this coincides with the fall in the incidence of appendicitis (Barker and Morris, 1988).

Barker *et al.* (1986) have suggested that there is a strong positive correlation between potato consumption and the incidence of appendicitis, and a clear negative correlation with the consumption of green vegetables and tomatoes. The suggestion is that these foods have different effects on the bacterial flora. The complexities of the interrelated roles of diet and life style are reviewed by Heaton (1987).

Heredity plays only a minor role in aetiology but there are a few remarkable family histories. Budd and Foulty (1977) record one which, in the course of two generations, produced 16 cases of acute retrocaecal appendicitis among a total of 20 offspring.

REFERENCES

Addiss, D. G., Shaffer, N., Fowler, B. S. *et al.* (1990) Epidemiology of appendicitis and appendectomy in the United States. *Am. J. Epidemiol.*, **132**, 10–25.

Andersson, R., Hugander, A., Thulin, A. *et al.* (1994) Indications for operation in suspected appendicitis and incidence of perforation. *BMJ*, **308**, 107–110.

Arnbjornsson, E., Asp, N.-G., Westin, S. I. (1982) Decreasing incidence of acute appendicitis, with special reference to the consumption of dietary fibre. *Acta Chir. Scand.*, **148**, 461–464.

Barker, D. J. P. (1985) Acute appendicitis and dietary fibre: an alternative hypothesis. *BMJ*, **290**, 1125–1127.

Barker, D. J. P. and Morris, J. (1988) Acute appendicitis, bathrooms and diet in Britain and Ireland. *BMJ*, **296**, 953–955.

Barker, D. J. P., Morris, K. and Nelson, N. (1986) Vegetable consumption and acute appendicitis in 59 areas of England and Wales. *BMJ*, **292**, 927–930.

Brown, J. J. M. (1956) Acute appendicitis in infancy and childhood. *J. R. Coll. Surg. Edin.*, **1**, 268–273.

Budd, D. C. and Foulty, W. J. (1977) Familial retrocaecal appendicitis. *Am. J. Surg.*, **133**, 670–671.

Burkitt, D. P. (1971) The aetiology of appendicitis. *Br. J. Surg.*, **58**, 695–699.

Fitz, R. H. (1886) Perforating inflammation of the vermiform appendix, with special reference to early diagnosis and treatment. *Am. J. Med. Sci.*, **92**, 321–346.

Gilmour, I. E. W. and Lowdon, A. G. R. (1952) Acute appendicitis. *Edin. Med. J.*, **59**, 361–373.

Heaton, K. W. (1987) Aetiology of acute appendicitis. *BMJ*, **294**, 1632–1633.

Hospital In-patient Enquiry (1989) *Series MB4 No 29*, Department of Health, HMSO, London.

Lett, H. (1914) Present position of acute appendicitis and its complications. *Lancet*, **i**, 295–302.

Lewis, F. R., Holcroft, J. W., Boey, J. *et al.* (1975) Appendicitis: a critical review of diagnosis and treatment in 1000 cases. *Arch. Surg.*, **110**, 677–682.

Lindgren, I. and Aho, A. J. (1969) Microangiographic investigations on acute appendicitis. *Acta Chir. Scand.*, **135**, 77–82.

Luckmann, R. (1989) Incidence and case fatality rates for acute appendicitis in California. *Am. J. Epidemiol.*, **129**, 905–918.

McBurney, C. (1889) Experience with early operative interference in cases of disease of the vermiform appendix. *N.Y. Med. J.*, **50**, 676–684.

Moynihan, B. G. A. (1896) Case of acute perforated appendicitis, followed by septic peritonitis: abdominal section: recovery. *Lancet*, **ii**, 1806–1808.

Pieper, R., Kager, L. and Nasma, P. (1982) Acute appendicitis: a clinical study of 1018 cases of emergency appendectomy. *Acta Chir. Scand.*, **148**, 51–62.

Registrar General for Scotland (1996) *Annual Report, 1995*, General Register Office, Edinburgh.

Riddell, J. S. (1900) Appendicitis. *Scot. Med. J.*, **6**, 214–222.

Scottish Health Statistics (1994) *The NHS in Scotland*, HMSO, Edinburgh.

Shaw, R. E. (1965) Appendix calculi and acute appendicitis. *Br. J. Surg.*, **52**, 451–459.

Shepherd, J. A. (1956) Lawson Tait and acute appendicitis. *Lancet*, **ii**, 1301–1302.

Smith, D. C. (1986) A historical overview of the recognition of appendicitis. *N.Y. State J. Med.*, 571–583; 639–647.

Wilkie, D. P. D. (1914) Acute appendicitis and acute appendicular obstruction. *BMJ*, **ii**, 959–962.

2.4 THE CLINICAL PICTURE

Acute appendicitis, when it presents in a typical manner in a young man, can be one of the easier clinical diagnoses to make. However, it will become clear that it can also present in ways that considerably obscure the true pathology and, as Wilkie (1931) has pointed out, it is not the typical case that is the dangerous one. Later, discussion of the differential diagnosis will also show that other conditions can closely resemble appendicitis: some of these require an operation but some require active medical, not surgical, treatment.

In the following pages, figures where given, are taken from the surveys of Lewis *et al.* (1975), Pieper *et al.* (1982) and Winsey and Jones (1967).

2.4.1 THE HISTORY

In a majority of patients an attack of acute appendicitis starts with pain around or just above the umbilicus. It may waken them from sleep, and varies from a dull ache to actual colicky pain; this arises from a degree of appendicular obstruction and is therefore referred, like intestinal colic, to the midline. After some hours there is often a characteristic shift of pain to the right iliac fossa (RLQ) as parietal peritoneal irritation develops from contact with the inflamed appendix. However, in some 25–30% of patients pain is felt solely and from the start in the RLQ. As local peritonitis develops patients notice that coughing and movement is painful, and when they travel to hospital they may notice sharp pain when the transport passes over humps in the road. Nausea and vomiting are common and anorexia is nearly always present.

An important 15–20% of patients complain of diarrhoea. Among 114 children with acute appendicitis, 20 had diarrhoea and 15 showed noticeable rectal tenderness: they all had an acutely inflamed pelvic appendix. The symptom of diarrhoea naturally arouses suspicion of gastroenteritis, but if it has been preceded by the onset of abdominal pain pelvic appendicitis must be suspected and abdominal and pelvic signs sought. (This needs to be remembered by family doctors, who may see only two or three patients with appendicitis in a year.)

It is sometimes said that headache does not accompany appendicitis, but this should not be regarded as a rule, and sometimes nausea or diarrhoea appear before the onset of pain. There may be a history of a similar previous attack: mild appendicitis certainly settles spontaneously, but can leave the patient with a fibrous stricture to complicate a further attack.

2.4.2 SIGNS

As always much will have been learnt about the condition of the patient during the history. Some will appear in near-normal health, others with incipient peritonitis will be tense and anxious, unwilling to move, weary and sunken-eyed after a long period of pain and vomiting.

Fever may be present in appendicitis, but is usually below 37.8°C. Higher temperatures will be found in established peritonitis and with some abscesses.

The **pulse rate** is commonly within normal limits, but tachycardia is always significant. When retroileal or pelvic appendicitis first presents the signs can be equivocal, but we have found a sustained tachycardia a vital early-warning sign which requires explanation.

Difficulty in movement in bed. If the patient is asked to sit up, about two-thirds find that this sharply aggravates the pain in the RLQ. Coughing may produce the same response, although Golledge *et al.* (1996) found that this was not a reliable sign. Others place reliance on asking the patient to stand, to rise on tiptoe and suddenly drop back on the heels, and noting the result.

Inspection of the tongue is always done but as many as one-third of patients have a clean tongue. The presence of furring and fetor oris depends very much on the duration of illness. The fauces should be inspected because tonsillitis is certainly associated with mesenteric and cervical lymphadenitis.

There is only one sign that is present in every case of acute appendicitis and that is local **tenderness**. It was McBurney, in 1889, who first made a particular point of this by stating 'I believe that in every case the seat of greatest pain, determined by the pressure of the finger, has been very exactly between an inch and a half and two inches from the anterior superior spinous process of the ilium on a straight line drawn from that process to the umbilicus'. It is necessary to remember that he made this statement after examining only 11 patients, and it is unfortunate that it has been repeated on countless occasions since then. The statement is correct for many patients, but in high retrocolic appendicitis the point of maximal tenderness can be inches above and lateral to McBurney's point while in some cases of pelvic appendicitis the only significant tenderness is elicited only by rectal examination. It is easy to expect that tenderness will be maximal over McBurney's point and, when this sign is absent, to omit to examine other possible sites (Figure 2.1).

Guarding. This involuntary tightening of the muscles of the abdominal wall over an area of parietal peritoneal irritation is a most valuable sign because it is more objective than tenderness. The patient must be lying flat and relaxed. The surgeon's warm hand is laid gently on the left lower quadrant and the fingers dip gently into it, far from the sore area. If there is complete painless relaxation of the musculature in this area, but there is perceptible tightening of the muscles when the hand is slowly moved to palpate over the RLQ, then the sign is positive, and it is found in 80–90% of patients with acute appendicitis (p. 50). When local peritonitis surrounds the appendix the guarding will be more marked and may amount to rigidity: as peritonitis spreads so will the area of rigidity extend.

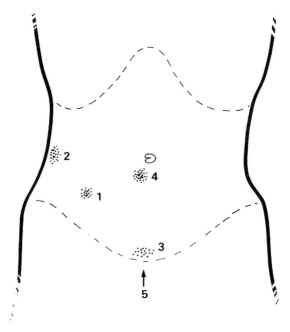

Figure 2.1 The site of tenderness in acute appendicitis depends on the position of the appendix. 1. Iliac. 2. Retrocaecal or retrocolic. 3. Pelvic. 4. Retroileal. 5. The tenderness of low pelvic appendicitis is only detected on rectal examination.

Rebound tenderness. This is another sign of peritoneal irritation and has the same source as pain on movement. When the signs of appendicitis are clear-cut it is neither necessary nor considerate to attempt to elicit this sign because it will not alter the decision to operate. In the group of patients with equivocal signs light abdominal percussion is a good way to predict whether a positive response is likely: if this produces little reaction then deep palpation some distance from the site of tenderness, followed by quick lifting of the hand can be tried. It is best to watch the patient's face when judging the result. We found that 75% of patients with acute appendicitis gave a positive response, compared with only 5% of patients with non-specific pain in the RLQ. Views vary on the value of this sign but Golledge *et al.* (1996) found in 100 patients with acute abdominal pain that it had a high degree of sensitivity and specificity among the 44 patients with proven appendicitis.

Sometimes an appendicular **mass** or abscess can be felt and these are considered on page p. 70.

Examination of the scrotum in males and **of the hernial orifices** in all patients is an integral part of abdominal examination that must never be omitted. There are several important reasons for this.

- Torsion of the testes sometimes presents with a complaint of pain in the RLQ, where there will be few signs. If there is not a firm routine of examining the scrotum serious testicular damage can occur before pain is complained of in the testis.

- The patient may complain of pain in a hernia although the primary disease is in the abdomen.
  - Acute appendicitis occasionally presents with the appendix lying in a hernial sac. Thomas *et al.* (1982) reported seven patients seen over eight years in two large hospitals. All complained of a painful lump in the right groin (three inguinal, four femoral) and only three complained of abdominal pain. All were thought before exploration to have a strangulated hernia.
  - If general peritonitis develops in a patient with a patent inguinal or femoral hernial sac, pus may enter the sac, cause pain and swelling which worries the patient more than the abdominal pain, and lead to a diagnosis of strangulated hernia. Cronin and Ellis (1959) saw two patients with abdominal pain and tender swollen inguinal hernial sacs. When explored the sacs contained only pus, and laparotomy revealed perforated appendices. Hartley *et al.* (1994) describe a woman of 79 with a crepitant swelling in the thigh; incision yielded faecal pus. Exploration revealed a perforated appendix strangulated in an obturator hernia.
  - Occasionally a phlegmonous appendicitis produces enough peritoneal serous exudate for it to distend an inguinal hernial sac: the patient complains of pain in the testis and a tender oedematous scrotum is found, with minimal abdominal signs (Bowen and Bruce, 1994).
- An important reason for never failing to examine the hernial sites is that a strangulated femoral hernia is easily missed in the groin of a well-covered patient: the swelling is often neither painful nor tender and the patient complains only of abdominal colic and vomiting. This is fully considered on page p. 215.

Rectal examination is an essential part of abdominal examination in some but not all patients. When the abdominal signs show clear evidence of acute appendicitis with local peritonitis it is not necessary to make a patient turn over and undergo an uncomfortable procedure that will not alter the decision to operate. On the other hand, when the diagnosis remains in doubt after full examination and a complaint of abdominal pain remains unexplained, then the case has not been fully assessed until a rectal examination has been performed. We can look back on a number of patients with pelvic appendicitis in whom the abdominal signs were equivocal but the rectal findings were conclusive. When a patient presents with diarrhoea and abdominal pain this examination is essential. It is described in detail because it is necessary to help the patient to distinguish the inevitable discomfort in the anal canal from true deep tenderness.

It is important to explain to the patient the reason for the examination, and to give time to it. In the left lateral position the buttocks must just overhang the side of the bed and the hips be fully flexed. It helps relaxation if the lubricated pulp of the index finger is first drawn firmly over the closed anus. Then, with the right index finger lying flat on the natal cleft, pointing anteriorly, the pulp is pressed flat against the anus, the distal interphalangeal joint is flexed and the patient is asked to strain down. The pulp will gradually sink into the relaxing anus and the flexed finger is then smoothly advanced into the rectal ampulla to its full length. All movements should then be stopped, and the patient should be reassured that the most uncomfortable part of the examination is over. At this point the patient should not feel any appreciable pain from the manoeuvre.

The finger is then straightened so that the nail and dorsum of the distal phalanx press on the pelvic peritoneum, first to the left then to the right. The response to this should be judged by watching the patient's face, and asking whether pain is felt – it is exacerbation of abdominal pain that is significant. It is a mistake to exert this pressure after rotating the finger and pressing forwards with the pulp, because this movement causes confusing discomfort in the anal canal. It should be possible to determine whether tenderness is felt more to the right or left, or widely over the pouch of Douglas. If a mass is felt the finger can be carefully rotated to allow more accurate palpation.

Dickson and Mackinlay (1985), who made a rectal examination on 103 children, and Dixon *et al.* (1991), who examined 395 children and adults, all with proven appendicitis, found anterior or right-sided rectal tenderness in between one-third and one-half of these patients. However, both surveys concluded that in over 90% of their patients the diagnosis was based on the history and abdominal signs, and rectal examination was not helpful. There is a strong case for having a rule that when, in a doubtful case, rectal examination is necessary, it is performed once only (especially in children) by the surgeon who will decide on management.

2.4.3   THE DIFFICULT APPENDIX

The pelvic and retrocaecal positions are two of the more common sites of the appendix, and when appendicitis occurs the presentation can be atypical.

In **pelvic appendicitis** diarrhoea is often a symptom, which can lead to suspicion of the much commoner gastroenteritis. The inflamed appendix lies sufficiently far away from the peritoneum of the anterior abdominal wall for guarding to be slight or absent, although there is deep tenderness. There is definite right-sided tenderness on rectal examination and occasionally a mass is felt. The appendix that lies relatively high in the pelvis is the most difficult variety because it does not stimulate abdominal guarding and yet lies rather too high for tenderness to be elicited in the adult by the rectal finger. Both abdominal and rectal findings are equivocal, and here close observation plays a vital role. After 2–3 hours the observer may find the patient a little anxious and uncomfortable, and the pulse has quickened. A rising white cell count and C-reactive protein can be helpful. Critical repetition of the abdominal and rectal findings then show tenderness to be more definite. In these circumstances it can be satisfactory but surprising to find a gangrenous appendix, in spite of the lack of clear-cut signs.

The proximity of the appendix to the ureter probably accounts for the fact that a midstream specimen of urine may contain as many as 50 white cells per high-power field. Brewster *et al.* (1994) remark that the absence of organisms in the film should raise doubts about a urinary infection, and give examples of occasions when this interpretation caused delay in diagnosis.

In **retrocaecal and retrocolic appendicitis** tenderness and guarding are found well out towards the flank, above the anterior iliac spine (Figure 2.1). This is a common form of appendicitis, and it must be remembered because the RLQ itself may be soft and not noticeably tender. These appendices lie close to or within the retroperitoneal aspect of the ascending colon, and so occasionally perforation causes a retroperitoneal abscess: these can present with a history of pain in the flank and groin for a week or two; nausea and anorexia may be absent and this late presentation is quite unlike acute appendicitis. An X-ray may show gas around the kidney. Exploration reveals the true cause, and if the appendix is perforated there should be a careful search for a faecolith (Turner and Daniell, 1984).

In **retroileal appendicitis** there can be difficulty in reaching a decision, however careful the examination. The patient complains of dull central or subumbilical pain, and loss of appetite. A shift of pain is unlikely. There may be diarrhoea and vomiting. Gentle palpation with the warm flat hand may show consistent deep tenderness some 2–3 cm below and lateral to the umbilicus, and there may be a little tightening of the rectus muscle compared to the left side. There can be reflex ileus of the terminal ileum, and this can give a picture after a day or two of small-bowel obstruction. Once again active observation is essential and, as in pelvic appendicitis, can show that a patient who is ill at ease, with a rising pulse but indeterminate signs, requires urgent operation.

Occasionally **neurological examination** is required. We saw a boy of 4 who woke from sleep at 4 am with acute abdominal pain, and there was some tenderness and a little guarding in the RLQ. It was only 4 hours later that he complained of a sore head, and neck stiffness was demonstrated. Lumbar puncture confirmed a diagnosis of meningitis.

Examination of the lungs is necessary because right-sided pneumonia with pleural involvement can cause pain referred into the right iliac fossa. In young children it must be remembered that shallow frequent respirations are a feature of diffuse peritonitis.

Chemical examination of the urine must never be omitted. When there is doubt over the diagnosis of appendicitis a urinary infection must be considered (although this is very unusual in young men). A quick and cheap test is the Ames Multistix 10 SG (Nitrostix), which tests for two markers of urinary infection (leucocyte esterase and nitrites). Woodward and Griffiths (1993) tested 133 samples and found that if both markers were absent an infection could be excluded. If the test is positive then a fresh clean-catch specimen must be obtained. If side-room microscopy is practised and infection is present an unspun shaken specimen will show more than 10 red or white cells per high-power field and bacteria will be seen shimmering in the film.

This result should lead to a careful review of physical signs because red and white cells are found to excess in some patients with appendicitis. Varshney *et al.* (1996) recorded this in 24 of 114 patients with retrocaecal appendicitis and in 22 the appendix was gangrenous or perforated. Acute right-sided pyelitis needs consideration as a differential diagnosis in pregnancy (p. 498).

2.5 INVESTIGATIONS

It is fairly general practice to estimate the serum electrolytes, and in adults the serum amylase, and to perform a full blood count. Plain abdominal radiography is of little help in the diagnosis of appendicitis because there are no certain signs apart from the rarely seen opaque faecolith. Barium enema has been used in diagnosis but is neither reliable nor appropriate.

The **white cell count (WCC)** is commonly requested and is a simple test that is universally available. Most patients with proven acute appendicitis show a leucocytosis – among more than 400 such patients a preoperative count of more than 14×10^9/l between 12 and 48 hours after onset of symptoms had a predictive value of 90% (McCombe and Gunn, 1991). However, a single count taken on admission still needs careful interpretation.

Allowance has to made for age, because in infancy the upper limit of a normal WCC is $15 \times 10^9/l$, and this figure gradually falls: above 15 years of age the normal limit is 10, or at the most $11 \times 10^9/l$. Then account must be taken, in the individual patient, of the fact that substantial surveys have shown that 20–30% of patients with proven appendicitis had a preoperative WCC within normal limits (although most showed neutrophilia; Bolton et al., 1975; Pieper et al., 1982; Goodman et al., 1995). Timing may play a part here, because Doraiswamy (1978) found that only 20 of 100 children with proven appendicitis had a leucocytosis during the first 24 hours of their illness.

In the other direction, 20% of patients who later prove to have had NSAP show, for some reason, a leucocytosis at the time of admission (Bolton *et al.*, 1975): C-reactive protein (CRP) is now commonly estimated at the same time as the WCC, at the time of admission. CRP is a non-specific phase protein that is synthesized in the liver and responds to tissue trauma, inflammation and infection: a noticeable rise can be detected in 6–8 hours and the peak is reached in 24–48 hours. The normal value is about 1 mg/l, and a report can be obtained in 15 minutes at a cost of £0.35. NSAP patients are usually observed because of their equivocal signs (p. 50) and it is then useful to repeat the WCC and CRP after several hours: a falling count or CRP is much against appendicitis while a rise in the two estimates would support the diagnosis. A CRP value over 15 mg/l is significant but, as in the case of white counts, the time after onset of symptoms can be significant (Davies *et al.*, 1991; Thompson *et al.*, 1992). However, it must be remembered that a single WCC taken in isolation can clearly be misleading, and when signs are at variance with the WCC or CRP the whole clinical picture must take precedence in reaching management decisions.

Fine catheter aspiration cytology of the peritoneal cavity depends on the fact that neutrophils are normally virtually absent from peritoneal fluid but they accumulate rapidly and widely in the presence of bacterial infection (Stewart *et al.*, 1988). Under local anaesthesia, a 14 FG intravenous cannula is introduced below the umbilicus and through it is passed a 3.5 Ch umbilical artery catheter, which is directed towards the tender area while suction is applied. The sample obtained is spread on a slide, stained and 500 cells are counted: if more than 50% are neutrophils the test is positive (Vipond *et al.*, 1990). The main value of the test is in doubtful cases and it may be of particular value when there are reasons, e.g. a pregnancy, to avoid operation. A positive result indicates infection, which may require operative treatment – or not, as in the case of salpingitis. Stewart (1991) has written a full review.

There has been growing interest in the use of grey-scale **ultrasonography** in the diagnosis of acute appendicitis since the technique was first described by Puylaert in 1986. Gentle graded compression is applied over the point of maximal tenderness, with the operator locating the appendix by finding a non-compressible, tubular, closed-end structure: parameters have been developed for wall thickness and overall diameter that are characteristic of appendicitis. Faecoliths, mesenteric adenitis and terminal ileitis may also be visualized.

This is an investigation which, used selectively, can provide helpful information, but it has its limitations. An expert operator is required to provide a reliable report, and such an opinion may not always be available. In about one-third of scans the appendix cannot be visualized. There is nothing to be gained by spending time on scanning patients who clearly require an operation, but in a doubtful case the changes characteristic of appendicitis, when seen, are specific. It is valuable in showing collections of fluid and gynaecological abnormalities. A meta-analysis encompassing over 3000 patients in 17 studies concluded that ultrasonography was helpful in patients with continuing abdominal symptoms and indeterminate clinical findings (Orr *et al.*, 1995). The clear result from a number of surveys is that the clinical findings must remain the principal guide to management and the ultrasound report must be interpreted with care: in some 10% of negative reports exploration on clinical grounds revealed an inflamed appendix (Wade *et al.*, 1993; Ramachandran *et al.*, 1996).

There can rarely be a reason for using **computed tomography**. Most cases of acute appendicitis arise in young people so, except in the event of unusual difficulty, they should not be exposed to the high dose of radiation involved in CT. Because CT has a high degree of accuracy in diagnosing or excluding appendicitis, it has been suggested that it can be used regularly, to reduce the number of negative appendicectomies and the consequent demands on hospital resources (Rao *et al.*, 1998). These aims can be safely achieved by careful bedside examination, and the practice of active observation, which can deliver a negative appendicectomy rate of 4–8% (p. 51).

The role of **laparoscopy** in the differential diagnosis of the acute abdomen, and especially of acute appendicitis, has received much attention. The increasing availability and refinement of the equipment, the success of laparoscopic cholecystectomy and the long experience of gynaecologists have combined to make general surgeons aware of the contribution that laparoscopy can make to diagnosis.

Experience suggests that in children and in adult men the value of laparoscopy in diagnosis is quite limited. When there are clear clinical indications to operate, either on admission or after observation, there are few occasions on which a surgical condition is not found, and the normal appendicectomy rate is well below 10%. Now that the merits of open and laparoscopic appendicectomy are seen to be fairly evenly balanced (p. 59), the open approach will continue to be widely used in this group. In woman of child-bearing age the contribution which laparoscopy can make to diagnosis is considerable and is fully discussed on p. 57. In some debatable situations laparoscopy has a part to play. In a patient with known inflammatory bowel disease who presents with possible appendicitis, the pathology could be terminal ileitis, which would be better treated medically. In an older person with acute central lower abdominal pain, this could arise from non-perforative sigmoid diverticulitis which, once identified, might settle on a medical regime.

REFERENCES

Bolton, J. P., Craven, E. R., Croft, R. J. *et al.* (1975) An assessment of the value of the white cell count in the management of suspected acute appendicitis. *Br. J. Surg.*, **62**, 906–908.

Bowen, J. and Bruce, J. (1994) Acute testicular pain: an unusual presentation of appendicitis. *Br. J. Surg.*, **81**, 776.

Brewster, S. F., Lovering, A. M. and McLoughlin, J. (1994) Pelvic appendicitis in young adult males masquerading as cystitis. *J. R. Coll. Surg. Edin.*, **39**, 119–120.

Cronin, K. and Ellis, H. (1959) Pus collections in hernial sacs: unusual complication of general peritonitis. *Br. J. Surg.*, **46**, 364–367.

Davies, A. H., Bernace, F., Salisbury, A. *et al.* (1991) C-reactive protein in right iliac fossa pain. *J. R. Coll. Surg. Edin.*, **36**, 242–244.

Dickson, A. P. and Mackinlay, G. A. (1985) Rectal examination and acute appendicitis. *Arch. Dis. Child.*, **60**, 666–667.

Dixon, J. M., Elton, R. A., Rainey, J. B. *et al.* (1991) Rectal examination in patients with pain in the right lower quadrant of the abdomen. *BMJ*, **302**, 386–388.

Doraiswamy, N. V. (1978) Progress of acute appendicitis: a study in children. *Br. J. Surg.*, **65**, 877–879.

Golledge, J., Toms, A. P., Franklin, I. J. *et al.* (1996) Assessment of peritonitis in appendicitis. *Ann. R. Coll. Surg. Engl.*, **78**, 11–14.

Goodman, D. A., Goodman, C. D. and Monk, J. S. (1995) Use of the neutrophil:lymphocyte ratio in the diagnosis of appendicitis. *Am. Surgeon*, **61**, 257–259.

Hartley, B. E. J., Davies, M. S. and Bowyer, R. C. (1994) Strangulated appendix in an obturator hernia presenting as gas gangrene in the thigh. *Br. J. Surg.*, **81**, 1135.

Lewis, F. R., Holcroft, J. W., Boey, J. *et al.* (1975) Appendicitis: a critical review of diagnosis and treatment in 1000 cases. *Arch. Surg.*, **110**, 677–682.

McBurney, C. (1889) Experience with early operative interference in cases of disease of the vermiform appendix. *N.Y. Med. J.*, **50**, 676–684.

McCombe, A. W. and Gunn, A. A. (1991) Laparotomy in the acute abdomen, *BMJ*, **303**, 1476.

Orr, R. K., Porter, D. and Hartmann, D. (1995) Ultrasonography to evaluate adults for appendicitis. *Acad. Emerg. Med.*, **2**, 644–650.

Pieper, R., Kager, L. and Nasman, P. (1982) Acute appendicitis: a clinical study of 1018 cases of emergency appendectomy. *Acta Chir. Scand.*, **148**, 51–62.

Puylaert, J. B. C. M. (1986) Acute appendicitis: ultrasound evaluation using graded compression. *Radiology*, **158**, 355–360.

Ramachandra, R., Sivit, C. J., Newman, K. D. *et al.* (1996) Ultrasonography as an adjunct in the diagnosis of acute appendicitis: a 4-year experience. *J. Pediatr. Surg.*, **31**, 164–169.

Rao, P. M., Rhea, J. T., Novelline, R. A. *et al.* (1998) Effect of computed tomography of the appendix on treatment of patients and use of hospital resources. *N. Eng. J. Med.*, **338**, 141–6.

Stewart, R. J. (1991) The acute abdomen: the role of peritoneal cytology. *Baillière's Clin. Gastroenterol.*, **5**, 667–689.

Stewart, R. J., Gupta, R. K., Purdie, G. L. *et al.* (1988) Fine catheter peritoneal cytology for the acute abdomen: a randomized controlled trial. *Austr. N.Z. J. Surg.*, **58**, 565–570.

Thomas, W. E. G., Vowles, K. D. J. and Williamson, R. C. N. (1982) Appendicitis in external hernia. *Ann. R. Coll. Surg. Engl.*, **64**, 121–122.

Thompson, M. M., Underwood, M. J., Dookeran, K. A. *et al.* (1992) Role of sequential leucocyte counts and C-reactive protein measurements in acute appendicitis. *Br. J. Surg.*, **79**, 822–824.

Turner, G. and Daniell, S. J. (1984) Lumbar abscess resulting from acute appendicitis. *J. R. Soc. Med.*, **77**, 884–885.

Varshney, S., Johnson, C. D. and Rangnekar, G. V. (1996) The retrocaecal appendix appears to be less prone to infection. *Br. J. Surg.*, **83**, 223–224.

Vipond, M. N., Paterson-Brown, S., Tyrell, M. R. *et al.* (1990) Evaluation of fine catheter aspiration cytology of the peritoneum. *Br. J. Surg.*, **77**, 86–87.

Wade, D. S., Morrow, S. E., Balsara, Z. N. *et al.* (1993) Accuracy of ultrasound in the diagnosis of acute appendicitis compared with the surgeon's impression. *Arch. Surg.*, **1993**; 1039–1046.

Wilkie, D. P. D. (1931) Observations on mortality in acute appendicular disease. *BMJ*, **i**, 253–253.

Winsey, H. S. and Jones, P. F. (1967) Acute abdominal pain in childhood: analysis of a year's admissions. *BMJ*, **i**, 653–655.

Woodward, M. N. and Griffiths, D. M. (1993) Use of dipsticks for routine analysis of urine from children with acute abdominal pain. *BMJ*, **306**, 1512.

2.6   DIFFERENTIAL DIAGNOSIS

Acute appendicitis presents a characteristic clinical picture sufficiently often to make it seem that diagnosis is straightforward, and Fitz in 1886 remarked that 'diagnosis in most cases is comparatively simple'. However, experience has taught some hard lessons and not only can appendicitis present in unusual ways (p. 44) but it can be imitated by a number of conditions and diseases. It is certainly the commonest organic cause of acute abdominal pain, but Tables 1.1–1.3 are a reminder that this symptom has many causes and that these vary with age and sex. In children and younger men there are few surgical imitators of appendicitis, but particularly in children confusion can arise from medical conditions such as constipation, urinary tract infection and gastroenteritis (Chapter 3), while in young women some of the disorders of the internal genitalia resemble appendicitis but only a few require surgical treatment (p. 56). In older men and women the spectrum of diseases that have to be considered is noticeably different. In patients of all ages the commonest cause of acute abdominal pain is the syndrome that can only be identified when other causes of pain have been excluded and the patient is ready for discharge; this is called acute non-specific abdominal pain, or NSAP.

2.6.1   ACUTE NON-SPECIFIC ABDOMINAL PAIN

Experience in Aberdeen in the 1960s led us to recognize that a number of children were being referred to hospital with a diagnosis of acute appendicitis who nevertheless settled, without treatment, within 24–36 hours of admission. An impressive example was seen when a colleague asked one of us to see his 6-year-old son at home. The signs of appendicitis were convincing and admission for operation was arranged. On a visit to the ward 3 hours later, on the way to theatre, the pain and tenderness were less and operation was postponed: next day the child had recovered. It was then decided to collect information on every child admitted to the Children's Hospital with acute abdominal pain during 1965, and full details were entered on a structured record form for each patient.

A total of 315 children were admitted and 135 (42.9%) appeared to have acute appendicitis and came to operation: this diagnosis was confirmed in 114 (36%) but the appendix was normal in 21 (15% of 135). A medical illness such as pneumonia was identified in 43 children (13.7%) and 18 (5.7%) required urgent operation for intussusception, band obstruction or blunt abdominal injury. In a large residual group of 119 (37.8%) no firm diagnosis was made and they left hospital after 24–48 hours (Winsey and Jones, 1967).

The latter group was larger than expected so the survey was continued over the following 2 years, and once again over 100 children each year settled quickly following admission. From this experience we had to conclude that, among children suspected of having appendicitis, about one-third would recover without treatment. We called this syndrome – identified after a period of observation – 'acute non-specific abdominal pain of childhood' (Jones, 1969); this was soon abbreviated to NSAP.

We had to consider whether these patients had in fact suffered a mild attack of appendicitis, which could recur. The records of 323 children were reviewed between 6 and 24 months after discharge and six had returned with acute appendicitis. Jess *et al.* (1982) considered this possibility and reviewed 230 NSAP patients after 5 years: eight had had an appendicectomy but only five had an acute appendix. It seems unlikely that many NSAP patients have true but resolving appendicitis.

Can patients with true early surgical disease, with equivocal signs on first examination, be distinguished from patients with NSAP? For a long time it was believed that operation should be performed forthwith in these doubtful cases lest perforation of the appendix should occur as a result of delay, but this resulted in 20–30% of appendices removed as a precaution being histologically normal. These patients derived no benefit from the operation and some suffered serious late complications, including adhesive small-bowel obstruction that required operative release (Pieper *et al.*, 1982).

When the symptoms and signs of patients with NSAP are compared with those who have appendicitis (Figure 2.2), some clear differences emerge, and it seemed reasonable to test whether a strictly controlled period of 'active observation' would allow more NSAP patients to be identified without acutely inflamed appendices being given time in which to perforate. In this regime patients are not allowed oral fluids and, if dehydrated, intravenous fluids are given. Hourly temperature and pulse recordings are kept, the WCC and CRP are estimated and the nursing staff keep a close watch on the patient. After 2–3 hours the surgeon who made the first examination returns to reassess the situation: in some patients the signs will have developed and operation is arranged. In others the situation remains equivocal, or has improved, and observation is continued. In another group investigations will have confirmed a medical disease and treatment can be started.

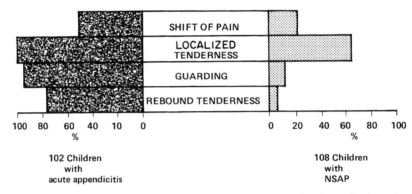

Figure 2.2 Percentage incidence of 4 symptoms and signs, at the time of admission, in 210 children with a final diagnosis of acute appendicitis in 102 and of NSAP in 108. (Reproduced with permission from Jones, 1969.)

Figure 2.3 illustrates this sequence as seen in a trial conducted on 363 consecutive admissions to the Royal Aberdeen Children's' Hospital in 1974/5 (Jones, 1976).

In 106 children operation was clearly needed at the time of admission, while active observation and necessary investigation were practised in the other 257. At the first re-examination 19 children were selected for operation and one more was found at the second assessment. One of these 20 appendices was perforated but recovery was uneventful and there was no death in this series. A total of 12 (10.5%) of the 114 appendices removed were normal, but nine of these patients had shown persistent tenderness and guarding. Eventually 108 (30%) were considered to have suffered from NSAP.

There have been several other trials of active observation, in adults as well as children, showing a much-reduced rate of negative appendicectomy (Table 2.1), and in a total of 1043 patients there was one death in a child admitted with advanced peritonitis.

O'Donnell (1985) gave observation an extended trial in Dublin: when the policy of operating when in doubt was changed to observation of patients with equivocal signs, the negative appendicectomy rate fell from 26% to 7%, so it seems that active observation is safe and effective.

The NSAP syndrome is now recognized in many countries as the commonest cause of acute abdominal pain (de Dombal, 1988). This being so, it is important to identify as many of these patients as possible without, as Hoffmann and Rasmussen (1989) remark, 'the

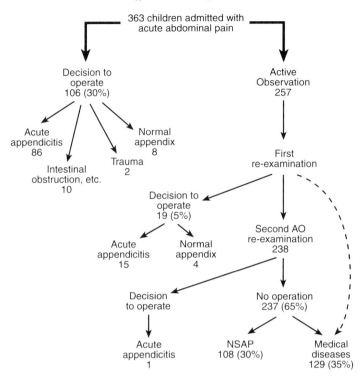

Figure 2.3 Outcome of the use of active observation in 363 consecutive admissions of children with acute abdominal pain. The dotted line indicates that diagnosis of some medical conditions is reached soon after admission.

Table 2.1 Outcome at laparotomy for suspected acute appendicitis, with and without use of active observation (A = adult; C = children; AA = acute appendicitis)

Reference	City	Age	?AA	Operation Proven AA	Other surgical emergency	No. normal appendix removed (%)
Trials of active observation						
White *et al.*, 1975	Baltimore	C	104	98	2	4 (4)
White *et al.*, 1975	Baltimore	A	74	67	2	5 (7)
Jones, 1976	Aberdeen	C	116	102	2	12 (10.5)
Thomson and Jones, 1986	Inverness	A+C	48	42	2	4 (8)
Dolgin *et al.*, 1992	New York	C	100	93	1	6 (6)
O'Donnell, 1983	Dublin	C	520	483	–	37 (7)
Driver and Youngson, 1992	Aberdeen	C	81	78	–	3 (4)
Active observation not used						
Jones, 1969	Aberdeen	C	462	398	6	58 (12.5)
White *et al.*, 1975	Baltimore	C	266	213	4	49 (18)
Lewis *et al.*, 1975	San Francisco	A+C	1000	772	22	188 (18)
O'Donnell, 1975	Dublin	C	3677	2694	–	983 (26.6)
Pieper *et al.*, 1982	Stockholm	A+C	1018	688	42	288 (28)

Gordian knot of appendicitis diagnosis [being] untied with the scalpel'. The question that remains to be answered is whether active observation, though carefully conducted, allows an unacceptable number of appendices to progress to perforation.

The 'better safe than sorry' approach is based on the belief that all acutely inflamed appendices are equally liable to perforate. The figures do not support this, and in fact show that patients with **perforative appendicitis** have distinctive features.

- In the five trials in Table 2.1 that provide perforation rates, 523 acutely inflamed appendices were removed, of which 92 (17.5%) were perforated. In 85 the signs must have been clear on admission because they were promptly operated on: only seven were removed after a period of observation and in two operation was delayed to allow resuscitation of the patient. All made a good recovery. This result is typical of a number of reports, which show that, because there is a mean delay of 40–50 hours before admission, the signs are by then quite evident: consequently the large majority of patients with perforated appendicitis will not be candidates for observation (Moss *et al.*, 1985; Temple *et al.*, 1995).
- The age of the patient has a major influence on the tendency to perforation. Incidence is high among the under-fives but then falls quickly, and between 10 and 40 years of age the risk of perforation is less than 10%, even when admission is delayed for 36 hours. After 40 the risk of perforation rises gradually to about 30% at 60, and it is over 50% after the age of 75. So, just at the age when appendicitis is most common, and active observation is most needed, the risk of perforation is at its lowest (Koepsell *et al.*, 1981; de Dombal, 1991; Luckmann, 1989).

These facts and figures give a numerical basis to the claim that active observation, when carefully conducted, is a safe and effective method of identifying most NSAP patients. What it does not do is to distinguish between the various inflammatory causes of acute pain in the lower abdomen: this is of particular importance in young women, and is considered on p. 56.

So far there is no clear explanation for the NSAP syndrome. Viral titres are rarely raised, and psychological tests show no differences compared to controls. Doshi and Heaton (1994) consider that as many as one-third of NSAP patients go on to show features of the irritable bowel syndrome. One very important fact must be remembered about patients who are over 50 years of age: 10% of **gastrointestinal cancers** first present with acute abdominal symptoms. In 3% the patient suffers an acute illness, such as bowel perforation or obstruction; another 3.5% have the carcinoma (usually of the colon) diagnosed during the admission; but 3.5% leave hospital with the NSAP label and continue for some months before the true diagnosis is made (de Dombal *et al.*, 1980).

The term NSAP is certainly not a diagnosis. Experience over some 30 years shows that, in the great majority of patients, it identifies a syndrome that has a characteristic pattern, is self-limiting and does not recur. Its recognition contributes significantly to the management of patients with acute abdominal signs.

2.6.2   ACUTE MESENTERIC ADENITIS

In the 1960s, when patients with suspected acute appendicitis were usually operated upon, some 10–20% of operations revealed a normal appendix; in a number, oedema and swelling of the lymph nodes in the ileocaecal mesentery was found, and this was considered to be the cause of the pain.

Mair *et al.* (1960) studied 93 children who had an operation for suspected acute appendicitis. In 17 the appendix was normal but the ileocaecal lymph nodes were swollen and oedematous and the mesentery was inflamed. A biopsy of the glands was taken and the juice was cultured for viral strains and organisms: the viral cultures were negative but in three children *Yersinia pseudotuberculosis* was cultured and the serology showed a marked rise in the titre.

Now that observation is more widely practised, relatively few of these cases are seen. In a typical case a child between 2 and 15 years of age complains of feeling unwell, with loss of appetite, nausea and central abdominal pain. Some complain of headache and sore throat, and there may be cervical lymphadenopathy. The temperature registers 38–40°C. In the abdomen the pain may shift to the RLQ, where there is some tenderness but only rarely guarding. Occasionally, persistent signs in the RLQ lead to laparotomy, but generally the picture is not typical of appendicitis.

Morrison (1981) suspected that mesenteric adenitis due to yersiniosis might be one of the contributors to the NSAP syndrome. In 24 NSAP patients, four developed strongly positive serology for *Y. pseudotuberculosis*, but so did two of 13 patients with proven acute appendicitis. All investigations for infection with adenovirus of *Yersinia enterocolitica* were negative.

As will be seen in the next section, all the major causes of acute bacterial enterocolitis can sometimes produce terminal ileitis and mesenteric adenitis, and in a minority of patients there are localizing signs in the RLQ. These require careful assessment (in which ultrasonography may be helpful) and close observation.

2.6.3 ACUTE GASTROENTERITIS

Family doctors are very familiar with this illness which, especially in summer and among children, causes acute diarrhoea and vomiting. Abdominal pain is not common but when it is associated with acute diarrhoea this is a danger signal. Family doctors in the UK now see only two or three cases of acute appendicitis in a year so it is necessary to be mindful of the rule that pelvic appendicitis must be suspected when diarrhoea is accompanied by abdominal pain (p. 40), or in infancy the possibility of intussusception (p. 98) must be considered.

The situation is further complicated by the fact that enteritis due to *Y. enterocolitica*, *Campylobacter* spp. and *Cryptosporidium* can be accompanied by a considerable degree of abdominal pain. Generally these patients do not present like appendicitis. There is malaise, fever of 39–40°C, headache, nausea and vomiting over a day or two. Then quite profuse diarrhoea, often blood-stained, commences and in about one-half of the cases there is generalized cramping abdominal pain. Ponka *et al.* (1981) studied 81 patients with *Campylobacter* enteritis in Finland and found that half showed diffuse abdominal tenderness, localized in the RLQ in seven. This persisted and, after observation, four patients had a laparotomy that revealed a normal appendix and some terminal ileitis. Puylaert *et al.* (1988) found ultrasonography to be helpful: they examined nine patients, all thought to have appendicitis, with immediate operation planned in five. Ultrasound failed to identify the appendix but showed abnormal thickening of the wall of the terminal ileum and enlarged mesenteric nodes: one operation went ahead and confirmed these findings. Perkins and

Newstead (1994) had a patient with *Campylobacter* enteritis that went on to signs of small-bowel obstruction: he had to be explored; 50 cm of terminal ileum was greatly thickened and inspissated faeces had to be squeezed through it into the caecum. The appearance of the ileum raised a doubt about Crohn's ileitis but mural biopsy did not confirm this and the patient slowly recovered. The differential diagnosis of these bacterial causes of terminal ileal thickening from Crohn's ileitis, neoplasms and endometriosis, all of which can look similar to the naked eye, is considered in full on p. 233.

2.6.4   OTHER INFLAMMATORY DISEASE IN THE RLQ

A number of surgical conditions can present with signs suggestive of acute appendicitis and, because they are unusual and have no distinctive features, are only recognized when the abdomen is opened. This is no disadvantage, because they all need surgical treatment, and they are considered in the section 'on finding a normal appendix' (p. 68). In older patients, diverticulitis of the sigmoid colon can present with signs in the right lower abdomen.

2.6.5   MEDICAL DISEASES

Diabetic ketoacidosis can present with acute abdominal pain. These patients have several distinctive features and these are fully considered on pages p. 114 and p. 537.

Infective hepatitis in the preicteric phase can cause acute upper abdominal pain. These patients are febrile and unwell, and the tenderness is chiefly over the liver: this could be confused with cholecystitis or a high retrocolic appendicitis. In daylight a touch of jaundice may be seen; the urine may contain a little bile and the liver function tests would show some changes. There should be some doubt about the whole picture, indicating the need for observation.

Meningitis occasionally presents with abdominal pain rather than headache. In any patient (most often a child or teenager) who is clearly unwell, not typical of appendicitis, pale but feverish and, most importantly, with a haemorrhagic non-blanching rash, meningitis must be suspected. If suspicion is high, intramuscular benzylpenicillin must be started (Granier *et al.*, 1998). Wylie *et al.* (1997) advise caution over the use of lumbar puncture for diagnosis.

Respiratory infections. The classical picture of a febrile, cyanosed and dyspnoeic patient with troublesome cough must not be expected. These patients, usually children, are not numerous but the lack of respiratory complaints can be misleading (p. 115).

2.6.6   URINARY TRACT PROBLEMS

The pain arising from a stone passing down the right ureter is distinctive: it is very intense and pain often radiates into the groin and scrotum or labia. The patient is restless. A plain X-ray is likely to show a stone in the ureter and an intravenous pyelogram can be very helpful (p. 478).

In acute infections, with pyelonephritis, the pain is felt mainly in the loin; there is high fever, malaise, headache and marked tenderness over the kidney. If the kidney is obstructed there can be a disturbing degree of guarding as well as tenderness over the kidney, and little sign of pus in the urine, but the whole picture is unlike appendicitis. The acute pyelitis of pregnancy can raise real doubts about the possibility of appendicitis (p. 498).

2.6.7   LEAKING DUODENAL ULCER

Occasionally a small perforation of a duodenal ulcer can allow irritant fluid to track down the paracolic gutter and cause pain and tenderness in the RLQ. This picture, which is now unusual, is very different to the rigid abdomen of a free perforation. If the onset of pain was very sudden and the whole of the right side of the abdomen is tender, this diagnosis might be suspected and X-rays after the injection of water-soluble contrast down a nasogastric tube can be helpful.

2.6.8   INTESTINAL OBSTRUCTION

Confusion can arise in two ways.

- The onset of acute obstructive appendicitis produces colicky periumbilical pain. Signs in the RLQ, inactive bowel sounds and normal hernial sites would favour a diagnosis of appendicitis.
- Acute appendicitis in the older patient can present after a day or two of pain with abdominal distension due to ileus. The picture can be confusing and is considered on page p. 75.

2.6.9   CHOLECYSTITIS

The majority of cases of appendicitis occur before the age of 40, but only some 10% of patients with acute cholecystitis are below this age. The pain of acute cholecystitis is usually localized to the right upper quadrant and tenderness is maximal right under the rib cage. Occasionally the caecum turns upwards and the appendix is subhepatic, so appendicitis can resemble cholecystitis. The history may be helpful, because appendicitis often commences with acute pain around the umbilicus. If there is doubt about this differential diagnosis, between 90 and 95% of acutely inflamed gallbladders contain stones, so ultrasonography can be very helpful.

2.6.10   PRIMARY TORSION OF THE GREAT OMENTUM

This is a rare condition that is likely to be difficult to distinguish from appendicitis. A portion of the omentum rotates around a pedicle and becomes infarcted. There is no explanation for this event, which occurs mostly on the right side. Tenderness is higher than is usual in appendicitis and can be acute. On opening the abdomen blood-stained fluid may be seen. If, as is likely, a gridiron incision has been used and the appendix is normal, the specimen is likely to be found by exploring the right upper abdomen. The pedicle is ligated and the mass removed (Chew *et al.*, 1995).

2.6.11   HAEMATOMA WITHIN THE RECTUS SHEATH

During activity, especially coughing, the right inferior epigastric artery is ruptured, and this produces an acutely tender area in the right lower quadrant. The rest of the abdomen is soft and not tender. The main step in reaching a diagnosis is to think of this unusual condition. It is most often seen during pregnancy (p. 499) or in patients on anticoagulants.

2.6.12   ACUTE LOWER ABDOMINAL PAIN IN WOMEN

There are particular difficulties over making a clinical diagnosis of acute appendicitis in women of child-bearing age: nowadays this includes even the youngest teenagers. The pelvic organs in the female often lie close to the appendix and both physiological and pathological changes in these organs cause symptoms that closely resemble appendicitis. Many of these conditions do not require surgical treatment (Table 1.2) and incidence varies considerably with age. This group of patients presents in several distinct ways, each calling for a different approach, and these provide a good example of the manner in which the surgeon caring for abdominal emergencies has to adjust management to circumstances.

- A small minority are already seriously ill on admission, because of either spreading peritonitis (most often due to perforated appendicitis) or, less commonly, an increasing haemoperitoneum (usually due to a ruptured ectopic pregnancy). The priority is to prepare the patient for the operation, which is urgently needed. Here a decision on timely practical management takes precedence over precise diagnosis. The peritonitis might be due to a late case of perforated peptic ulcer, and the bleeding be due to a ruptured splenic artery aneurysm, but the priority is to start intensive treatment and to operate to deal with the cause of the emergency – whatever the laparotomy may reveal this to be.
- In another group, quite often seen in accident and emergency departments, the diagnosis is usually clear. The patient is in the first trimester of pregnancy and has started to lose blood and clots *per vaginam* and experience lower abdominal pain. This is characteristic of an incomplete or threatened miscarriage, and these patients are considered further in Chapter 12.

  Patients with known and established pregnancy and acute lower abdominal pain, with no vaginal loss, may have an emergency unconnected with the pregnancy, such as appendicitis or torsion of an ovarian cyst, or one of the later complications of pregnancy such as red degeneration in a fibroid (Chapter 12).
- There remain a large number of women who are in normal health when they suffer the onset of acute lower abdominal pain. This is a group in which reaching a correct diagnosis can make a material difference to the line of management. The range of conditions is wide; fewer than one-third require surgical correction and nearly one-half recover without active treatment (Table 1.2). Active observation will be much used, and it is helpful to remember that it is in this group that the number of cases of appendicitis going on to perforation is at its lowest (p. 52).

The first step is to establish whether the patient is pregnant because, though few harbour an ectopic pregnancy, it is potentially a dangerous condition and it is necessary to be forewarned. More than 80% will be between 15 and 50 years of age and, in addition to their natural anxiety about their condition, they are very likely to have social concerns – children left at home or fear of pregnancy. Some may be shy to respond to necessary questions, and all will appreciate a gentle line of enquiry.

The issue of possible pregnancy can usually be settled by a slide test on the urine for chorionic gonadotrophin or estimation of beta-hCG in serum. If the history and the test confirm a pregnancy then the most likely possibility is that an early normal pregnancy is complicated by an unconnected emergency such as appendicitis, of which there will be the usual symptoms and signs. A patient with an unruptured ectopic pregnancy has usually had lower abdominal discomfort and dyspareunia over several days, some amenorrhoea or menstrual irregularity, and 90% see a little vaginal loss of blood. These signals are very important because they warn that pelvic examination can disturb a tubal pregnancy and lead to serious bleeding (p. 493). As soon as an ectopic pregnancy is a real possibility the advice of a gynaecologist should be sought. Transvaginal pelvic ultrasonography can be helpful – if an intrauterine pregnancy is seen then a tubal pregnancy can be more or less ruled out. Laparoscopy should clarify the diagnosis, and many gynaecologists now treat an unruptured tubal pregnancy through the laparoscope (Magos *et al.*, 1989). The role of the lone general surgeon is considered in Chapter 12, as are other treatment options.

Among the majority who are not pregnant there will be many who, under observation, show the steady improvement characteristic of the NSAP syndrome. In another substantial group there will be persistent symptoms and signs of inflammation in the lower abdomen, and the main question will be whether appendicitis or pelvic inflammatory disease (PID) is the cause. One requires operative treatment, the other urgent and well-chosen administration of antibiotics, perhaps intravenously, to minimize tubal damage (p. 515). In 85% of cases PID presents in the 14 days after the last menstrual period, and often there has been pain and some vaginal discharge over 2–3 days: on pelvic examination movement of the cervix is exceptionally painful. However in the individual patient purely clinical differentiation of these two conditions is not clear-cut. Ultrasonography by an experienced radiologist can help, but as many as one-third of appendices are not visualized. There is a strong case for performing diagnostic laparoscopy in women who, after a period of observation, have persisting signs in the lower abdomen, because precision of diagnosis is achieved. Leape and Ramenovsky (1980), in children, and Deutsch *et al.* (1982), in women aged 18–50 years, showed that if laparoscopy was performed on patients with equivocal signs in the RLQ they were able to cancel one-third of the laparotomies that previously they would have undertaken. In about half these patients an acutely inflamed appendix is seen and in about one-third there are signs of salpingitis, a ruptured graafian follicle or torsion of an ovarian cyst.

Recent reports (Spirtos *et al.*, 1987; Paterson-Brown and Vipond, 1990) tend to emphasize the reduction in the negative appendicectomy rate that follows terminating the laparoscopy when no surgical lesion is identified. The question must be asked as to whether it is correct to leave an apparently normal appendix *in situ* when the examination has been carried out under general anaesthesia and a laparoscopic appendicectomy could be carried out. There is a strong case for this. It must be remembered that when macroscopically normal appendices are submitted to microscopy, some 15–20% show mucosal ulceration, with pus in the lumen (Grunewald and Keating, 1993; Kollias *et al.*, 1994), and of 40 carcinoids of the appendix removed at operation for acute appendicitis only four had looked abnormal to the surgeon (Parkes *et al.*, 1993).

REFERENCES

Chew, D. K., Holgersen, L. O. and Friedman, D. (1995) Primary omental torsion in children. *J. Pediatr. Surg.*, **30**, 816–817.

De Dombal, F. T., Matharu, S. S., Staniland, J. R. *et al.* (1980) Presentation of cancer to hospital as 'acute abdominal pain'. *Br. J. Surg.*, **67**, 413–416.

de Dombal, F. T. (1988) The OMGE Acute Abdominal Pain Survey. *Scand. J. Gastroenterol.*, **33** (Suppl. 144), 35–42.

De Dombal FT (1991) *Diagnosis of Acute Abdominal Pain*, 2nd edn, Churchill Livingstone, Edinburgh.

Deutsch, A. A., Zelikovsky, A. and Reiss, R. (1982) Laparoscopy in the prevention of unnecessary appendicectomies: a prospective study. *Br. J. Surg.*, **69**, 336–337.

Dolgin, S. E., Beck, A. R. and Tartter, P. I. (1992) The risk of perforation when children with possible appendicitis are observed in hospital. *Surg. Gynecol. Obstet.*, **175**, 320–324.

Doshi, M. and Heaton, K. W. (1994) Irritable bowel syndrome in patients discharged from surgical wards with nonspecific abdominal pain. *Br. J. Surg.*, **81**, 1216–1218.

Driver, C. P. and Youngson, G. G. (1995) Acute abdominal pain in children: a 25-year comparison. *Health Bull.*, **53**, 167–172.

Fitz, R. H. (1886) Perforating inflammation of the vermiform appendix, with special reference to early diagnosis and treatment. *Am. J. Med. Sci.*, **92**, 321–346.

Granier, S., Owen, P., Pill, R. *et al.* (1998) Recognizing meningococcal disease in primary care. *BMJ*, **316**, 276–9.

Grunewald, B. and Keating, J. (1993) Should the 'normal' appendix be removed at operation for appendicitis? *J. R. Coll. Surg. Edin.*, **38**, 158–160.

Hoffmann, J. and Rasmussen, O. O. (1989) Aids in the diagnosis of acute appendicitis. *Br. J. Surg.*, **76**, 774–779.

Jess, P., Bjerregaard, B., Brynitz, S. *et al.* (1982) Prognosis of acute nonspecific abdominal pain. *Am. J. Surg.*, **144**, 338–340.

Jones, P. F. (1969) Acute abdominal pain in childhood, with special reference to cases not due to acute appendicitis. *BMJ*, **i**, 284–286.

Jones, P. F. (1976) Active observation in the management of acute abdominal pain in childhood. *BMJ*, **ii**, 551–553.

Koepsell, T. D., Inui, T. S. and Farewell, V. T. (1981) Factors affecting perforation in acute appendicitis. *Surg. Gynecol. Obstet.*, **153**, 508–510.

Kollias, J., Harries, R. H. C., Otto, G. *et al.* (1994) Laparoscopic vs. open appendicectomy for suspected appendicitis: a prospective study. *Austr. N.Z. J. Surg.*, **64**, 830–835.

Leape, L. L. and Ramenofsky, M. L. (1980) Laparoscopy for questionable appendicitis: can it reduce the negative laparotomy rate? *Ann. Surg.*, **191**, 410–413.

Lewis, F. R., Holcroft, J. W., Boey, J. *et al.* (1975) Appendicitis: a critical review of diagnosis and treatment in 1000 cases. *Arch. Surg.*, **110**, 677–682.

Luckmann, R. (1989) Incidence and case fatality rates for acute appendicitis in California. *Am. J. Epidemiol.*, **129**, 905–918.

Magos, L., Baumann, R. and Turnbull, A. C. (1989) Managing gynaecological emergencies with laparoscopy, *BMJ*, **299**, 371–374.

Mair, N. S., Mair, H. J., Stirk, E. M. *et al.* (1960) Three cases of acute mesenteric lymphadenitis due to *Pasteurella pseudotuberculosis*. *J. Clin. Path.*, **13**, 432–439.

Morrison, J. D. (1981) Yersinia and viruses in acute nonspecific abdominal pain and appendicitis. *Br. J. Surg.*, **68**, 284–286.

Moss, J. G., Barrie, J. L. and Gunn, A. A. (1985) Delay in surgery for acute appendicitis. *J. R. Coll. Surg. Edin.*, **30**, 290–293.

O'Donnell, B. (1985) *Abdominal Pain in Children*, Blackwell Scientific Publications, Oxford, pp. 6, 57.

Parkes, S. E., Muir, K. R., Sheyyal, M. A. I. *et al.* (1993) Carcinoid tumours of the appendix in children, 1956–1986: incidence, treatment and outcome. *Br. J. Surg.*, **80**, 502–504.

Paterson-Brown, S. and Vipond, M. N. (1990) Modern aids to clinical decision-making in the acute abdomen. *Br. J. Surg.*, **77**, 13–18.

Perkins, D. J. and Newstead, G. L. (1994) *Campylobacter jejuni* enterocolitis causing peritonitis, ileitis and intestinal obstruction. *Austr. N.Z. J. Surg.*, **64**, 55–558.

Peiper, R., Kager, L. and Nasman, P. (1982) Acute appendicitis: a clinical study of 1018 cases of appendectomy. *Acta Chir. Scand.*, **148**, 51–62.

Ponka, A., Pitkanen, T. and Kosunen, T. U. (1981) *Campylobacter* enteritis mimicking acute abdominal emergency. *Acta Chir. Scand.*, **147**, 663–666.

Puylaert, J. B. C. M., Lalisang, R. I., van der Werf, S. D. J. *et al.* (1988) *Campylobacter* ileocolitis mimicking acute appendicitis: differentiation with graded-compression ultrasound. *Radiology*, **166**, 737–740.

Spencer, P. A. S. (1990) Pneumonia, diagnosed on the abdominal radiograph, as a cause for acute abdomen in children. *Br. J. Radiol.*, **63**, 306–308.

Spirtos, N. M., Spirtos, T. W., Poliakin, R. I. *et al.* (1987) Laparoscopy – a diagnostic aid in cases of suspected appendicitis. *Am. J. Gynecol.*, **156**, 90–94.

Telfer, S., Fenyo, G., Holt, P. R. *et al.* (1988) Acute abdominal pain in patients over 50 years of age. *Scand. J. Gastroenterol.*, **23** (Suppl. 144), 47–50.

Temple, C. L., Huchcroft, S. A. and Temple, W. J. (1995) The natural history of acute appendicitis: a prospective study. *Ann. Surg.*, **221**, 278–281.

Thomson, H. J. and Jones, P. F. (1986) Active observation in acute abdominal pain. *Am. J. Surg.*, **152**, 522–525.

White, J. J., Santillana, M. and Haller, J. A. (1975) Intensive in-hospital observation: a safe way to decrease unnecessary appendectomy. *Am. Surgeon*, **41**, 793–798.

Winsey, H. S., Jones, P. F. (1967) Acute abdominal pain in childhood: analysis of a year's admissions. *BMJ*, **i**, 653–655.

Wylie, P. A. L., Stevens, D., Drake, W. *et al.* (1997) Epidemiology and clinical management of meningococcal disease in West Gloucestershire. *BMJ*, **315**, 774–779.

2.7   TREATMENT

The best treatment for acute appendicitis is prompt appendicectomy. The source of trouble is removed, further attacks are prevented and, when the appendix is perforated, the source of continuing peritoneal contamination is removed. In patients with a palpable appendicular mass conservative treatment is often appropriate, but sometimes an abscess requires drainage (p. 70).

There have been suggestions that appendicitis could be treated by bed rest and antibiotics but in practice, because outcome is uncertain, this line of treatment is confined to situations in which safe surgery is impractical, e.g. on a ship at sea far from land and without a surgeon. In a trial in 20 patients of a regime of intravenous fluids with cefuroxime and metronidazole, 19 recovered but one required laparotomy for spreading peritonitis: over the following 12 months, seven developed recurrent appendicitis, in some cases within weeks (Eriksson and Granstrom, 1995).

2.7.1   CHOICE OF METHOD

Until the mid-1980s the accepted method of performing appendicectomy was by open operation. Since then it has been demonstrated that the acutely inflamed appendix can be safely removed by laparoscopic techniques, and there have been sufficient trials comparing open appendicectomy (OA) with the laparoscopic operation (LA) to allow some judgements to be made (Tate, 1996).

At first it seemed that, although the operation took longer, patients having LA required less analgesia, resumed drinking and eating sooner, had a shorter hospital stay and returned to full activity earlier than their counterparts who had an OA. These outcomes naturally led to a critical examination of the results of OA, and recent prospective randomized studies show that there is little difference in the outcomes of the two methods (Kollias *et al.*, 1994; Hassen and Cade, 1996). The cost of LA tends to be greater because generally the operation takes longer. LA can be technically more difficult, and conversion to OA is necessary in up to 20% of cases (Tate, 1996). If disposable equipment is used this increases the cost. On a busy receiving day it takes longer to sterilize laparoscopic equipment. Wound infections are, with proper precautions, equal for the two methods. Now that speedy postoperative discharge after operation for uncomplicated appendicitis is general, it is difficult to recoup the extra costs of LA.

In the light of these studies there is little advantage is using LA in children and in grown men. With careful clinical assessment and observation the negative appendicectomy rate is rarely above 5%, so there is little diagnostic advantage is using laparoscopy (Mutter *et al.*, 1996). Most children are thin, their recuperative powers are great and the disparity in size between patients and equipment tends to favour the use of OA. There can however be an advantage in using LA in obese men because the extent of the incision can be large in comparison to three or four puncture wounds, which heal quickly.

The advantage of using laparoscopy in young women is real and has been discussed on p. 57. Laparoscopy cannot be safely used in established pregnancy (Chapter 12), and the wide exposure obtainable at laparotomy is preferable in general peritonitis (p. 146).

As emergency surgery is increasingly performed during the daytime, in dedicated theatres, emergency appendicectomy will be seen to provide an excellent opportunity for supervised practical training in the techniques of open and of laparoscopic surgery.

2.7.2   THE OPEN OPERATION

In the majority of patients a muscle-splitting or muscle-cutting incision, sited over the appendix, is appropriate, and most often a McBurney/McArthur type of incision is used. If access proves to be inadequate it is easy to extend the incision into a muscle-cutting one, which will allow good exposure of a retrocolic appendix, Meckel's diverticulum, caecal diverticulitis or Crohn's disease of the ileocaecal angle. Right hemicolectomy and ovarian cystectomy can be performed through a muscle-splitting incision that has been properly extended. If it is found that the patient actually has a perforated peptic ulcer, or perforated sigmoid diverticulitis then the incision must be closed, and good exposure obtained by making a suitable vertical incision. When an advanced pelvic appendicitis is suspected it is easier and safer to operate through a vertical incision. Many pelvic appendices are gangrenous and adherent, but unperforated: using the tip of a sucker as a dissector, these can be teased out still intact, and this can be very difficult to achieve through a gridiron incision.

2.7.2.1   Making the incision

McBurney and McArthur published their descriptions of a gridiron muscle-splitting incision simultaneously in 1894: a little reading of the two papers shows that McArthur was the first to use it, but he has received little of the credit.

The sterile towels should be placed so that both the anterior superior iliac spine and the umbilicus are visible. McBurney suggested that the incision should run nearly at right angles to the line joining the iliac spine to the umbilicus, and about 2 cm internal to the iliac spine. This oblique incision allows for extension if the exposure is inadequate; it is more difficult

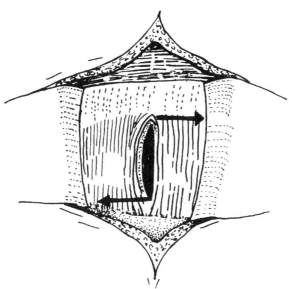

Figure 2.4 Surgeon's eye view of a gridiron incision. Retractors separate the split fibres of external oblique and reveal the split in internal oblique and transversus: extension of this incision is achieved downward by cutting these two muscles along the lateral edge of the rectus sheath. Extension upward is obtained by cutting the two muscles from the lateral end of the split in them, for as far as is necessary.

to extend a transverse (Lanz) skin incision. The external oblique is then split in the line of its fibres. It is usually easiest to start the split in internal oblique and transversus by incising the lateral edge of the rectus sheath, opening this up by spreading the tip of a pair of scissors, and then prolonging the split laterally. Opening a short length of the rectus sheath is harmless and improves the exposure. The two index fingers, or retractor blades, are then inserted into the split and widely separated to secure the maximum benefit of the incision.

A gridiron incision, however widely retracted, gives only limited access to the right iliac fossa. When simple acute appendicitis is present, and the caecum is mobile, this exposure is completely adequate. When, as often happens, the posterior wall of the caecum is extraperitoneal it can be difficult to bring it, and so the appendix, up to the surface. It is important in these circumstances not to struggle on with a poor exposure, because extension of the wound is easy and harmless. If the appendix lies behind the caecum and ascending colon the incision should be extended upwards by dividing the muscles and peritoneum at the lateral end of the muscle split (Figure 2.4).

Even a cut of 2 cm produces a surprising improvement in exposure. If downward extension is needed, to reach a pelvic appendix or pathological ovary, it is best to cut down the lateral edge of the rectus sheath.

When faced with a stout patient, or where experience suggests that the operation will be technically difficult, there is much to be said for using the incision described by Rutherford Morison in 1901. This is an oblique muscle-cutting incision, in the same line as McBurney's, which cuts the internal oblique and transversus instead of splitting them. The length of the cut is variable. The skin incision is usually 10–12 cm long and so is the split in external oblique. A central incision in the muscles of about 5 cm is usually sufficient and can be made without much bleeding if the diathermy needle is used. If it is found that more room is needed then the incision in the muscles can be extended and this can be made, without harm, on the occasions when an ileocaecal resection is found to be necessary. When extending downwards it is wise to remember the anatomy of the inferior epigastric artery and vein.

2.7.2.2 Technique of appendicectomy

On opening the peritoneum, the first viscus seen will probably be small intestine. If there is much fluid this should be sucked away, a specimen placed in a jar for culture, and a bacteriological swab specimen taken from the surface of the inflamed appendix. Two Czerny's retractors should be inserted under the upper and lower edges of the peritoneum and lifted a little as well as being pulled horizontally. If caecum is still covered by small intestine it should be sought by sliding the finger down into the lateral paracolic gutter. It is a mistake to start pulling out small intestine. Occasionally the sigmoid colon presents, with prominent appendices epiploicae. At this stage protect the wound edges with swabs soaked in chlorhexidine 0.5%.

The colour of the caecum (grey–blue) and the taenia coli are both quite characteristic. When seen, the caecum should be picked up and its mobility assessed by hooking the index finger under the anterior taenia and using it as a handle to gently ease the caecum out of the wound. If it comes up readily this is useful because this must reveal the base of the appendix. It is then an easy matter to run the finger gently along the appendix to the tip. If the tip is free then it should be possible to deliver the whole appendix on to the surface. If the body and tip of the appendix are not free, as is often the case in retrocaecal and pelvic appendicitis, then a pause is needed to decide on the approach.

An adherent pelvic appendix may be surrounded by a small abscess, which is contained within adjacent coils of intestine. If this is found it will be helpful to extend the incision downwards. Then proceed to free the appendix with the sucker, as already described, and gently ease the appendix up into the incision. If it is perforated and no faecolith can be felt, search for one in the abscess cavity.

If exploration shows that the appendix is in the retroileal position, extend the incision as necessary and try to deliver the ileocaecal area on to the surface. Turn the bowel over so as to expose the undersurface of the ileocaecal mesentery and free the appendix, using the sucker as dissector to catch any spillage of pus.

Gentleness and patience are life-saving qualities when removing a tense unruptured gangrenous appendix. By taking time over securing a good exposure, and judicious manipulation, many of these appendices can be removed intact. If rupture does occur then highly infective faecal pus is spilled, and this must be minimized by suction and antibiotic washout. If omentum is firmly adherent to an inflamed appendix then it should not be disturbed because it may be sealing off a perforation. Detach the affected piece of omentum from the rest of the great omentum by ligation and division of appropriate bunches of tissue.

In the case of retrocaecal and retrocolic appendicitis, a different approach to mobilization is needed. Here the appendix is often bound to the back of the bowel by fibrous tissue, and early use of blunt dissection is not appropriate. Enlargement of the incision is nearly always necessary to secure proper exposure. Experience shows that readiness to extend, where indicated, allows the operation to go forward neatly and quickly, with the minimum of handling of the colon and contamination of the wound.

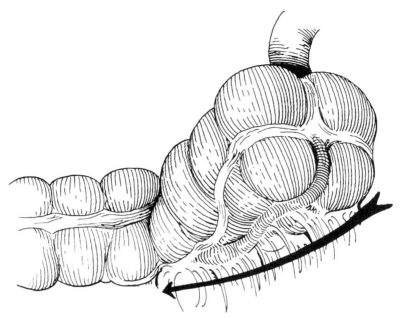

Figure 2.5 Mobilization of the caecum by dividing the peritoneum of the lateral paracolic gutter. Blunt dissection in the bloodless plane behind the caecum allows it to be drawn up, out of the incision.

The degree of fixation of the colon varies greatly. In some cases fixation is minimal, and then the caecum and much of the ascending colon can be exteriorized. The best method is to draw the caecum out of the abdomen, using the taenia, and then to hold it in a swab and gently pull inferiorly, making a side-to-side movement of the hand at the same time. When as much progress has been made as is possible, then the caecum can be turned back, over the right upper abdomen, and the appendix can be inspected: the mobility of the colon may be sufficient for the whole length of the appendix to be exposed. More often there is adherence of the caecum and ascending colon to the posterior abdominal wall. Then the first step is to divide the peritoneum at the point where it leaves the lateral aspect of the colon and becomes the parietal peritoneum of the paracolic gutter, as is done at the start of right hemicolectomy (Figure 2.5). This produces a marked increase in mobility, allowing the posterior aspect of the caecum and colon to be freed from retroperitoneal adhesions until the bowel can be drawn out sufficiently to reveal the whole length of the appendix.

The next step is to cut with scissors along the lateral side of the appendix. Because the mesentery of the retrocaecal appendix is medial, there is this avascular plane laterally, which can be divided to mobilize the appendix and allow a view of the mesentery (Figure 2.6).

This is not a free mesentery, and the vessels are quite short. The tip of the appendix can be drawn laterally and the vessels can be freed on its medial side, isolated, ligated in continuity and divided. Working toward the base, the appendicular vessels are tied off successively in several places until the base is reached. The appendix can then be removed.

The other way of tackling the difficult retrocolic appendix is to perform **retrograde appendicectomy**. This can be helpful when a high retrocolic appendix is obviously inflamed

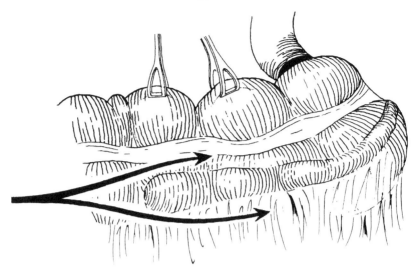

Figure 2.6 Mobilization of the retrocaecal appendix. The lower arrow indicates the bloodless peritoneal sheet, which can be safely divided to mobilize the appendix. The upper arrow shows the line along which the short mesentery is divided.

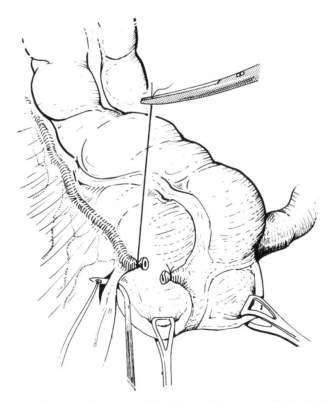

Figure 2.7 Retrograde appendicectomy. The base of the appendix is tied off and divided between two ligatures. As the distal ligature is drawn upward the mesentery is displayed.

but it is not easy to see the tip. The base of the appendix is isolated and tied off on the caecum and on the appendix, and the appendix is divided between the ligatures. The ligature on the appendix can be used to draw it away from the caecum (Figure 2.7), and this reveals the mesentery, which can be tied off in segments. Gradually the appendix is eased away from the ascending colon until the tip is revealed.

2.7.2.3 The mesentery

It is not unusual to see the mesentery being clamped with artery forceps and divided, and then the resultant bunch of tissue tied off behind the forceps. Sooner or later, an oedematous and friable mesentery will crack with this treatment, the artery forceps will drop off and a briskly bleeding tear of the mesentery will have to be dealt with. Once this event has been experienced a solution will be sought, and it is strongly recommended that artery forceps should never be applied to the appendicular – or any other – mesentery. If the mesentery is thin, it is easy to see the vessels and to choose a suitable site for ligation. The mesentery is incised (Figure 2.8), the ligature drawn through with artery forceps and the first hitch gently tightened on the mesentery (Figure 2.9).

If the oedematous tissues of the mesentery fragment as the ligature tightens it is most unusual for the artery to cut through, so the mesentery can be safely divided beyond the ligature. Other branches of the artery are dealt with in the same way, until the whole appendix is freed. In the very unusual event of the artery cutting through, the bleeding point should be oversewn.

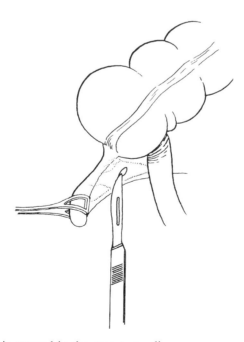

Figure 2.8 A window is created in the mesoappendix.

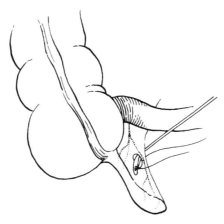

Figure 2.9 A ligature is passed and the appendicular artery is tied off.

Before closing the abdomen, always check the ligatures on the appendicular artery. We have a vivid memory of a girl who had a straightforward emergency appendicectomy. In a darkened ward her pallor was not noticed until, 6 hours later, her pulse could barely be felt. She had a tumid, tender abdomen and was gravely hypotensive. After resuscitation the abdomen was reopened, much blood was sucked out and the bleeding cut end of the appendicular artery was secured.

2.7.2.4 Removing the appendix

It is necessary to take out the whole length of the appendix from tip to base. The anterior taenia coli extends down to the base, and is a good guide to it (Figure 2.7). This is another place where an unwise crush with artery forceps can result in the oedematous appendix being cut straight through. It is recommended that a 0 polyglyconate ligature should be tied around the base without preliminary crushing, and that the appendix should be held lightly with forceps and divided beyond the ligature. Traditionally the open end of the appendix base is cleansed with a swab soaked in antiseptic or cauterized, but there is no evidence that this is useful. Next, the appendix is placed in a sterile dish and opened from end to end with sterile scissors and dissecting forceps (which are then discarded). There are two reasons for doing this.

- If the appendix is perforated and contains no faecolith, consider whether the faecolith may have been shed into the bed of the appendix. If this is possible it must be sought, because if it is left *in situ* a faecolith can give rise to a chronic discharging sinus.
- On a number of occasions we have seen a reddened appendix, coated with fibrin, which on opening showed a normal mucosa. Clearly another cause for the surface inflammation had to be found, and search revealed that the appendix had been lying alongside either an inflamed Meckel's diverticulum or an area of acute diverticulitis in the sigmoid colon. Making a routine of opening up the appendix at this juncture takes less than a minute: it is always of interest and occasionally is a vital step in reaching a true diagnosis.

2.7.2.5 The appendix stump

It may seem obvious that the whole appendix must be removed, but the reminder needs to be given because **recurrent appendicitis** can occur in a stump only 2–3 cm long. This, as we can confirm, produces a confusing picture, with a patient providing a convincing history and in spite of the scar of appendicectomy all the signs of appendicitis. In a recent example, Milne and Bradbury (1996) saw a patient with lower abdominal peritonitis who had had a laparoscopic appendicectomy 18 months previously. Exploration revealed a perforated retrocaecal appendix. They removed an appendix 3.2 cm long, with two metallic clips at the tip: at the previous operation an appendix 4.5 cm long had been removed.

There has always been controversy over whether the ligated stump should be left alone or buried. Most often the stump was surrounded by a purse-string suture, the stump inverted and the suture tied over the top. The theory was that this left a smooth serosal surface, rather than the devascularized stump, and it was hoped that fewer adhesions would form. Charles Mayo opposed burying the stump in the 1930s, although it continued to be used on countless occasions. Now, there are a number of extensive trials that have shown that there is no detectable advantage in the extra step of burying the stump – in fact there are more examples of postoperative ileus when this is done (Kingsley, 1969; Engstrom and Fenyo, 1985).

Sometimes the whole appendix is so oedematous that the ligature applied around the base cuts through the wall: it usually occludes the lumen but this cannot be relied on, and it is then reasonable to close the caecal wall over the stump with a few Lembert sutures or a Z-stitch, which tuck the stump down into a shallow trench, and tack omentum over it. If there is doubt about the security of the closure a drain must be left down to the stump for several days. In everyday practice inversion of the stump has now been widely abandoned, with no perceptible disadvantage, and it avoids two unusual complications of this practice.

Mayo in 1934 stated that he had often seen a collection of pus in the closed cavity containing the septic stump when attending post-mortem examinations, and that these collections occasionally burst. A few days into an uneventful convalescence the patient is suddenly seized with acute pain and there are signs of peritonitis in the RLQ. On exploration pus is found in a messy septic area around the exposed appendix stump. Thomas (1974) reported four such cases. The other complication arises when a chronic abscess forms the apex of an intussusception of the caecum, which can progress to become a palpable mass in the epigastrium. La Salle *et al.* (1980) found 19 reports of this event, and a mass was felt in 13. They presented between 3 days and 6 years after appendicectomy, and in 12 a right hemicolectomy was required.

2.7.2.6 Failed appendicectomy

Appendices that have been inflamed on previous occasions can present serious problems with adhesions to adjacent structures. This is a situation in which an inexperienced surgeon should ask for help, rather than press on in an inflamed and vascular field. In the exceptional case, when such help is not available, it may well be safer to establish drainage and retire, and arrange for interval appendicectomy.

2.7.2.7   On finding a normal appendix

There will be occasions when exploration reveals a normal appendix. There are then a number of possibilities to be sought, which can conveniently be divided into those that can be dealt with through a gridiron incision, and those that will require a fresh incision to be made. The first step is to withdraw the terminal ileum. This may reveal acute lymphadenitis in the ileocaecal mesentery (p. 52), or acute Meckel's diverticulitis (p. 104), or rarely acute terminal ileitis (p. 249). Acute caecal diverticulitis (p. 74) and jejunal diverticulitis (p. 256) are other unusual possibilities. If the caecum is tensely distended an obstructing carcinoma of the ascending colon with secondary appendicitis (p. 74) must be sought: occasionally the carcinoma lies more distally.

In the female the next step would be to inspect the pelvis, where the right ovary and fallopian tube may show one of a number of changes (pp. 510 and p. 491). All these possibilities can generally be dealt with by extending the original incision.

If all these conditions can be excluded and there is no sign of abnormal fluids or pus, then it must be assumed that the patient has the NSAP syndrome. The appendix is removed and the abdomen closed.

There are a number of other conditions, which can present with signs in the right lower quadrant, that cannot be explored though a gridiron incision.

- **Perforated duodenal ulcer**. Some brown or bilious free fluid will be seen, and exploration upwards will reveal more fluid. A swab on a holder passed upwards is likely to return covered in bile and fibrin. The appendix must be removed and a fresh vertical incision made.
- **Acute diverticulitis**. It is not unusual for some of the sigmoid colon to lie to the right of the midline so, in the presence of inflammatory changes, signs will develop in the RLQ. The indurated inflamed colon is likely to be felt and seen, and an appropriate decision must be made on how to proceed, depending on the extent of the sepsis (p. 311).
- Finding a blood-stained effusion would suggest either **intestinal ischaemia** or **acute pancreatitis**. Pure blood in a female would suggest an unusually free bleed from a ruptured ovarian follicle (p. 513) or a tubal pregnancy (p. 493), both of which could be explored through extension of the gridiron incision. Another possibility could be unsuspected blunt trauma.
- We have in the past been caught out by **acute obstruction of a hydronephrotic kidney**. This can cause a surprising amount of tenderness and guarding over the right abdomen and flank. The flank tenderness might suggest that an ultrasonic scan should be the first step, but if this situation is encountered *via* a gridiron incision then the appendix must be removed and the incision closed. Before doing anything further it is essential to learn more about the state and function of both kidneys.

2.7.2.8   Drainage

Intraperitoneal drainage is no longer a feature of practice and it is generally acknowledged that a tube cannot drain the general peritoneal cavity. The one exception arises when an acutely inflamed appendix cannot for some reason be removed and should be drained through a closed system.

Thorough lavage of the surroundings of a perforated appendix and layers of the wound with tetracycline (1 mg/ml) in warm physiological saline is highly effective. (In children and pregnant women use cefotaxime 1 mg/ml). There is rarely any indication for drainage of the area. Wound drainage, also much used in the past, is rarely indicated. Good operative technique, with use of an adequate incision and protection of the wound edges with chlorhexidine-soaked swabs, and careful removal of the appendix, can all contribute to prevention of contamination. With good technique and tetracycline lavage Longland *et al.* (1971) showed that the wound infection rate could be kept below 4%, and in 230 consecutive appendicectomies Krukowski *et al.* (1988) recorded a rate of 2.6%.

2.7.2.9   Closure

When an acutely inflamed appendix has been removed through a muscle-splitting incision and the peritoneum has been closed with a running absorbable suture (e.g. 2/0 polydioxanone) only a few more absorbable sutures are required in the muscle layers, because this incision tends to close itself. Careful repair of any muscle-cutting extension is important. A subcuticular skin closure is used. It is good practice to infiltrate the incision with bupivacaine 0.25%.

2.7.3   THE LAPAROSCOPIC METHOD

2.7.3.1   Port sites

A variety of port sites can be used for laparoscopic appendicectomy but the sites described permit good access for the majority of patients and can be supplemented by an additional port if exposure is problematic. A 10 mm supraumbilical port is inserted either after inducing a pneumoperitoneum with a Veres needle or by direct cut-down on the peritoneum, according to preference. A second 10 mm port is inserted in the left lower quadrant, under the 'bikini line', under direct vision, taking care to avoid the inferior epigastric vessels. A 5 mm port is inserted in a similar site on the right side. The laparoscope is then removed from the umbilical port and reinserted through the LLQ port. The operator then manipulates the instruments through the RLQ and umbilical ports with the camera ideally positioned between the operating ports. When access is poor, usually in the obese or those with organizing advanced inflammation, inserting an additional 5 mm port in the right hypochondrium below the costal margin allows additional manipulation or retraction.

   Alternatively, the three ports can be inserted in the umbilicus, LLQ and RUQ with the laparoscope remaining in the umbilical port. This alternative position gives good depth perception and optimal ergonomics with the minor disadvantage of a more visible port-site puncture scar

2.7.3.2   Mobilization of the appendix

The appendix (or if very inflamed the mesoappendix) is held in an atraumatic grasper in the left hand. Laparoscopic appendicectomy differs from conventional appendicectomy in that the mesoappendix is normally dissected off the appendix with hook diathermy rather than ligated at its base. The rationale for this is to reduce the bulk of the resected appendix to allow easy extraction through a 10 mm port. Often the small vessels entering the appendix wall are satisfactorily dealt with by diathermy alone but if there is active bleeding from the mobilized mesoappendix it may be clipped or ligated with an Endo-loop (Ethicon Ltd) at its base to secure haemostasis. Once skeletonized the appendix base is ligated with a size 1 chromic catgut or other absorbable loop ligature close to the caecum. A second loop or clip is applied distally before division of the base. The divided appendix is extracted through the umbilical port.

Some, for whom cost and the requirement for a 12 mm port must be a minor concern, prefer the convenience of an endoscopic stapler for transection of the appendix and mesoappendix. This device may not be appropriate when the appendix base is significantly diseased.

The laparoscopic approach permits thorough lavage of the peritoneum and pelvis with tetracycline solution.

2.7.3.3 Closure

It is not normally necessary to close the fascial layers of unextended 10 mm ports and the skin can be closed with one or two interrupted 4/0 subcuticular absorbable suture material. We have never drained the abdomen after a laparoscopic appendicectomy.

2.7.3.4 Conversion to open operation

If the technical difficulty encountered during the laparoscopic dissection exceeds the level of experience of the operating team the procedure should be converted to a conventional approach without hesitation or concern over recrimination.

2.7.4 POSTOPERATIVE MANAGEMENT

This has changed considerably, spurred on by the results of laparoscopic surgery. It is now clear that patients who have either open or laparoscopic removal of non-perforated appendicitis can be started on oral fluids and light diet from the time of recovery from the general anaesthetic, that over 70% can return home on the day after the operation, and that most are back at work or school in 7–10 days (Ramesh and Galland, 1993). Patients with perforation and peritonitis naturally have to stay longer. The treatment of the patient with general peritonitis is considered on p. 149.

2.7.5 MANAGEMENT OF THE APPENDICEAL MASS

Although well known it is fairly unusual for appendicitis to present as an inflammatory mass. In adults this is only seen in 3–4% of patients (Lewis *et al.*, 1975), although in children a mass is felt in as many as one-third of patients (Puri *et al.*, 1981). The mass may consist of the inflamed appendix surrounded by oedematous adherent omentum and intestine, and this is known as a phlegmon. For an abscess to form there has to be a balanced progression of inflammation so that, when the appendix perforates, the adhesions between the surrounding omentum and viscera are sufficiently firm to prevent a spreading peritonitis.

Most patients with an abscess have been ill for 5–6 days, and fever and the WCC are higher than usual. Because the inflammation is confined the rest of the abdomen is easily examined, and the progress of the mass can readily be followed by clinical examination. (The exceptions to this statement are infants, in whom diagnosis is often difficult and delayed, and the mass is quite often only felt under anaesthesia; p. 94.)

Over the years some surgeons have favoured an operative approach, but there is now a fairly general consensus in favour of conservative management, unless there are clear signs that this is failing. A close watch is kept, with 4-hourly recordings, twice-daily clinical review, light diet (with intravenous fluids if necessary) and rest, although the patient need not be confined to bed. Some favour giving antibiotics; others believe that this can weaken but not abolish bacterial growth in a closed cavity and lead to a chronic abscess. Hoffman *et al.* (1991) withheld antibiotics in 28 patients with an abscess, and they all settled over the space of a month (mean 10 days). In an earlier series (Hoffman *et al.*, 1984) 59 patients were similarly treated but given antibiotics; 12 showed signs of increasing tenderness and rising temperature, and these had open drainage of the abscess. Bagi and Dueholm (1987) performed an ultrasound scan on 40 patients with a mass – nine with a phlegmon, 31 with an abscess. Some 21 patients settled but 17 required percutaneous drainage and three needed open operation, two for perforation of the abscess and one for small-bowel obstruction. In a review of the subject, Nitecki *et al.* (1993) consider that computed tomography (CT) can provide a more accurate picture of the mass, and that CT-guided drainage has a high success rate. In our experience this has not proved to be necessary and is only indicated if an abscess becomes more tender, with a swinging fever, and there seems to be a real risk of perforation and peritonitis. In the past, this was treated by open drainage, through a muscle-cutting incision placed well to the lateral side of the mass, entering the cavity extraperitoneally, gently breaking down any loculi with the finger, washing out the cavity and removing any faecolith. A wide, soft drain was introduced and the layers of the incision were closed around it with absorbable sutures. The tube was left *in situ* for about 10 days to allow a track to form. Occasionally, a faecal fistula would become established – as can happen after percutaneous drainage – but these are usually of low output and they can heal spontaneously. The sinus must not be allowed to heal until a sinogram shows that the cavity has closed. Such a course may still be appropriate in an isolated situation.

Occasionally, one operates for a probable perforated appendicitis, with a 36–48-hour history: because of the degree of guarding a mass is not felt until anaesthesia has been induced. In these circumstances, in the years beyond infancy, we have chosen to proceed and one finds that the mass consists of oedematous omentum wrapped around a swollen appendix, which is often gangrenous. Some care and a good exposure are needed to remove the appendix, and the attached omentum, without rupturing it, and this is a situation in which skilled assistance may be needed.

Now that a majority of appendiceal masses are managed conservatively, careful follow-up is needed. There are two reasons for this.

• The appendix remains *in situ* so recurrent appendicitis is a possibility. In the past this was considered to be a real threat and it was common to perform interval appendicectomy after 2–3 months. Sometimes a small fibrosed remnant was all that could be found, although some appendices were still candidates for recurrent inflammation. Now, a more selective policy is practised. In a review of 329 patients treated conservatively, only 13.7% returned with recurrent appendicitis, mostly during the first year, and very few arose beyond 2 years (Nitecki *et al.*, 1993). The situation needs to be explained to the patient: some will feel safer to have the appendix removed, and it may be a wise course for those who live in remote places or who often undertake international travel. For the remainder it seems reasonable to keep them under review for a year, with a warning to report any untoward symptoms promptly.

- Each report of a series of adult patients includes a few in whom the true cause of the mass was not appendicitis. In children who remain well there is no need for further investigation, but in older patients thought must be given to the possibility of occult disease. A previously silent carcinoma of the proximal colon, or ileocaecal Crohn's disease, are possibilities. It is wise to wait at least 8 weeks before performing a barium enema, otherwise misleading appearances may be seen (Hoffmann *et al.*, 1984). Other investigations, such as colonoscopy with biopsy, may be needed if there is continuing concern.

2.7.6 SEPTIC COMPLICATIONS

Once a major cause of postoperative morbidity and mortality, the septic complications of acute appendicitis have, with modern methods of treatment, become relatively unusual. Some patients with perforated appendicitis will form a residual abscess, and these are considered in Chapter 4.

Pylephlebitis, once a much-feared complication, is now very rarely seen. A septic thrombus in the appendicular veins led to portal pyaemia, and the lodgement of septic thrombi in the liver. These went on to form scattered abscesses, which in the days before antibiotics were virtually untreatable. The warning sign occurred several days after admission, when the patient began to suffer rigors with high fever. The liver might be tender, liver function tests slightly deranged, and a blood culture was often positive. Should these warning signs be encountered, intensive parenteral antibiotic therapy would be likely to arrest the process.

2.7.7 LATE COMPLICATIONS

Small-bowel obstruction may be a problem in some patients making a slow recovery from perforated appendicitis. The question then arises whether the obstruction is due to paralytic ileus or to early adhesive obstruction. This difficult differential diagnosis is considered on p. 195.

2.7.7.1 Acute small-bowel obstruction

Acute small-bowel obstruction occurring some time after appendicectomy requires careful handling. With the history of a previous laparotomy, adhesions are much the most likely cause, and the patient is likely to be placed on nasogastric suction and intravenous fluids. The important fact to remember is that this is rarely effective in this situation. Meagher *et al.* (1993) reviewed 330 admissions for small-bowel obstruction occurring after a laparotomy. In 34 patients the previous operation was an appendicectomy, and in six the operation had been on the ovary or fallopian tube. Only two of these 40 patients settled and 38 required division of adhesions, 32 being band obstructions: nine resections were needed for ischaemic bowel. A total of 95% of this group needed adhesiolysis, compared with only 53% of the other 290 patients.

2.7.7.2 Infertility

This has been said to be a complication of perforated appendicitis in girls. However, several papers make this claim but lack information on the sperm count of the husband. Puri *et al.* (1984) studied 59 married women 10 or more years after appendicectomy for a perforated appendix. Of these, 50 had borne a child, and detailed study of the other nine did not yield clear evidence that their fertility was impaired. This issue remains open, but it is only reasonable to seek to forestall the development of pelvic peritonitis and to treat it vigorously when it occurs.

REFERENCES

Bagi, P. and Dueholm, S. (1987) Non-operative treatment of the ultrasonically evaluated appendiceal mass. *Surgery*, **101**, 602–605.

Engstrom, L. and Fenyo, G. (1985) Appendicectomy: assessment of stump invagination versus antibiotic therapy for acute appendicitis. *Br. J. Surg.*, **72**, 971–972.

Eriksson, S. and Granstrom, L. (1995) Randomized controlled trial of appendicectomy versus antibiotic treatment for acute appendicitis. *Br. J. Surg.*, **82**, 166–169.

Hassen, A. H. S. and Cade, R. J. (1996) A prospective trial of open vs. laparoscopic appendicectomy. *Austr. N.Z. J. Surg.*, **66**, 178–180.

Hoffman, J., Lindhard, A. and Jensen, H.-E. (1984) Appendix mass: conservative management without interval appendicectomy. *Am. J. Surg.*, **148**, 379–382.

Hoffman, J., Rolff, M., Lomborg, V. *et al.* (1991) Ultraconservative management of the appendiceal mass. *J. R. Coll. Surg. Edin.*, **36**, 18–20.

Kingsley, D. P. E. (1969) Some observations on appendicectomy with particular reference to technique. *Br. J. Surg.*, **56**, 491–496.

Kollias, J., Harris, R. H. C., Otto, G. *et al.* (1994) Laparoscopic vs open appendicectomy for suspected appendicitis: a prospective study. *Austr. N.Z. J. Surg.*, **64**, 830–835.

Krukowski, Z. H., Irwin, S. T., Denholm, S. *et al.* (1988) Preventing wound infection after appendicectomy: a review. *Br. J. Surg.*, **75**, 1023–1033.

La Salle, A. J., Andrassy, R. J., Page, C. P. *et al.* (1980) Intussusception of the appendix stump. *Clin. Pediatr.*, **19**, 432–435.

Lewis, F. R., Holcroft, J. W., Boey, J. *et al.* (1975) Appendicitis: a critical review of diagnosis and treatment in 1000 cases. *Arch. Surg.*, **110**, 677–682.

Longland, C. J., Gray, J. G., Lees, W. *et al.* (1971) The prevention of infection in appendicectomy wounds. *Br. J. Surg.*, **58**, 117–119.

McArthur, L. L. (1894) Choice of incisions of the abdominal wall; especially for appendicitis. *Chicago Med. Reporter*, **7**, 289–292.

McBurney, C. (1894) Incision made in the abdominal wall in cases of acute appendicitis, with a description of a new method of operating. *Ann. Surg.*, **20**, 38–43.

Mayo, C. W. (1934) Appendicitis. *Southwestern Med.*, **18**, 397–403.

Meagher, A. P., Moller, C. and Hoffmann, D. C. (1993) Nonoperative treatment of small bowel obstruction following appendicectomy, or operation on the ovary or tube. *Br. J. Surg.*, **80**, 1310–1311.

Milne, A. A. and Bradbury, A. W. (1996) 'Residual' appendicitis following incomplete laparoscopic appendicectomy. *Br. J. Surg.*, **83**, 217.

Morison, R. (1901) Diagnosis and treatment of abscess in connection with the vermiform appendix. *Lancet*, **i**, 533–535.

Mutter, D., Vix, M., Bui, A. *et al.* (1996) Laparoscopy not recommended for routine appendectomy in men: results of a prospective randomized study. *Surgery,* **120**, 71–74.

Nitecki, S., Assalia, A. and Schein, M. (1993) Contemporary management of the appendiceal mass. *Br. J. Surg.,* **80**, 18–20.

Puri, P., Boyd, E., Guiney, E. J. *et al.* (1981) Appendix mass in the very young child. *J. Pediatr. Surg.,* **16**, 55–57.

Puri, P., Guiney, E. J., O'Donnell, B. *et al.* (1984) Effects of perforated appendicitis in girls on subsequent fertility. *BMJ,* **288**, 25–26.

Ramesh, S. and Galland, R. B. (1993) Early discharge from hospital after appendicectomy. *Br. J. Surg.,* **80**, 1192–1193.

Tate, J. J. T. (1996) Laparoscopic appendicectomy. *Br. J. Surg.,* **83**, 1169–1170.

Thomas, M. P. (1974) Burst appendectomy stump abscess. *Austr. N.Z. J. Surg.,* **44**, 47–49.

2.8 EMERGENCIES IN THE PROXIMAL COLON AND ACUTE APPENDICITIS

Acute appendicitis frequently has an obstructive basis, and an unusual cause is **carcinoma of the colon**. A carcinoma of the caecum may directly infiltrate the base of the appendix, or an annular carcinoma in the ascending colon can, in the presence of a competent ileocaecal valve, produce a tense closed-loop obstruction of the caecum, with secondary acute appendicitis.

The individual surgeon will only rarely encounter this latter situation: Miln and McLaughlin (1969) saw two examples in the course of treating 329 patients with appendicitis over 2 years. In a personal case it was immediately apparent that the situation was unusual because the caecum was so tensely distended that it could not be delivered through the gridiron incision. The incision was extended, a tight annular carcinoma of the ascending colon was found, with secondary appendicitis, and a right hemicolectomy performed. The obstructing carcinoma can lie in a more distal part of the colon, and then a change of incision may be needed to obtain access.

A more difficult situation can arise if a carcinoma of the caecum directly infiltrates and obstructs the base of the appendix. The thickening of the caecal wall can understandably be mistaken for oedema due to the appendicitis, and this could lead to delay in diagnosis. Waller and Glasgow (1977) explored a patient with a gangrenous appendix wrapped in omentum and stuck to the caecum. When the mass was separated from caecum it broke away, leaving an open hole in the thickened caecal wall. A biopsy was taken from the edge and the defect closed. The biopsy came from a carcinoma and 9 days later an early carcinoma of the caecum, 2 cm in diameter, was removed. It would be preferable to take a frozen section and proceed.

Acute caecal diverticulitis is another unusual condition that presents as acute appendicitis. Only one or two examples will be seen for every 100 cases of diverticulitis of the distal colon and, unlike this common variety, these diverticula tend to be solitary and most often lie in the posterior wall of the caecum. If a diverticulum becomes obstructed by a faecolith, an abscess can form and produce an inflammatory mass outside the wall of the caecum. At exploration, the appendix is normal and, because the situation is unusual, the first thought is that the mass must be a carcinoma. However, with a short history, in a relatively young and fit patient, and with the signs of an inflammatory mass, there should be more than a suspicion that it is not a carcinoma.

In Williams' (1960) well-illustrated report of ten cases, four patients were below the age of 31, and the eldest was 55. We have seen five such cases and, on the first occasion, when we were unaware of the condition, it seemed best to proceed to ileocaecal resection. We now recognize that the acute presentation of an inflammatory mass which, as Williams shows, usually has a smooth-edged and elastic-feeling ulcer at its centre, is quite unlike the induration and nodularity that would be found in a carcinomatous ulcer. Anscombe *et al.* (1967) also saw ten patients, and in the first seven a resection was performed. Then two patients were treated by appendicectomy and a course of antibiotics, followed by close follow-up, and they remained well. In another patient the anterior caecal wall was opened, with full precautions, and a biopsy was taken from the ulcer edge: this case also settled. Local excision is sometimes possible. As Williams remarks, 'the greatest aid (in diagnosis) is an awareness of the condition', and this knowledge will encourage the surgeon to explore the situation, and to favour a conservative line of management.

This approach is particularly relevant in centres with a large Asian population, in whom right-sided colonic diverticulitis is more common than the left-sided variety. Harada and colleagues in Hawaii (1993) reported a series of 90 patients, 78% of whom were Asian in origin. Right hemicolectomy or caecectomy was performed in 49 but in 39 patients in whom the diagnosis was clear and there was no abscess present they performed either appendicectomy alone or diverticulectomy. Only four of the 29 patients undergoing appendicectomy had recurrent symptoms and they recommended this conservative approach provided the diagnosis is appreciated.

Acute terminal ileitis and **Crohn's disease** are considered in Chapter 6.

REFERENCES

Anscombe, A. R., Keddie, N. C. and Schofield, P. F. (1967) Solitary ulcers and diverticulitis of the caecum. *Br. J. Surg.*, **54**, 553–557.

Harada, R. N. and Whelan, T. J. Jr (1993) Surgical management of caecal diverticulitis. *Am. J. Surg.*, **166**, 666–669.

Miln, D. C. and McLaughlin, I. S. (1969) Carcinoma of proximal large bowel associated with acute appendicitis. *Br. J. Surg.*, **56**, 143–144.

Waller, D. G. and Glasgow, M. (1977) Acute appendicitis in association with non-obstructive carcinoma of the caecum. *Postgrad. Med. J.*, **53**, 234–236.

Williams, K. L. (1960) Acute solitary ulcers and acute diverticulitis of the caecum and ascending colon. *Br. J. Surg.*, **47**, 351–358.

2.9 ACUTE APPENDICITIS IN OLDER PATIENTS

Increasing attention is rightly being given to the abdominal emergencies that occur in older patients. There are several reasons for this. They now account for 25–30% of all surgical emergency admissions (Telfer *et al.*, 1988; Irvin, 1989; Eskelinen *et al.*, 1995), they suffer from some conditions which are rarely seen in younger patients and, most importantly, common emergencies present in unfamiliar guise. Finally, many of these patients were not fit before the emergency arose and they require not only skilful diagnosis and surgery but vigilant after-care if they are to survive.

Table 1.3 shows that beyond the age of 50 the incidence of acute abdominal diseases changes considerably, cholecystitis becoming at least as frequent as appendicitis, and intestinal obstruction, pancreatitis and diverticular disease all becoming much commoner than in younger patients. Vascular mishaps (ruptured aortic aneurysm, mesenteric ischaemia) and the complications of alimentary tract cancer, which are barely seen before 50, present in significant numbers.

The presentation of acute appendicitis illustrates some of these points. Fewer than 10% of all cases arise in patients over 60 years of age, but it is often a serious condition. In 35% the appendix has perforated, compared with a perforation rate of 10% below the age of 60. An important factor is that the elderly are often rather tolerant of abdominal pain: they take an antacid, they hope it will settle and delay seeking advice. As a consequence the mean delay between onset of pain and coming to operation is over $3\frac{1}{2}$ days (Sherlock, 1985). The blood supply to the appendix becomes poorer with advancing age and this may account for the fact that the risk of perforation in a patient over 60, seen only 12 hours after the onset of pain, is over 30% (de Dombal, 1991).

The clinical picture is at first rather low-key. General abdominal discomfort, with some gaseous distension, are early features, and a shift of pain is unusual. Temperature and pulse rate are often normal, and the distension – which is due to a measure of ileus – makes it more difficult to demonstrate tenderness and guarding over the appendix: this picture can suggest intestinal obstruction, possibly of neoplastic origin. In about one-quarter a mass is palpable. Acute cholecystitis and colonic diverticulitis are not uncommon at this age and must figure in the differential diagnosis. It is wise to record an ECG, and to pay close attention to the state of the lungs. While investigations are proceeding active preoperative preparations can go forward, treating dehydration and possible bacteraemia, and any cardiorespiratory problems.

The operation can be technically difficult and is likely to require at least the supervision of an experienced surgeon. Palpation under the anaesthetic may reveal a mass. This finding, and the localization of signs to the RLQ, would make it right to commence with a gridiron incision. If this reveals an inflamed appendix this approach will allow the patient easier movement and breathing, even if the incision has to be extended to improve access. However, if there is doubt about the diagnosis it is better to start with a vertical incision, which allows for a thorough laparotomy.

A vital part of the treatment comes after the operation, when these patients require expert nursing care, at first in a high-dependency unit, with at least a twice-daily visit from the surgical team. The combination of diffuse peritonitis in a patient with respiratory problems will require a period in the intensive care unit. It is now almost unheard of for death to occur among patients under the age of 50. The risk of death in 60-year-olds is about 2%, and this rises to 7% in patients who are 80 or more years of age (Telfer *et al.*, 1988). Taylor, writing in 1935 on appendicitis in the aged, said: 'there are two great dangers: general peritonitis which is the result of the disease, and pneumonia which is the result of the treatment'. In spite of advances in a number of areas, these remarks still emphasize two major aspects of the care of these patients.

REFERENCES

De Dombal, F. T. (1991) *Diagnosis of Acute Abdominal Pain*, 2nd edn, Churchill Livingstone, Edinburgh.
Eskelinen, M., Ikonen, J. and Lipponen, P. (1995) The value of history-taking, examination and computer assistance in the diagnosis of acute appendicitis in patients more than 50 years old. *Scand. J. Gastroenterol.*, **30**, 349–355.
Irvin, T. T. (1989) Abdominal pain: surgical audit of 1190 emergency admissions. *Br. J. Surg.*, **76**, 1121–1125.

Sherlock, D. J. (1985) Acute appendicitis in the over-sixty age group. *Br. J. Surg.*, **72**, 245–246.

Taylor, H. (1935) Appendicitis in the aged. *Lancet*, **ii**, 937–939.

Telfer, S., Fento, G., Hold, P. R. *et al.* (1988) Acute abdominal pain in patients over 50 years of age. *Scand. J. Gastroenterol.*, **23**(Suppl. 144), 47–50.

2.10 NEOPLASMS OF THE APPENDIX AND ACUTE APPENDICITIS

One of the important reasons for submitting all excised appendices for histological examination is that over 80% of appendicular neoplasms are not identified until they reach the laboratory (Deans and Spence, 1995). This is because most of these appendices are acutely inflamed, so the neoplasm (which is usually small) goes unnoticed in the theatre. They are also rare and consequently are not expected.

2.10.1 CARCINOIDS

Carcinoids account for 80% of appendicular neoplasms and are found about once in every 200 appendices examined. The female-to-male ratio is about 4:1. Apart from childhood, they are found at all ages, with a mean age of presentation of 30 years. It is very unusual for there to be any specific symptoms, and appendices that are not removed as an emergency are incidentally removed during a laparotomy. Anderson and Wilson (1985) reported on 147 carcinoids removed in Northern Ireland during 1970–1981. They found that 139 (94%) were less than 1 cm in diameter, and that only 7% arose in the proximal one-third of the appendix. This means that appendicectomy alone provides adequate removal for the large majority, and there is no record of metastases occurring from tumours less than 1 cm in diameter. Six of the 147 patients had a tumour 1–1.5 cm in diameter and, after simple appendicectomy, they had remained well for 2–14 years. Only two patients, aged 67 and 71, had a tumour more than 1.5 cm in diameter, and they showed signs of metastasis and died soon afterwards.

The surgeon faced with a report on a carcinoid between 1 cm and 2 cm in diameter will find it helpful to discuss the situation with the pathologist. Generally, if the tumour is under 1.5 cm and the resection line is clear then the risk of a right hemicolectomy may well be greater than the risk of recurrence. Closeness of the tumour to the base, invasion of the mesoappendix and cellular pleomorphism would make resection advisable. (Deans and Spence, 1995). If the carcinoid is more than 1.5 cm diameter and the patient is fit then right hemicolectomy with radical removal of the ileocaecal lymph nodes is necessary.

2.10.2 ADENOCARCINOMA

Adenocarcinoma of the appendix is a rarity, having an incidence of 1 in 1000 appendicectomies. Like carcinoid, most patients have no symptoms and the tumour is only discovered when appendicectomy is performed for appendicitis or as an incident in another operation, but the outlook is much more serious. As in colorectal cancer, an older age group is affected, and in 25% of cases lymph node metastasis has already occurred (Ferro and

Anthony, 1985). Some patients present with an adherent mass and are already beyond cure, and if the appendix has perforated early recurrence is fairly certain (Gilhome *et al.*, 1984). Right hemicolectomy should be performed whenever it offers a chance of complete removal. Even so, the prognosis seems to be rather worse than for colorectal cancer.

2.10.3 BENIGN TUMOURS

Benign tumours of the appendix are mostly cystadenomas, which produce an excessive secretion of mucus that can accumulate to form a mucocele: if this should rupture it causes localized pseudomyxoma peritonei. Cystadenomas are liable to become cystadenocarcinomas, and these tumours, should they rupture, cause generalized pseudomyxoma peritonei. Recent reviews suggest that, although the ovary is involved in this condition, the appendix is the primary site (Sugarbaker, 1994).

A mucocele can be discovered at operation for acute appendicitis, and if it is unruptured great care should be taken to ensure that it does not burst during removal. These patients remain well (Landen *et al.*, 1992). Cystadenocarcinoma with generalized pseudomyxoma causes abdominal distension that is dull to percussion, without shifting dullness. Sometimes it is complicated by spontaneous haemorrhage, or by intestinal obstruction. This is a rare and serious situation, which has been reviewed by Sugarbaker (1994). A combination of extensive radical surgery and intraperitoneal chemotherapy with 5-FU has given promising results.

REFERENCES

Anderson, J. R. and Wilson, B. G. (1985) Carcinoid tumours of the appendix. *Br. J. Surg.*, **72**, 545–546.

Deans, G. T. and Spence, R. A. J. (1995) Neoplastic lesions of the appendix. *Br. J. Surg.*, **82**, 299–306.

Ferro, M. and Anthony, P. P. (1985) Adenocarcinoma of the appendix. *Dis. Colon Rectum*, **28**, 457–459.

Gilhome, R. W., Johnston, D. H., Clark, J. *et al.* (1984) Primary adenocarcinoma of the vermiform appendix. *Br. J. Surg.*, **71**, 553–555.

Landen, S., Bertrand, C., Maddern, G. J. *et al.* (1992) Appendiceal mucoceles and pseudomyxoma peritonei. *Surg. Gynecol. Obstet.*, **175**, 401–404.

Sugarbaker, P. H. (1994) Pseudomyxoma peritonei. *Ann. Surg.*, **219**, 109–111.

2.11 CROHN'S DISEASE CONFINED TO THE APPENDIX

Occasionally an acutely inflamed appendix shows histological evidence of Crohn's disease (CD). Allen and Biggart (1983) reported on 14 patients, seen over a period of 20 years, who presented as typical acute appendicitis and who had a thickened and inflamed appendix removed. No one developed an abdominal faecal fistula, and only two later showed further signs of CD. Ewen *et al.* (1971) reported on 185 patients with CD, among whom were three who had an emergency appendicectomy: within 4 years two had developed signs of ileocaecal CD.

It seems that appendicectomy can, occasionally, appear to eradicate CD, but all these patients must be considered to be at risk and carefully followed up.

REFERENCES

Allan, D. C. and Biggart, J. D. (1983) Granulomatous disease in the vermiform appendix. *J. Clin. Path.*, **36**, 632–638.
Ewen, S. W. B., Anderson, J., Galloway, J. M. D. *et al.* (1971) Crohn's disease confined to the appendix. *Gastroenterology*, **60**, 853–857.

2.12 APPENDICITIS AND OTHER ABDOMINAL EMERGENCIES IN PATIENTS WITH AIDS

Many patients with AIDS complain of abdominal pain. This is often associated with gastroenteritis due to cryptosporidiosis or *Campylobacter* spp. infection, while others experience discomfort from enlargement of the liver and spleen. In the small proportion in whom an emergency appears to require surgical correction, particular care is needed over diagnosis and selection of appropriate treatment because the complications of AIDS leave many in a poor state to withstand an operation. In the early days of care of AIDS patients emergency surgery carried a mortality of 50–70%, but this has now fallen to as low as 11% (Lowy and Barie, 1994).

Davidson *et al.* (1991) reviewed 26 patients who required an emergency laparotomy. Cytomegalovirus (CMV) infection produced toxic megacolon in five patients and one colonic perforation, all requiring total colectomy and ileostomy. Ileal lymphoma caused a perforation and two obstructions requiring resection and anastomosis. In others adhesions and volvulus caused small-bowel obstruction. Six patients presented characteristic evidence of acute appendicitis, and had an uneventful operation and recovery.

A diagnosis was reached in these patients by following standard lines of examination and investigation: the indications for emergency operation are not different in these patients but are applied with special care. Davidson *et al.* (1991) found that surgery for the complications of CMV infection, and for acute appendicitis, generally had a good outcome, but prognosis is more reserved on visceral perforation or haemorrhage due to Kaposi's sarcoma or lymphoma. They observed normal healing of anastomoses and incisions, but remarked that exceptional care had been taken over technical details and pre- and postoperative care.

Whitney *et al.* (1992) and Saviez *et al.* (1996) reviewed 34 patients with AIDS admitted with suspected acute appendicitis. They noted a tendency towards delay before admission, and consequently a perforation rate as high as 40% and consequent diffuse peritonitis. Two-thirds had fever over 38.5°C, and some had rigors. The WCC was generally below 10 000. Saviez *et al.* (1991) reported 17 HIV-positive patients with suspected appendicitis: in 11 who did not have AIDS ten had acute appendicitis, but among the six AIDS patients only two had proven acute appendicitis, and they found CT scanning and laparoscopy helpful in differential diagnosis.

Acute cholecystitis occurs in this relatively young population because of infection by *Cryptosporidium* or CMV. Ultrasound can yield valuable information, and Tanner *et al.* (1994) draw attention to the particular advantages of laparoscopic surgery in HIV-positive patients.

REFERENCES

Davidson, T., Allen-Mersh, T. G., Miles, A. J. G. *et al.* (1991) Emergency laparotomy in patients with AIDS. *Br. J. Surg.*, **78**, 924–926.

Lowy, A. M. and Barie, P. S. (1994) Laparotomy in patients infected with human immunodeficiency virus: indications and outcome. *Br. J. Surg.*, **81**, 942–945.

Saviez, D., Lironi, A., Zurbuchen, P. *et al.* (1996) Acute right iliac fossa pain in acquired immunodeficiency: a comparison between patients with and without AIDS. *Br. J. Surg.*, **83**, 644–646.

Tanner, A. G., Hartley, J. E., Darzi, A. *et al.* (1994) Laparoscopic surgery in patients with human immunodeficiency virus. *Br. J. Surg.*, **81**, 1647–1648.

Whitney, T. M., Macho, J. R., Russell, T. R. *et al.* (1992) Appendicitis in acquired immunodeficiency syndrome. *Am. J. Surg.*, **164**, 467–471.

2.13   RARITIES

2.13.1   DIVERTICULUM OF THE APPENDIX

A diverticulum of the appendix is occasionally seen and, strangely, the diverticulum can become inflamed while the appendix itself remains unaffected. Delikaris *et al.* (1983) record ten cases, six having a peridiverticular abscess secondary to perforation.

2.13.2   TORSION OF THE APPENDIX

This is also very uncommon. There is no explanation for its occurrence. The patient complains of severe mid-abdominal colic and vomiting. Gangrene soon sets in, with signs of peritonitis in the RLQ. This sounds and looks very like acute obstructive appendicitis, the pathology is in many respects comparable, and the diagnosis can only be made when the appendix is exposed. Torsion occurs anticlockwise, and there is a short length of normal appendix proximal to the twist. Merrett *et al.* (1992) review the subject.

2.13.3   DUPLICATION OF THE APPENDIX

This is exceptionally rare. There may be two appendices arising from a common base, or there is one normal appendix with one arising from another part of the colon. Kjossev and Losanoff (1996) describe a man of 32 with acute pain and signs of local peritonitis in the left upper quadrant. Working through a midline incision, they found and removed a normal appendix in the RLQ, and a gangrenous appendix 8 cm long at the splenic flexure.

2.13.4   THE LEFT-SIDED APPENDIX

There are two distinct anatomical peculiarities that result in the appendix lying to the left of the midline. **Situs inversus**, or **transposition of the viscera**, occurs once in 6000–8000 individuals. There is a good clinical account by Holgersen *et al.* (1970) of a girl of 12 years who presented with pain and tenderness in the left iliac fossa. She was observed, and tenderness increased. A chest X-ray showed dextrocardia and the liver on the left, so a gridiron incision was made and an inflamed appendix was removed. It seems likely that examination of the heart will suggest the diagnosis. Blegan (1949) warned that pain is sometimes felt in the right lower quadrant, but the signs will clearly be on the left side.

Malrotation of the midgut results in the colon lying to the left of the midline, and is described in detail on page p. 208. Owen-Smith (1969) could only find two cases comparable to the case that he describes. A boy of 9 complained of acute pain in the left upper quadrant, but there was tenderness and guarding in both iliac fossae. He was explored through a right gridiron incision, and the caecum could not be found. On extending the incision a lump was felt in the left abdomen and an inflamed appendix was removed: the terminal ileum entered the caecum from the right (p. 109).

REFERENCES

Blegan, H. M. (1949) Surgery in situs inversus. *Ann. Surg.*, **129**, 244–259.

Delikaris, P., Teglbjaerg, P. S., Fisker-Sorensen, P. *et al.* (1983) Diverticula of the vermiform appendix. *Dis. Colon Rectum*, **26**, 374–376.

Holgersen, L. O., Kuehner, C. R. and Stanley-Brown, E. G. (1970) Acute appendicitis in a child with complete situs inversus. *J. Pediatr. Surg.*, **5**, 379–380.

Kjossev, K. T. and Losanoff, J. E. (1996) Duplicated vermiform appendix. *Br. J. Surg.*, **83**, 1259.

Merrett, N. D., Lubowski, D. Z. and King, D. W. (1992) Torsion of the vermiform appendix: a case report and review of the literature. *Austr. N.Z. J. Surg.*, **62**, 981–983.

Owen-Smith, M. S. (1969) Acute left-sided appendicitis. *Br. J. Surg.*, **56**, 233–234.

3

Emergency abdominal surgery in infancy and childhood

3.1 INTRODUCTION

3.1.1 PRINCIPLES OF CARE

Paediatric surgery is not just a miniaturized form of adult practice. It ranges across the surgical specialties. It deals with conditions rarely seen in older patients and calls for skill in communication, not merely sufficient to obtain a history from the young, but also a clinical manner sufficiently reassuring and patient to gain agreement to the examination of a painful lump or tender abdomen in a suspicious youngster.

It is of paramount importance that any surgeon undertaking an operation on an infant or young child has already gained considerable experience in adult surgery and with older children. Operations on the young demand certain skills, in terms of tissue handling and finesse with smaller structures, that are not readily obtained by the trainee surgeon dealing with adult general surgery.

The need to acquire these skills is real because for the foreseeable future the pressure of numbers and the facts of geography mean that emergency care for children outwith the neonatal period must continue to be provided in district hospitals (Table 3.1) by general surgeons and anaesthetists with a specific paediatric interest and additional training. Clearly, complex clinical problems and all neonatal surgical problems (postconceptual age < 44 weeks) should be treated by paediatric surgeons in regional referral centres.

Table 3.1 Admission of children to surgical wards – England (Reproduced from Department of Health, 1995)

Specialty providing care	0–4 years	5–15 years	Total
General surgery	25 826	58 551	84 377
Paediatric surgery	27 927	21 065	48 992

Emergency Abdominal Surgery. Edited by Peter F. Jones, Zygmunt H. Krukowski and George G. Youngson. Published in 1998 by Chapman & Hall, London. ISBN 0 412 81950 3.

The pattern of training in the UK is progressively towards specialization, with the consequence that fewer trainees will be exposed to paediatric surgery in basic training, and in higher training a narrower spectrum of experience will be obtained with possibly no exposure to children's surgery. It is, therefore, crucial that adequate training is provided for those surgeons who subsequently wish to operate on children.

Several contemporary reports (Children Act, 1995; Department of Health, 1991; Scottish Office/Home and Health Department, 1995) emphasize the need for provision of a suitable environment, with care provided by dedicated staff, i.e. children's nurses in a paediatric ward, wing or hospital; similarly, operations should be performed in an appropriate environment by anaesthetists and surgeons with the necessary expertise and previous training. This environment must allow good provision for temperature control and facilities for careful measurement of fluid balance. Precise haemostasis is particularly important in small children and fluid losses require to be carefully recorded, as does the specific prescription of postoperative fluid administration regimes and medication dosages.

3.1.2 PERIOPERATIVE MANAGEMENT

High-quality care includes good communication with parents, the child and other team members. Recent legislation (Children Act, 1995) instructs doctors on the need to provide children with the details of their care when they are capable of understanding the nature and consequences of the treatment. They also have the legal right to consent to such treatment and in this circumstance parental consent is not a prerequisite. It is my practice, however, to try to obtain the assent of both parent and child.

Preoperative care involves the appropriate clinical assessment, investigation, diagnostic considerations and instigation of treatment. When this requires surgery, early collaboration with anaesthetic staff helps decide issues such as the fasting status, appropriate medications, intravenous fluid regimes before theatre, and the need, if any, for blood or blood products for transfusion intraoperatively, with consequent preoperative cross-matching.

Pain control is as relevant preoperatively as it is after surgery and, providing clinical evaluation is not compromised, analgesia should be provided when preoperative preparations are being made. An infusion of morphine is usually effective. Administer an i.v. bolus of 100mcg/kg, and continue 10 mcg/kg/h in 5% dextrose or 0.9% saline. In infants under 6 months the dose is reduced to 5mcg/kg/h with a similar reduction in the loading dose.

A nasogastric tube must be passed if there is any concern over gastric stasis or dilatation. It is not a kindness to avoid the discomfort of this procedure if the consequence is aspiration on induction of anaesthesia.

A brief discussion of the postoperative care that is planned, including the strategy for pain control, provides considerable reassurance for most children, as does identifying yourself as their surgeon.

Intraoperative care, other than the detail of the planned procedure, includes warming of all intravenous fluids, control of the temperature and humidity in the theatre, judicious use of warming and cooling mats and, importantly, good lighting. My strong preference is to use a halogen-powered headlight, which, since it is coaxial with the surgeon's line of sight, provides optimal illumination.

In paediatric operative technique, haemostasis is of prime importance and many paediatric surgeons use bipolar diathermy for sharp dissection as well as haemostasis.

Postoperative orders should be written following completion of the operation note and should indicate the following:

- the oral intake allowed (if any);
- the maintenance intravenous fluid and its rate: 4% glucose/0.18% saline at a rate of 2 × body weight (kg) + 10 = ml/h;
- replacement of losses: (drainage, vomit, nasogastric aspiration) measured 4-hourly and replaced in hourly aliquots by 0.9% saline + KCl (10 mmol/500 ml);
- additional replacement fluid (if continuing resuscitation is necessary) given as albumin solution (10–20 ml/kg) over 4 h;
- requirements for postoperative antibiotics: cefotaxime (30 mg/kg/dose) and metronidazole (7 mg/kg/dose) is an effective regimen against gut organisms;
- the recording of pulse rate, blood pressure, oxygen saturation by oximetry, fluid balance and urine output and blood sugar measurement (in the first year of life the sensitivity of the non-myelinized component of the CNS to hypoglycaemia requires 6-hourly bedside estimation of the blood glucose level);
- postoperative investigations and special care plans (e.g. free drainage or 4-hourly aspiration of nasogastric tubes and care of drains and catheters).

3.1.3   FLUID AND ELECTROLYTE THERAPY IN INFANCY AND CHILDHOOD

Simplicity is the key to understanding, and thus to minimizing the risk of error in prescribing. This is particularly true in the fluid management of babies and children, where the inexperienced surgeon may feel inclined to devolve fluid management to the paediatrician sharing in the child's medical care. Medical conditions are seldom associated with the degree of flux of extracellular fluid found in surgical illness, and the responsibility for the care of fluid balance rightly rests with the operating surgeon. Uncertainty in fluid management indicates a lack of expertise in postoperative care and suggests that operative responsibility should be transferred to a more experienced unit.

The general principles of fluid shifts and management apply to children as they do to adults. With the exception of the neonatal period (which this chapter excludes from further consideration), approximately 60% of the body weight of children is water (i.e. 600 ml/kg body weight) of which two-thirds is intracellular fluid (ICF), the remainder (200 ml/kg) is extracellular fluid (ECF). The total body water fluctuates by only 1–2% per day and is thus closely controlled.

Circulating blood volume is 80 ml/kg – an important figure to remember, particularly when managing the traumatized child. Modulation occurs *via* carotid and aortic baroreceptors, atrial and great vein volume receptors and the renin–angiotensin–aldosterone mechanism, as well as through the effect of antidiuretic hormone (ADH) and the process of osmoregulation, controlled through the pituitary/hypothalamic axis.

Fluid management is best considered in three phases:

1. Maintenance fluids
2. Replacement of continuing losses
3. Resuscitation/restoration of deficit.

Maintenance fluids

Maintenance fluids can be calculated from a number of equations; a simple one is:

$$(2 \times \text{body weight in kg}) + 10 = \text{ml/h}.$$

This is a conservative regime but suitable for use in the postoperative period when ADH is usually active and other losses are being measured and actively replaced.

Administration of maintenance fluids has three aims:

- to replace insensible losses through sweat, respiration, normal gastrointestinal losses (total 20 ml/kg/d);
- for replacement of essential urine output;
- to maintain a modest diuresis and tissue hydration.

An alternative formula in more widespread usage is:

Body weight	*Fluid requirement* (ml/kg/h)
First 10 kg	4
Second 10 kg	2
Subsequent kg	1

The type of fluid given should reflect the body's fluid composition of ICF and ECF. An isotonic solution of 4% glucose and 0.18% sodium chloride approximates to this and also provides 160 kcal of energy per litre. In infancy the need to maintain the blood glucose level is such that a solution of 10% dextrose/0.18% NaCl may be required instead.

Electrolyte requirements are: sodium and chloride 2 mmol/kg/d and potassium 1 mmol/kg/d. Sufficient potassium is provided by the addition of 10 mmol KCl into 500 ml of the maintenance solution.

Replacement fluids

Abnormal losses (vomit, nasogastric tube losses, stomal and drain losses) share the same solute content as plasma, i.e. approximately 140 mEq NaCl/l, and such measured losses are best replaced by an equivalent volume of 0.9% NaCl (150 mmol/l). Maintenance fluid (4% glucose/0.18% saline solution), on the other hand, contains 30 mmol/l sodium and 30 mmol/l chloride and is thus unsuitable for replacement therapy. Simply increasing the rate of maintenance of glucose/saline to cater for losses results in dilutional hyponatraemia. It is therefore good practice to have two separate solutions in the postoperative period, i.e. maintenance and replacement. KCl (10 mmol/500 ml) is added to the 0.9% saline solution which approximates to the content of potassium in gastric (5–20) and intestinal (5–15) secretions, and sweat (6–15 mmol KCl/l). Diarrhoea can have a high potassium content (34–150 mmol/l) which requires careful monitoring.

Deficit therapy

Losses of body fluids should be replaced at a rate equal to the rate of loss. Hypovolaemia from haemorrhage requires urgent replacement with blood, plasma or plasma substitute.

Dehydration, by contrast, is a gradual process and in general is not detected until it is greater than 5% (50 ml/kg) of the total body weight. The degrees of severity used clinically are:

Mild	5%	Dry mouth, reduced urine output, decreased skin turgor
Moderate	10%	As above + sunken eyes, tachycardia
Severe	> 10%	As above + tachypnoea, drowsiness, irritability.

Once dehydration exceeds 5%, intravenous fluid replacement is required. In all types of dehydration the fluid lost is extracellular in type and should be replaced with physiological saline. If it is not, dilutional hyponatraemia will occur. This volume should be given in addition to the maintenance solution over a 24-hour period.

Thus a 10 kg child with a 7.5% deficit requires:

- maintenance (2 × body weight + 10) = 30 ml, 4% glucose/0.18 NaCl/h; plus
- replacement of deficit (7.5 × wt × 10) = 750/24 = 31 ml/h NaCl.

In practice this can be given as 0.45% NaCl/4% glucose at 61 ml/h. All fluids require potassium at physiological replacement levels.

In hyponatraemic states, infusion of 0.45% saline will correct the situation over 24 hours.

Hypernatraemic dehydration, however, requires cautious correction and is an exception to the above regime. In view of the excess loss of water over solute, the readministration of water should be in the form of 0.45% saline, replacing the deficit over 48 hours, giving the maintenance at three-fifths normal requirement. This prevents rapid re-entry of intracellular water and reduces the risk of cerebral oedema.

Hypovolaemia

Children with sudden, significant blood loss require urgent vascular access by the intravenous or the intraosseous route. Fluid therapy should be commenced as a bolus of 20 ml/kg in the form of crystalloid or colloid. The specification of the fluid is probably less important than the volume used, although current practice seems to lean towards the use of albumin solution until blood is available.

3.1.4   PHYSIOLOGICAL INDICES IN CHILDHOOD

The following equations/parameters may be of value to surgeons in training when first dealing with children. These equations are of particular value in the emergency and resuscitation situation, when precise indices may be unavailable.

Weight (kg) = 2 × (age + 4)
Blood pressure (systolic) = 80 + (2 × age in years)
Blood volume = 80 × weight (kg)
Urine output = 1 ml/kg/h
Insensible fluid losses = 20 ml/kg/d.

Vital signs

Age	Respiratory rate	Systolic blood pressure	Heart rate
< 1	30–40	70–90	110–160
2–5	25–30	80–100	95–140
5–10	20–25	90–110	80–120
> 10	15–20	100–120	60–100

Fluid challenge in hypovolaemia

Crystalloid 20 ml/kg – assess response – give colloid – 20 ml/kg

Endotracheal tube sizes

Tube size = age/4 + 4 = internal diameter (mm)
Oral length (cm) = age/2 + 12
Nasal length (cm) = age/2 + 15

REFERENCES

Scottish Office/Home and Health Department (1993) *At Home in Hospital. A Guide to the Care of Children and Young People*, HMSO, Edinburgh.
Children Act (1995) *The Children (Scotland) Act 1995*, HMSO, Edinburgh.
Department of Health (1991) *Welfare of Children and Young People in Hospital*, HMSO, London.

3.2 PYLORIC STENOSIS

Infantile hypertrophic pyloric stenosis remains a common surgical problem and is one of the most frequently performed procedures to be carried out in infancy by non-specialist surgeons.

Controversy exists over the quality of care provided for infants with pyloric stenosis by non-specialist surgeons. Brain (Brain and Roberts, 1996) from Norwich supports the case for management by paediatric surgeons, citing improvement in the results in his hospital after the appointment of a specialist surgeon. The contrary view has also been recently expressed (Saunders and Williams, 1990).

As with all surgery, the commitment to care and attention to detail provided by an experienced doctor is more important than the designation given that individual and his team.

The global incidence of this condition varies, but the median overall incidence of 2–3 cases per 1000 live births seems to predominate in the UK. The condition is less common in breast-fed babies, and it is remarkable that little progress has been made in revealing and understanding its aetiology. Recent work suggests a role for nitric oxide in the mechanism of hypertrophic change (Vanderwinden *et al.*, 1992) but the precise cause remains obscure.

The child is typically a first-born male of 4–6 weeks of age, who presents with a history of projectile non-bilious vomiting in the first, second or, less commonly, the third month of life. Diagnosis rests on history and palpation of the pyloric lump during a test feed, when gastric peristalsis may also be present on inspection. A test feed of warmed dextrose/ electrolyte solution is preferable to milk, which will curdle in the stomach.

It is best to sit to the left of the child, opposite the mother or nurse feeding the infant, with the child's legs and head supported and relaxed. The fingers of the left hand should gently palpate the upper abdomen from midline into the right upper quadrant. Identification of the pyloric olive on palpation is unmistakable and if doubt exists then it should be assumed that the pyloric lump has not been palpated. Time should be allowed for this examination since 4–5 minutes can pass before the characteristic lump is suddenly felt.

Some infants can be irritable during feeds, in part because of gastric distension and in part because of oesophagitis. These babies settle rapidly with the passage of a size 8 FG nasogastric tube and the test-feed examination will be more rewarding with the tube on free drainage during the feed. Indeed, if there is difficulty in palpating a tumour in a child in whom the history and biochemical investigation indicate pyloric stenosis, passing a nasogastric tube assists palpation by keeping the stomach decompressed during the feed.

Failure to palpate a pyloric olive can occur and may be addressed by repeating the test feed the following day, allowing the infant milk feeds in the interim. This will usually be diagnostic. Alternatively an abdominal ultrasound examination (Neilson and Hollman, 1994) will help define the diagnosis. This technique is extremely reliable, and often replaces the repeat test feed when the diagnosis is suspected, but not confirmed, on initial clinical examination.

Barium meal is occasionally used in some centres for diagnostic purposes but more often the contrast study is requested to establish the presence of, and evaluate the details of, suspected gastro-oesophageal reflux which then reveals the pyloric stenosis.

Pyloric stenosis can be especially difficult to diagnose when it complicates the postoperative course of another neonatal operation such as repair of an oesophageal atresia or diaphragmatic hernia, and in these instances recourse to some modality of imaging is often needed. My practice, however, in the uncomplicated cases, is to depend entirely upon clinical diagnosis by palpation and not commence the incision until I have felt the pyloric tumour.

Preparation for surgery

The electrolyte status and hydration of the child are important preoperative considerations and any abnormality must be corrected prior to surgery. Infusion with 0.45% saline/4% dextrose solution with added potassium (10–20 mmol/500 ml) should be given to correct any biochemical abnormality, along with the appropriate volume of replacement fluid (0.9% saline with added KCl) for replacement of any on-going nasogastric fluid losses. While the sodium and potassium concentration must be in the normal range prior to surgery, the bicarbonate concentration may be slower to return to normal and should not, in itself, defer the operation. Deranged biochemistry is usually correctable over a 24-hour period, allowing the procedure to proceed on the following day.

The operation

The original description of the condition by Hirschsprung in 1888 and the successful procedure by Ramstedt in 1911 remain the most influential early contributions. Ramstedt performed his operation first on the son of a local noble. He had intended to carry out Fredet's extramucosal pyloroplasty but the appearances following pyloromyotomy led him to believe, correctly, that the procedure of pyloromyotomy would suffice.

Although this condition may now be treated laparoscopically, there is no significant benefit and the traditional approach remains the mainstay of treatment. Laparotomy is performed through a transverse muscle cutting or muscle-splitting approach in the right upper quadrant at a point two-thirds of the way between xiphisternum and umbilicus. This is sufficiently low to provide good access to the pylorus and yet sufficiently high to allow the liver to act as an obturator of the abdominal contents when it comes to closing the abdomen.

A circum-umbilical incision has been described recently and offers the advantage of a superior cosmetic result (Tan and Bianchi, 1986).

The pyloric olive can be delivered atraumatically, by gentle traction on the omentum, which first delivers the transverse colon. Further traction on the gastrocolic omentum delivers the greater curve of stomach and then the pyloric tumour, which comes easily into the wound. This is preferable to grasping with Babcock's forceps.

With the left index finger gently compressing the duodenal fornix so as to flatten the duodenum against the lateral margin of the olive (Figure 3.1), an incision is made on the antero-superior part of the lump in a curvilinear fashion extending on to the antrum but stopping precisely at the lateral margin of the pyloric muscle.

There is potential hazard in extending the incision distally because the duodenal fornix becomes abruptly superficial and may be inappropriately entered. A Denis Browne spreader is used to separate the muscular margins of the incision, after the superficial scalpel incision has been deepened with the tip of a haemostat forceps (Dunhill) or tissue dissector (Ash). The integrity of the prolapsing mucosa should be tested by asking the anaesthetist to insufflate the stomach with air through the nasogastric tube and watching the mucosal surface for evidence of perforation. Any perforation, should it occur, should be treated with an omental patch using 6/0 or 7/0 polydioxanone to oversew the defect and subsequent deferment of oral feeds. The pyloromyotomy can be considered complete when paradoxical motion of the two sides of the split can be easily produced. Haemorrhage from the margins of the split is extremely

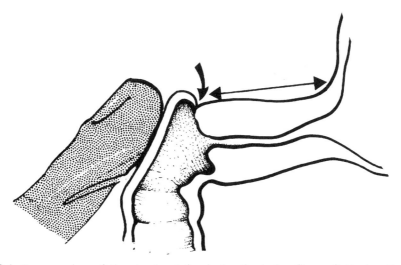

Figure 3.1 Compression of the duodenal fornix by the index finger flattening the fornix against the pyloric tumour.

uncommon (Eriksen and Anders, 1991) but the possibility exists; if it occurs it usually settles with compression with a swab after the lump has been returned to the peritoneal cavity.

Mass closure with a continuous absorbable 3/0 monofilament suture (polydioxanone) is associated with extremely low morbidity in terms of wound sepsis and dehiscence (Rao and Youngson, 1989).

Infiltration of the regional nerves (T9 and T10) with 0.25% bupivacaine solution (0.5 ml/kg) often suffices for postoperative analgesia.

Other operative techniques have been used, such as balloon dilatation (Hayashi *et al.*, 1990) and laparoscopic pyloromyotomy (Najmaldin and Tan, 1995) but have not been widely embraced because of the efficacy of the classic Ramstedt procedure.

Postoperative care

Recovery is usually uncomplicated, with wound sepsis or wound dehiscence being extremely rare in modern practice. Pain management is well catered for by intraoperative nerve block, but rectal paracetamol (15 mg/kg) can be used to supplement the block if the baby does not tolerate handling.

A variety of strategies exist for postoperative feeding, all designed to minimize postoperative vomiting, reduce consequent oesophagitis and mucosal bleeding, and facilitate early discharge from hospital. Turnock and Rangecroft (1991), in studying 100 infants, found that babies in whom feeding was deferred for 18 hours following operation had fewer vomits. Wheeler and his colleagues, however, in Southampton (1990), in a prospective trial of three feeding regimes, found no difference in the incidence of vomiting and concluded that vomiting was independent of the regime chosen. The simplicity of one of the regimes they described – nil orally for 24 hours, with the nasogastric tube *in situ*, followed by subsequent institution of full-strength milk feeds – is highly satisfactory and has much to commend it because it reduces the work of the nurses and handling of the infant.

Any persistent small vomits can be attributed to secondary gastro-oesophageal reflux, managed by placing the baby in a semi-reclining position and thickening the feed.

REFERENCES

Brain, A. J. L. and Roberts, D. S. (1996) Who should treat pyloric stenosis: the general or specialist pediatric surgeon. *J. Pediatr. Surg.*, **31**, 1535–1537.

Eriksen, C. A. and Anders, C. J. (1991) Audit of results of operations for infantile pyloric stenosis in a district general hospital. *Arch. Dis. Child.*, **66**, 130–133.

Hayashi, A. H., Giacomantonio, J. M., Lau, H. Y. *et al.* (1990) Balloon catheter dilatation for hypertrophic pyloric stenosis. *J. Pediatr. Surg.*, **25**, 1119–1121.

Najmaldin, A. and Tan, H. L. (1995) Early experience with laparoscopic pyloromyotomy for infantile hypertrophic pyloric stenosis. *J. Pediatr. Surg.*, **30**, 37–38.

Neilson, D. and Hollman, A. S. (1994) The ultrasonic diagnosis of infantile hypertrophic pyloric stenosis: technique and accuracy. *Clin. Radiol.*, **49**, 246–247.

Rao, N. and Youngson, G. G. (1989) Wound sepsis following Ramstedt pyloromyotomy. *Br. J. Surg.*, **76**, 1144–1146.

Saunders, M. P. and Williams, C. R. (1990) Infantile hypertrophic pyloric stenosis: experience in a district general hospital. *J. R. Coll. Surg. Edin.*, **35**, 36–38.

Shanbhogue, L. K., Sikdar, T., Jackson, M. *et al.* (1992) Serum electrolytes and capillary blood gases in the management of hypertrophic pyloric stenosis. *Br. J. Surg.*, **79**, 251–253.

Tan, K. C. and Bianchi, A. (1986) Circumumbilical incision for pyloromyotomy. *Br. J. Surg.*, **73**, 399.

Turnock, R. R. and Rangecroft, L. (1991) Comparison of postpyloromyotomy feeding regimens in infantile hypertrophic pyloric stenosis. *J. R. Coll. Surg. Edin.*, **36**, 164–165.

Vanderwinden, J. M., Mailleux, P., Schiffmann, S. N. *et al.* (1992) Nitric oxide synthase activity in infantile hypertrophic pyloric stenosis. *N. Engl. J. Med.*, **27**, 511–515.

Wheeler, R. A., Najmaldin, A. S., Stoodley, N. *et al.* (1990) Feeding regimens after pyloromyotomy. *Br. J. Surg.*, **77**, 1018–1019.

3.3 ABDOMINAL PAIN

3.3.1 HISTORY AND EXAMINATION IN CHILDREN

After head injury, abdominal pain is one of the commonest reasons for a child to be admitted to hospital. To achieve this admission the child needs to convince a number of adults, including his parents, teachers, carers, family doctor or admitting doctor, that the pain is sufficiently severe to warrant hospitalization and a considerable time may lapse in some children before admission is arranged. In a study recently carried out in North-east Scotland, of 335 children with abdominal pain admitted to hospital over a 1-year period, 78 had appendicitis. Of this group, 70% had symptoms for 24 hours or less, 20% had been in pain for 24–48 hours and 4% had pain exceeding 48 hours: 6% had had symptoms for 4 days or more (Driver and Youngson, 1995).

The lack of correlation between a symptom and its anatomical source is a problem for those dealing with children and this applies increasingly with age. This difficulty is reflected in a study (Winsey and Jones, 1967) which indicated that only 40 out of every 100 children admitted to hospital with abdominal pain have a surgical cause. Constitutional upset from systemic infectious illnesses such as measles or rubella or totally unrelated inflammatory illnesses such as otitis media and tonsillitis may be responsible for the apparent symptom of abdominal pain in the younger child, and emphasize the need for a full clinical examination.

While some coexisting symptoms such as headache or nausea are non-specific and not necessarily those of a surgical illness, certain symptoms are pathognomonic of a surgical condition. One such is bilious vomiting, which must always be attributed to a surgical cause and the only task for the clinician is to define the cause of the obstruction.

Constructing a history for a child with abdominal pain can be a challenging task. Sources of information include the admitting physician and the parents as well as the child; other important clues may be non-verbal, such as the spontaneity of movement and, in particular, the interaction between the parent and child. The examining doctor must not only have, but must show patience in history-taking. The greater the agitation of parent and child, the greater the benefit from a display of patience. An unhurried clinical approach accrues significant benefits in what otherwise may be an unforgiving situation. Contrary to practice in adult surgery, I find benefit in not discussing the symptoms with the child during physical examination of the abdomen, but rather focusing discussion on areas of interest to the child such as schoolteachers, classmates, sports, music, etc. (this requires a contemporary outlook on the part of the doctor, if not to be considered outdated by the child!). The relative merits of television characters, sports teams and teachers may require tact.

A child with peritonitis will have signs of tenderness and guarding, but peritoneal irritation displays itself in other ways: reluctance to move, cough, laugh or even cry. Young children may be distressed by some conventional clinical techniques, such as attempting to elicit rebound tenderness (p. 42). Conversely, the child who holds her abdomen with her forearm crossed over the hypochondrium and who elevates her right shoulder in response to abdominal palpation, indrawing her abdomen as she does so, will seldom have peritoneal irritation.

It should not be assumed that, just because a child is asleep when approached, intraperitoneal sepsis is absent. Indeed, a gentle hand under the sheet of the bed can often elicit guarding in a sleeping child although, more often than not, the examination will arouse the child.

The most testing situation of all is the restive infant or toddler, clasping his mother. His distress, pain and fear of his new environment will make compliance with examination limited. It is difficult in these circumstances to elicit abdominal signs and those signs that are found need care in interpretation. A display of friendly concern to his mother will often gain a modicum of the infant's confidence. Any attempt, however, to remove him from his mother's arms may instantly destroy that confidence and the doctor must find some way to maintain this physical contact with his mother throughout the examination, even if this requires examination of the child from behind as he cuddles his mother.

The aphorism that no abdominal examination is complete until the genitalia have been examined bears repetition in children. Torsion of the testis in particular, may present as lower abdominal pain and the need to establish the state of descent of the testis is part of the abdominal examination of every boy. Examination of the external genitalia of a girl is often considered difficult or inappropriate by many doctors; however this is a simple manoeuvre and is easily achieved in toddlers by lifting the heels above the abdomen. This needs to be done gently if there is peritoneal irritation and inspection is the only component of examination tolerated by most girls. Older girls should be examined in the left lateral position and may even require examination under anaesthesia (EUA) if there is an absolute need for the examination to be completed. EUA however is preferable to inappropriate examination, when, for example, haematocolpos is the suspected diagnosis and inspection of the hymen is required for confirmation.

For details of rectal examination, see Chapter 2, p. 43.

3.3.2   ACUTE APPENDICITIS – CHILDHOOD ISSUES

The diagnosis and management of childhood appendicitis shares many of the features of the adult condition outlined in Chapter 2. The presentation in childhood is in some ways simpler, because diagnostic options are fewer and the incidence of the disease in childhood is relatively high. In a study of 649 children admitted to hospital in Aberdeen with abdominal pain (Driver and Youngson, 1995), 30% (192) had appendicitis and the other surgical conditions comprised intussusception (15), adhesive intestinal obstruction (6), trauma including splenic and liver laceration (14). Of the 192 with appendicitis, only 20 were aged 5 years or under (Table 2.1, p. 51).

The behaviour of appendicitis is different in the very young, with the frequency of perforation increasing with the youth of the child. This may in part derive from difficulties of communication, which poses obstacles to early diagnosis and prompt intervention in children less than 5 years of age. The progression from an inflamed state to perforation of the appendix with peritonitis is measured in hours rather than days, and obstructive appendicitis due to a faecolith progresses more rapidly to a state of perforation than when catarrhal inflammation of the lymphoid component is responsible (Anderson *et al.*, 1994).

Although the increased rate of perforation may, in part, be due to the relative delay in diagnosis in the young, the omentum in children under 5 seldom seems capable of restricting sepsis to one quadrant; hence diffuse peritonitis is a common finding in children under 5 years with appendicitis.

Active observation (p. 50) retains primacy as the diagnostic tool in early management, even with the liberal application of abdominal ultrasound examination in emergency practice. Clinical examination will, in many children, give clear evidence of the need to operate and, in the more doubtful case, active observation will be adopted as a safe and effective management process. Ultrasound examination does, however, have particular value if pelvic or retroileal appendicitis is suspected, where free fluid may be seen in the rectovesical pouch, or, on a rare occasion, the thickened appendix itself may be visualized.

In the doubtful case, recognition of the lack of specificity of abdominal signs as indicators of appendicitis emphasizes the need for repeated clinical assessment before deciding to operate. Consistency of the clinical findings is in itself reassuring that the correct decision has been made, be that operative or conservative. Similarly a trend in evolution of signs, either receding or reinforcing the need for operation, also points the way to correct decision-making. Jones (1969) clearly demonstrated the contribution which time and repeated observation makes to diagnostic accuracy. Using this technique as the main guide, surgeons at Royal Aberdeen Children's Hospital, in a 1-year period, removed only two normal appendices from 83 children being treated for appendicitis.

Coexisting disease processes in childhood such as acute lymphoblastic leukaemia and cystic fibrosis present very difficult diagnostic and management issues although, in reality, the main problem centres on the question of diagnosis and the need to operate. The ability of the body to develop an appropriate immune and inflammatory response is severely compromised in leukaemia, and, although the existence of typhlitis (enteritis of the ileocaecal region) complicating treatment with chemotherapy is a well-recognized event (p. 544), suspicion of appendicitis should prompt appendicectomy, supported by haematological treatment such as bone marrow stimulation and transfusion of the appropriate blood elements and factors.

There are no universally recognized laboratory investigations diagnostic of appendicitis. The combination of an elevated white cell count and measurement of C-reactive protein (Thompson *et al.*, 1992), or indeed, C-reactive protein by itself (Oosterhouse *et al.*, 1993; Albu *et al.*, 1994) enhances the clinical diagnosis of appendicitis (p. 46). Radiological studies will, on occasion, contribute to the diagnosis, with abdominal ultrasound making the major contribution in this regard. Active observation, however, still remains predominant in the diagnostic process.

Operation

It is generally agreed, in the management of childhood appendicitis, that delaying an operation, to avoid surgery between 24.00 and 06.00 hours, does not increase the incidence of perforation or other morbidity (Surana *et al.*, 1993). There are important qualifications to this approach, however, which include the provision of rehydration therapy, pain relief and systemic antibiotics during this time, and that firm arrangements are made for appendicectomy the following morning.

The surgeon in training will find that the combination of tissue elasticity and relative non-fixation of the right colon usually allows an easier delivery of the caecum and appendix in children than in adults. Hence the need to perform any incision other than a muscle-splitting gridiron type of approach is uncommon.

The operative strategy at the children's hospital in Aberdeen for the last 6 years, in 429 patients, has comprised appendicectomy without stump inversion, thorough peritoneal lavage with an antibiotic solution (cefotaxime 1 mg/ml), primary wound closure without drainage, subcuticular skin closure and one-dose perioperative antibiotic administration (cefotaxime and metronidazole) in non-perforated appendicitis. The duration of antibiotic treatment in ruptured appendicitis depends on progress and generally extends to a minimum of 3 days. This regime has a prospectively recorded wound sepsis rate of 2% and no mortality.

Postoperative analgesia is facilitated by intraoperative injection of bupivacaine (0.25 ml/kg) into the regional nerves at the lateral margin of the muscle incision (Wright, 1993).

There are occasions when the appendix may be difficult to find and deliver. The principles involved in mobilization and wound extension are outlined in Chapter 2. If the appendix is unduly high, consider the possibility of coexisting malrotation. In this rare situation an apparent postoperative ileus may in fact be obstruction and on two occasions I have had to perform urgent re-laparotomy for volvulus (p. 107).

There is disagreement over what constitutes an acceptable 'normal' appendicectomy rate, for fear of missing the diagnosis (Chapter 2). If clinical doubt exists over the need to operate, revisit your patient, rethink the case and then make a decision. That decision should be to operate or to revisit again. The option of not operating is only entertained when the patient is deemed not to have appendicitis.

Laparoscopic appendicectomy in childhood is an alternative technique that has yet to supplant open operation. While many reports attest to the safety of this operation (Najmaldin, 1995), a French study of 406 operations, 200 of which were laparoscopic (Varlet *et al.*, 1994), indicated that the peroperative complication rate was higher in laparoscopic appendicectomy, although the postoperative morbidity was reduced. The possibility of intraoperative haemorrhage from the appendicular vessels, diathermy injury or intestinal injury during establishment of the pneumoperitoneum is a disincentive for the many paediatric surgeons in whose hands the open procedure remains controlled and precise.

Postoperative recovery following appendicectomy can be expected to be rapid with discharge on the second or third day in uncomplicated cases.

Opinion is still varied on the management of the appendix mass. In the unusual event of absence of signs of peritoneal irritation, treatment with intravenous antibiotic should cater for three prime pathogens – *Escherichia coli*, *Streptococcus milleri* and *Bacteroides fragilis*. A combination of cefotaxime, metronidazole and ampicillin is effective against this flora. The intravenous route of metronidazole may be replaced by rectal administration after the first dose. Conversion to oral antibiotic coincides with restoration of oral intake following resolution of ileus.

Sequential ultrasound examination is of value in assessing the response of any non-operated appendix mass to treatment, but progress must also be monitored clinically and the decision to continue with conservative management must be revised if progressive signs of peritoneal irritation are recognized. In the event of peritoneal signs coexisting with the mass, an operative approach should be undertaken; it must be recognized that this will be a technically challenging operation that requires optimal operating conditions, and neither operation nor anaesthesia should be delegated to someone junior.

Another controversy that prevails is over the use of intraperitoneal drainage, with some surgeons, particularly in North America, favouring such an approach. Lund and Murphy (1994), reviewing a 10-year experience of perforated appendicitis, quote a low incidence of morbidity (7.7%) using a protocol employing immediate appendicectomy, peritoneal lavage with antibiotic solution, transperitoneal drainage and a 10-day course of intravenous antibiotics. Current practice in the UK does not follow this pattern and intraperitoneal drainage is seldom employed following definitive treatment of intraperitoneal sepsis.

REFERENCES

Albu, E., Miller, B. M., Choi, Y. *et al.* (1994) Diagnostic value of C-reactive protein in acute appendicitis. *Dis. Colon Rectum*, **37**, 49–51.

Anderson, R., Hugander, A., Thulm, A. *et al.* (1994) The indications for operation in suspected appendicitis and incidence of perforation. *BMJ*, **308**, 107–110.

Driver, C. P. and Youngson, G. G. (1995) Acute abdominal pain in children: A 25 year comparison. *Health Bull.*, **53**, 167–172.

Jones, P. F. (1969) Acute abdominal pain in childhood with special reference to cases not due to appendicitis. *BMJ*, **i**, 284–286.

Jones, P. F. (1976) Active observation in the management of acute abdominal pain in childhood. *BMJ*, **i**, 551–553.

Lund, D. P. and Murphy, E. U. (1994) Management of perforated appendicitis in children: a decade of aggressive treatment. *J. Pediatr. Surg.*, **29**, 1130–1133.

Najmaldin, A. (1995) Minimal access surgery in paediatrics. *Arch. Dis. Child.*, **72**, 107–109.

Oosterhuis, W. P., Zwinderman, A. H. and Teeuwen, M. (1993) C reactive protein in the diagnosis of acute appendicitis. *Eur. J. Surg.*, **159**, 115–119.

Surana, R., Quinn, F. and Puri, P. (1993) Is it necessary to perform appendicectomy in the middle of the night in children? *BMJ*, **306**, 1168.

Thompson, M. M., Underwood, M. J., Dookeran, K. A. *et al.* (1992) Role of sequential leucocyte counts and C-reactive protein measurements in acute appendicitis. *Br. J. Surg.*, **79**, 822–824.

Varlet, F., Tardieu, D., Limonne, B. *et al.* (1994) Laparoscopic versus open appendectomy in children – comparative study of 403 cases. *Eur. J. Pediatr. Surg.*, **4**, 333–337.

Winsey, H. S. and Jones, P. F. (1967) Acute abdominal pain in children, analysis of a year's admissions. *BMJ*, **i**, 653–655.

Wright, J. E. (1993) Controlled trial of wound infiltration with bupivacaine for postoperative pain relief after appendicectomy in children. *Br. J. Surg.*, **80**, 110–111.

3.3.3   NON-SPECIFIC ABDOMINAL PAIN

The studies which led to the recognition of NSAP as an entity were largely made in children's hospitals and the subject is reviewed in Chapter 2.

3.3.4   SURGICAL CONDITIONS

3.3.4.1   Intussusception

Incidence

Intussusception is a relatively uncommon event comprising 8–9 cases per 100 000 population of children per year or 1.5–2 cases per 1000 live births, but it remains a dangerous illness with 33 children dying from this condition in England and Wales between 1984 and 1989

(Stringer *et al.*, 1992). The presentation can be variable according to the type and location of the intussusception and is perhaps at its most threatening when it occurs outwith the classical age of presentation of 2 months to 2 years.

The commonest age of occurrence is between 5 and 7 months and two-thirds of all cases happen in the first year of life. About 20% occur after age 2 and it is this group, often associated with other abdominal pathology, that accounts for delay in diagnosis and hence morbidity and mortality.

There is a slight male predominance in this condition (65–70%). The peak incidence occurs in early summer when enteric viruses are more active.

Aetiology

Hyperplasia of the lymphoid element of the distal small bowel can occur in response to the changing antigenic content of foodstuffs on weaning, or reactive swelling in response to an enteric viral infection (adenovirus) with associated mesenteric adenitis. As a result the thickened Peyer's patch becomes caught up in the peristaltic mechanism and is propelled down-stream; (the word derives from *intus*, meaning 'within', and *susceptum*, meaning 'caught up').

Other lead points include any form of enteric 'mass', including Meckel's diverticulum, duplication enteric cyst, adenomata of the small bowel and – an especially important cause – B-cell lymphoma of the gut. This last disease process will often produce chronic low-grade intussusception with an insidious presentation which is entirely different from the acute variety. Intussusception involving such lead points invariably affects older children, resulting on occasion in delay of the diagnosis.

Postoperative intussusception is a condition seen exclusively in children and occurs in the postoperative period, after any abdominal operation but most commonly after intestinal anastomosis, when disordered peristalsis, in conjunction with intestinal oedema, may result in small-bowel intussusception. This condition presents as a small-bowel obstruction and can be a difficult diagnostic challenge.

In all cases of intussusception, as the bowel is propelled through the distal lumen, the feeding mesentery is compressed by the entrapping bowel. The danger in intussusception is that this results in mucosal ischaemia with ulceration and bleeding. If allowed to remain uncorrected, this will progress to ischaemic necrosis and infarction of the tip of the intussusceptum, perforation and dramatic deterioration of the child's condition.

The enveloping layer is hardly ever rendered gangrenous by the process.

Types

There are four main types of intussusception (Strang, 1959).

(a) Ileocolic

In this type a swollen Peyer's patch in the ileum is the lead point and passes through the ileocaecal valve to progress through the colon for a variable distance (Figure 3.2). This is the commonest type, accounting for more than half of cases.

(b) Ileocaecal

The ileocaecal valve constitutes the lead-point in this type, which accounts for approximately one-third of cases (Figure 3.3). The remaining types account for about 5% of cases each.

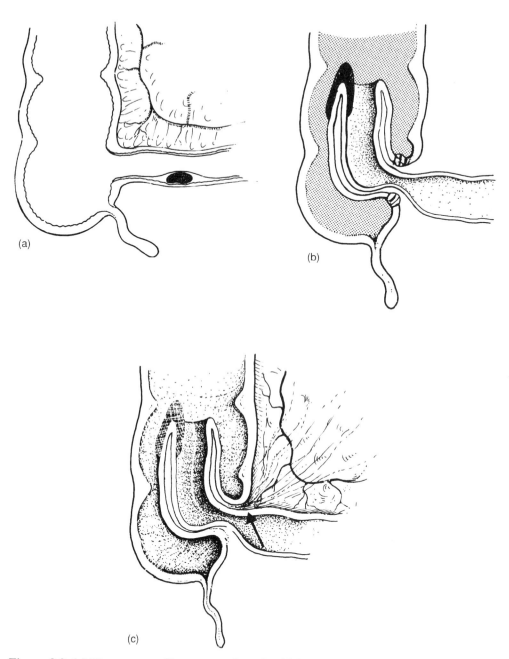

(a)

(b)

(c)

Figure 3.2 **(a)** The process of intussusception of a thickened patch of lymphoid tissue in the terminal ileum. **(b)** Through the ileocaecal valve and then downstream for a variable distance through the colon in the most common type – ileocolic intussusception. **(c)** Compression of the small-bowel mesentery makes this type susceptible to ischaemic perforation.

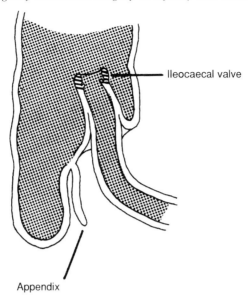

Appendix

Figure 3.3 Ileocaecal intussusception is more easily reduced and less likely to ischaemic necrosis because of the wide neck of the intussusception being colon. This type accounts for about one-third of cases.

(c) Caecocolic
This form of intussusception is loose and reduced without difficulty. The apex is the caput caeci and they mostly occur in children over 2 years of age.

(d) Ileoileal
These are variable in presentation but often present as a small-bowel obstruction such as is seen in postoperative intussusception. There is no rectal bleeding in this variety nor is there a mass. Imaging is frequently unhelpful and management should be through prompt operative intervention on suspicion of the diagnosis.

Clinical presentation

The history is the crucial and most influential factor in alerting the clinician to the possibility of intussusception. The onset of symptoms is abrupt, often preceded by a respiratory illness. The infant starts to cry forcibly and strain. The mother will tell you that her baby is in pain. The child may vomit and during attacks of pain will attempt to curl up by flexing hips and knees. He will then become calm and may even fall asleep. During sleep, the infant will often appear pale and listless. Such episodes recur every 20 minutes or so, the pain attacks lasting approximately 20 minutes themselves. Generally the longer the history, the poorer the general appearance of the infant between attacks.

Diarrhoea is often present and should not be considered incompatible with the diagnosis. MacDonald and Beattie (1995), reviewing 100 cases of intussusception presenting to the Accident and Emergency Department of the Hospital for Sick Children, Edinburgh, found that the complaint of diarrhoea tended to lead to a diagnosis of gastroenteritis and referral to the paediatricians rather than the surgeons. Only 42% of cases were correctly diagnosed within 3 hours of admission and 50% were admitted to the medical as opposed to the surgical service. However the presence of blood in the stool along with mucus, the so-called 'redcurrant jelly' stool, will point the clinician more directly to the diagnosis but is only seen in about 60% of children.

Early in the course of the condition, vomiting may be present but this is reflex in origin and will only contain altered foodstuffs. As the condition proceeds the vomiting will become more bile-stained.

During episodes when the baby falls asleep, in the mother's arms, opportunity should be taken to perform gentle abdominal examination, with the mother still holding the baby (attempts to place him in his cot will awaken and unsettle him/her). A palpable mass can be felt in approximately 70% of cases. The mass is most easily palpable lying in the upper abdomen across the epigastrium, unless it falls under the left lobe of the liver. In this instance the mass becomes palpable as the bowel contracts but this will promptly produce pain and the opportunity for palpation will be brief before the child becomes unsettled again.

Rectal examination is essential in this condition and on occasion the intussusceptum will be palpable in the rectum. This often causes alarm but does not necessarily prejudice the responsiveness of the condition to treatment. The presence of blood on the examining finger is a strong pointer to the diagnosis.

The abdominal mass is palpable in approximately 60–70% of cases, with blood being in the rectum in a similar proportion. A number of cases, therefore, do not fit the classical picture.

Babies who do not scream and remain pale and floppy (10%) should be considered to be in a more advanced stage of the illness and in need of urgent resuscitation from their intestinal obstruction and septicaemia.

Investigation

Plain X-ray of the abdomen should be taken in all cases, if for no other reason than to exclude intestinal perforation. The target sign (two concentric circular radiolucent lines superimposed on the right kidney) is seen in about two-thirds of cases, although a soft tissue mass is the commonest sign to be seen. Signs of small-bowel obstruction may be present but are uncommon except in the ileoileal type (Ratcliffe *et al.*, 1992).

A high level of confidence now exists among paediatric radiologists in their ability to diagnose intussusception by abdominal ultrasound, with a sensitivity of 98.5% and a specificity of 100% being reported in a series of 130 children with intussusception (Shanbogue *et al.*, 1994).

Treatment

Volume replacement with infusion of plasma, antibiotic administration and analgesia will stabilize most sick infants. The current practice in most paediatric centres is to attempt pneumostatic reduction of the intussusception. Exceptions to this are those children with signs of peritonitis or radiological signs of perforation in whom a decision must be made to proceed to laparotomy. Air reduction can be expected to reduce approximately 80% of intussusceptions (Markovitz and Meyer, 1992). Whereas hydrostatic techniques previously used generated steady pressures of 80–100 cmH$_2$O, air reduction provokes high, sharp pressure peaks which appear to be more effective in the reduction process (Zambuto *et al.*, 1995).

Recurrence after initial reduction should not dissuade the clinician from further attempts at non-operative reduction, but failure to reduce should elicit the suspicion of the presence of a lead point. Puri and Guiney in Dublin (1985) treated 292 children with intussusception and found a lead point in 27. In 13 this was a Meckel's diverticulum, four had Henoch–Schönlein purpura and in ten there was a tumour (either benign or in one case malignant). The children with lead points as a cause of the intussusception are older than other children with this condition.

Operation

As with most abdominal approaches in infancy, good exposure is achieved through a transverse muscle-cutting abdominal incision. A right-sided incision, cutting rectus abdominis at or immediately above the level of the umbilicus, will provide ample exposure of the abdomen in general and the intussuscepted right colon in particular. There is seldom gross distension of the small bowel, but if there is, deflation should be achieved in the standard fashion by retrograde milking into the stomach with nasogastric aspiration of the gastric content. In most instances it is possible to approach the intussusception directly.

Reduction is achieved using some traction on the small bowel but mainly by squeezing the apex of the intussuscepted bowel back into position. A warmed moist pack should be applied to the colon prior to attempting this manoeuvre and care must be taken to ensure reduction is slow and steady, avoiding any splitting of the muscular coat of the bowel (Figure 3.4).

Once the bowel is completely reduced the viability of the intussusception must be thoroughly evaluated. Perforation, particularly at the mesenteric aspect of the ileocaecal valve, must be carefully looked for; ischaemic colour change does need patient management with application of warm towels to the bowel (p. 199).

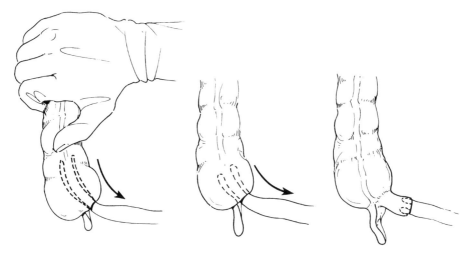

Figure 3.4 Reduction of the intussusception by compression of the colon distal to the intussusception and gentle traction on the ileum.

Restoration of normovolaemia and control of sepsis with a broad-spectrum antibiotic (cefotaxime 30–50 mg/kg and metronidazole 7 mg/kg) are important intraoperative considerations and should be given before resection of ischaemic bowel. The presence of lead points may be quite obvious but lymphomatous change in thickened small bowel requires vigilance.

The indications for resection are those for any bowel of doubtful viability. In addition there is a mandatory case for resection if a lead point is encountered, irrespective of the nature of the lead point. Particular care must be taken after reduction to palpate any polyp because bowel oedema makes this easy to miss.

The anastomotic techniques used following resection are outlined in Chapter 1. Resection techniques in infancy follow the same principles, employing finer sutures, and my preference is 4/0 braided nylon (Nurolon) in children and 6/0 PDS (polydioxanone) in infants.

Recurrence after resection is rare and postoperative management requires no specific alteration from the care afforded any infant following bowel resection.

REFERENCES

Macdonald, I. A. and Beattie, T. F. (1995) Intussusception presenting to a paediatric accident and emergency department. *J. Accident Emergency Med.*, **12**, 182–186.

Markowitz, R. I. and Meyer, J. S. (1992) Pneumatic versus hydrostatic reduction of intussusception. Radiology, **183**, 623–624.

Puri, P. and Guiney, E. (1985) Small bowel tumours causing intussusception in childhood. *Br. J. Surg.*, **72**, 493–494.

Ratcliffe, J. F., Fong, S., Cheong, I. *et al.* (1992) The plain abdominal film in intussusception: the accuracy and incidence of radiographic signs. *Pediatr. Radiol.*, **22**, 110–111.

Shanbhogue, R. L., Hussain, S. M., Meradji, M., *et al.* (1994) Ultrasonography is accurate enough for the diagnosis of intussusception. *J. Pediatr. Surg.*, **29**, 324–327.

Strang, R. (1959) Intussusception in infancy and childhood. *Br. J. Surg.*, **46**, 484–495.

Stringer, M. D., Pledger, G. and Drake, D. P. (1992) Childhood deaths from intussusception in England and Wales, 1984–9. *BMJ*, **304**, 737–739.

Zambuto, D., Bramson, R. T. and Blickman, J. G. (1995) Intracolonic pressure measurements during hydrostatic and air contrast barium enema studies in children. *Radiology*, **196**, 55–58.

3.3.4.2 Meckel's diverticulum

Johann Meckel (the younger) was Professor of Anatomy and Surgery at Halle when, in 1809, he first described the anomaly that subsequently assumed his name. He correctly identified that this structure was a remnant of the yolk sac (Meckel, 1838) and identified three characteristics as a prerequisite to the diagnosis.

- It has the same structure as the adjacent bowel.
- It arises from the antimesenteric side of the ileum.
- It has a dedicated separate blood supply from the adjacent bowel known as the omphalomesenteric artery.

A Meckel's diverticulum (MD) may be a blind-ended saccule of bowel (85%) or it may be attached to the umbilicus. It is said that most diverticula lie some 2 feet (60 cm) proximal to the ileocaecal valve, but as many as 25% lie higher up the ileum, with some descriptions referring to jejunal MDs. The unattached MD can vary significantly in its length and be of

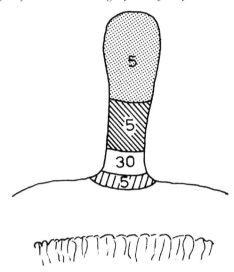

Figure 3.5 Distribution of acid-producing mucosa within Meckel's diverticulum as first described by Cobb (1936). This demonstrates the potential extension of the ectopic gastric mucosa into ileum.

a variety of shapes. The fundus may be hollow or solid and even contain ectopic pancreatic tissue. It is important to be familiar with the distribution of gastric mucosa as first described by Cobb (1936) who examined the location of the gastric mucosa in 45 MDs (Figure 3.5). In a significant proportion, gastric mucosa extends as far as the base of the diverticulum and this has a bearing on the choice of operative procedure recommended.

The attached MD has a variety of potential connections:

- patent vitellointestinal duct with faecal fistula (2%; Figure 3.6);
- partial patency of the duct resulting in a sinus at the umbilicus, which may secrete mucus or bleed occasionally with a 'raspberry' tumour (1%; Figure 3.7);
- the band from the MD develops a secondary connection, usually to the adjacent mesentery: a meso-diverticular band (5–10%; Figure 3.8).

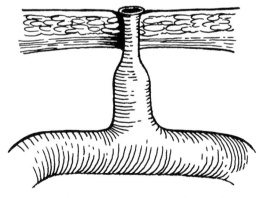

Figure 3.6 Patency of the vitellointestinal duct with a faecal fistula.

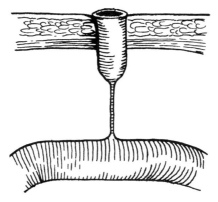

Figure 3.7 Partial patency of the duct with a distal sinus, which may produce intermittent purulent discharge.

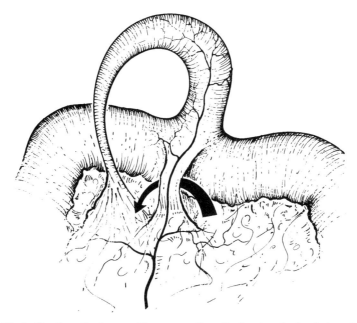

Figure 3.8 Meckel's diverticulum with a mesodiverticular band. An internal hernia may occur in the 'window' produced by the omphalomesenteric artery shown by the arrow.

Clinical presentation

This common congenital anomaly of the small intestine occurs in about 2% of the population and can present as an emergency in one of several ways or can be found incidentally during the course of an unrelated abdominal operation. The three main presentations are intestinal obstruction (40–50%), peptic ulceration (25%) and acute inflammation (20%).

The presence of heterotopic gastric mucosa in the lumen, or a band indicating a persistent remnant of the vitellointestinal duct, are responsible for these presenting features. The gastric mucosa may be responsible for bleeding consequent on ulceration of the adjacent small bowel, or even for perforation of the bowel.

Diverticulitis with subsequent perforation will produce an illness almost identical to appendicitis, save for the lack of a shift of the pain to the right iliac fossa.

(a) Intestinal obstruction

Intussusception may occur with the diverticulum acting as the lead point as outlined above, and since the intussusception is ileoileal, small-bowel obstruction is the commonest presentation. Persistence of the fibrous band, which was once vitellointestinal duct, produces the most serious presentation, with volvulus of the adjacent small bowel pivoting on the band that extends from the MD to the umbilicus. This process of volvulus can on occasion involve significant lengths of bowel. Moreover, bowel infarction can occur by entrapment of small bowel in the hiatus produced by the omphalomesenteric artery. Brookes (1954) described five cases where this event resulted in thrombosis of the omphalomesenteric artery with ischaemia of the diverticulum. The MD is occasionally so long as to make a knot with another part of the bowel and a rare mechanism of obstruction is stricture due to cicatricial peptic ulceration at the mouth of the diverticulum.

(b) Peptic ulceration

Heterotopic gastric mucosa, which secretes hydrochloric acid and pepsin, is found in 20–40% of all MDs. MD containing such mucosa is often identified by thickening of the diverticulum and, on sectioning these lesions, the gastric mucosa is readily identifiable as a white plaque-like sheet extending along the wall of the diverticulum. Extension into the adjacent ileum is exceedingly rare. The ulceration produced by the acid, however, is commonly at the neck of the MD, or a few millimetres downstream in the ileum.

With a bleeding MD, the child is usually asymptomatic but for the presence of fresh blood *per rectum*. The rate of bleeding is usually sufficiently brisk to differentiate it from bleeding from other causes, e.g. intussusception or colonic polyp; indeed, such is the pace of blood loss that intravenous fluid administration is required for resuscitation. It is worth remembering, however, that the process that produces the bleeding can progress to perforation of the intestine with associated peritonitis.

In the event of the bleeding being less brisk, investigation is required to identify the cause. Contrast study of the colon will eliminate other causes and isotope scanning with ^{99m}Tc pertechnetate to localize ectopic gastric mucosa is useful when a positive result is obtained (Berquist *et al.*, 1976).

(c) Acute inflammation

Acute inflammation of a MD produces an illness very similar to acute appendicitis, but the pain persists in the periumbilical area, with no shift to the right lower quadrant. Nonetheless, the child is frequently managed as a case of appendicitis. At operation, however, suspicion of the diagnosis is aroused by the normal appearance of the appendix and the presence of purulent fluid in the abdomen (hence the importance of careful laparotomy when a normal appendix is discovered). As in appendicitis, perforation can occur following obstruction of the lumen but the distinction from perforation secondary to peptic ulceration can only be made by histology. Diverticulitis can also be caused by impaction of foreign bodies, such as swallowed fish bones, which go on to perforate.

Late complications of MD include neoplastic change including carcinoid, adenocarcinoma and leiomyosarcoma (Leijonmark *et al.*, 1986). Littré's hernia, a condition first described in 1719 by Alexis Littré, occurs when a MD enters either an inguinal or femoral hernia, subsequently becoming strangulated.

Operation

Two specific issues must be addressed at operation. These are management of the omphalomesenteric artery and the extent of resection of the bowel adjacent to the MD. The vascular supply may be separated from the adjacent mesentery and ligated, but is more easily controlled in many other cases by simply under-running the artery and vein with a fine Prolene stitch.

Some surgeons advocate clamping the base of the MD and oversewing the defect. However this practice does not cater for the possibility of extension of the gastric mucosa beyond the junction of MD and ileum and risks leaving residual acid-bearing mucosa with the potential for recurrence of ulceration. Removal of a wedge of healthy ileum is to be commended particularly when surgery is performed for bleeding. An open technique permits examination of the bowel mucosa and identification of any distal ulcer and bleeding point. It is therefore preferable to extend the resection and carry out diverticulectomy with adjacent resection of small bowel by the technique described in Chapter 1.

Incidental diverticulectomy

There is no consensus on the merit or otherwise of removal of a MD found incidentally during the course of another operation. This probably indicates that there is no single policy appropriate, but that several factors need be considered. These include:

- the nature of the original operation, which may make a non-essential enterotomy potentially hazardous;
- the risk of complication arising in the particular MD; risk is elevated if the diverticulum is long with a broad base and if there is palpable ectopic gastric mucosa;
- the risk of complications, which is greatest in the first 30 years of life;
- the balance of risk between the likely natural history and the expectation of complication following surgery.

Several contradictory works have been produced on this aspect of MD. Cullen *et al.* (1994), in a large epidemiological study performed in Minnesota over a 54-year review period, compared the morbidity and mortality accompanying surgery for complicated MD (12% and 2% respectively) with the morbidity and mortality associated with incidental diverticulectomy (2% and 1%) and concluded that MD encountered by chance at surgery should be removed for most patients regardless of age. Similarly, the experience of Dutch surgeons (Bemelman *et al.*, 1995) in 136 patients treated for MD was that the lifetime risk of illness is such that diverticulectomy should be performed when the MD is encountered incidentally.

However surgeons from the academic unit in Leeds (Kashi and Lodge, 1995), following 43 patients over an 8-year period who had MD diagnosed during laparotomy, found a complication rate of 26% in the 35 who had diverticulectomy performed. In 21 of the 35 the MD was an incidental finding. However in eight patients in whom the MD was left *in situ*, none developed early or late complications. Such a retrospective study, however, must inevitably contain a substantial bias in terms of selection.

From this conflicting experience, a large MD, with clinical suggestion of the presence of heterotopic gastric mucosa, found early in life, should on balance be resected.

REFERENCES

Bemelman, W. A., Hugenholtz, E., Heij, H. A. *et al.* (1995) Meckel's diverticulum in Amsterdam: experience in 136 patients. *World J. Surg.*, **19**, 734–736.

Berquist, T. H., Nolan, N. G., Stephens, D. H. *et al.* (1976) Specificity of ^{99m}Tc pertechnetate in scintigraphic diagnosis of Meckel's diverticulum: review of 100 cases. *J. Nucl. Med.*, **17**, 465–469.

Brookes, V. S. (1954) Meckels diverticulum in children: a report of 43 cases. *Br. J. Surg.*, **42**, 57–68.

Cobb, D. B. (1936) Meckel's diverticulum with peptic ulcer. *Ann. Surg.*, **103**, 747–768.

Cullen, J. J., Kelly, K. A., Moir, C. R. *et al.* (1994) Surgical management of Meckel's diverticulum. An epidemiologic, population-based study. *Ann. Surg.*, **220**, 564–568.

Kashi, S. H. and Lodge, J. P. (1995) Meckel's diverticulum: a continuing dilemma? *J. R. Coll. Surg. Edin.*, **40**, 392–394.

Leijonmark, C. E., Bonman-Sandelin, K, Frisell J. *et al.* (1986) Meckel's diverticulum in the adult. *Br. J. Surg.*, **73**, 146–149.

Meckel, J. F. (1838) *Manual of Descriptive and Pathological Anatomy*, (ed. G. Henderson), London, p. 385.

3.3.4.3 Duplication cysts

Duplications, a term first used by Fitz in 1884, are cystic or tubular malformations that lie alongside or close to the alimentary tract and have a similar muscular and mucosal structure. They are seen most often within the intestinal mesentery, sharing its blood supply, but may lie in the posterior mediastinum or beside the stomach or rectum.

The majority are cystic, variable in size and sometimes palpable. Tubular duplications communicate with the lumen of the gut, often in contact with the intestinal wall. Many duplications communicate with the lumen of the gut, and 30% contain ectopic gastric mucosa, so a peptic ulcer may form, causing rectal bleeding or perforation and peritonitis (Basu *et al.*, 1960).

Duplications are not often seen outside childhood, and then are unusual, but they can cause some demanding emergency situations. A mesenteric cyst may cause volvulus or kinking of small bowel or provide the lead point of an intussusception. As in MD, only a small number are diagnosed preoperatively, by either ultrasonography or isotope techniques (Teele *et al.*, 1980; Waterston *et al.*, 1980).

Peptic ulcer haemorrhage in association with a tubular duplication can present technical difficulties, because the duplication can be as much as 100 cm long and may lie beside the whole length of the small bowel. Severe rectal haemorrhage, or perforation and spreading peritonitis, may demand attention. If there is enough length of small bowel above and below the duplication and the ulcer, resection and anastomosis can be performed. If this is not feasible, resection of the ulcer and anastomosis of the distal end of the duplication to the stomach may be a useful measure (Jewett et al., 1983) that avoids further trouble.

In the case of tubular jejunoileal duplications that extend into the lesser sac, a full dissection should be performed to ensure that the duplication does not extend through the diaphragm. It should also be assumed that this variety of duplication coexists with an oesophageal duplication found in the posterior mediastinum. These, if not diagnosed, may cause dysphagia, respiratory distress or haemoptysis. Mediastinal duplications can also be associated with defects in the cervical and thoracic spine, with the duplication rarely extending into the spinal canal, a so-called neuroenteric cyst (Bentley and Smith, 1960).

Malignant transformation of the lining of duplication cysts is well documented in the adult literature (Hickey and Corson, 1981).

Treatment is by the resection technique most appropriate to the site of the cyst. For the majority, this will be resection and end-to-end anastomosis.

REFERENCES

Basu, R., Forshall, I. and Rickham, P. P. (1960) Duplications of the alimentary tract. *Br. J. Surg.*, **47**, 477–484.
Bentley, J. F. R. and Smith, J. R. (1960) Developmental posterior enteric remnants and spinal malformations. *Arch. Dis. Child.*, **35**, 76–86.
Hickey, W. F. and Corson, J. M. (1981) Squamous cell carcinoma arising in a duplication of the colon: Case report and literature review of squamous cell carcinoma of the colon and malignancy complicating colonic duplication. *Cancer*, **47**, 602–609.
Jewett, T. C., Walker, A. B. and Cooney, D. R. (1983) A long-term follow-up on a duplication of the entire small intestine treated by gastroduplication. *J. Pediatr. Surg.*, **18**, 185–188.
Teele, R. L., Henschke, C. I. and Tapper, D. (1980) The radiographic and ultrasonic evaluation of enteric duplication cysts. *Pediatr. Radiol.*, **10**, 9–14.
Waterston, T., Lyall, M. H., Longrigg, N. *et al.* (1980) Diagnosis of intestinal duplication by $^{99}Tc^m$-Pertechnitate scanning. *Br. J. Surg.*, **67**, 419–420.

3.3.4.4 Malrotation

A disturbance to the sequence of return of the intestine into the abdominal cavity during fetal development will result in poor fixation of the duodenum and colon, normally retroperitoneal structures. Moreover the disordered return results in abnormal location such that both the colon and duodenum are malrotated (Figure 3.9).

The stability of the small bowel and mesentery in normal rotation rests upon the distance between points of fixation, X and Y, the duodenojejunal and ileocaecal junctions respectively (Figure 3.10(a)). The reduction in this distance because of the location of the D/J flexure to the right of the midline (point X) and the placement of the caecum under the liver (point Y) results in approximation of these two points and a predisposition to twisting around this narrow, unstable axis (Figure 3.10(b)). Sir Norman Dott first documented the clinical consequences of this embryological anomaly in 1923.

Condensation of the peritoneal bands attaching caecum to the retroperitoneum can compress the duodenum as they pass across it and are known as Ladd's bands, which are responsible for the alternative presentation of bile vomiting (Ladd, 1932).

Although this condition may exist undetected throughout life (0.2%), it is generally accepted that the natural history of this condition is sufficiently lethal to recommend surgery upon diagnosis, irrespective of the symptoms present. Some 55% of cases present within the first week of life and 80% in the first month of life, placing these cases within the domain of paediatric surgeons, but the remainder occur sporadically throughout childhood and may even present in adult life (Berardi, 1980).

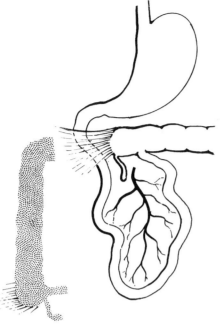

Figure 3.9 Malrotation of the duodenum and colon with Ladd's bands compressing the duodenum (the stippled area indicates the usual location of caecal peritoneum).

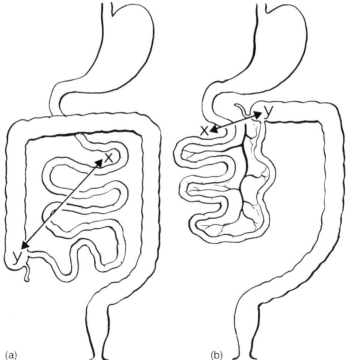

(a)   (b)

Figure 3.10 (a) Normal rotation. **(b)** Approximation of the malrotated D/J flexure (point X) to the high malrotated caecum (point Y) produces a narrow pedicle around which volvulus of the small-bowel mesentery will occur.

Clinical presentation

Presentation in the neonatal period is by bilious vomiting with intermittent intestinal obstruction. Alternatively, strangulating midgut volvulus can present with a progressive intestinal obstruction progressing to peritonitis and occasionally altered blood *per rectum*. In the older child the presentation can be quite insidious with chronic abdominal pain, intermittent bile vomiting or failure to thrive (Janik and Ein, 1979; Yanez and Spitz, 1986) but is usually accompanied by bile vomiting and excruciating abdominal colic.

In acute strangulated midgut volvulus the significance of bile in the vomit is again emphasized as an important feature of this illness. Such children are invariably significantly hypovolaemic and require substantial volume transfusion with plasma. Septicaemia is an important feature of midgut volvulus and its early appearance in small-bowel obstruction is strongly suggestive of the diagnosis. The combination of the severity of pain with marked hypovolaemia highlights the urgency of the situation.

The abdominal findings are seldom as impressive as the degree of pain that the volvulus produces. The accompanying tachycardia, poor capillary refill, and paradoxical lowering of peripheral temperature point to circulatory failure consequent to the hypovolaemia and septicaemia.

If signs of peritonitis are established, this indicates advanced ischaemia of the gut, which may not be a salvageable situation. Bowel sounds tend to be active and obstructive in the early phase of the illness, but laparotomy must not await the appearance of signs of peritonitis if volvulus is suspected.

Investigation

Plain erect X-ray of the abdomen typically shows a gasless abdomen with a ground-glass appearance in the mid-abdomen, with only a little stomach gas as the isolated feature. In the few children presenting with bilious vomiting only, the lesser degree of urgency allows investigation. Contrast studies are diagnostic, with a barium examination of the upper gastrointestinal tract, showing a corkscrew appearance to the duodenum, with the D/J flexure to the right of the midline. A barium enema shows the caecum to assume a high subhepatic position with a medial 'take-off' of the ileum. Ultrasound of the mesenteric vessels will demonstrate abnormal relationship of the superior mesenteric artery and vein to each other (Pracros *et al.*, 1992).

Treatment

Volvulus requires prompt aggressive resuscitation with plasma infusion and broad-spectrum antibiotic cover. Haemodynamic monitoring is of considerable value in fluid management. Blood should be cross-matched in preparation for surgery and baseline evaluation of haematological and biochemical indices made. The result of these, however, should not defer surgery unless any severe abnormality can be rapidly corrected, particularly in relation to the plasma potassium concentration.

The operation is carried out through a long transverse incision. In the case of volvulus without infarction, the first finding is one of milky free fluid, with the fluid having a high chyle content because of the obstructed lymphatics in the mesentery. Similarly the veins in the mesentery are usually very enlarged and engorged as a result of chronic obstruction. Blood-stained fluid is an ominous sign, indicative of intestinal infarction and necrosis.

The volvulus occurs in a clockwise fashion and therefore should be reduced by counterclockwise rotation. Patience must be exercised before passing judgement on the viability of the bowel and indeed this is also the time that reperfusion of ischaemic tissue renders the patient rather unstable. Systemic perfusion must be optimized before decisions are made on local tissue perfusion.

Having untwisted the mesentery, attention is now directed to the narrow base of the midgut. The peritoneal folds that cross from caecum to gallbladder and liver, compressing the duodenum, are divided by sharp dissection. This mobilizes the right colon. The duodenojejunal flexure is similarly divided by sharp dissection, freeing the ligament of Treitz from the duodenum and straightening the duodenal loop. Any residual thickened and shortened peritoneum over the origin of the superior mesenteric artery is divided. This last manoeuvre requires great care to avoid injury to the crucial site of vascular supply of the midgut. Moreover, many thickened lymphatics are present at this point and coagulated with diathermy. Infarcted bowel is resected as is appropriate.

This ingenious procedure, first described by Ladd and bearing his name, is completed by placing the bowel in a state of non-rotation with the right colon on the left-hand side of the peritoneal cavity and the small bowel to the right of the abdomen (Figure 3.11).

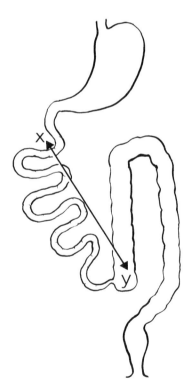

Figure 3.11 The arrangement of the intestine following Ladd's procedure. The caecum is placed in the left lower quadrant and the distance between caecum (Y) and malrotated duodenum (X) renders the small-bowel axis stable.

This manoeuvre is preceded by performing appendicectomy, which arguably helps fix the caecum in its new position but certainly precludes the diagnostic difficulties that would accrue from appendicitis developing in the left iliac fossa. No fixation of the bowel is required.

The abdomen is then closed in the standard fashion with a mass suture technique using PDS to the muscle layers and subcuticular suture to skin.

REFERENCES

Berardi, R. S. (1980) Anomalies of midgut rotation in the adult. *Surg. Gynecol. Obstet.*, **151**, 113–116.

Dott, N. M. (1923) Anomalies of intestinal rotation: Their embryology and surgical aspects, with report of 5 cases. *Br. J. Surg.*, **11**, 251–286.

Janik, J. S. and Ein, S. H. (1979) Normal intestinal rotation with non-fixation: a cause of chronic abdominal pain. *J. Pediatr. Surg.*, **6**, 670–674.

Ladd, W. E. (1932) Congenital obstruction of the duodenum in children. *N. Engl. J. Med.*, **206**, 277–283.

Pracros, J. P., Sann, L. and Genin, G. (1992) Ultrasound diagnosis of midgut volvulus: the 'whirlpool' sign. *Pediatr. Radiol.*, **22**, 18–20.

Yanez, R. and Spitz, L. (1986) Intestinal malrotation presenting outside the neonatal period. *Arch. Dis. Child.*, **61**, 682–685.

3.3.4.5 Omental infarction

This is a rare cause of acute onset of abdominal pain, which generally presents with an illness almost identical to appendicitis. The findings on opening the abdomen that suggest this diagnosis are the presence of a normal appendix, with serosanguinous free fluid. This condition is discussed further in Chapter 2.

3.3.4.6 Acute cholecystitis

Cholecystitis can be secondary to cholelithiasis or acalculous in origin. Cholelithiasis has been considered to be rare in childhood in the past, but the last two decades have seen a significant increase in the incidence of this condition. Prolonged parenteral nutrition dating from neonatal life, ileal resection or ileal disease, gallbladder stasis and hereditary haemolytic diseases leading to cholelithiasis are causes that are almost exclusively confined to childhood. The greatest rise in incidence, however, is in the incidence of idiopathic biliary calculi and non-haemolytic stones (Holcomb, 1993; Rescorla and Grosfeld, 1992). All these conditions are amenable to the newer techniques of cholecystectomy, so the hazards of open cholecystectomy are now obsolete and laparoscopic cholecystectomy has the prime role in management of gallbladder disease. This technique is as applicable to children as it is to adults and has been shown to be as safe, if not even superior, in terms of postoperative hospitalization and reduced levels of pain (Kim *et al.*, 1995).

Acalculous cholecystitis can complicate other conditions such as enteric fever due to *Salmonella typhi* (Tsakayannis *et al.*, 1996), a condition seen more commonly in the Indian subcontinent than Europe, and the condition can also complicate the recovery from major trauma, possibly as a consequence of biliary sludge from haematoma breakdown (Raunest *et al.*, 1992; Imhoff, 1992). Assessment uses ultrasound to assist in the diagnosis and, although milder forms may settle with gut rest and antibiotic treatment, necrosis of the gallbladder wall is likely to develop in most cases. The surgeon therefore should have a low threshold for operation, either cholecystectomy if there is necrosis in the wall and the dissection in the porta hepatis so permits, or cholecystostomy if the gallbladder is only thickened.

REFERENCES

Holcomb, G. W. III (1993) Laparoscopic cholecystectomy. *Semin. Pediatr. Surg.*, **2**, 159–167.

Imhof, M., Raunest, J., Ohmann. C. *et al.* (1992) Acute acalculous cholecystitis complicating trauma: a prospective sonographic study. *World J. Surg.*, **16**, 1160–1165.

Kim, P. C., Wesson, D., Superina, R. *et al.* (1995) Laparoscopic cholecystectomy versus open cholecystectomy in children: which is better? *J. Pediatr. Surg.*, **30**, 971–973.

Raunest, J., Imhof, M. and Rauen, U. (1992) Acute cholecystitis: a complication in severely injured intensive care patients. *J. Trauma*, **32**, 433–440.

Rescorla, F. J. and Grosfeld, J. L. (1992) Cholecystitis and cholelithiasis in children. *Semin. Pediatr. Surg.*, **1**, 98–106.

Tsakayannis, D. E., Kozakewich, H. P. and Lillehei, C. W. (1996) Acalculous cholecystitis in children. *J. Pediatr. Surg.*, **31**, 127–130.

3.3.5   NON-SURGICAL CONDITIONS

3.3.5.1   Primary peritonitis

This is predominantly a condition of girls (85%) in whom a pathogen enters the peritoneal cavity through an obscure route to establish peritonitis, without any intra-abdominal structure being responsible for the infection; it is responsible for only 1–2% of cases of peritonitis in childhood and is found most often in the 3–8-year age group.

While the incidence is now low, this condition was much commoner in previous years and was associated with significant morbidity and occasional mortality (McCartney and Fraser, 1922).

Aetiology

Two organisms, *S. pneumoniae* and *E. coli*, are now responsible for the majority of cases, although previously haemolytic *Streptococcus* was predominant (McDougal *et al.*, 1975). The genital tract has in the past been incriminated as the portal of infection in the female, with poor hygiene associated with low socioeconomic status implicated as risk factors, with the finding at operation, if performed, of reddening of the fallopian tubes supporting this hypothesis. However, both preceding upper respiratory tract and urinary tract infection have been cited as a source of sepsis.

The presence of ascitic fluid is an important antecedent in this condition. Kimber and Hutson, from the Royal Children's Hospital in Melbourne, reviewed 26 cases of primary peritonitis over a 5-year period from 1989–1994 and found that six (23%) had a major underlying medical condition which included nephrotic syndrome, liver cirrhosis and alpha-1-antitrypsin deficiency.

Clinical presentation

Primary peritonitis should be considered when the degree of toxaemia exceeds the expectation of the clinician, based on the abdominal findings. The pain is rapid in onset. There is a high fever from the outset, and the constitutional upset is marked. Haematological findings show an elevated white cell count with marked neutrophilia; there is elevation of the C-reactive protein and blood culture will be diagnostic, with a pure growth of *S. pneumoniae* being reported.

The clinical findings of lower abdominal peritonitis proceeding to generalized peritonitis lead to most children being operated on for suspected appendicitis. At operation, soapy purulent fluid is found covering the surface of pelvic organs, intestine and other viscera. The fallopian tubes are often red and, on occasion, pus can be expressed from the ostia of the tubes. After careful exploration of the contents of the abdomen to exclude a primary intra-abdominal cause, the surgeon should perform thorough peritoneal lavage with a ceph-alosporin solution, as described in the section on appendicectomy, and close the abdomen.

There is current controversy as to whether or not the appendix should be removed, although previously, the consensus view was to perform appendicectomy. However recent operative procedures in paediatric surgery that use the appendix as a conduit for catheterization and other purposes make this decision less straightforward, although my practice is to remove the appendix.

While primary peritonitis appearing in a previously healthy child is usually managed surgically, if the child is recognized as having an underlying medical condition causing ascites, or has a ventriculoperitoneal shunt *in situ*, it is entirely proper to consider this diagnosis from the outset and manage the condition medically by administration of analgesia and high-dose intravenous penicillin. In those cases of primary peritonitis complicating ascites, the response to antibiotic is prompt, but a full 7-day course is recommended.

REFERENCES

Kimber, C. P. and Hutson, J. M. (1996) Primary peritonitis in children. *Austr. N.Z. J. Surg.*, **66**, 169–170.
McCartney, J. E. and Fraser, J. (1922) Pneumococcal peritonitis. *Br. J. Surg.*, **9**, 479–489.
McDougal, W. S., Izart, R. and Zollinger, R. M. (1975) Primary peritonitis in infancy and childhood. *Ann. Surg.*, **181**, 310–313.

3.3.5.2   Pancreatitis

Trauma to the abdomen, particularly blunt abdominal trauma from cycle handlebar injury, is recognized as one of the main causes of pancreatitis in childhood (Young, 1984); otherwise it is rare in childhood in comparison to adult practice. Childhood pancreatitis is virtually always of the benign, oedematous variety unlike the lethal condition often seen in adults. Haddock *et al.* (1994) studied the outcome of pancreatitis affecting 49 children from three centres in Scotland over a 10-year period which confirmed the benign nature of this disease. When it has a fatal outcome this is because it complicates other multisystem disease such as haemolytic uraemic syndrome.

Non-traumatic pancreatitis is caused by a number of different diseases in children, including viral infection, notably mumps, or less frequently Coxsackievirus infection. Cystic fibrosis and hyperlipidaemia are metabolic causes. Congenital abnormalities of the pancreatobiliary tree such as choledochal cyst or pancreas divisum are also possible causes. Familial pancreatitis, pancreatitis secondary to cholelithiasis and idiopathic pancreatitis are all possible but rare causes of childhood pancreatitis.

The clinical presentation in those children where trauma has not been a feature includes onset of progressively severe upper abdominal pain, often radiating through to the back and virtually always associated with a disproportionately severe amount of vomiting. This history should prompt the measurement of the serum amylase level. Whereas mild elevation is seen in viral illness without pancreatitis, when this is present there is significant elevation.

Management of this group is initially supportive with intravenous fluid administration, gut rest and appropriate analgesia. This last provision may, on occasion, require pethidine given by patient-controlled analgesia infusion pump.

Ultrasound may show evidence of diffuse pancreatic swelling and reveal an underlying cause in the pancreas and biliary tree.

Increasingly a case is being made for more aggressive anatomical investigation. This is not required when an infective illness is the cause, but if there is doubt as to the origins of the pancreatitis or it is traumatic in origin, then a strong case can be made for early ERCP following contrast-enhanced CT scan of the abdomen.

Rescorla *et al.* (1995) highlighted the importance of early identification of ductal disruption as a guide to management, but the treatment of blunt pancreatic injury remains controversial. A conservative policy of gut rest, parenteral nutrition and infusion of octeotride, a somatostatin analogue that reduces bile and pancreatic fluid production, has been shown to be an effective strategy.

The operative approach, distal pancreatectomy, the preferred option in adult practice, is frequently associated with splenectomy, a procedure to be strenuously avoided in childhood because of the potential legacy of overwhelming post-splenectomy sepsis.

The present climate therefore favours a conservative policy in childhood. In the last two children with traumatic pancreatitis treated in the surgical unit in Aberdeen Children's Hospital, the ERCP was extremely influential in directing the management along conservative lines in the first instance. The laceration in the pancreas was seen to be to the right of the superior mesenteric axis, i.e. in the head of the pancreas. Ductal disruption was identified a few centimetres from the sphincter of Oddi and, although one case was complicated by a pseudocyst that required cystogastrostomy, the outcome was entirely satisfactory in both cases.

Identification of a congenital anomaly of the biliary tree as the cause for the pancreatitis requires the appropriate corrective surgery.

REFERENCES

Haddock, G., Raine, P. A. M., Couper, G. *et al.* (1994) Acute pancreatitis in children. *J. Pediatr. Surg.*, **29**, 719–722.

Rescorla, F. J., Plumley, D. A. and Sherman, S. (1995) The efficacy of early ERCP in pediatric pancreatic trauma. *J. Pediatr. Surg.*, **30**, 336–340.

Young, D. G. (1984) Abdominal trauma in children. *Austr. N.Z. J. Surg.*, **54**, 439.

3.3.5.3 Medical conditions

Diabetic ketoacidosis

This serious complication of diabetic destabilization may, in a previously undiagnosed child, present with acute abdominal pain and signs that can suggest acute appendicitis, and the child is referred to a surgical ward (Valerio, 1979). The history of a progressive deterioration over several days, the characteristic deep acidotic breathing and the smell of acetone in the breath (if it can be appreciated) should lead at once to estimation of the blood sugar (because a urine sample can be hard to obtain on account of the dehydration). Diagnosis and management are fully considered in Chapter 15.

It should always be kept in mind, however, that diabetic patients develop surgical conditions of the abdomen just as often as the non-diabetic. In a known diabetic the onset of control of the diabetic state may indicate the presence of intra-abdominal pathology.

Respiratory illnesses

Tonsillitis and acute otitis media in the toddler can present with abdominal pain. This may be due to poor localization of symptoms due to communication difficulties in this age group, but the lower abdominal tenderness may also be due to associated mesenteric adenitis.

Pneumonia is a classical example of an extra-abdominal condition that can simulate the acute abdomen, with the very clear need to identify this condition and avoid surgery. Ravichandran and Burge (1996) identified 19 children, from 1168 admitted with abdominal pain to the paediatric surgical unit at Southampton over a 6-year period, who had pneumonia as the sole cause of their symptoms. Although the correct diagnosis was made on review of the X-rays, one patient had a negative laparotomy.

The mechanism of the symptom production is not clear and the concept of referred pain from the diaphragmatic pleura is refuted by Burge. He reported that the pneumonia affected the upper and middle lobes in 41% and that left-sided pneumonia could be associated with right-sided pain. He confirmed that blood cultures and white-cell count were unhelpful. In any child with abdominal pain, fever and no identifiable cause for the pain, the child should be asked to cough, the chest should be examined clinically, the respiratory rate should be counted (bear in mind that tachypnoea can be seen in peritonitis) and a chest X-ray that includes the bases should be taken. The radiograph must be seen by the surgeon and, preferably, also by the radiologist prior to any diagnostic label being given to the patient.

Systemic infection

The prodrome associated with a number of infections such as measles or rubella may present with abdominal pain: rehydration and antipyretic management has a surprisingly beneficial effect on the pain. More specific infections may have a clearer relation to the pain, such as stretching of the liver capsule in cases of infective hepatitis, or L1 or L2 nerve root pain in Herpes zoster infection. Urinary tract infection, particularly when complicated by a right-sided pyelonephritis as a consequence of vesicoureteric reflux, may simulate retrocaecal appendicitis. A particularly difficult diagnosis in the very young patient is the child with meningitis, where irritability to touch may simulate abdominal tenderness. Associated septic ileus may also be a misleading feature, suggestive of the primary pathology residing in the abdomen.

Infective hepatitis is another, though now infrequent, cause of abdominal pain simulating appendicitis. In the preicteric phase nausea is intense and an important symptom. The pain is usually subcostal, and may originate from stretching of the liver capsule as the liver enlarges, but the precise mechanism of pain production is unclear. Bilirubin is present in the urine and the derangement in liver function tests points to the diagnosis.

All these cases demand consideration and appropriate investigations to identify the prime cause of the symptom and avoid unnecessary laparotomy.

Mesenteric adenitis

The combination of abdominal pain, pyrexia and peripheral lymphadenopathy should point to a diagnosis of mesenteric adenitis although this diagnosis is often applied to children where the diagnosis could just as well be NSAP. The diagnosis is more correctly applied to lymphadenopathy as a consequence of infection with *Yersinia enterolitica* (p. 53) although other pathogens, viral as well as bacterial, produce inflammation or suppuration of the mesenteric lymph nodes and presumably the lymphoid tissue of the gut. The associated peritoneal reaction produces signs in many children that are indistinguishable from appendicitis and the diagnosis is more often than not, made at operation.

Enterocolitis

Several enteric bacterial and viral pathogens, including Rotavirus, Astrovirus, Adenovirus, *Salmonella*, *Campylobacter* and *Cryptosporidium*, can cause severe colicky pain and fever prior to the appearance of diarrhoea, which makes for diagnostic uncertainty and often simulates a surgical condition.

The bacterium *E. coli* serotype O157 is, however, a particularly virulent organism, which, through its cytopathic effects on the colon, produces a haemorrhagic colitis. This presentation with pain and bloody stool in a young child less than 5 years of age can mimic an intussusception and inappropriate diagnostic laparotomy is occasionally performed. Friedland *et al.* (1995) report the value of colour Doppler ultrasound in evaluating the characteristically avascular and thickened colonic wall produced by the O157 *E. coli*. However the main concern with this disease process is the legacy of the verotoxin. This toxin can produce acute tubular necrosis and is the commonest cause of acute renal failure in children. The toxin also induces severe haemolysis and thrombocytopenia, i.e. the haemolytic uraemic syndrome.

The organism is usually acquired from uncooked meat or unpasteurized dairy products and the condition has two forms, an endemic and an epidemic type that has been responsible for several outbreaks throughout Scotland in recent years (Abu-Arafeh *et al.*, 1991).

Management of this illness is supportive, with peritoneal dialysis and transfusion of blood products until resolution of renal failure occurs.

Feeding disorders

Infants receiving formula milk may present with irritability, a poorly established feeding pattern, prolonged crying and disordered sleep. The weary mother of such a child often attempts to settle her child by feeding but, by doing so, may overfeed, thus producing gastro-oesophageal reflux, oesophagitis and hence the above symptoms. This situation is compounded if the mother introduces cow's milk prematurely into the child's diet, which should be deferred until after 12 months of age.

Recognition allows correction by establishing the correct volume of feed, nursing the child in a semi-erect position, in a reclining seat, and adding Gaviscon to the feeding regime (1 ml Gaviscon liquid after each bottle).

A caloric content of 0.6 kcal/ml of formula and an energy requirement of 100 kcal/kg body weight is required for adequate growth in the first few months of life; the appropriate feeding regime will therefore comprise 150 ml of formula per kg divided into six four-hourly feeds for the first few weeks and thereafter five 5-hourly feeds.

This management strategy is often so successful by itself as to obviate confirmation by other diagnostic means; however, if the baby shows evidence of failure to thrive, or fails to settle on this regime, contrast study of the upper gastrointestinal tract should be performed.

Henoch–Schönlein purpura (HSP)

Enteritis is one of the four main features of this illness, which typically declares itself with a purpuric rash and consequently is usually admitted to paediatric medical wards. The rash is over the extensor aspects of the limbs and the trunk, accompanied by arthralgia and nephritis. Surgeons should be aware that testicular pain can be a feature in some boys and present as an acute scrotum.

The diagnosis is straightforward when one of the recognized features precedes the abdominal pain associated with the enteritis. On rare occasions, however, the enteritis and pain precede the rash. This is diagnostically challenging because the features of the illness are very similar to other causes of enteritis, notably Crohn's disease or, indeed, in some cases to intussusception.

The surgeon must remember that, although the enteritis is managed conservatively with gut rest and intravenous fluids, intussusception of the small bowel can occur and present with rectal bleeding and small-bowel obstruction. Such cases are not responsive to hydrostatic or pneumostatic reduction and require operative management.

The indication for intervention can be difficult to establish on clinical grounds alone. Connelly and O'Halpin (1994) and Couture and his colleagues in Montpellier in France (1992) emphasized the reliability of high-frequency ultrasound not only in determining intestinal involvement in HSP but also in detecting surgical complications such as ileoileal intussusception and perforation.

Prior to the development of sophisticated ultrasound examination, resort to laparotomy was often the only reliable method of excluding intussusception in a child with vomiting and abdominal pain in association with HSP. Martinez-Frontilla *et al.* (1988) report 54 children from the children's hospital in Denver, 13 of whom had signs of peritoneal irritation. In seven laparotomy was carried out (only one child had a rash at that time) and four had subserosal haemorrhage. Three of the children required resection of bowel, two for gangrenous intussusception and one for perforation of the terminal ileum. Such is the difficulty in distinguishing between enteritis with subserosal oedema and haemorrhage, and intussusception, that laparotomy can be the only recommendation when doubt persists.

This condition can, on occasion, recur, and when that happens treatment with corticosteroids may be indicated.

Abdominal migraine

In families with a strong history of migraine it is not unusual for abdominal pain to coexist with the headache (Abu-Arafeh and Russell, 1995). Precipitating factors include trigger foods such as caffeine (in effervescent drinks like cola), cheese and chocolate. Children with these symptoms may periodically suffer an acute exacerbation and be admitted to hospital. There are no physical signs but a careful family history and dietary history allows confident diagnosis. Management is by dietary exclusion of the trigger foods and, if necessary, administration of pizotifen.

Helicobacter gastritis

Extensive studies have been made to evaluate the contribution of this organism to the cause of abdominal pain in children where no identifiable cause has been demonstrated, but as yet no consistent role for this organism has been found.

REFERENCES

Abu-Arafeh, I., Smail, P., Youngson, G. G. *et al.* (1991) Haemolytic uraemic syndrome in the defined population of North-East Scotland. *Eur. J. Paediatr.*, **150**, 279–281.

Abu-Arafeh, I. and Russell, G. (1995) Prevalence and clinical features of abdominal migraine compared with those of migraine headache. *Arch. Dis. Child.*, **72**, 413–417.

Connolly, B. and O'Halpin, D. (1994) Sonographic evaluation of the abdomen in Henoch–Schoenlein purpura. *Clin. Radiol.*, **49**, 320–323.

Couture, A., Veyrac, C., Baud, C. *et al.* (1992) Evaluation of abdominal pain in Henoch–Schoenlein syndrome by high frequency ultrasound. *Pediatr. Radiol.*, **22**, 12–17.

Friedland, J. A., Herman, T. E. and Siegel, M. J. (1995) *Escherichia coli* O157: H7-associated hemolytic–uremic syndrome: value of colonic color Doppler sonography. *Pediatr. Radiol.*, **25**(Suppl. 1), S65–S67.

Martinez-Frontanilla, L. A., Silverman, L. and Meagher, D. P. Jr (1988) Intussusception in Henoch–Schoenlein purpura: diagnosis with ultrasound. *J. Pediatr. Surg.*, **23**, 375–376.

Ravichandran, D. and Burge, D. M. (1996) Pneumonia presenting as acute abdominal pain in children. *Br. J. Surg.*, **83**, 1706–1708.

Valerio, D. (1976) Acute diabetic abdomen in childhood. *Lancet*, **i**, 66–68.

3.4 GASTROINTESTINAL HAEMORRHAGE

Haemorrhage from the gastrointestinal tract in children is comparatively rare in comparison to adult medicine but when it does occur it is more likely to be slow rather than acute sudden blood loss. Bleeding from oesophageal varices and Meckel's diverticulum are exceptions to that generalization.

3.4.1 UPPER ALIMENTARY TRACT BLEEDING

3.4.1.1 Oesophagitis

Oesophagitis consequent on primary gastro-oesophageal reflux is a common problem in the first year of life and usually settles with treatment of the reflux. It seldom produces vomiting of pure blood, presenting more commonly as vomit streaked with fresh blood or as vomit containing 'coffee-grounds'. Stress ulceration occurs most often in children in intensive care, with burns and severe head injury being the major associated causes. Ranitidine, an H_2-receptor antagonist, is effective in reducing blood loss by reducing acid secretion and is often used pre-emptively. The endocrine side-effects of cimetidine led Kelly (1994) in the Liver Unit in the Children's Hospital in Birmingham to recommend ranitidine for treatment of children with severe oesophagitis, peptic ulceration and for prophylaxis of stress ulceration.

3.4.1.2 Oesophageal varices

The childhood causes of oesophageal varices differ from those in adults in that liver function can be remarkably well preserved, particularly in the large majority who have portal vein occlusion. Cystic fibrosis, portal vein obliteration, and cirrhosis complicating biliary atresia are other causes of portal hypertension and oesophageal varices in children (Stringer *et al.*, 1994). In biliary atresia, however, the concomitant liver disease may dictate the need for liver transplantation, particularly when portal hypertension and liver cirrhosis coexist.

Variceal haemorrhage is treated according to standard practice, with balloon tamponade using paediatric Sengstaken–Blakemore tubes (with the oesophageal balloon inflated to a pressure of $40 \text{cmH}_2\text{O}$), octeotride infusion to reduce portal blood flow, and subsequent sclerotherapy (p. 369). Endoscopic band ligation (Karrer *et al.*, 1994; Cano *et al.*, 1995) and transjugular intrahepatic portosystemic shunting, TIPPS (LaBerge *et al.*, 1992; 1993), provide new alternatives to the traditional surgical methods of decompressing the portal system by either open portosystemic anastomosis, using mesocaval, distal lienorenal, or portocaval shunts or by the Suguira devascularization of the oesophagus (Suguira and Futagawa, 1984; Belloli *et al.*, 1992; Idezuki *et al.*, 1994).

Treatment with propranolol has been recommended as maintenance therapy in portal hypertension in childhood (Plevris *et al.*, 1994) but has little place in the acute management. Pre-emptive injection sclerotherapy is similarly not recommended and endoscopic treatment should be reserved until haemorrhage has occurred.

Management of children with variceal haemorrhage is challenging. Close cooperation with intensivists and paediatric anaesthetists is essential. Secure venous access and invasive haemodynamic monitoring through multilumen central venous access are prerequisites. Balloon tamponade is not readily tolerated in the conscious child and the sedation required makes ventilatory support the safe option.

Once haemorrhage has been arrested, and stability maintained, these children should be transferred to a regional paediatric liver unit.

3.4.1.3 Peptic ulceration

As in the adult population this is an increasingly rare disease entity. Haemorrhage in childhood is rarely significant and, with current pharmacological treatment with proton pump inhibition, H_2-receptor antagonists and endoscopic injection techniques for arrest of haemorrhage, surgical intervention in childhood is seldom required. Peptic ulcer diathesis is seldom the cause of bleeding ulcers in children but when it does occur there is often a strong family history of onset of duodenal ulceration and the condition is restricted to late childhood/early adolescence (Kumar and Spitz, 1984). Stress ulceration is more likely to be the cause of brisk bleeding and diagnosis depends heavily upon flexible oesophago-gastroduodenoscopy. In the presence of stigmata of recent haemorrhage, adrenaline injection can be made into the ulcer base (p. 355).

3.4.2 LOWER GASTROINTESTINAL TRACT BLEEDING

3.4.2.1 Introduction

Whereas upper gastrointestinal bleeding is rare in childhood, rectal bleeding and other lower gastrointestinal bleeds are relatively more common. Henoch–Schönlein purpura, intussusception and Meckel's diverticulum, as outlined previously, are all causes of lower gastrointestinal bleeding. Other causes include anal fissure, colonic polyps, perianal cellulitis, enterocolitis, rectal prolapse and inflammatory bowel disease.

3.4.2.2   Anal fissure

This is the commonest cause of rectal bleeding in children under 1 year of age and the second most common in those above 1 year, the commonest in this group being juvenile polyps of the rectum (Spencer, 1964). Constipation is a predisposing feature and the combination of painful defaecation and bright red blood on the stool suggests the diagnosis and inspection will confirm the diagnosis. Parting the buttocks and inspecting the anus with the child in the left lateral position is sufficient to allow visualization of the fissure in either the 6 or 12 o'clock position extending from the anal verge to the dentate line. There is often an associated sentinel pile or skin tag to be seen in the adjacent tissues. Digital examination has no place in the diagnosis because it will cause severe pain.

With the use of appropriate doses of laxative and the exercise of patience, most cases will resolve spontaneously. Anal stretch is occasionally required. Lateral sphincterotomy is not indicated for anal fissure in childhood and chemical sphincterotomy with glyceryl trinitrate has yet to be evaluated in a paediatric setting.

3.4.2.3   Perianal cellulitis

Grant *et al.* (1993) in the Royal Hospital for Sick Children in Edinburgh described this condition in 20 children reviewed over an 8-year period. Increased recognition and appreciation of the condition, however, has unmasked a higher incidence than this. Group A *Streptococcus* infection in the perianal tissues causes perianal discomfort and bleeding, and maceration of the perianal skin, with superficial fissuring at many sites.

Bacteriological culture of the mucous discharge evident in the anal canal results in a profuse growth of the pathogen. A protracted course (6 weeks) of either penicillin V or co-amoxiclav is needed to eradicate the infection.

3.4.2.4   Rectal prolapse

Constipation with straining is the commonest cause of rectal prolapse, the typical age affected being 2–3 years. Bleeding occurs when the prolapse has not been promptly reduced and becomes congested. Most cases of prolapse are partial-thickness and can be manually reduced with pressure from the flat of the palm. Reduction is best performed as soon as possible after the prolapse has occurred and certainly before oedema of the prolapse makes such reduction difficult. Recurrence is common until the constipation responds to laxatives; the use of a training seat helps youngsters to reduce the tendency to strain.

All children with rectal prolapse should have a sweat test to rule out cystic fibrosis, which may be asymptomatic and unsuspected. Neurological abnormalities associated with prolapse are usually apparent on physical examination. If the prolapse is recurrent and no other cause is evident then colonoscopy should be performed to exclude rectal polyps.

Although most cases will resolve without treatment, when there is failure to improve injection sclerotherapy can be performed, as reported in a series of 100 cases by Wyllie (1979).

3.4.2.5   Colonic polyps

The association between intestinal polyps and abnormal mucocutaneous pigmentation was first described by Peutz in 1921. In 1941 Jeghers and his associates established the syndrome in 22 cases, ten of which were their own. The disease is inherited in a mendelian dominant gene of high penetrance. These polyps may bleed or produce intussusception but, more commonly, the cause of polypoidal bleeding is from a juvenile polyp, which is a hamartomatous condition of the upper rectum. The polyps are usually solitary but can be multiple and present with fresh blood streaking the outside of the stool. Ulceration of the surface of the polyp produces episodes of bleeding, which can continue until such time as the polyp is removed or autoamputation of the polyp occurs. This latter phenomenon occurs in 10–20% of cases.

Diagnosis can be made on digital examination of the rectum in many cases but the majority are diagnosed on colonoscopy or sigmoidoscopy and coincident removal with snare electrocautery is straightforward. It should be remembered that approximately one-quarter of cases have more than one polyp.

The aetiology of this condition is unknown and, while most hamartomatous conditions are present from birth, the presence on histological examination of fingers of smooth muscle infiltrating the stalk suggests that this lesion may share some of the features of solitary rectal ulcer seen in adults. Juvenile polyps are not malignant and when solitary hold no premalignant risk.

3.4.2.6 Haemorrhagic enterocolitis

As outlined above (p. 116) several enteric infections cause pain and many also produce rectal bleeding. *Campylobacter* and *E. coli* O157 are notable examples. The early phase of infection with *E. coli* is characterized by bloody diarrhoea before the main features of haemolytic uraemic syndrome develop in approximately 5–10% of infected patients.

3.4.2.7 Inflammatory bowel disease

The incidence of childhood inflammatory bowel disease is increasing in many countries in the world. Many of the features of presentation reflect those of the adult condition and are described in Chapters 6 (p. 228) and 7 (p. 319). In addition to the enteric symptoms, failure to thrive with growth arrest is an important feature in childhood and may itself be influential in management decisions.

Ulcerative colitis

If there is protracted bleeding or failure to respond rapidly to medical therapy, then the poor long-term outlook favours early surgical intervention.

As in adult life, children may present with a severe attack, which requires expert medical care and constant joint medical and surgical watch for irreversible complications that require total colectomy or ileostomy: these are outlined in Chapter 7, p. 324. At the emergency operation, the rectum may be brought out as a mucous fistula but, if a rectal stump is preferred, closure should be with polydioxanone and sufficient length should be left to allow ready recognition at the restorative procedure to follow. It is therefore not usually necessary to divide the inferior mesenteric artery.

A generous spout to the ileostomy is advised to avoid the complications of stoma leakage in the active child.

Catch-up growth should be well established before proceeding to restorative proctectomy.

Crohn's disease

This condition is increasingly diagnosed in young children. This is because of either a change in the characteristics of the disease or a new awareness on the part of clinicians, leading to earlier diagnosis.

Extraintestinal manifestations, such as perianal disease, may occur and these in some cases, as in adults, can precede the gut symptoms. Involvement of colon or rectum can result in rectal bleeding, as can the presence of a fissure, although in Crohn's disease this is often painless in comparison to the more common variety unassociated with Crohn's disease.

Similarly, cheilosis, lip oedema and oral ulceration may herald the onset of the disease, with biopsy of the mouth occasionally disclosing granulomata that confirm the diagnosis. Genital oedema can occur in boys and is a difficult management problem.

Severe acute Crohn's colitis is not significantly different to acute ulcerative colitis, and is treated in the same way. If urgent operation becomes necessary, close inspection of the whole small bowel is necessary, but evidence of Crohn's enteritis is not often found in these patients.

If enteritis is extensive there will be great reluctance to operate. Localized disease may present with small-bowel obstruction or as ileocaecal enteritis (Chapter 6, p. 228) and will be treated in the same way as in adults. There will, if possible, be even more emphasis on a conservative attitude to resection, and preference for strictureplasty. The longitudinal enterotomy is closed transversely, as in pyloroplasty, with sutures of 4/0 polydioxanone (Telander, 1995).

REFERENCES

Belloli, G., Campobasso, P. and Musi, L. (1992) Suguira procedure in the surgical treatment of bleeding esophageal varices in children: long-term results. *J. Pediatr. Surg.*, **27**, 1422–1426.

Cano, I., Urruzuno, P. and Medina, E. (1995) Treatment of esophageal varices by endoscopic ligation in children. *Eur. J. Pediatr. Surg.*, **5**, 299–302.

Grant, H. W., Bisset, W. H., Mackinlay, G. A. *et al.* (1993) Perianal cellulitis in children caused by group A streptococcus. *Pediatr. Surg. Int.*, **8**, 410–416.

Idezuki, Y., Kokudo, N. and Sanjo, K. (1994) Sugiura procedure for management of variceal bleeding in Japan. *World J. Surg.*, **18**, 216–221.

Karrer, F. M., Holland, R. M. and Allshouse, M. J. (1994) Portal vein thrombosis: treatment of variceal hemorrhage by endoscopic variceal ligation. *J. Pediatr. Surg.*, **29**, 1149–1151.

Kelly, D. A. (1994) Do H_2 receptor antagonists have a therapeutic role in childhood? *J. Pediatr. Gastroenterol. Nutrit.*, **19**, 270–276.

Kumar, D. and Spitz, L. (1984) Peptic ulceration in children. *Surg. Gynecol. Obstet.*, **159**, 63–66.

LaBerge, J. M., Ring, E. J. and Lake, J. R. (1992) Transjugular intrahepatic portosystemic shunts: preliminary results in 25 patients. *J. Vasc. Surg.*, **16**, 258–267.

LaBerge, J. M., Ring, E. J. and Gordon, R. L. (1993) Creation of transjugular intrahepatic portosystemic shunts with the wallstent endoprosthesis: results in 100 patients. *Radiology*, **187**, 413–420.

Losty, P. D., Lynch, M. J. and Guiney, E. J. (1994) Long term outcome after surgery for extrahepatic portal vein thrombosis. *Arch. Dis. Child.*, **71**, 437–440.

Plevris, J. N., Elliot, R. and Mills, P. R. (1994) Effect of propranolol on prevention of first variceal bleed and survival in patients with chronic liver disease. *Aliment. Pharmacol. Ther.*, **8**, 63–70.

Spencer, R. (1964) Gastrointestinal haemorrhage in infancy and childhood. *Pediatr. Surg.*, **55**, 718–734.

Stringer, M. D., Heaton, N. D., Karani, J. *et al.* (1994) Patterns of portal vein occlusion and their aetiological significance. *Br. J. Surg.*, **81**, 1328–1331.

Suguira, M. and Futagawa, T. (1984) Esophageal transection with para-esophageal devascularization in the treatment of esophageal varices. *World J. Surg.*, **8**, 673–679.

Telander, R. L. (1995) Surgical management of Crohn's disease in children. *Curr. Opin. Pediatr.*, **7**, 328–334.

Wyllie, G. G. (1979) The injection treatment of rectal prolapse. *J. Pediatr. Surg.*, **14**, 62–64.

3.5   INGESTED FOREIGN BODIES

Inhaled and ingested foreign bodies are a cause of significant morbidity and mortality in young children, with 70% of patients being 3 years of age or younger. Of 449 children in the USA whose deaths were attributable to choking on man-made objects, the commonest cause was choking on balloons (29%). Of 165 children in the same study (Rimell *et al.*, 1995), who were treated by endoscopy for ingested foreign bodies, coins proved to be the most common (60 children). Not all coins require removal but those impacted in the proximal or middle oesophagus require prompt removal. Children with distal oesophageal coins may spontaneously clear the coin from the oesophagus and so can be observed for 24 hours before being subjected to endoscopy (Connors *et al.*, 1995). All children suspected of swallowing a coin should, therefore, have an X-ray to confirm location.

A number of techniques are available for clearance of a foreign body from the oesophagus. They often entail flexible or rigid oesophagoscopy (Kelley *et al.*, 1993) but Foley catheter retrieval under fluoroscopy without anaesthesia is successful in about 90% of impacted foreign bodies if the duration of impaction is less than 3 days. This success rate drops to less than 50% if the object (usually a coin) is *in situ* for more than this time period (Schunk *et al.*, 1994).

Disc battery ingestion requires a management policy identifying those children at risk from corrosive injury; removal is indicated if the battery lodges in the oesophagus or if there is more than one battery in the gastrointestinal tract.

Ingestion of a single battery is effectively treated without removal, by H_2-receptor antagonist therapy (to avoid acid digestion of the outer case of the battery) and catharsis using laxative (Lavelle-Jones *et al.*, 1992). The presence of more than one battery requires endoscopic removal using a basket snare.

An extensive review of 2382 cases of ingestion of cylindrical and button batteries (Litovitz and Schmitz, 1992) confirmed the progressive decline in intervention for battery removal for sites other than the oesophagus. Oesophageal retention depends upon size, with cylindrical batteries being predominant but neither battery diameter nor the presence of symptoms reliably predicts oesophageal battery position. No patients in this large series had evidence of mercury poisoning. Attempts at enforced vomiting as a mechanism for battery removal must be discouraged, as this is never successful and may merely convert a gastric position to an oesophageal position.

Most other ingested foreign bodies pass through the gastrointestinal tract uneventfully. Even sharp objects such as drawing pins, tacks and open safety pins can be left to make a safe passage through the gut. Such is the high expectation of spontaneous passage that, following confirmation of the presence of a foreign body in the gastrointestinal tract by X-ray, no further X-ray needs to be taken, but spontaneous passage should be confirmed by stool examination; normal diet is allowed in the interim. Spitz (1971) found that the average time for the passage of rounded objects was 5 days and sharp-ended ones 7 days.

REFERENCES

Connors, G. P., Chamberlain, J. M. and Ochsenschlager, D. W. (1995) Symptoms and spontaneous passage of esophageal coins. *Arch. Pediatr. Adolesc. Med.*, **149**, 36–39.

Kelley, J. E., Leech, M. H. and Carr, M. G. (1993) A safe and cost-effective protocol for the management of esophageal coins in children. *J. Pediatr. Surg.*, **28**, 898–900.

Litovitz, T. and Schmitz, B. F. (1992) Ingestion of cylindrical and button batteries: an analysis of 2382 cases. *Pediatrics*, **89**, 747–757.

Lavelle-Jones, M., Lyall, M. H., McCollum, P. *et al.* (1992) Disc battery ingestion: a review and a management plan. *J. R. Coll. Surg. Edin.*, **37**, 120–122.

Rimell, F. L., Thome, A. Jr and Stool, S. (1995) Characteristics of objects that cause choking in children. *J.A.M.A.*, **274**, 1763–1766.

Schunk, J. E., Harrison, A. M. and Corneli, H. M. (1994) Fluoroscopic Foley catheter removal of esophageal foreign bodies in children: experience with 415 episodes. *Pediatrics*, **94**, 709–714.

Spitz, L. (1971) Management of ingested foreign bodies in childhood. *BMJ*, **iv**, 469–472.

3.6 ABDOMINAL TRAUMA

Trauma is the commonest cause of death in childhood and the teenage years. The care of abdominal trauma in childhood has, since the 1980s, increasingly emphasized the importance of conservative management. This is particularly appropriate in splenic and hepatic injury, for which paediatric surgeons have demonstrated the efficacy of non-operative management.

Blunt abdominal trauma causes the majority of abdominal injuries, with most occurring in road traffic or bicycling accidents. A significant number of injuries occur during recreation and a high level of suspicion is required to detect non-accidental or intentional injury.

The history of the mechanism of the injury is always useful in anticipating the likely injuries. Children secured in the back seat of cars involved in high velocity deceleration accidents, who are restrained by a lap belt, risk lumbar spine and visceral injury (Lane, 1994). Bicycle handlebar injuries are particularly associated with pancreatic and duodenal damage (Schimpl *et al.*, 1992).

Reception of traumatized children and subsequent evaluation with primary and secondary surveys, concurrent resuscitation and stabilization are now standardized and taught in paediatric resuscitation courses. These regimes place priority on airway care, cervical spine immobilization and the establishment of adequate circulating blood volume. The surgeon who takes care of children must be familiar with these protocols, be prepared to continue them and be familiar with all aspects of the child's care and assessment carried out up to the point at which the surgeon takes over.

Intra-abdominal injury may be manifest by the systemic response to hypovolaemia but haematological and biochemical evaluation, particularly the serum amylase, can point to pancreatic, small bowel, mesenteric or solid organ injury. Clinical examination, particularly in the younger child may be difficult and non-contributory, and increasingly radiological imaging together with ongoing transfusion requirements for the maintenance of normovolaemia, direct the management of the case.

Abdominal ultrasound is particularly useful in identifying free fluid or blood in the peritoneal cavity (Akgur *et al.*, 1993). Computed tomography, supplemented with intravenous or luminal contrast, remains the most sensitive imaging technique in the measurement of solid organ injury or intestinal perforation for which there is no immediate clinical indication for laparotomy (Albanese, 1996).

Solid organ injury can be safely managed by conservative non-operative methods, even when injury results in moderate blood loss, and studies from the department of surgery at the Hospital for Sick Children in Toronto have pointed to the effectiveness of such a strategy in splenic injury (Ein *et al.*, 1978) and hepatic injury (Giacomantonio *et al.*, 1984). The guidelines subsequently developed by this team of surgeons (Wesson *et al.*, 1981) suggest that patients can be safely managed by blood transfusion to approximately half blood volume (40 ml/kg body weight) before laparotomy for continued bleeding is necessary. The protocol emphasizes the need for surgery to arrest ongoing haemorrhage rather than as a response to the demonstration of intraperitoneal blood (Haller *et al.*, 1994).

When laparotomy is essential for liver injury, the emphasis is to control haemorrhage by packing, with subsequent debridement of non-viable tissue considered at a later stage (Losty *et al.*, 1997; see Chapter 10). If massive bleeding can be stopped by packing then, if possible, transfer to a more expert team should be sought where these unusual injuries can receive the advantages of multidisciplinary care.

Morse and Garcia (1994) in a review of 120 children with splenic injury in Cincinnati, and Haller *et al.* (1994) from Baltimore, in a review of 2900 children, have validated the safety of the conservative approach to splenic and hepatic injury from blunt abdominal trauma, particularly with regard to the concern that some concomitant injury may be overlooked.

The management of splenic and liver injuries, the effects of splenectomy, blunt injuries to the intestines and seat-belt injuries are considered in detail in Chapter 10. Injuries to the urogenital tract are examined in Chapter 11.

REFERENCES

Akgur, F. M., Tanyel, F. C. and Akhan, O. (1993) The place of ultrasonographic examination in the initial evaluation of children sustaining blunt abdominal trauma. *J. Pediatr. Surg.*, **28**, 78–81.

Albanese, C. T., Meza, M. P. and Gardner, M. J. (1996) Is computed tomography a useful adjunct to the clinical examination for the diagnosis of pediatric gastrointestinal perforation from blunt abdominal trauma in children? *J. Trauma*, **40**, 417–421.

Ein, S. H., Shandling, B. and Simpson, J. S. (1978) Nonoperative management of traumatised spleen in children. *J. Pediatr. Surg.*, **13**, 117–119.

Giacomantonio, M., Filler, R. M. and Rich, R. H. (1984) Blunt hepatic trauma in children: experience with operative and nonoperative management. *J. Pediatr. Surg.*, **19**, 519–522.

Haller, J. A. Jr, Papa, P., Drugas, G. *et al.* (1994) Nonoperative management of solid organ injuries in children. Is it safe? *Ann. Surg.*, **219**, 625–628.

Lane, J. C. (1994) The seat belt syndrome in children. *Accident Anal. Prevent.*, **26**, 813–820.

Morse, M. A. and Garcia, V. F. (1994) Selective nonoperative management of pediatric blunt splenic trauma: risk for missed associated injuries. *J. Pediatr. Surg.*, **29**, 23–27.

Losty, P. D., Okoye, B. O., Walter, D. P., *et al.* (1997) Management of blunt liver injury in children. *Br. J. Surg.*, **84**, 1006–1008.

Schimpl, G., Schmidt, B. and Sauer, H. (1992) Isolated bowel injury in blunt abdominal trauma in childhood. *Eur. J. Pediatr. Surg.*, **2**, 341–344.

Wesson, D. E., Filler, R. M., Ein, S. H. *et al.* (1981) Ruptured spleen – when to operate? *J. Pediatr. Surg.*, **16**, 324–326.

3.7 EXTERNAL HERNIA

3.7.1 INGUINAL HERNIA

While incarceration of an infant hernia is a common event, strangulation and ischaemic necrosis of the contents is a rarity. The incidence of incarceration of inguinal hernias is highest in the first few months of life with newborns being at the greatest risk. Some 69% of episodes occur in the first year of life and the remaining 31% between 1 and 15 years (Rowe and Clatworthy, 1970).

In spite of the frequency of episodes of incarceration, gangrene and perforation of small bowel is extremely uncommon (1.4%) and many series report no cases of intestinal resection. Thus the great majority of cases of incarceration can be managed by manipulative reduction as a preliminary to scheduled repair 48 hours later.

Diagnosis is usually simple, with the reported onset of inguinal or inguinoscrotal swelling in an unsettled infant. Bowel sounds may be high-pitched. The mass is usually smooth and can, on occasion, transilluminate because of associated entrapped fluid. Such a case should be distinguished from a tense hydrocele by clinical examination and, if necessary, an ultrasound examination. If left unattended, the hernia may become firmer, with reddening of the overlying skin, and vomiting will eventually turn faeculent following initial bilious vomits. The testes are usually normal but in some infants the hernia compresses the spermatic cord, causing irrecoverable damage in 3–4% of testes (Puri *et al.*, 1984).

The differential diagnosis includes lymphadenitis of the inguinal nodes, which are usually more laterally placed in the groin, and a tense hydrocele of the cord. There are usually no associated findings in these cases and of particular value is performance of a rectal examination, by which the internal ring can be palpated and comparison made with the opposite side. Raine and Young (1986) also used this technique to ensure complete reduction of small bowel after an episode of incarceration.

Torsion of an undescended testis may simulate an incarcerated hernia but again, on rectal examination, the deep ring should be clear of contents.

Management

The management of an incarcerated inguinal hernia without signs of strangulation is non-operative. Some surgeons elect to sedate the infant with rectal administration of diazepam and elevate the cot end or apply gallows traction to the legs: the infant is observed for 1–2 hours to allow for spontaneous reduction. There is a real risk, however, of apnoea after such sedation and others, myself included, prefer to attempt manipulative reduction of the contents by exerting steady pressure on them by squeezing the sac.

If reduction is achieved, repair is carried out electively 48 hours later, which allows cord oedema to settle in the interim. The infant must not be discharged to await elective repair since recurrent incarceration is likely in the interim.

Operation

When the hernia cannot be reduced, or there is reddening of the skin over a large hernia with signs of small-bowel obstruction – suggestive of strangulation – then speedy resuscitation and operation are needed. It must be recognized that this is not an easy operation, the more so because it is particularly likely to occur in babies under 3 months of age (Smith, 1954), and should only be undertaken by a surgeon experienced in elective inguinal herniotomy in infancy. Concurrent illness may have resulted in increased straining and it is equally important that these infants are in the care of an anaesthetist with paediatric experience.

The difficulties inherent in this operation are much increased if the oedematous, friable, delicate hernial sac is approached through the groin. The abdominal preperitoneal approach (Jones and Towns, 1983) is safer and easier to perform, and should be preferred unless, under the relaxation induced by the anaesthetic, the hernia reduces before the operation has begun – then the groin approach can be used.

The incision is the Fowler–Weir incision often used for appendicectomy. It runs medially from a point just internal to the anterior superior iliac spine, and stops short of the midline, over rectus sheath. External oblique is split to reveal the lateral edge of the rectus sheath, which is incised. This opening is enlarged by splitting the anterior rectus sheath medially and the internal oblique and transversus laterally, working first with scissors and then using the index fingers to widen the gap in the muscles, as in a gridiron incision. The transversalis fascia is then opened and this reveals the surface of the peritoneum. If the lower half of the incision is now retracted the distended neck of the inguinal hernial sac will be seen entering the deep inguinal ring (Figure 3.12). If it is suspected that bowel is caught in the hernia it is

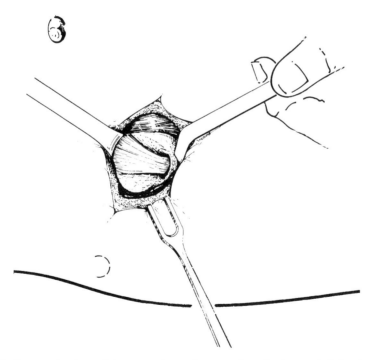

Figure 3.12 Surgeon's view of the preperitoneal approach to the internal abdominal ring. The anterior superior iliac spine and umbilicus are indicated. The muscle-splitting incision is held open, with the lateral edge of the rectus abdominis retracted medially. The neck of the oblique hernial sac is entering the internal ring. It can readily be opened proximal to the ring, and this allows strangulated bowel to be secured before withdrawal from the inguinal canal.

a good move to open the peritoneum at the neck of the sac and place a Babcock forceps on the bowel so that it is not lost when reduced.

At this stage the contents of the hernial sac often reduce, but when there is strangulation the contents have to be released, and to do this it is helpful to dissect under the skin of the lower side of the incision, superficial to external oblique, and to expose and incise the external abdominal ring. This may release the bowel. If not, the inguinal canal can be dilated by passing a blunt curved artery forceps gently through the peritoneal incision, alongside the bowel, down the canal: then the jaws are opened to dilate the canal and allow withdrawal of the bowel, through the peritoneal incision, for inspection and assessment of viability (p. 199).

It is uncommon for the bowel to be non-viable. Smith (1954) made a full review of the subject and concluded that about 4% of irreducible hernias contained a gangrenous bowel requiring resection. In the event of this being needed it is easy to perform resection because this incision gives direct access to the peritoneal cavity.

It then remains to separate the neck of the hernial sac from the spermatic vessels and vas. If the sac is gently elevated on curved artery forceps it is relatively easy to identify the vessels (coming from behind) and the vas (as it rises from the pelvis to lie on the postero-medial aspect of the hernial sac). Once these two structures have been identified and drawn to one side (Figure 3.13), an artery forceps is placed across the hernial sac and the sac is divided below it: the forceps is lifted up, rotated once and the neck of the sac is ligated with thread.

The remainder of the sac is best left alone. If the peritoneum has had to be opened this incision should be closed with a running suture of 4/0 PDS. This peritoneum, though thin, is quite strong, in contrast to the friable oedematous sac that is encountered in the usual approach through the inguinal canal. The split muscles are sutured and these wounds heal strongly.

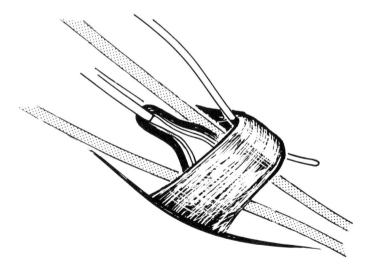

Figure 3.13 The empty hernial sac has been drawn up into the wound and supported on artery forceps. The testicular vessels and the vas have been separated from the sac, and the neck of the sac is ready for division and ligation.

About 65% of irreducible hernias occur on the right so if the muscle-splitting incision is used parents should be warned that the appendix has not been removed, because the scar could cause confusion if suspicion of acute appendicitis arises later in life.

This approach also confers considerable benefit in access for orchidopexy in cases of impalpable testis (Youngson and Jones, 1991). Familiarity with this muscle-splitting approach can be obtained during orchidopexy, thus providing confidence for the demanding task of repairing the incarcerated infant hernia.

If the testis is exposed at any time, more commonly during the groin approach, the discoloration that is invariably present in the testis should not tempt the surgeon into orchidectomy because restoration of normal testicular function and size is usual; after any hernia operation the surgeon must, however, ensure a scrotal position of the testis at the end of the procedure, and where a satisfactory position cannot be obtained, then concomitant orchidopexy should be carried out.

Special considerations

There is an increasing incidence of survival following premature birth. Approximately 15% of infants with a birth weight of less than 2000 g have an inguinal hernia. Walsh (1962) found seven of 28 infants under 1500 g (28%) to have hernias and the incidence approaches 60% as the birth weight decreases to 500 g (Nakayuma and Rowe, 1989). Surgery for inguinal hernia repair in such infants carries so significant a risk of postoperative apnoea that some high-risk babies are operated upon under spinal anaesthesia (Webster *et al.*, 1991). It is now standard practice to repair inguinal hernias in these babies before they are discharged home from neonatal special care units since the need for repair outweighs the operative risk.

Steward (1982) reviewed 71 infants undergoing herniotomy and found that 13 of the 33 premature babies had intraoperative or postoperative respiratory complications, with six requiring bag/mask ventilation for apnoea. Among the 38 full-term babies, only one developed respiratory complications.

The reason for this particular predisposition to respiratory problems is not clear but possibly involves fatigue of the diaphragm and intercostal muscles and the response of the ventilatory control mechanism to anaesthesia. It is clear, however, that such babies should receive monitoring of their respiratory function, with surveillance for episodes of apnoea. It is current practice in our unit to maintain measurement of oxygen saturation for a 24-hour period for babies of birth weight of less than 2.5 kg, up to 46 weeks gestational age. The exact duration of this risk is unclear but in very low birth-weight babies, monitoring is instituted for a 24-hour period until they exceed 60 weeks post-conceptual age.

3.7.2 FEMORAL HERNIA

Femoral hernia is comparatively rare in childhood, accounting for fewer than 1% of all paediatric groin hernias. Tam and Lister (1984) recorded an incidence of 0.2%, with others quoting an incidence ranging from 0.4–1.1%. The peak incidence in childhood is in the 5–10 age group (Radcliffe and Stringer, 1997). Contrary to the situation in incarcerated inguinal hernia, there is no place for attempts at manipulative reduction of an incarcerated femoral hernia and the preperitoneal approach outlined above provides excellent exposure of the femoral canal, allowing incision, if need be, of the lacunar ligament to achieve reduction of the content of the sac without risk to an aberrant obturator artery. Moreover, if intestinal resection is required, it is an uncomplicated procedure through this high approach.

Radcliffe and Stringer documented ten cases from Leeds over an 11-year period and describe the diagnostic difficulties. The hernia can be misdiagnosed as an inguinal hernia and indeed the authors suggest that if, during exploration for an inguinal hernia, no sac can be identified, then the surgeon should explore the femoral ring. The elements of femoral hernia repair include reduction of contents, excision of the sac and repair of the femoral canal using a non-absorbable suture.

Apart from misdiagnosis as inguinal hernias, femoral hernia can also be mistaken for suppurative lymphadenitis or encysted hydrocele.

3.7.3   OTHER HERNIAS

Strangulation of an umbilical hernia is extremely uncommon in childhood, and the expectation is for this hernia to disappear spontaneously with growth. Surgery, if performed at all, should be on the basis of cosmetic considerations and thus should be deferred until school age. Similarly, epigastric hernia although not uncommonly symptomatic, never produces complications such as incarceration and hence it only requires elective repair of the tiny midline defect, along with protruding preperitoneal fat.

REFERENCES

Jones, P. F. and Towns, G. M. (1983) An abdominal extraperitoneal approach for the incarcerated inguinal hernia of infancy. *Br. J. Surg.*, **70**, 719–720.
Nakayuma, D. K. and Rowe, M. I. (1989) Inguinal hernia and the acute scrotum in infants and children. *Pediatr. Rev.*, 1187–1193.
Puri, P., Guiney, E. J. and O'Donnell, B. (1984) Inguinal hernia in infants. The fate of the testis following incarceration. *J. Pediatr. Surg.*,**19**, 44–46.
Radcliffe, G. and Stringer, M. D. (1997) Reappraisal of femoral hernia in children. *Br. J. Surg.*, **84**, 58–60.
Raine, P. A. M. and Young, D. (1986) Incarcerated inguinal hernia in infants. *BMJ*,**293**, 296.
Rowe, M. I. and Clatworthy, H. W. (1970) Incarcerated and strangulated hernia in children. *Arch. Surg.*, **101**, 136–139.
Smith, I. (1954) Irreducible inguinal hernia in children. *Br. J. Surg.*, **42**, 271–274.
Steward, D. J. (1982) Preterm infants are more prone to complications following minor surgery than are term infants. *Anesthesiology*, **56**, 304–306.
Tam, P. K. H. and Lister, J. (1984) Femoral hernia in Children. *Arch. Surg.*, **119**, 1161–1164.
Walsh, S. (1962) The incidence of external hernias in premature infants. *Acta Paediatr.*, **51**, 161.
Webster, A. C., McKishnie, I. *et al.* (1991) Spinal anaesthesia for inguinal hernia in high risk neonates. *Can. J. Anaesth.*, **38**, 281–286.
Youngson, G. G. and Jones, P. F. (1991) Management of impalpable testis. Long term results from the preperitoneal approach. *J. Pediatr. Surg.*, **26**, 618–620.

3.8   TESTICULAR TORSION

There are two variants of this condition, one occurring in the neonatal period and the other occurring throughout childhood with a peak incidence around puberty. This latter type of torsion occurs because of a bilateral congenital abnormality of the tunica vaginalis (Figure 3.14).

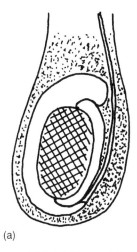
(a)

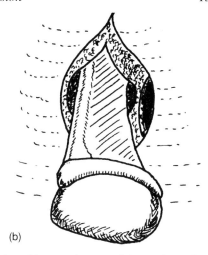
(b)

Figure 3.14 (a) Normal fixation of the testis is produced by attachment of the tunica at head and tail of the epididymis. (b) In the 'clapper-bell' anomaly the tunica surrounds the testis so that the testis is suspended by the vascular pedicle.

3.8.1 NEONATAL TORSION

This variety of torsion occurs when the testis is recently descended and still mobile, and the torsion is in the cord, above the tunica. It may take place *in utero*, in which case there is absorption of the testis (testicular regression syndrome). Neonatal torsion accounts for approximately 10% of cases of torsion. Either testis may be involved. Bilateral torsion may occur either in asynchronous or metachronous fashion.

The clinical presentation is one of a hard, swollen testis in a term baby. The infant is invariably asymptomatic in spite of the noticeably blue appearance of the swollen scrotum. The features are usually present from birth but are not always noticed until the second or third day of life.

Controversy exists over the merits of exploration, with advocates indicating the possibility of subsequent metachronous torsion (Stone *et al.*, 1995). However, because success in testicular salvage is so rare, many surgeons urge a conservative approach and believe that the other side does not need fixation.

3.8.2 TESTICULAR TORSION

The testis hangs free within the tunica vaginalis, suspended on the cord and free to rotate. Torsion seems to occur quite spontaneously and the abrupt onset of pain even occurs during sleep. The pain is usually intense although it may, on occasion, be only a dull ache and radiate into the groin and lower abdomen. It is associated with reflex vomiting and abdominal pain may well be the admitting diagnosis; hence the importance of genital examination in all children with abdominal pain (Cass *et al.*, 1980).

The diagnosis is made on the history and a relatively high and horizontal lie of the opposite testis. The pain is often so severe that compliance with the examination is limited.

The sequelae of torsion are initially venous congestion with lymphatic obstruction resulting in hardness and oedema, with ultimate obstruction to arterial inflow. The rate of this process is dependent upon the number of twists on the cord, with two or three complete turns (720°) resulting in infarction in under 6 hours, whereas a single 360° turn may be tolerated for up to 12 hours (Sonde and Lapides, 1961). Speed is therefore a priority in management, although Williamson (1976) found that fewer than 50% of patients are treated within 10 hours and only 30% within 6 hours.

Detorsion may occur spontaneously and historically attempts have been made to untwist the testis (Nash, 1893), but now exploration of the testis with intraoperative detorsion is recommended rather than attempting to manipulate the scrotum of an awake child.

The implications of torsion as regards subsequent fertility are varied. Puri *et al.* (1985) found that, of 18 patients who suffered testicular torsion prior to the age of 12 years and had an apparently non-viable testis returned to the scrotum, the testis was subsequently impalpable in 12 and very small in 4; yet of five of these patients who had married, all had one or more children and of the unmarried men, all bar one had a normal sperm count. This contradicts the concerns of Krarup (1978) and Thomas and Williamson (1983), who suggested that testicular injury from torsion produced autoimmunization with subsequent contralateral sympathetic orchitis.

Differential diagnosis

While fever and vomiting frequently coexist with torsion they also occur in epididymitis, which is a condition usually found in association with urinary tract infection in infants and should prompt the thorough investigation of the urinary tract. Epididymitis is seen only occasionally with 12 cases documented in 1500 male emergency admissions to the Royal Aberdeen Children's Hospital in recent years, while 30 cases of testicular torsion were treated.

The only safe rule is to assume that an acutely painful swollen testicle in a boy or adolescent is due to torsion.

Torsion of the appendix testis can simulate testicular torsion. The pain is often present for several days duration prior to admission to hospital, in contradistinction to torsion of the testis, where the severity of pain results in prompt hospitalization. The age group is also younger in torsion of the appendix testis, with the peak age group being around 4 years.

The appendix of the testis described by Morgagni in 1761 (also known as the hydatid) is a remnant of the upper end of the müllerian duct. Because it is pedunculated, it is subject to torsion. Colt (1922), an assistant to Professor Marnoch in Aberdeen, first described torsion of the appendix testis in 1922 in a 14-year-old boy with a painful hemiscrotum of 6 days duration. He removed the torted appendix testis.

The presence of a visible blue dot on the upper pole of the testis can be seen on transillumination in many cases, and confirms the diagnosis. The degree of swelling and erythema that this lesion produces is surprisingly significant and when diagnostic doubt exists exploration is the only policy. Otherwise the condition can be managed conservatively with a few days bed rest and appropriate levels of analgesia and will settle in a few days.

Ultrasound examination is of value as a diagnostic tool, with the infarcted appendix being readily identifiable in many examinations. The degree of swelling in the epididymis and the surrounding reactive fluid may on occasion point towards an ultrasound diagnosis of epididymo-orchitis. A total of 30 cases of torsion of the hydatid of Morgagni have been seen in the previously identified cohort of 1500 boys referred to above.

Surgeons should also recognize that testicular pain can be the first presenting feature of Henoch–Schönlein purpura and predate the rash.

Treatment

Testicular torsion should be treated by urgent scrotal exploration through a midline scrotal incision, entering the subdartos space on each side of the raphe. The tunica vaginalis is opened first on the rotated side and the testis is untwisted. It should be removed if frankly necrotic, but the operator should recognize that severe venous congestion will also give rise to significant blue discoloration. Three-point fixation is carried out with a non-absorbable suture; 4/0 Prolene is a suitable suture. This is also done on the contralateral side, which is also subject to torsion on account of the bilateral nature of the tunical morphology. All reported cases of recurrent torsion after fixation have involved the use of absorbable sutures (Thurston and Whitaker, 1983). An alternative operative strategy is to create a subdartos pouch as in performing an orchidopexy for undescended testis (Shanbogue and Miller, 1987).

When dealing with torsion of an undescended testis, the usual operative approach through the inguinal canal should be used, although the surgeon will invariably find that the testis is irrevocably damaged by the torsion.

3.8.3 IDIOPATHIC SCROTAL OEDEMA

Idiopathic scrotal oedema presents with thickening and reddening of the scrotal skin, the underlying testis being palpably normal. Moreover the appearance is distinctly worse than the mild discomfort which is all that boys experience. Scrotal exploration has no place in the management of this condition, which can be differentiated from testicular torsion by noting the posterior extension of the erythema and induration into the perianal region. Indeed, the red oedema may also spread to groin and down thigh.

The precise aetiology remains unclear but one proposal is that the condition derives from an allergic response to the presence of threadworms and is often provoked by the death of the threadworms following treatment, the erythema then advancing from the perirectal tissues anteriorly outwith the deep fascia (Nicholas, 1970). Seven cases have been seen in Aberdeen in the cohort of boys referred to above.

REFERENCES

Cass, A. S., Cass, B. P. and Veeraraghavan, K. (1980) Immediate exploration of the unilateral acute scrotum in young male subjects. *J. Urol.*, **24**, 829–832.

Colt, G. H. (1922) Torsion of the hydatid of Morgagni. *Br. J. Surg.*, **9**, 64–65.

Krarup, T. (1978) The testis after torsion. *Br. J. Urol.*, **50**, 43–46.

Nash, W. G. (1893) Acute torsion of the spermatic cord; reduction; immediate relief. *BMJ*, **i**, 42–43.

Nicholas, J. L. (1970) Idiopathic edema of scrotum in young boys. *J. Urol.*, **67**, 847–850.

Puri, P., Barton, D. and O'Donnell, B. (1985) Prepubertal testicular torsion; subsequent torsion. *J. Pediatr. Surg.*, **20**, 598–601.

Shanbogue, L. K. and Miller, S. S. (1987) Subcutaneous dartos pouch fixation for testicular torsion. *Br. J. Surg.*, **74**, 510.

Sonde, L. P. and Lapides, J. (1961) Experimental torsion of the spermatic cord. *Surg. Forum*, **12**, 502–504.

Stone, K. T., Kass, E. J. and Cacciarelli, A. A. (1995) Management of suspected antenatal torsion: what is the best strategy? *J. Urol.*, **153**, 782–784.

Thomas, W. E. G. and Williamson, R. C. N. (1983) Diagnosis and outcome of testicular torsion. *Br. J. Surg.*, **70**, 213–216.

Thurston, A. and Whitaker, R. (1983) Torsion of the testis after previous testicular surgery. *Br. J. Surg.*, **70**, 217.

Williamson, R. C. N. (1976) Torsion of the testis and allied conditions. *Br. J. Surg.*, **63**, 465–476.

3.9 OVARIAN EMERGENCIES

3.9.1 OVARIAN TUMOURS

Ovarian cysts and tumours are infrequently seen during childhood. Of 1000 female emergency admissions to the Children's Hospital in Aberdeen, only 19 symptomatic cases of ovarian pathology have been identified, of which only four were due to malignant tumour. These rare tumours are observed throughout infancy and childhood; Groeber (1963) documented an increase in incidence with age, 17% occurring between birth and age 4 years, 28% in the 5–9-year age group and 55% during adolescence.

A significant proportion of ovarian masses are not neoplastic. Huffman (1981) reports that, in a collected series of 2567 patients under 16 years, 23% were non-neoplastic (follicular and corpus luteal cysts); but 32% of the neoplasms found in this review of world literature were malignant. The presentation of most cases of ovarian pathology is with abdominal pain and, because of the abdominal position of the ovary in childhood, a neoplastic condition will tend to present as an abdominal mass. On suspicion of ovarian pathology, investigation should be by pelvic ultrasound, with measurement of human chorionic gonadotrophin (beta-hCG) and alpha-fetoprotein, with subsequent magnetic resonance scanning. Urgent collaboration with a paediatric oncologist should take place. Laparotomy may be required urgently if haemorrhage or signs of peritonitis are present; otherwise laparotomy should be planned in consultation with the oncologist, according to the appropriate protocol of the national children's cancer authority. In the UK this is the United Kingdom Children's Cancer Study Group (UKCCSG).

3.9.2 MID-CYCLE AND PELVIC PAIN

Mid-cycle pain and premenstrual pain may cause some concern when they first start in adolescence, until the nature of the pain is appreciated. Such symptoms are self-limiting and should be treated with simple analgesia. The incidence of physiological ovarian cysts is probably greater than is generally appreciated. Cohen *et al.* (1992) report an incidence of 68% in 101 healthy prepubertal girls and this ultrasonic finding should not be accepted as necessarily the cause of pelvic pain if the cysts are small (< 9 mm). The abrupt onset of severe pelvic pain should prompt a provisional diagnosis of torted ovarian cyst. In this circumstance, ultrasound diagnosis is particularly reliable (Stark and Seigel, 1994). If at operation the ovary appears still viable and there are no clear signs of malignancy, a conservative operative approach with detorsion and subsequent cystectomy has been recommended as good practice (Zweizig *et al.*, 1993).

REFERENCES

Cohen, H. L., Eisenberg, P. and Mandel, F. (1992) Ovarian cysts are common in premenarchal girls: a sonographic study of 101 children 2–12 years old. *A.J.R.*, **161**, 89–91.

Groeber, W. R. (1963) Ovarian tumors during infancy and childhood. *Am. J. Obstet. Gynecol.*, **86**, 1027–1035.

Huffman, J. W. (1981) Ovarian tumors in children and adolescents, in *The Gynecology of Childhood and Adolescence*, 2nd edn, (eds Huffman *et al.*), W. B. Saunders, Philadelphia, pp. 257–317.

Stark, J. E. and Siegel, M. J. (1994) Ovarian torsion in prepubertal and pubertal girls: sonographic findings. *A.J.R.*, **163**, 1479–1482.

Zweizig, S., Perron, J., Grubb, D. *et al.* (1993) Conservative management of adnexal torsion. *Am. J. Obstet. Gynecol.*, **168**, 1791–1795.

4

Peritonitis

4.1 INTRODUCTION

When King Edward VII suffered from perforated appendicitis in 1902, the hospital mortality for appendicitis with peritonitis was 75%. Nowadays, the overall mortality of the commonest cause of diffuse peritonitis, acute appendicitis, is very low (p. 36) and it may seem that the threat of general peritonitis is slight. However, mortality among patients whose appendicitis is complicated by peritonitis is still five to ten times higher than among those operated on before perforation, and a report from Montreal on 176 patients with general peritonitis (Bohnen *et al.*, 1983) showed that, although no one died from acute appendicitis, among 48 patients with peritonitis due to perforation of small or large bowel, 50% died: when peritonitis developed as a complication of gastrointestinal surgery the mortality was 60%. A more contemporary report from Vienna (Koperna and Schulz, 1996) on outcome on 92 patients, almost half of whom had postoperative peritonitis, revealed an overall mortality of 18.5%. There was a clear relationship with the APACHE II score: patients scoring less than 15 had a mortality of 4.8% whereas those scoring 15 or above had a mortality of 46.7%.

Such disturbing results occur in spite of modern surgery and intensive care. It is particularly important to achieve earlier diagnosis, especially in the fist few days after operation, to anticipate situations in which the natural defences of the peritoneal cavity will be overwhelmed. This avoids inducing the exaggerated immunological cascade of events that results in the self-perpetuating intraperitoneal inflammatory response which leads to multiorgan failure and death.

Peritoneal defences are very considerable and are both mechanical and chemically (cytokine) mediated. Small amounts of infected fluid, debris and bacteria can be rapidly cleared from the peritoneum. Contaminating material is swept up to the subdiaphragmatic space along the paracolic gutters to large lacunae opening into specialized lymphatic channels in the diaphragm. In the past familiar complications of acute appendicitis were subphrenic and pelvic abscesses and Autio (1964) showed that, if 10 ml of radio-opaque material is placed beside the caecum at the time of appendicectomy and radiographs are taken subsequently, the contrast travels upwards along the paracolic gutter to lie above the liver, and also trickles downwards into the pelvis. If the volume exceeds the defensive capacity infection tends to localize as a residual abscess in the familiar locations.

Emergency Abdominal Surgery. Edited by Peter F. Jones, Zygmunt H. Krukowski and George G. Youngson. Published in 1998 by Chapman & Hall, London. ISBN 0 412 81950 3.

When inflammation develops gradually the peritoneum has effective methods of localization. The inflammation quickly inhibits the fibrinolytic activity of peritoneal exudate, enabling adjacent omentum and loops of bowel to adhere and surround the inflamed organ. Should the affected organ then perforate, the pus is localized, forming an appendicular or other form of intraperitoneal abscess. These defence mechanisms are less effective at extremes of age and older patients, in particular, tend to present with more advanced and diffuse peritoneal sepsis (Watters *et al.*, 1996). Thus an intraperitoneal abscess may be considered a relatively successful response of the peritoneal defence system, in contrast to a diffuse peritonitis, which is consequently associated with a higher mortality.

Generalized peritonitis occurs when the capacity of the peritoneum to localize infection is overwhelmed and is conventionally classed as primary or secondary. Recent developments suggest that a group of patients develop 'tertiary' peritonitis.

Primary peritonitis arises because of haematogenous spread to the peritoneal cavity in the absence of perforation of a hollow viscus. This may complicate ascites in, for example, cirrhosis or nephrotic syndrome and can be a problem associated with CAPD.

Secondary peritonitis is the result of contamination of the peritoneum by perforation of a hollow viscus. Intraperitoneal leakage of bile, urine or blood, which in themselves are relatively non-irritant, could possibly be infected by haematogenous spread but the disruption of a viscus responsible for the initial leak would class these as secondary. The bacteriology of the normal GI tract, the changes in microflora induced by the underlying disease process and the influence of therapy, particularly antibiotics, dictate the nature of the infecting organisms.

Tertiary peritonitis occurs in some patients as a result of modification of the normal response to peritonitis by aggressive therapy. Although virulent organisms have been eliminated this results in the overproduction of peritoneal cytokines, which initiate an ongoing inflammatory response in the absence of virulent microorganisms (Wittman *et al.*, 1996). Such a state is highly lethal and contemporary management should be alert to the danger of inducing this state by inappropriate therapy. Aborting this cycle is difficult and the key to emergency surgery is a short but effective plan of action such that a prolonged stay in ITU with the increased risk of tertiary disease is avoided.

Bacteriology

Pathogenic organisms reach the peritoneal cavity by one of four routes: perforation of the gastrointestinal or biliary tract; through the female genital tract; by penetration of the abdominal parietes; or by haematogenous spread; and knowledge of the source permits informed prediction of the likely organisms. The description of bacteria as 'aerobes' and 'anaerobes' remains in common currency, although these should now be more correctly termed 'facultative' and 'obligate anaerobes' respectively.

Primary or 'spontaneous' peritonitis is now uncommon except in patients with nephrosis or ascites secondary to hepatic disease. Streptococci, pneumococci and, less often, *Haemophilus* spp. are the common pathogens.

Although the gastrointestinal tract is the source of organisms in most cases of secondary peritonitis, there are important differences between the bacteriology of established peritonitis and that of the intact gut lumen. The complex equilibrium in the intact gut is lost when intestinal contents escape into the peritoneum and only a few of the many hundreds of species of bacteria, familiar as the common pathogens, proliferate. Most bacterial species disappear spontaneously within a short time of inoculation unless the common pathogens are eliminated by antibiotics to present an opportunity for proliferation of the rarer and low-virulence organisms. The normal distribution of bacteria in the fasting gut is altered by pathological processes that may be associated with peritonitis, including high gastric pH, small-bowel obstruction and vascular insufficiency. The Gram-negative aerobic, coliform organisms, particularly *Escherichia coli* and, to a lesser extent, *Pseudomonas* and *Proteus* species, and the anaerobic *Bacteroides* species, particularly *B. fragilis*, account for the vast majority of secondary bacterial peritonitis.

There is a wealth of fascinating information on the development and progression of peritonitis available from experimental work in animals which relates well to the pattern of disease in humans (Bartlett *et al.*, 1978). Most secondary intra-abdominal infections are polymicrobial and it is difficult to induce peritonitis experimentally by injecting a single species. The synergism between the common aerobic and anaerobic bacteria is well illustrated by the manner in which the aerobes, particularly *E. coli*, reduce oxygen tension and facilitate growth of obligate anaerobes. The number of organisms required to establish peritonitis is reduced by various naturally occurring adjuvant substances and by foreign materials. When sterile, blood, bile and urine can accumulate to a dramatic degree yet evoke a negligible inflammatory response, whereas intense chemical peritonitis is induced by gastric or duodenal perforation or the enzymatic digestion of activated pancreatic juice. The addition of even a single species of pathogenic organism to any of these fluids transforms the situation from one of simple fluid loss to that of potentially lethal bacterial peritonitis. Sterile particulate foreign material alone does not induce peritonitis and experimental injection of sterilized faeces results only in small sterile abscesses. Inoculation of fresh faeces, however, is the most reliable method of inducing fatal peritonitis in experimental animals and reflects a similar relationship in man.

There is a biphasic pattern in the bacteriology of peritonitis with the aerobic, coliform organisms predominating in the initial phase following initial inoculation. This is characterized by a stage of diffuse peritonitis, bacteraemia and high mortality. The second phase developing over a few days is characterized by formation of abscesses, predominance of anaerobes and lower mortality (Bartlett *et al.*, 1978). Giving antibiotics against the aerobes reduces mortality but has no effect on abscess formation; anti-anaerobic agents alone have no impact on mortality or bacteraemia but surviving animals have few abscesses; and finally, combining antibacterial activity against both aerobes and anaerobes reduces both mortality and abscess formation.

In man, although every peritoneal collection of fluid secondary to perforation of the gut eventually becomes infected, the mix and concentration of organisms during the first 24–48 hours is related to the source of the perforation (Lorber and Swenson, 1975). Most duodenal perforations (75%) show no growth in the peritoneal fluid, compared with 50% of gastric perforations, in which hypochlorhydria is often present. Small-bowel perforations, however, are often secondary to obstruction, which predisposes to proliferation of intraluminal organisms and, as a result, the concentration of organisms recovered is increased and the spectrum of bacteria approximates that of the colon. Perforated appendicitis or colonic disease are the commonest causes of diffuse peritonitis but the variety and concentration of bacteria in the peritoneum is remarkably small. It is unusual for the peritoneal fluid to grow more than six species even though the initial inoculum must have contained hundreds of organisms.

Ascending genital tract infection in the female may lead to pelvic peritonitis and, occasionally, gonococcal infection causes generalized peritonitis (Curtis–Fitz-Hugh syndrome). Rupture of a tubo-ovarian abscess, however, is more likely to lead to contamination with a variety of organisms including gonococci, streptococci, *Bacteroides* and *Chlamydia*. Penetrating abdominal trauma carries skin organisms into the peritoneal cavity and penetration of any hollow viscus will, of course, release the regional bacterial flora.

A spreading generalized bacterial peritonitis has two major effects on the subject: loss of extracellular fluid and bacterial contamination.

Loss of extracellular fluid

As the infection spreads through the peritoneal cavity a protein-rich exudate is produced, with extensive fibrinous plaques that cause adjacent viscera to adhere to each other. This prevents the usual easy movement of one piece of bowel on other and introduces a measure of mechanical obstruction, to which is added the inhibition of peristalsis that occurs in the presence of infection, i.e. neurogenic ileus (p. 258).

As a consequence, extracellular fluid is lost to the patient in the formation of the purulent exudate, in the sequestration of intestinal secretions within aperistaltic small bowel and through the repeated vomiting which is characteristic of the ileus of general peritonitis. With this naturally goes a cessation of normal drinking, so the losses cannot be made good. Theron and Wilson (1949) made blood volume studies in 35 patients with severe peritonitis and found that in more than half there was a 20–30% reduction. Pledger and Buchan (1969) showed that among 204 children who died from acute appendicitis in England and Wales the most frequent identifiable cause of death was failure to correct hypovolaemia in peritonitis.

It is worth remembering that the surface area of the peritoneum is roughly equal to the skin surface area of $1.5–2.0\,m^2$. The reaction of the peritoneum to injury can reasonably be compared to the effects of a scald on the skin, so general peritonitis may lead to fluid losses comparable to those of an extensive burn.

Bacterial contamination

A gastroduodenal perforation produces its instantaneous irritant effect because of its acid content, which sets up a chemical peritonitis. Comparatively few organisms escape, principally staphylococci and streptococci, and it takes 24–48 hours for a significant purulent peritonitis to develop. Duodenal perforations, with a relatively high acid content, may be almost sterile at first.

Small-bowel perforations produce a mixed infection in which *E. coli* is likely to predominate (although there is a much heavier inoculation of anaerobes if obstruction is also present; p. 185). The common perforations of the appendix will produce initially a rich growth of faecal aerobes such as *E. coli* and *Streptococcus faecalis* and it is at this stage that Gram-negative bacteraemia may occur. Anaerobes do not grow well in the relatively vascular peritoneum, but if the infection becomes localized in an abscess then anaerobes grow more freely, helped by the oxygen requirements of the aerobes.

Perforations of the large bowel cause a highly dangerous inoculation of the peritoneum, rich in aerobes and anaerobes, along with the foreign matter in faeces which assists bacterial growth. *Bacteroides* spp. are the principal anaerobes, especially *B. fragilis*, and *E. coli* the dominant aerobe. Although many different bacterial species can be recovered by thorough bacteriological examination of fresh peritoneal contaminant the practical significance of these is small. *Candida albicans* can usually be recovered from faeces but assumes serious significance only when antibiotics have been continued too long, having overcome bacterial contamination.

The risk of bacteraemia is a real one. The absorption of particulate matter from the peritoneal cavity occurs mostly through the lymphatics on the undersurface of the diaphragm, and thence to the mediastinal nodes and lymphatics *via* the lymphatic duct. Hau *et al.* (1979) found that bacteria injected into the peritoneum of dogs appeared in thoracic lymph in about 6 minutes and in the blood stream in 12 minutes. Lorber and Swenson (1975) found that, among 76 patients with peritonitis, 30% had a positive blood culture, usually for *B. fragilis* or *E. coli*.

If bacteraemia is due to virulent organisms, and suitable parenteral antibiotic treatment is delayed, then the serious complication of bacteraemic or septic shock is likely to develop. This is a particular problem of emergency surgery and may occur when bowel is strangulated, or when the urethra is catheterized or dilated, as well as in established alimentary tract perforation (which may be due to disease, trauma or postoperative misadventure). It is a diagnosis that must be considered whenever a surgical patient becomes ill, with unexplained restlessness and confusion, tachycardia, tachypnoea and hypotension, and in whom there is no suspicion of major internal haemorrhage. Speedy diagnosis and appropriate treatment are essential if this serious situation is to be reversed; this depends on thinking of the diagnosis, because there are no pathognomonic signs.

All forms of surgical shock are due to the volume of the circulating blood being less than the capacity of the vascular bed. In septic shock there may be an element of hypovolaemia, but the principal cause is vasodilatation and increased capillary permeability due to the endotoxins released by Gram-negative bacteria. The consequences are hypotension, impaired perfusion of vital organs, and cellular hypoxia with metabolic acidosis. The kidneys are particularly sensitive to the effects of septic shock. So are the lungs where septal oedema and alveolar collapse lead to hypoxaemia, notwithstanding the development of hyperventilation, which is a most important early sign of pulmonary insufficiency in a patient with peritonitis.

The clinical syndrome of septic shock may come on suddenly, for example an hour or two after urethral instrumentation, or more gradually as a faecal peritonitis develops. The patient feels shivery and unwell, but is mentally alert. There is usually a fever of 38–40°C and the skin is warm and flushed. There is almost always a tachycardia, and often some tachypnoea. Urine output is usually normal at this stage, provided blood pressure is maintained.

This warm phase is followed by a cold hypotensive stage, when the patient is cool, slightly confused and oliguric. Very energetic steps have to be taken if this situation is to be reversed.

4.2 PRIMARY PERITONITIS

This is now a fairly unusual condition. In the course of a year at the Aberdeen Children's Hospital 100–120 patients with acute appendicitis are seen, but only one or two with primary peritonitis (p. 112). The incidence in adult practice is even lower and when Armitage and Williamson (1983) surveyed Bristol hospitals over a 5-year period only six cases were identified: four in children and two in adults. The latter were both elderly women who presented with diffuse peritonitis and were thought to have perforated diverticulitis; both had ovarian tumours and these were presumably secondary infections of pre-existing ascites, probably haematogenous in origin. A striking feature of these patients is that although they have a diffuse peritoneal exudate, they are not as ill as one would expect, and the effusion is odourless, which strongly suggests that it is not due to alimentary tract leakage. Occasionally a pre-existing condition will permit a non-operative diagnosis of primary peritonitis but when the diagnosis is made or suspected at laparotomy an immediate Gram stain of the exudate is useful.

Bacterial peritonitis complicating ascites in a cirrhotic patient is a serious event for the individual, and seems to be increasing in incidence (Crossley and Williams, 1985). In these cases symptoms of abdominal pain and fever should arouse suspicions. Symptoms and signs may be slight, and a diagnostic aspiration of 20 ml of ascitic fluid should be performed whenever there is doubt. Normally ascitic fluid contains fewer than 300 white cells/mm^3: if more than 250/mm^3 are polymorphs an infection must be diagnosed. While awaiting cultures, which generally yield *E. coli*, the most useful antibiotic is considered to be cefotaxime (Crossley and Williams, 1985).

A rare form of primary peritonitis occurs in association with the presence of an intrauterine contraceptive device (p. 514).

4.3 SECONDARY PERITONITIS

4.3.1 AETIOLOGY

Infection of the peritoneum is generally due to a breach in the alimentary canal, which can be the result of intrinsic disease or external trauma. In women, the genital tract is an important portal of entry for pelvic inflammatory disease.

There are many causes of a leak from the gastrointestinal tract and incidence varies considerably. In Northern Europe, North America and Australasia the likely causes are:

- acute appendicitis (p. 36);
- perforated peptic ulcer (p. 163);
- acute colonic diverticulitis (p. 308);
- perforation of neoplasms, e.g.
  - small-bowel lymphoma (p. 233)
  - colorectal carcinoma (p. 266);
- inflammatory bowel disease (p. 319);
- gangrene of the intestine, e.g.
  - volvulus (pp. 208 and p. 289)
  - adhesive strangulation (p. 193)
  - mesenteric vascular occlusion (p. 525)
  - 'gangrene of the colon' (p. 331);
  - necrotizing enterocolitis (p. 252);
- acute obstructive cholecystitis (p. 401);
- other rare causes of intestinal perforation (p. 252).

In tropical and subtropical countries typhoid fever and amoebiasis are likely causes (p. 254).

In all parts of the world trauma is an increasingly important cause, due to either penetrating or blunt injury (pp. 418–20).

Unhappily, an important cause of peritonitis is postoperative leakage, due to either breakdown of an anastomosis, ischaemia or accidental damage. This is the most lethal form of general peritonitis, with a mortality as high as 60% (Bohnen *et al.*, 1983).

Patients undergoing continuous ambulatory peritoneal dialysis are liable to peritonitis (p. 137).

4.3.2   CLINICAL PICTURE

The almost instantaneous onset of a generalized chemical peritonitis, characteristic of perforated peptic ulcer, is well known. A similar picture can develop quickly when acute obstructive appendicitis perforates within hours of onset, or the wall of an abscess gives way. Although the patient looks pale and is obviously in great pain, the patient with a perforated peptic ulcer does not, as is sometimes said, show signs of shock. The severe stimulus to the peritoneum is chemical rather than bacterial and produces the intense response from the sensitive parietal peritoneum that produces the classical rigidity of the overlying abdominal wall musculature. These patients generally show neither fever nor tachycardia, and are normotensive because they arrive quickly in hospital, before significant hypovolaemia can develop.

Onset may be more gradual, and this slow progressive onset is typical of acute appendicitis in the elderly, who often present with the signs of peritonitis with paralytic ileus, and may be thought to have a mechanical small-bowel obstruction (p. 183). Blunt injury of the bladder or small bowel can lead to a similar picture (pp. 418 and p. 488).

Somewhat speedier is the presentation of spreading faecal peritonitis from perforated diverticular disease, and it is not surprising, considering the severity of the bacterial contamination, that these patients look dehydrated and toxic. There is generally a history of pain and vomiting over a day or two, so there is usually fever and tachycardia, the blood pressure may be low, and the abdomen is likely to be diffusely and acutely tender and guarded, with few or no bowel sounds. There is usually tenderness on rectal palpation of the pouch of Douglas. In the elderly it may already be apparent that there are respiratory or cardiac complications, and renal function may also be affected, as this situation merges into the picture of septic shock. Sepsis is a major cause of adult respiratory distress syndrome, and anyone in these circumstances with tachypnoea should have a chest X-ray and estimation of blood gases.

Richardson *et al.* (1983) found diagnostic peritoneal lavage helpful when peritonitis is suspected in a patient who is unconscious or too ill to give a history. They regard the test as positive if the return from a 1 litre lavage contains more than 500 white cells/mm^3 or if bile is present. There was only one false positive in 138 patients. More recently, peritoneal cytology has had some popularity as a diagnostic aid in peritonitis but more usually in milder forms of disease as an aid to decision-making for or against operation.

4.3.3   TREATMENT

There is no question of rushing these ill patients to theatre: surgery is an integral part of treatment but it must be wisely timed, after a period of a few hours of active preparation to optimize resuscitation.

In anyone (and especially in an elderly person) who is seriously ill and suspected of being in early septic shock, there is everything to be said for immediate admission to the intensive therapy unit when available. In addition to expert nursing and monitoring, the anaesthetists are immediately involved in the resuscitation and in the timing of laparotomy.

(a) Water, electrolyte and protein replacement

For reasons already outlined these losses can be considerable. At the time of placement of a wide-bore intravenous cannula, blood is removed for culture, biochemical and haemato-logical analysis. Then an infusion mixing electrolyte and colloid solutions can be commenced. Hartmann's solution is useful because it not only replaces electrolytes but also helps to correct metabolic acidosis, which is likely to be present.

An adult of 70 kg with diffuse peritonitis is likely to have been ill for a day or two, and during that time will have vomited, and drunk very little. A water deficit of 5–6 litres is probable, and this makes it reasonable to run the infusion fairly fast. A 500 ml aliquot can be infused every 20–30 minutes for 1.5–2 hours, mixing Hartmann's and colloid, either human albumin solution or a synthetic colloid according to local protocol. As a general rule no more than 1 litre of synthetic colloid should be infused in a 24-hour period because, if septic shock should develop with a coagulation problem, the synthetic material may affect clotting and cross-matching of blood.

In the elderly with peritonitis it is relatively easy to induce pulmonary oedema, and over-dosage of electrolyte solutions in any patient who is seriously ill with peritonitis is liable to produce 'shock lung'. It is therefore wise in all such ill and elderly patients to measure CVP, but it is unwise to risk a pneumothorax by using the infraclavicular route for insertion of the central line, particularly before initial volume replacement has improved venous filling sufficiently to allow safe cannulation. Provided readings do not exceed 8–10 cmH$_2$O, a careful estimate of the fluid dosage required by the individual has been made and a mixture of electrolyte and colloid solutions is given, then fluid overload should be avoided.

(b) Antibiotic treatment

Antibiotic treatment must commence whenever there is a suspicion of bacteraemia or a clinical diagnosis of bacterial peritonitis. At this early stage this has to be based on clinical judgement. It is probably unnecessary in a patient with an early and typical perforation of a duodenal ulcer, in whom the peritoneal fluid is initially sterile, but it is mandatory, for instance, in an ill, feverish child who has had a perforated appendix for several days, and in anyone believed to have faecal peritonitis.

It is possible to give firm recommendations on the principles of antibiotic treatment although it is more difficult to be dogmatic on the choice of specific agents because there are many agents and combinations of equivalent efficacy, albeit with large variations in cost. The final decision should be based on an institutional policy based on known bacterial sensitivities. It is crucial that the aerobic coliforms, predominantly *E. coli*, and the anaerobic bacteroides, particularly *B. fragilis*, are covered. Concerns about the role of the enterococci (*S. faecalis*) have largely been resolved and it is unnecessary to provide cover for these bacteria.

Although some authorities consider aminoglycosides obsolete in the management of peritonitis (Wittman *et al.*, 1996) this is not our experience and gentamicin remains the first choice agent for its rapid bactericidal action against coliforms: 100% of *E. coli* cultured from patients not previously exposed to antibiotics are sensitive to gentamicin in our hospital. We have relied on a short (3-day) course of antibiotics for surgically treated peritonitis for a number of years (Krukowski and Matheson, 1988) and the modern regime of a loading dose of 7 mg/kg body weight and once-daily administration of gentamicin means that only two serum levels require to be checked during treatment. Concerns over nephro- and ototoxicity have not been realized over many years but an effective alternative is a third-generation cephalosporin (cefotaxime or ceftrioxanone).

There is still no anti-anaerobic antibiotic to rival the safety, efficacy and economy of metronidazole and the combination of this with either gentamicin or a third-generation cephalosporin is sufficient initial, and usually all the antibiotic therapy required following surgical elimination of the source of sepsis from the peritoneal cavity. Indeed the long half-life of metronidazole means that a twice-daily dose (500 mg i.v.) may suffice when postoperative contamination is minimal.

Arguments for monotherapy in peritonitis are not supported by objective evidence, partly because of the difficulty in organizing randomized trials comparing equivalent groups of patients and also because of the prohibitive cost of some of these agents, which are more appropriately reserved for second-line therapy.

As indicated above we have long believed that if the cause of the peritonitis is effectively dealt with at operation, antibiotic treatment is not required for more than 3–4 days and this clinical observation is receiving increasing support (Schein *et al.*, 1994).

(c) Ventilation

In any patient with severe generalized peritonitis there is poor diaphragmatic movement and some impairment of tissue perfusion, and oxygen should be given *via* a face mask. Older patients generally require estimation of blood gases.

(d) Temperature reduction

Children are particularly liable to run a high fever, and tepid sponging can be helpful.

(e) Analgesia

Patients with peritonitis are anxious and in pain, and it is both safe and humane to give adequate analgesia, e.g. morphine, which may need to be by slow intravenous injection to ensure absorption if tissue perfusion is poor (p. 17).

It is wise to consult the anaesthetist over choice and dose of analgesic. Such early consultation with the anaesthetist who will be responsible during the operation is most desirable anyway, because in ill patients it can be difficult to choose the best time for surgery, and it is valuable for the anaesthetist to have seen the response to preoperative treatment.

(f) Renal function

Particularly in older patients a close watch must be kept on the lungs for signs of oedema. Cardiac irregularities such as atrial fibrillation may appear and require treatment. Renal function needs very careful monitoring with measurement of hourly output *via* a urethral catheter, and the aim should be 1 ml/kg body weight/h. If in the adult this is less than 20–30 ml/h it is useful to measure osmolality. The use of large doses of steroid is no longer recommended in septic shock. Although there is debate about the value of a low-dose infusion of dopamine in improving renal function in the critically ill (Duke and Bersten, 1992) this still appears to be of value in the prevention of renal impairment if used early, when urine flow remains poor after adequate fluid resuscitation. As ever, anticipation of problems and pre-emptive action are always preferable to late intervention once the complication is established.

4.3.4 OPERATION

Ideally, systolic blood pressure should be above 100 mmHg and urine output over 40 ml in the hour when the anaesthetic is commenced. In faecal peritonitis, where abdominal cleansing is a vital part of resuscitation, it may be necessary to go ahead when it is judged the response is as good as can be obtained.

The **choice of operative procedure** depends on the pathology. There is no difficulty in deciding on appendicectomy or cholecystectomy for a gangrenous perforated organ. In intestinal perforations and injuries this decision can be more difficult and is discussed in the appropriate places.

Peritoneal lavage and debridement is still a controversial issue. It is difficult not to be impressed with Kennedy's description, in 1905, of the methods of Price in Philadelphia, who was an enthusiastic advocate of thorough peritoneal lavage with volumes of warm water and saline, and of equally thorough debridement. His mortality for cases of peritonitis was said to be less than 1%. Burnett *et al.* (1957) give a vivid description of their first case, in 1942, of an apparently hopelessly advanced case of appendicular peritonitis: thorough cleansing of every part of the abdomen with many pints of sulphanilamide in warm saline was followed by a smooth recovery. They stress the need to separate each loop of small bowel so that interloop abscesses are found and dispersed. Lavage with large amounts of warm saline removes gross faecal contamination and effectively dilutes the bacterial population. However, this effect is only temporary unless an antibiotic is added to the saline: this delivers a high concentration throughout the peritoneum, at a much higher level than can come *via* the blood stream.

Hudspeth, in 1975, repeated this advice, and paid particular attention to the removal of as many fibrinous plaques as possible, calling this thorough mechanical cleansing 'radical surgical debridement'. He treated 92 patients with advanced generalized peritonitis without a death. Subsequently a randomized trial of conventional with Hudspeth's radical debridement showed no advantage (Polk and Fry, 1980). The good results reported by Hudspeth are now generally attributed to the relatively low-risk group of patients treated by him rather than to the radical, and traumatic, debridement.

The addition of an antibacterial substance to the lavage fluid has been used by a number of surgeons since Burnett used sulphanilamide in 1942. In 1957 he was using penicillin and streptomycin. In 1967 Noon *et al.* were using kanamycin and bacitracin, and they were particularly impressed with its effect in reducing wound infections. Stewart and Matheson (1978) began to use tetracycline (1 mg/ml) in warm physiological saline in 1966 and were able to show that there were fewer septic complications and wound infections than with conventional treatment. We have shown that tetracycline at this concentration is lethal to all aerobic and anaerobic intestinal bacteria (Krukowski *et al.*, 1986). Very extensive use of tetracycline lavage in Aberdeen, both for prophylaxis and therapy over almost 30 years has shown that the method is apparently harmless and strikingly effective.

Orr *et al.* (1983) showed that after lavage of the peritoneum with several litres of tetracycline solution the levels in the serum never approached toxic levels (maximum 7 μg/ml). There is no evidence that tetracycline induces adhesion formation at the concentrations used clinically in the treatment of peritonitis but the experimental work of Phillips and Dudley (1984) suggested that tetracycline lavage should be limited to cases of material bacterial contamination.

Contemporary opinion no longer favours postoperative irrigation of the peritoneum, with or without antibiotic in the solution, although in the past Fowler (1975) and Stephen and Loewenthal (1979) thought it had been beneficial in cases of faecal peritonitis. On the only occasion on which we employed it (Krukowski and Matheson, 1984) we encountered serious problems with the overgrowth of fungi. Our impression after extensive use of intraoperative lavage is that it is so effective that postoperative lavage is not needed. The only exception seems to be in a severe cases of necrotizing pancreatitis when, correctly speaking, the drainage is of the retroperitoneum rather than the peritoneal cavity *per se*.

The basis of our surgical approach is:

1. A long vertical incision to allow access to all parts of the abdomen and every effort made to avoid contamination and inoculation of the abdominal parietes by infected peritoneal content. Elevation of the wound and aspiration of fluid through a small initial opening in the peritoneum prevents flooding of the operative field. Mechanical wound protection should be used (p. 20).

2. Pus and debris is aspirated and mopped out. It is important to send pus for inoculation on to aerobic and anaerobic media, although by the time the results are available the patient ought to be well on the road to recovery. A Gram film gives a good idea of the nature and severity of contamination and if there are no organisms present, as can occur with duodenal perforation, antibiotic use can be minimized.

3. The peritoneum is irrigated with warm saline containing 1 mg/ml tetracycline until the return is clear.

4. In diffuse peritonitis there is usually considerable gaseous distension of small bowel, and it helps to decompress this. The best method is to withdraw all the small bowel from the abdomen and carefully to separate each loop from its neighbour. This often releases collections of pus trapped between loops of bowel and mesentery. There are often fibrinous plaques, which can be gently removed although, if the sepsis is long established, debridement that causes excessive trauma and bleeding should be abandoned. The small-bowel content is carefully emptied by retrograde stripping to the stomach for aspiration by the anaesthetist (p. 191). This manoeuvre, although very useful, has a number of potential hazards. Do not be too ambitious with the first pass along the bowel, and it may be sensible to milk the bowel gently hand over hand first before returning to strip the contents between index and middle finger. If the bowel is very distended start close to the duodenojejunal flexure and work progressively back to the terminal ileum. This avoids the risk of overdistension of friable proximal small bowel, which can disrupt if handled roughly. Avoidable perforations of small bowel are a disaster in this type of surgery. Make sure that the anaesthetist is aware that a large volume of fluid is returning to the stomach and that this can be aspirated before a flood

of gastric content refluxes up into the mouth and pharynx, increasing the risk of contamination of the airway on extubation at the end of the operation.

5. It is important not to forget the subdiaphragmatic and subhepatic spaces, the paracolic gutters and the pelvis. These areas often trap fibrin and debris. Much dirty fibrin can be recovered by sweeping gauze swabs over the upper surface of the liver and under the domes of the diaphragm.

6. This is usually the stage at which any resection is performed, and if stomata are required the incisions are made and the bowel exteriorized. The details of these procedures, and the choice of operation, are fully discussed in, for example, the sections on colonic injuries and perforated diverticular disease. If the peritoneum remains grossly inflamed after thorough toilet and lavage, the patient is unstable and perfusion poor, there should be considerable caution about performing an anastomosis. This is most likely to apply in postoperative patients in whom there has been delay in intervening following anastomotic leakage. Under these circumstances it is generally unwise to attempt to salvage the anastomosis and it is best to dismantle the join, resect back to healthy bowel and form an enterostomy and a mucous fistula, or, in the case of an anterior resection of rectum, perform a Hartmann's closure of the rectal stump. Such postoperative peritoneal sepsis is the most lethal type of peritonitis, with a mortality which approaches 50%. An important factor is undoubtedly delay in diagnosis and our more recent experience suggests that early diagnosis and intervention can salvage an anastomotic leak when this is due to a small defect, caused by a minor technical problem, rather than ischaemia of the bowel (Watson *et al.* in preparation).

7. Finally, the whole abdominal cavity and its contents receive a final lavage with the tetracycline solution with a small amount left in the abdomen. The small bowel is carefully replaced in an orderly fashion and overlaid with omentum if possible.

8. The abdominal incision is closed with a mass suture of polydioxanone and after further irrigation of the subcutaneous space the skin is closed. With the use of lavage of the incision we have not found that delayed primary suture of the skin is necessary (p. 21). Injection of 20 ml of 0.5% bupivacaine into each side of a long incision dramatically reduces immediate postoperative pain.

4.3.5 PLANNED REOPERATION

With the above policy our reoperation rate for recrudescent peritoneal sepsis after 'dirty' surgery is low (Krukowski and Matheson, 1988) but the adverse effect of reoperation on mortality was also clear. A few patients with diffuse peritonitis due to faecal soiling or, and this ought to be even more uncommon, delay in diagnosis of a disrupted surgical suture line present late, with evidence or septic shock, and sometimes remote organ failure. Prognosis is poor in these patients, but this is made worse by the fact that, following laparotomy, there is a likelihood of continued intraperitoneal suppuration, particularly if the initial operation has been tentative.

The initial operation should be definitive and adequate to treat virtually every patient presenting for their first operation for peritoneal sepsis, although some surgeons, who must have a different referral pattern to ours, suggest that 10–15% of patients require more radical therapy (Wittmann *et al.*, 1996). For the general surgeon not catering for a tertiary referral practice there will be only a small number of patients in whom either sepsis cannot be eliminated or there is a certainty of recurrence and who represent a particular challenge. An aggressive surgical approach is necessary to salvage these patients and, in truth, it is likely to be effective only in younger patients because the adverse effect of chronic diseases of the elderly, allied to such severe sepsis, result in high APACHE II scores, which correlate well with adverse outcome (Knaus *et al.*, 1985).

There are a number of alternative approaches to this dilemma, which may be summarized as: laparotomy 'on demand', 'planned relaparotomy' or 'laparostomy'.

There is some evidence that, in this small group in whom sepsis cannot be eliminated at the first operation, waiting for a clinical indication to re-explore the abdomen is associated with poorer outcome than the more radical alternative approaches. A number of these patients deteriorate postoperatively and succumb without re-operation. They are described as having become 'too ill' to tolerate another operation, although post-mortem examination reveals potentially treatable sepsis (Barendregt *et al.*, 1992). The decision for further surgery should be made at the time of laparotomy and the choice made between closing the abdomen temporarily or leaving the abdomen open.

Penninckx and colleagues (1983), after definitive treatment and peritoneal debridement, closed the abdomen in one layer with drainage. After 48–72 hours in ITU the abdomen was deliberately re-opened, further loculi of pus sought and drained and further peritoneal lavage performed. In 22 of 31 patients so treated further foci of sepsis had formed and were drained at the second laparotomy. Some required a third planned exploration. They contrast the nine (29%) deaths in this group with eight (73%) deaths in 11 other patients who only had their second laparotomy when they had become severely septic, after the delay of a week or so. The interval between operations in 'planned relaparotomy' is debated and current opinion favours 24 hours.

There are however problems associated with 'planned relaparotomy'. There is evidence that repeated operation itself may aggravate the inflammatory cycle that leads to 'tertiary peritonitis' and multiple organ failure (Waydhas *et al.*, 1996) and although the process can be repeated there is a limit to how often the abdominal wall will tolerate this procedure. If relaparotomy proves necessary on more than one occasion an alternative strategy may prove necessary. Indeed, the alternative of leaving the abdomen open is preferred by some as the first line of therapy in patients judged to be in this high-risk category.

If the abdomen is left completely open, 'laparostomy' (Mughal *et al.*, 1986), this allows ready access to all quadrants of peritoneum, albeit for only a few days, until progressive adhesion and granulation tissue formation restricts access. While simple and effective in preventing reaccumulation of major collections of suppuration this method also has deficiencies. If it is successful over a period of several days the wound edges contract and retract preventing primary closure or making this so tight as to risk inducing 'abdominal compartment syndrome' (Schein *et al.*, 1995). This may be overcome by a sliding graft of the anterior abdominal wall in which the lateral margin of the rectus sheath is divided longitudinally along its length. The anterior sheath is mobilized off the muscle and the resulting mobilized thick layer of skin, fat and anterior sheath can be approximated in the midline achieving biological cover of the exposed viscera. The large defect resulting from leaving the entire anterior aspect of the rectus muscle exposed heals remarkably quickly by a combination of contraction and epithelialization such that on those occasions on which we have had to use this manoeuvre no skin grafting has been necessary.

Furthermore when laparostomy is employed exposed bowel is liable to fistulation, and suture lines can leak. If this disaster occurs it defies early repair and precludes closure of the abdomen. Under these circumstances open management must proceed until such time as skin grafting of the granulating surface can take place. Grafting can proceed once the output from fistulae can be controlled. The somatostatin analogue octreotide can be invaluable in reducing fistula output in this situation.

A variation on laparostomy is to insert a synthetic mesh to cover the exposed viscera and some stitch in a zip fastener to facilitate subsequent reopening of the abdomen. The mesh prevents excessive retraction of the abdominal muscles, excessive tension and intra-abdominal pressure and can be left *in situ* when incorporated in granulation tissue, although the zipper must be removed and if possible the edges of the mesh sutured.

We have no experience of the zipper technique, which appears unaesthetic. On those occasions when the abdomen has had to be left open because of excessive intra-abdominal pressure we prefer to cover the exposed intra-abdominal viscera or mesh, if this has been necessary to replace deficient abdominal wall, with a sliding graft of the anterior abdominal wall rather than use prosthetic material.

4.3.6 POSTOPERATIVE CARE

An important decision will have to be made at the end of the operation over transfer of the patient to the intensive therapy area. In advanced peritonitis it may be vital to continue respiratory assistance for 24–48 hours and, in the elderly particularly, the heart and kidneys may need particularly close observation.

Nasogastric suction *via* an Andersen-type tube is useful in aspirating swallowed air. Intravenous fluids need to be particularly carefully supervised, to give enough but to avoid the risk of overloading.

Systemic antibiotic treatment will generally be continued. When gentamicin is used as a once-daily dose only, trough ($< 3\,\mu g/ml$) levels need be estimated, and the timing of dosage calculated from a nomogram. With these precautions, and the fact that administration can usually be stopped after 3 days, there should be no adverse effect on renal function.

In older patients, it is vital to keep a close clinical and radiographic watch on the respiratory tract. Abdominal pain and distension limit diaphragmatic movements, so secretions can easily accumulate and physiotherapy is exceptionally important. Blood gases should be checked in any patient not clearly making quick progress. Unexplained tachypnoea and hypoxaemia are indications for careful review with the intensive therapy unit.

Sedation needs to be carefully used. It is an important part of care to give these patients a good sleep at night, and if progress is satisfactory recordings that disrupt sleep must be minimized. By day analgesics should be timed to precede periods of physiotherapy. Although now fairly familiar, it still is a little surprising to see how often a patient with a severe peritonitis will make steady progress after the cause of sepsis has been removed, the peritoneum thoroughly cleansed and effective antibiotic treatment provided. This is reflected in the general appearance and behaviour, the recordings, the softening of the abdomen and the return of bowel sounds and passage of flatus.

However, knowing the extent of contamination, a very close watch is kept for two major complications of general peritonitis: so-called paralytic ileus (p. 258) and residual abscesses. There is no precise time at which it can be said that a state of paralytic ileus exists. However, if on the fourth postoperative day the patient with peritonitis looks ill, has a distended silent abdomen and high nasogastric aspirates, and has passed no flatus *per rectum*, it is wise to presume that ileus exists.

The first consideration must be to establish whether there is a mechanical element in the obstruction. Wind pains and peristaltic sounds suggest a kink but the plain abdominal film gives most help, because in neurogenic ileus there is considerable gas and fluid distension of the large as well as the small bowel: if an adhesion is causing a small bowel kink then gas will be absent from the large bowel.

If a diagnosis of neurogenic ileus is made it is important to check fluid and electrolyte balance. Significant anaemia should be corrected. A residual abscess, especially in the pelvis, may be forming. If all these checks and corrections have been carried out then for a further day or two it is necessary to await developments. The phase of aperistalsis may cease for no apparent reason and a normal if slow recovery take place. On or about the sixth day, if there is no easing of the obstruction, it is time to commence parenteral nutrition. It is better to commence at this stage rather than allow the patient's condition to deteriorate visibly: even at best it will be some days before a reasonably nourishing diet can be taken by mouth.

At the twice-daily visits the situation is reviewed, particularly with a view to detecting mechanical obstruction or residual abscess (see below). Other details of treatment and the indications for pharmacological stimulation in neurogenic ileus are fully considered on pp. 258–60.

4.3.7   RESULTS

These are difficult to analyse because there are many variables. However the study of Bohnen *et al.* (1983) remains relevant. They saw 176 consecutive patients in Montreal with free pus or gastrointestinal content in the peritoneum. They made a useful division into three categories:

1. patients with acute appendicitis or perforated duodenal ulcer – this should be a relatively low-risk group and there were no deaths among 40 patients with appendicitis; however, there were seven deaths among the 28 duodenal ulcer patients (25%);
2. patients with perforation of other organs, i.e. stomach, small and large bowel; 24 of 48 patients (50%) died, 15 from sepsis;
3. a total of 60 patients who developed peritonitis after abdominal surgery – for example, 14 had a leaking anastomosis, nine a leaking duodenal stump; there were 36 deaths (60%).

Age is a material factor, the mortality under 50 years being 17%, and over 50 years 45%. Other factors are advanced malignant disease and delay in diagnosis and treatment. Bohnen *et al.* make the important point that evidence of organ failure (such as deteriorating blood gases, rising serum bilirubin and/or creatinine, platelets below $60\,000/mm^3$, hypotension, gastroduodenal bleeding) needs to be given particular attention in the postoperative group, among whom occult abdominal sepsis is likely but difficult to detect. If the surgeon responds quickly to deterioration, with a careful search for an abscess, it may be possible to drain it and stop the deterioration.

We reported (Koruth *et al.*, 1985) 93 consecutive patients in Aberdeen and Inverness who required emergency surgery for lesions of the distal colon, of whom 39 had peritonitis (16 faecal, 23 purulent). All save three had a resection and thorough debridement and tetracycline lavage, and there was one death. Among the three not resected one died before operation could be performed. Wound infection occurred in 6%. A mortality of around 5% in a group of patients with peritonitis of colonic origin, and of an average age of over 70 years, is distinctly encouraging, and suggests that these methods, when employed by experienced surgeons, are soundly based. However, this group was somewhat biased in so far as all became fit enough to be operated upon. Among 276 consecutive patients with peritonitis treated on the same lines, overall mortality was 7.9% (Krukowski *et al.*, 1986).

The increasing age of patients undergoing emergency surgery for peritonitis means that the overall reduction in mortality to which surgeons aspire may be confounded by the coincidental degenerative diseases of the elderly. The strong correlation between high APACHE II scores and mortality suggests that there will always be a number of patients for whom the insult of generalized peritonitis will remain lethal.

4.4   POSTOPERATIVE PERITONEAL ABSCESS

Residual abscesses are no longer the lethal condition they used to be, and it was surprising to see how much pus could accumulate when drained at an open operation. The appearance of a swinging fever a few days after operation, which continues and tends to become higher, is highly suggestive. A postoperative abscess should be sought by clinical examination and appropriate scans. If subphrenic there is likely to be a reactive pleural effusion on the affected side with tenderness on percussion or springing of the lower ribs. An interloop abscess may be apparent as an area of localized tenderness and rectal examination may reveal the characteristic tender bulge of a pelvic abscess presenting through the anterior rectal wall.

A localized abscess as a result of inadequate primary treatment of sepsis should now be a rare event and simple drainage suffices in the absence of intestinal leakage. Once suspected, it is important to pursue the possible diagnosis of an intraperitoneal abscess. If there is a suture line or anastomosis present integrity must be confirmed by contrast radiology either as an enema, orally or down a nasogastric tube. If anastomotic leakage is demonstrated this must be treated to eliminate continuing peritoneal contamination; usually this will require laparotomy and dismantling of the anastomosis. If this is not necessary, for a localized leak in an otherwise intact anastomosis, or not possible, e.g. a duodenal stump leak, sump drainage must be provided. If the contrast study shows no leak then either an ultrasound scan or CT of the abdomen is performed. This has transformed the management of postoperative abscesses in that a substantial collection can be localized accurately and, once found, drained. Nowadays this would most often be percutaneous ultrasound guided drainage without recourse to open operation. Although this has transformed management of a localized abscess percutaneous drainage is inadequate treatment for diffuse sepsis secondary to major anastomotic dehiscence. Furthermore beware inadvertent bowel puncture, which can occur in the hands of even the most skilled radiologist.

REFERENCES

Armitage, T. G. and Williamson, R. C. N. (1983) Primary peritonitis in children and adults. *Postgrad. Med. J.*, **59**, 21–24.

Autio, V. (1964) The spread of intraperitoneal infection. *Acta Chir. Scand. Suppl.*, **321**, 1–31.

Barendregt, W., de Bower, H. and Kubat, K. (1992) The results of autopsy of patients with surgical disease of the digestive tract. *Surg. Gynecol. Obstet.*, **175**, 227–232.

Bartlett, J. G., Onderdonk, A. B., Louie, T. J. *et al.* (1978) A review: lessons from an animal model of intra-abdominal sepsis. *Arch. Surg.* **113**, 853–857.

Bohnen, J., Boulanger, M., Metkins, J. L. *et al.* (1983) Prognosis in generalized peritonitis. *Arch. Surg.*, **118**, 285–290.

Burnett, W. E., Brown, G. R., Rosemond, G. P. *et al.* (1957) The treatment of peritonitis using peritoneal lavage. *Ann. Surg.*, **145**, 676–682.

Crossley, I. R. and Williams, R. (1985) Spontaneous bacterial peritonitis. *Gut*, **26**, 325–331.

Duke, G. I. and Bersten, A. D. (1992) Dopamine and renal salvage in the critically ill patient. *Anaesth. Intensive Care*, **20**, 277–302.

Fowler, R. (1975) A controlled trial of intraperitoneal cephaloridine administration in peritonitis. *J. Pediatr. Surg.*, **10**, 43–50.

Hau, T., Ahrenholz, D. H. and Simmons, R. L. (1979) Secondary bacterial peritonitis: the biologic basis of treatment. *Curr. Probl. Surg.*, **16**, 1–65.

Hudspeth, S. (1975) Radical surgical debridement in the treatment of advanced generalized bacterial peritonitis. *Arch. Surg.*, **110**, 1233–1236.

Kennedy, J. W. (1905) Appendicitis: the earliest and complete removal of the appendix. *Surg. Gynecol. Obstet.*, **1**, 216–220.

Knaus, W. A., Draper, E. A., Wagner, D. P. *et al.* (1985) APACHE II: a severity of disease classification system. *Crit. Care Med.*, **13**, 818–829.

Koperna, T. and Schulz, F. (1996) Prognosis and treatment of peritonitis. Do we need new scoring systems? *Arch. Surg.*, **131**, 180–186.

Koruth, N. M., Krukowski, Z. H. and Youngson, G. G. *et al.* (1985). Intraoperative colonic irrigation in the management of left-sided large bowel emergencies. *Br. J. Surg.*, **72**, 708–711.

Krukowski, Z. H. and Matheson, N. A. (1984) Peritonitis. *Surgery (Oxford)*, **1**, 260–267.

Krukowski, Z. H. and Matheson, N. A. (1988) Infection after abdominal surgery: a ten year computerised audit. *Br. J. Surg.*, **75**, 857–861.

Krukowski, Z. H., Koruth, N. M. and Matheson, N. A. (1986) Antibiotic lavage in emergency surgery for peritoneal sepsis. *J. R. Coll. Surg. Edin.*, **31**, 1–6.

Lorber, B. and Swenson, R. M. (1975) The bacteriology of intra-abdominal infections. *Surg. Clin. North Am.*, **55**, 1349–1354.

Mughal, M. M., Bancewicz, J. and Irving, M. H. (1986) 'Laparostomy': a technique for the management of intractable intra-abdominal sepsis. *Br. J. Surg.*, **73**, 253–259.

Noon, G. P., Beall, A. C., Jorden, G. L. *et al.* (1967) Clinical evaluation of peritoneal irrigation with antibiotic solution. *Surgery*, **62**, 73–78.

Orr, G., Thomson, H. J. and Reid, T. M. S. (1983) Serum tetracycline level following peritoneal lavage. *Br. J. Surg.*, **70**, 563.

Penninckx, F. M., Kerremans, R. P. and Lauwers, P. M. (1983) Planned relaparotomies in the treatment of severe generalized peritonitis from intestinal origin. *World J. Surg.*, **7**, 762–766.

Phillips, R. K. S. and Dudley, H. A. F. (1984) The effect of tetracycline lavage and trauma on visceral and peritoneal ultrastructure and adhesion formation. *Br. J. Surg.*, **71**, 537–539.

Pledger, H. G. and Buchan, R. (1969) Deaths in children with acute appendicitis. *BMJ*, **iv**, 466–470.

Polk, H. C. and Fry, D. E. (1980) Radical peritoneal debridement for established peritonitis. *Ann. Surg.*, **192**, 350–355.

Richardson, J. D., Flint, L. M. and Polk, H. C. (1983) Peritoneal lavage: a useful diagnostic adjunct for peritonitis. *Surgery*, **94**, 826–829.

Schein, M., Assalia, A. and Bacchus, H. (1994) Minimal antibiotic therapy in emergency abdominal surgery: a prospective study. *Br. J. Surg.*, **81**, 989–991.

Schein, M., Wittmann, D. H., Apprahamian, C. *et al.* (1995) Abdominal compartment syndrome; the physiological and clinical consequences of elevated intra-abdominal pressure. *J. Am. Coll. Surg.*, **180**, 745–753.

Stephen, M. and Loewenthal, J. (1979) Continuing peritoneal lavage in high-risk peritonitis. *Surgery*, **85**, 603–606.

Stewart, D. J. and Matheson, N. A. (1978) Peritoneal lavage in appendicular peritonitis. *Br. J. Surg.*, **65**, 54–56.

Theron, P. H. and Wilson, W. C. (1949) Blood changes in peritonitis. *Lancet*, **i**, 172–178.

Watson *et al.* (in preparation)

Watters, J. M., Blakslee, J. M., March, R. J. *et al.* (1996) The influence of age on the severity of peritonitis. *Can. J. Surg.*, **39**, 142–146.

Waydhas, C., Nast-Kolb, D., Trupka, A. *et al.* (1996) Post-traumatic inflammatory response, secondary operations and late multiple organ failure. *J. Trauma*, **40**, 624–630.

Wittman, D. H., Schein, M. and Condon, R. E. (1996) Management of secondary peritonitis. *Ann. Surg.*, **224**, 10–18.

4.5 EXTERNAL HERNIA AND PERITONITIS

When general peritonitis occurs in a patient with a patent but empty hernial sac, the patient may complain of the tense tender hernia and be admitted as a strangulated hernia.

Cronin and Ellis (1959) described five patients, four with an inguinal and one with a paraumbilical hernia, who all complained principally of their painful hernia. In two, perforated appendicitis was the source of peritonitis, one had a perforated duodenal ulcer and one biliary peritonitis. The last two presented a week after the laparotomy and had the pus drained and the sac excised. The first two were primarily explored as strangulated inguinal hernias, and only when pus was drained from the sac was a laparotomy done and the appendix found to be the source of the peritonitis

Edwueme (1973) reported 13 similar cases from Kampala, Uganda, including six in which a strangulated Richter's hernia had perforated and caused peritonitis. Thomas *et al.* (1982) showed that the tender inguinal or femoral hernia may contain acutely inflamed appendix. They collected seven such cases seen in Bristol and Exeter hospitals over 8 years, and all were diagnosed as strangulated hernias. This event may occur in infancy (p. 126).

Several of these patients also had abdominal pain but it is easy to concentrate on the obvious signs in the hernia. This is a rare event, but if it is suspected the abdominal incision can be planned to allow preperitoneal repair of the hernia. Systemic antibiotics and thorough lavage will play an important part in preventing infection of the inguinal canal.

REFERENCES

Cronin, K. and Ellis, H. (1959) Pus collections in hernial sacs: unusual complication of general peritonitis. *Br. J. Surg.*, **46**, 364–367.
Edwueme, O. (1973) Strangulated external hernia associated with general peritonitis. *Br. J. Surg.*, **60**, 929–933.
Thomas, W. E. G., Vowles, K. D. J. and Williamson, R. C. N. (1982) Appendicitis in external herniae. *Ann. R. Coll. Surg. Engl.*, **64**, 121–122.

4.6 STARCH PERITONITIS

In the 1940s it became apparent that talc powder, which was dusted on to surgical gloves to make them easier to draw on to the hand, had an irritant action on the peritoneum that often led to adhesion formation. Experiments suggested that starch powder would be a suitable substitute, because it appeared to be completely absorbed over the space of 12–14 days after laparotomy. Considering the number of laparotomies performed by surgeons using surgical gloves dusted with starch powder, it is clear that the claim for the relative harmlessness of starch was correct. However, there are a few patients who are sensitized to starch, and in them quite a severe peritoneal reaction can occur. Furthermore, current practice recommends powder-free gloves to abolish even this small risk (Sternlieb *et al.*, 1977).

In a typical case the patient makes a normal recovery from laparotomy for some 10–14 days and then develops malaise, nausea and abdominal pain. The abdomen looks distended and is diffusely tender. Because of the rarity of starch sensitivity this picture can look very much like a complication of the laparotomy, such as late anastomotic leakage, and may easily lead to a second laparotomy. There is usually a considerable amount of straw-coloured fluid present and numerous small white nodules are seen (which can easily be mistaken, after resection of a carcinoma, for metastases). Microscopy of the centrifuged fluid, or of a nodule, under polarized light will show the Maltese cross appearance typical of starch granuloma. If the diagnosis is suspected, it is valuable to perform paracentesis and examine the fluid under polarized light.

The peritoneal reaction settles with time, but it can be a worrying period until there are clear signs of improvement. Intradermal injection of a small quantity of starch powder in these patients shows an intense inflammatory reaction after 3–6 days (Grant *et al.*, 1982). Unfortunately, this delay is too long to be of much practical help when one is worried about the reason for the peritoneal reaction. If the diagnosis can be confirmed, resolution is hastened by administration of corticosteroids. With the introduction of starch-free gloves this unusual complication of laparotomy is likely to disappear altogether.

REFERENCES

Grant, J. B. F., Davies, J. D., Espiner, H. J. *et al.* (1982) Diagnosis of granulomatous starch peritonitis by delayed hypersensitivity skin reactions. *Br. J. Surg.*, **69**, 197–199.
Sternlieb, J. J., McIlrath, D. C., van Heerden, J. A. *et al.* (1977) Starch peritonitis and its prevention. *Arch. Surg.*, **112**, 458–461.

5

Emergencies in the upper alimentary tract

5.1 BOERHAAVE'S SYNDROME OR BAROGENIC RUPTURE OF THE OESOPHAGUS

5.1.1 BACKGROUND

Boerhaave's syndrome is a surgical emergency characterized by the sudden onset of abdominal or chest pain and breathlessness, in which patients rapidly become extremely ill and, unless diagnosed and treated quickly, death is the usual outcome. The first case was described by Hermann Boerhaave in 1724 (Derbes and Mitchell, 1955). Boerhaave of Leiden, one of the most prominent physicians in Europe at that time, was summoned to see the Grand Admiral of Holland who habitually induced vomiting after eating to excess. On the day Boerhaave was called to see him he felt a 'horrible pain' in the epigastrium after vomiting. Boerhaave gave a vivid description of the Admiral's distress, which contrasted strongly with the complete absence of physical signs. The Admiral died and Boerhaave performed an autopsy, when he found a distended stomach and fluid smelling of roast duck in both pleural cavities. A large tear was noted in the lower third of the oesophagus. During the succeeding 200 years the condition continued to be lethal and it is not clear who first reported survival but Barrett is usually given credit for the first successful transthoracic repair of barogenic rupture of the oesophagus (Barrett, 1947).

Barogenic rupture of the oesophagus is thought to occur as a result of a sudden increase in intra-oesophageal pressure. Most commonly this will result from an episode of vomiting or retching. Other less common causes include weightlifting (Griffith, 1932), labour (Kennard, 1950) and even defaecation (Lawson *et al.*, 1974). There is often a history of chronic alcohol ingestion (Kinsella *et al.*, 1948). The incidence is not known but in the Highlands of Scotland, with a population of approximately 200 000, 13 patients have been treated in the past 13 years.

5.1.2 THE RUPTURE

Oesophageal rupture usually occurs in the left lower oesophagus, but ruptures may also occasionally be seen on the right side, and even less commonly in the cervical oesophagus

Emergency Abdominal Surgery. Edited by Peter F. Jones, Zygmunt H. Krukowski and George G. Youngson. Published in 1998 by Chapman & Hall, London. ISBN 0 412 81950 3.

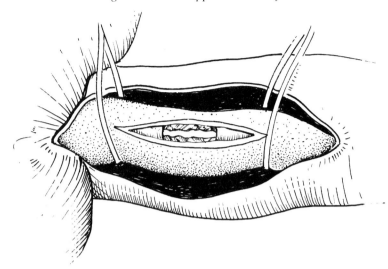

Figure 5.1 The ruptured oesophagus, as seen through a left thoracotomy. The defect in the pleura has been extended. The tear in the mucosa is often longer than the tear in the oesophageal musculature.

or in the intra-abdominal portion of oesophagus (Walsh, 1979). The rupture is generally 2–6 cm long but it is important to note that the tear in the mucosa (Figure 5.1) may be longer than the defect in the muscle fibres (Hughes, 1981). This can have implications when the surgeon is repairing the defect.

The pathogenesis of this condition has fascinated investigators for more than a century. In 1884 Mackenzie described experiments on cadaver oesophagus that necessitated filling the oesophagus with water after tying off the distal end. The oesophagus consistently ruptured longitudinally at the lower end. A more realistic experiment was performed on cadavers by Bodi *et al.* (1954), when oxygen was introduced into the stomach under pressure with the pylorus tied off. Eventually the oesophagus ruptured longitudinally in its lower third on the left side. It was noted that mucosa herniated through the muscle layers before rupture occurred. It was suggested that this tendency for the oesophagus to rupture may be exacerbated in some individuals by cricopharyngeus spasm as a result of incoordination of the vomiting reflex because of persistent vomiting (Bodi *et al.*, 1954).

5.1.3   CLINICAL PRESENTATION

Although oesophageal rupture is a thoracic emergency, it frequently presents with upper abdominal signs and symptoms. The typical patient is male, between 40 and 60 years old and has recently had a meal. More than 70% of patients will give a history of vomiting before the onset of pain (McFarlane and Munro, 1990). Sudden severe pain is often felt in the epigastrium or behind the sternum going through to the back. The pain is constant, relentless and very distressing. It may also spread towards the shoulders but not below the umbilicus. The patient feels short of breath and may look pale and cyanosed. Signs of shock usually supervene including peripheral vasoconstriction, low blood pressure and tachycardia.

Tenderness and guarding in the upper abdomen is a feature. The lower abdomen is usually relaxed. Chest signs include crepitus on the chest wall or at the root of the neck and clinical features of a pleural effusion or pneumothorax. A mediastinal crunch heard on auscultation of the praecordium is a helpful clinical sign of mediastinal emphysema (Hamman, 1934). Within a few hours there is a striking degree of surgical shock.

The diagnosis is often elusive and was made on admission in only two out of 14 cases in a recent study (Walker et al., 1985). The consequences of delay in diagnosis are very serious for the patient. Using collected data from the literature it has been shown that the mortality rate increases from 20% if the diagnosis is made within 6 hours to more than 50% if a diagnosis is delayed beyond 24 hours after the onset of symptoms (McFarlane and Munro, 1990).

Presentation at laparotomy

A patient with Boerhaave's syndrome may sometimes present with upper abdominal symptoms and signs and as a result have a laparotomy with a provisional diagnosis of perforated duodenal ulcer (two out of 13 patients in our series). In such circumstances it is important for the surgeon to perform a thorough laparotomy. If nothing obvious is found at operation it is crucial to examine the hiatus carefully to look for extravasated gastrointestinal content. The phreno-oesophageal membrane should be divided and lifted up with an artery forceps to allow dissection of the plane between the phreno-oesophageal membrane and the lower oesophagus. Since in most cases the tear is situated in the left lower oesophagus it is common to find blood-stained or bile-stained fluid with some food debris as soon as dissection of the lower oesophagus is undertaken.

5.1.4 INVESTIGATIONS

A chest radiograph should be done on admission if spontaneous rupture of the oesophagus is suspected. Gas is sometimes seen in the mediastinum outlining the mediastinal pleura (Walker *et al.*, 1985), and it may be visible in the soft tissues of the neck. Eventually in many cases a hydropneumothorax is seen on a chest radiograph (Walker *et al.*, 1985). If the chest radiograph is negative, it should be emphasized that a repeat chest radiograph a few hours after the first one is sometimes useful in the patient who has upper abdominal pain and there is a suspicion of either oesophageal perforation or peptic ulcer perforation.

The definitive diagnostic investigation is a water-soluble contrast study (Parkin, 1973). If there is difficulty in obtaining a contrast swallow because of the condition of the patient, fibre-optic endoscopy may be done with minimal air insufflation. We have used this method successfully in one patient who required intermittent positive pressure ventilation (IPPV) soon after admission. Alternatively, a nasogastric tube is passed into the stomach and slowly withdrawn while water-soluble contrast medium (e.g. gastrografin) is injected as the patient is screened by the radiologist. When the tip of the tube passes the rupture, extravasation is seen (Kerr, 1962). Serum amylase is usually normal but aspirate taken from a pleural effusion may well show a high amylase content. ECG in cases presenting with chest pain is an essential investigation. Liver function tests, including serum protein levels, are useful for baseline estimations. We have not found it necessary to resort to CT scanning in these patients to make a diagnosis.

5.1.5   DIFFERENTIAL DIAGNOSIS

Awareness of the possibility of Boerhaave's syndrome is the key to making the correct diagnosis in a patient presenting with upper abdominal or chest pain after vomiting or retching.

It is an unusual condition so more common disorders such as perforated peptic ulcer will be considered first. The sudden onset and site of pain in both disorders may be similar but the abdominal findings on examination are generally different. Upper abdominal tenderness and guarding are often found in Boerhaave's syndrome whereas in perforated peptic ulcer generalized tenderness and board-like rigidity are the usual features. The erect chest film will be useful in differentiating between the two conditions in many patients. The patient with a ruptured oesophagus rapidly becomes much more shocked than is usually seen in a perforated peptic ulcer.

Other possible diagnoses that will require to be considered include myocardial infarction, acute pancreatitis, acute dissection of the aorta, spontaneous pneumothorax and pulmonary embolus. These diagnoses will be less likely if the ECG, serum cardiac enzyme levels, serum amylase, chest radiograph and ventilation/perfusion lung scan and abdominal ultrasound are normal. Frequently it is only at this stage when initial investigations are negative that the clinician considers the possibility of spontaneous rupture of the oesophagus, particularly when faced with a patient who appears to be deteriorating rapidly.

5.1.6   MANAGEMENT

(a) Resuscitation

The spectrum of severity of illness at the time of presentation varies a great deal. Patients presenting with barogenic rupture of the oesophagus are often in poor condition as a result of delay in diagnosis, with resulting systemic sepsis. In these circumstances broad spectrum antibiotic therapy (e.g. a cephalosporin, a penicillin and metronidazole) to cover both aerobic Gram-positive and Gram-negative infection and anaerobic infection will be necessary. Hypotension may be a feature, resulting from hypovolaemia and poor cardiac output. These problems will require treatment with intravascular volume replacement and possibly inotropes. A number of our patients already had established adult respiratory distress syndrome at the time of presentation; a pleural effusion may be present which requires chest drainage. IPPV has been essential in a minority of our patients after admission. Monitoring using central venous pressure and Swan–Ganz catheters and arterial lines may be necessary and a urinary catheter must be inserted. These patients are best managed in an intensive therapy unit or high-dependency unit. Collaboration with the intensive therapy specialist and anaesthetist is very important in making decisions regarding both the resuscitation and eventual treatment of the patient, particularly the decision to operate.

In contrast, patients presenting acutely within a few hours of onset of symptoms may be haemodynamically stable and after administration of analgesia, investigation can be undertaken expeditiously over the succeeding few hours. If a diagnosis of oesophageal rupture is made, antibiotics should be commenced preoperatively and intravenous fluids administered. A chest drain should be inserted if there is evidence of a pleural effusion.

(b) Operative technique

Most patients with Boerhaave's syndrome should be managed surgically. In patients whose general condition is good, operation should be undertaken after initial resuscitation. Even in patients who present late but who have responded well to resuscitation, the consensus view is that surgery should be undertaken when shock has been successfully managed, mainly because there is often considerable improvement in the patient's condition after operation.

Thoracotomy or laparotomy?

If there is extensive contamination of the pleural cavity and the posterior mediastinum, there is no doubt that access in these circumstances is best achieved through a left thoracotomy. Our own practice is to perform a left thoracotomy through the seventh interspace after incising the periostium over the upper aspect of the eighth rib and then reflecting the periostium so that the pleural space is entered immediately above the rib. After the inferior pulmonary ligament is divided, debridement of the posterior mediastinum is carried out meticulously. Because we have added gastrostomy and feeding jejunostomy as an essential element in our routine management of patients with Boerhaave's syndrome, after completion of the thoracotomy we also make a short midline abdominal incision to allow insertion of a 24 FG Foley catheter into the stomach for drainage and a 14 FG Foley catheter into the upper jejunum for enteral feeding.

Although it was not our usual practice, two of 13 patients in our series had a laparotomy and no thoracotomy. One of these patients presented with oesophageal rupture secondary to gastrointestinal haemorrhage and, after excision of a gastric ulcer, the tear in the oesophagus was repaired and drained through the hiatus. In another patient who presented with oesophageal rupture and cardiogenic shock secondary to myocardial infarction, it was thought to be less traumatic for the patient to have a laparotomy rather than a thoracotomy. This was performed 2 weeks after admission. Drainage of the posterior mediastinum and suture of the oesophageal defect was possible through the hiatus and a feeding jejunostomy and gastrostomy was fashioned.

Should the oesophagus be repaired?

There is a tendency for the edges of the oesophageal rupture to be friable and sutures may cut out. This has resulted in some surgeons avoiding any attempt at primary repair and instead relying on adequate drainage of the mediastinum (Patton *et al.*, 1979). Our own view is that there is little to be lost by attempting to repair the rupture, even if more than 24 hours have elapsed after the rupture has taken place. All ten patients who had operation in our series had suture of the defect in the oesophagus performed. In five of these, primary healing occurred but the other five had some breakdown of the sutured oesophageal wound. If adequate drainage is provided (in our experience) the resulting fistula eventually heals.

Methods for suturing the oesophagus

The longitudinal tear in the mucosa may be longer than the defect in the muscle layers (Hughes, 1981). It is therefore important to inspect the rupture carefully and extend the incision in the musculature, if necessary, to gain adequate access to the mucosal defect. Some authors advocate closing the mucosa with absorbable suture material followed by closure of the muscle layer in one or two further layers of interrupted sutures (Hughes, 1981). In our experience the tissues may be very friable and separating the layers of the oesophagus has met with considerable difficulty. Although initially we tended to use single-layer interrupted sutures of 3/0 polyamide, more recently we have found a continuous suture technique through all layers of the oesophagus using continuous 3/0 monofilament polydioxanone on a 26 mm round-bodied needle to be very satisfactory. The advantage of monofilament suture material is that it tends not to cut so easily through the friable oesophageal tissue surrounding the rupture.

Other techniques

Because of unsatisfactory results with primary closure in some surgeons' hands many additional techniques for reinforcement of the repair have been described. These include fundoplication (Finley *et al.*, 1980), gastric patch (Thal and Hatafuku, 1964) and intercostal pedicle graft (Dooling and Zick, 1967).

If it is thought necessary to reinforce the repair, intact stomach is very useful material since the blood supply is so good and the stomach is easily mobilized. Creation of a controlled oesophageal fistula by T-tube drainage has been found to be a reliable method of management by some surgeons (Harrison *et al.*, 1976). Other surgeons have advocated exclusion of the oesophagus (Urschel *et al.*, 1974). If there is extensive necrosis of the oesophagus then total oesophagectomy with exteriorization of the cervical oesophagus and closure of the oesophagogastric junction and gastrostomy may be life-saving (Mayer *et al.*, 1977). We have no experience in using any of the reinforcing methods in closing the oesophageal defect.

Thoracoscopic repair

In the last 8 years many operations that were previously dealt with by conventional open surgery have been attempted using minimal access techniques. Repair of spontaneous rupture of the oesophagus is no exception. Scott and Rosin in 1995 described a patient who presented with a 12-hour history of severe chest pain after vomiting. After resuscitation the patient was operated on using video thoracoscopy performed through the left chest. The pleural cavity was thoroughly washed out using the thoracoscopic technique and after mobilizing the oesophagus it was possible to repair the rupture using interrupted polyglactin sutures. The patient made a straightforward recovery. Further experience is required before a judgement can be reached about the place of thoracoscopic intervention in treating patients with Boerhaave's syndrome.

Decompression of the upper gastrointestinal tract

Decompression using a nasogastric tube is only useful in the short term for patients who have oesophageal repair for spontaneous rupture: as a long-term measure it is uncomfortable for the patient and encourages gastro-oesophageal reflux. We prefer to insert a gastrostomy tube for this purpose.

Drainage

There is fairly general agreement that good drainage is vital for a successful outcome. This is best achieved by inserting under-water seal drains in both the mediastinum and the appropriate pleural cavity.

(c) Conservative treatment

The contrast swallow is helpful not only in making a diagnosis of barogenic rupture but also in determining whether the leak is (1) localized to the mediastinum or (2) involves either pleural cavity. In the unusual situation when there is a localized leak conservative treatment has been advocated as the management of choice. Cameron *et al.* (1979) suggested that conservative management is appropriate if the following circumstances pertain.

1. The rupture should be well contained within the mediastinum on contrast swallow examination. There should be free drainage back into the oesophagus from the rupture.
2. Minimal symptoms should be present.
3. There should be minimal evidence of sepsis.

In our own experience of managing 13 patients with Boerhaave's syndrome, one male patient was diagnosed to have a localized rupture (diagnosed 2 days after a negative laparotomy in another hospital for suspected duodenal ulcer) and was treated successfully using a conservative approach.

It is crucial to stress that although this approach may find widespread acceptance, localized leak represents an uncommon form of Boerhaave's syndrome. Conservative management of such patients will include continued broad-spectrum antibiotic therapy, nasogastric drainage to prevent gastric content refluxing into the posterior mediastinum and nutritional support. Repeat contrast radiological study 1 week after commencing therapy will be useful to see if the leak has remained localized. Conservative management using these methods will only be necessary for a few weeks in most patients with localized leak.

Another group of patients with Boerhaave's syndrome who are best managed conservatively are those with intrapleural leak who are too ill to be considered for surgical intervention, particularly those who present more than 24 hours after the onset of symptoms. Only small numbers of such patients have been reported in the literature and any form of treatment in this group, who are already severely debilitated, is likely to be associated with higher mortality. Our experience consists of managing five patients conservatively who presented late with intrapleural leak. One of these patients presented with multisystem organ failure from rupture of the oesophagus. She was in a very poor condition and it was felt that the only possible way to manage her was conservatively. A further patient presented with chest wall gangrene secondary to spontaneous oesophageal rupture a few years after left thoracotomy for resectable bronchial carcinoma. The only surgical intervention necessary on this patient was drainage of an abscess in his previous thoracotomy wound, insertion of a chest drain and later debridement of the chest wall. Although the hospital stay for both patients was prolonged ($3\frac{1}{2}$ months for the patient with multisystem organ failure) both made a good recovery. A further three patients were initially managed conservatively but surgical intervention was carried out at a later date. In one of these, operation was required for secondary bleeding from the oesophageal tear. The other two were operated on after some weeks of conservative treatment in the belief that, although their condition had improved, their recovery would be hastened by closure of the oesophagopleural fistula. Since that time we have increased experience of conservative management and it is possible that if similar patients presented now, we would continue conservative therapy.

The communication between the oesophagus and pleural cavity is a continued source of mediastinal and intrapleural sepsis in patients with Boerhaave's syndrome who are treated conservatively. It has been suggested that the application of stenting techniques may be a means of extending the role of conservative management. Agarwal and Miller (1995) reported the use of an Atkinson tube to seal an oesophagopleural fistula resulting from spontaneous rupture of the oesophagus. A covered metal expandable stent has also been used to seal the oesophageal leak in a patient who presented with delayed diagnosis but its use is not currently recommended by the manufacturers for benign conditions.

(d) Nutritional support

Most patients with Boerhaave's syndrome will require nutritional support during their stay in hospital. It is useful to consider how long nutritional support may be required at the outset of treatment since this may have a bearing on the chosen route for providing nutrition. If the patient is being treated conservatively for a localized oesophageal leak and it is anticipated that oral feeding will be possible within 2–3 weeks, parenteral nutrition using peripheral access may be all that is necessary. Alternatively, patients who have an intrapleural leak with multisystem organ failure will require many weeks or months of nutritional support and provision should be made for long-term feeding.

Although total parenteral nutrition (TPN) has been used as a short-term measure for some of our patients, we have increasingly used the enteral route *via* a jejunostomy when long-term feeding is anticipated. The cost of providing enteral nutrition is less and the enteral route avoids the catheter-related problems of TPN. There is an increasing awareness of the need to preserve gut mucosal integrity as a barrier to translocation of bacteria and endotoxin (Deitch, 1994). The presence of nutrients in the gut lumen appears to be the most important stimulus for maintaining gut integrity while TPN has been shown to be associated with mucosal atrophy (Alverdy *et al.*, 1985) and promotes bacterial translocation. There is now convincing evidence that postoperative septic complications are diminished with enteral compared to parenteral nutrition (Moore *et al.*, 1992).

5.1.7   OUTCOME

Although up to the middle of the 20th century Boerhaave's syndrome was a lethal condition, since then the outlook has gradually improved, although many recent series still fail to achieve acceptable results. We have treated 13 patients over the past 13 years without mortality. It is of interest that other reports with mortality rates of 10% or less over the past 25 years emphasize the value of treatment using primary closure of the oesophageal rupture, good drainage and antibiotic therapy (Finley *et al.*, 1980; Richardson *et al.*, 1985; Sabanthan *et al.*, 1994). This is a condition that taxes the diagnostic and therapeutic judgement of the surgeon. It is not common, and the outcome very much depends on awareness of Boerhaave's syndrome and the quality of management.

REFERENCES

Agarwal, P. K. and Miller, S. E. P. (1995) Spontaneous rupture of the oesophagus: case report of a delayed diagnosis and subsequent management. *J. R. Soc. Med.*, **88**, 149–150.

Alverdy, J. C., Chi, H. S. and Sheldon, G. F. (1985) The effect of route of parenteral nutrition on gastrointestinal immunity: the importance of enteral stimulation. *Ann. Surg.*, **202**, 681–684.

Barrett, N. R. (1947) Report of a case of spontaneous perforation of the oesophagus successfully treated by operation. *Br. J. Surg.*, **35**, 216–218.

Bodi, T., Fanger, H. and Forsythe, T. (1954) Spontaneous rupture of the esophagus. *Ann. Intern. Med.*, **41**, 553–562.

Cameron, J. L., Kieffer, R. F., Hendrix, T. R. *et al.* (1979) Selective nonoperative management of contained intrathoracic esophageal disruptions. *Ann. Thorac. Surg.*, **27**, 404–408.

Deitch, E. A. (1994) Bacterial translocation: the influence of dietary variables. *Gut Suppl.*, **1**, S23–S27.

Derbes, V. J. and Mitchell, R. E. (1955) Hermann Boerhaave's *Atrocis nec descripti prius morbi historia*. The first translation of the classic case report of rupture of the esophagus with annotations. *Bull. Med. Libr. Assoc.*, **43**, 217–239.

Dooling, J. A. and Zick, H. R. (1967) Closure of an esophagopleural fistula using only intercostal pedicle graft. *Ann. Thorac. Surg.*, **3**, 553–557.

Finley, R. J., Pearson, F. G., Weisel, R. D. *et al.* (1980) The management of non-malignant intrathoracic esophageal perforations. *Ann. Thorac. Surg.*, **30**, 575–583.

Griffith, R. S. (1932) Spontaneous rupture of the esophagus. *Pennsylvania Med. J.*, **35**, 639.

Hamman, L. (1934) Spontaneous mediastinal emphysema. *Bull. Johns Hopkins Hosp.*, **64**, 1–21.

Harrison, M. W., Lindell, T. D. and Brant, B. (1976) Surgical treatment of late esophageal perforations. *Am. Surgeon*, **42**, 488–491.

Hughes, L. E. (1981) Spontaneous oesophageal perforation. *Br. J. Surg.*, **68**, 294.

Kennard, H. W. H. (1950) Rupture of the esophagus during childbirth. *BMJ*, **i**, 417.

Kerr, I. H. (1962) A method of demonstrating the site of a perforation of the oesophagus. *Br. J. Radiol.*, **35**, 255–260.

Kinsella, T. J., Morse, R. N. and Hertzog, A. J. (1948) Spontaneous rupture of the esophagus. *J. Thorac. Surg.*, **17**, 613–631.

Lawson, R. A. M., Butchart, E. G., Soriano, A. *et al.* (1974) Spontaneous rupture of the oesophagus. *J. R. Coll. Surg. Edin.*, **19**, 363–369.

McFarlane, G. A. and Munro, A. (1990) The changing face of the management of ruptured oesophagus: Boerhaave's Syndrome. *Gullet*, **1**, 16–23.

MacKenzie, M. (1884) *Diseases of the Ear, Nose and Throat*, vol. 2, J. A. Churchill, London, p. 160.

Mayer, J. E., Murray, C. A. and Varco, R. L. (1977) The treatment of esophageal perforation with delayed recognition and continuing sepsis. *Ann. Thorac. Surg.*, **23**, 568–573.

Moore, F. A., Feliciano, D. V., Andrassy, R. J. *et al.* (1992) Early enteral feeding, compared with parenteral reduces postoperative septic complications. The results of a meta-analysis. *Ann. Surg.*, **216**, 172–183.

Parkin, G. J. S. (1973) The radiology of perforated oesophagus. *Clin. Radiol.*, **24**, 324–332.

Patton, A. S., Lawson, D. W., Shannon, J. M. *et al.* (1979) Re-evaluation of the Boerhaave Syndrome. A review of fourteen cases. *Am. J. Surg.*, **137**, 560–565.

Richardson, J. D., Martin, L. F., Borzotta, A. P. *et al.* (1985) Unifying concepts in treatment of esophageal leaks. *Am. J. Surg.*, **149**, 157–162.

Sabanthan, S., Eng, J. and Richardson, J. (1994) Surgical management of intrathoracic oesophageal rupture. *Br. J. Surg.*, **81**, 863–865.

Scott, H. J. and Rosin, R. D. (1995) Thoracoscopic repair of a transmural rupture of the oesophagus (Boerhaave's Syndrome). *J. R. Soc. Med.*, **88**, 414–415.

Thal, A. P. and Hatafuku, T. (1964) Improved operation for an esophageal rupture. *J.A.M.A.*, **188**, 826–828.

Urschel, H. C., Razzuk, M. A., Wood, R. E. *et al.* (1974) Improved management of esophageal perforation: exclusion and diversion in continuity. *Ann. Surg.*, **179**, 587–591.

Walker, W. S., Cameron, E. W. J. and Walbaum, P. R (1985) Diagnosis and management of spontaneous transmural rupture of the oesophagus (Boerhaave's Syndrome). *Br. J. Surg.*, **72**, 204–207.

Walsh, P. V. (1979) Rupture of the abdominal oesophagus: a review. *Br. J. Surg.*, **66**, 601–606

5.2 PERFORATED PEPTIC ULCER

5.2.1 BACKGROUND

Little was written about perforated ulcers of the stomach and the duodenum until, in the 19th century, autopsies were increasingly being performed and it became clear that this was the cause of death in a number of young women who had collapsed with abdominal pain. It is believed that Kriege in 1892 was the first medical practitioner to describe the successful management of a case. He summoned Heissner, a surgeon, (by telegram!) to a man of 41 whom Kriege believed had suffered a perforation. The patient was operated on at home by candlelight when, after a long search, a gastric perforation was sutured. The patient's convalescence was complicated by an empyema, which was drained. This successful case was followed quickly by others and in the UK both Morse of Norwich and MacLaren of Carlisle described successful surgical management of gastric ulcer perforation in 1894. In the same year Dean (1894) from the London Hospital was the first to describe successful suture of a perforated duodenal ulcer. An interesting feature of perforated peptic ulcer at this time was the fact that most of the patients who presented with the condition were females in their late teens or early twenties. They were often domestic servants and the perforation tended to occur high on the lesser curve of the stomach.

This preponderance of young women gave way to a steadily rising incidence of duodenal ulcerations in men. Throughout the first half of the 20th century the incidence of perforated peptic ulcer increased, and was closely followed in Glasgow. The annual incidence (per 100 000 of the population) was 11 in 1924, 19 in 1930, 30 in 1940 and 32 in 1950. Thereafter the incidence declined to 24 per 100 000 in 1971 (Illingworth *et al.*, 1944; MacKay, 1966, 1977). In Oxford, equivalent figures were 10 per 100 000 in 1960 and 7 per 100 000 in 1972–1982 (Watkins *et al.*, 1984). Although changing patterns have also been seen in other countries the trends have not always been in the same direction. In Hong Kong there was a 46% increase in the number of perforations treated between 1970 and 1980 (Koo *et al.*, 1983).

The introduction of H_2-receptor antagonists in 1976 gave clinicians an effective treatment for peptic ulcer for the first time and since then proton pump inhibitors have been introduced. More recently, treatment for *Helicobacter pylori* has changed the pattern of management for these patients. A recent study by Jibril *et al.* (1994) has shown a continued decline in perforated duodenal ulcer in Scotland. In 1975 the rate was 27 per 100 000 of the population whereas in 1990 the perforation rate was down to 15 per 100 000 of the population. In recent years perforated peptic ulcer has become a relatively unusual emergency.

Sex incidence

Since the beginning of the 20th century perforated duodenal ulcer has mainly been a disease of men but recently the male:female ratio has been falling. In 1924–1933 the ratio of males to females in Glasgow was 19:1 whereas by 1964–1973 the ratio had fallen to 4.4:1 (MacKay, 1977). In the recent study by Jibril *et al.* (1994) a further change has been demonstrated between 1975 and 1990. The male:female ratio of duodenal ulcer perforations was 3.7:1 in 1975 whereas in 1990 it was 1.5:1.

Age at perforation

Perforation of the stomach or duodenum in childhood or the early teens is a rarity. However in a study by Hendry *et al.* (1984) from Aberdeen it was demonstrated that out of a total of 398 perforated ulcers 4.5% were males between 14 and 20 years and 6.4% were between 21 and 30. Between 1960 and 1980 the incidence of perforation fell in men of all ages in the UK but in women over 65 there was a rise of 200% (Walt *et al.*, 1986). This rise has continued in women aged 65 and over, with rates increasing from 21 per 100 000 to 41 per 100 000 between 1975 and 1990 in Scotland (Jibril *et al.*, 1994).

5.2.2 *HELICOBACTER PYLORI* AND PERFORATED PEPTIC ULCER

Marshall and Warren first emphasized the potential importance of S-shaped spiral bacteria in the stomach of patients with gastritis in 1983. The following year the same authors reported that these *Campylobacter*-like organisms could be found in the gastric antrum of 95–100% of patients with active duodenal ulcer and in 70% of patients with gastric ulcer (Marshall and Warren, 1984). The organism was renamed *Helicobacter pylori* (HP) in 1989. Since then it has become generally accepted that HP is a major factor in the aetiology of peptic ulcer. Eradication of the organism leads to healing of the ulcer in most patients and also reduces the risk of recurrence: the relapse rate of peptic ulcer at 12–18 months was 65% in patients who remained HP-positive but only 3% in those who became HP-negative (Bell and Powell, 1993).

The relationship between perforated peptic ulcer and *Helicobacter* infection has also been recently investigated. Reinbach and colleagues (1993) from Glasgow reported a low prevalence of *Helicobacter* infection of 47% in a series of patients with acute duodenal ulcer perforations, which was not significantly higher than the general population. However, Ng *et al.* (1996) in Hong Kong found that 70% of their 70 patients with perforated duodenal ulcers had infection with HP; a possible explanation may lie with the percentage of patients in each series who were taking non-steroidal anti-inflammatory drugs (NSAIDs). In the Glasgow series, more than 40% of patients were taking NSAIDs whereas in the Hong Kong series only 18% were taking these drugs. It is well known that only a small percentage of patients with perforated ulcer due to NSAIDs are HP-positive and it has been suggested that HP infection and NSAID usage may be two different causes of perforated peptic ulcer (Ng *et al.*, 1997). If the patients taking NSAIDs were excluded from each series the percentage of patients who have *Helicobacter* infection would be broadly similar and of the same order as patients with non-perforated duodenal ulcer. Thus it seems likely that HP is an important aetiological factor in perforated peptic ulcer.

5.2.3 NON-STEROIDAL ANTI-INFLAMMATORY DRUGS IN PERFORATED PEPTIC ULCER

It has been suggested that the dramatic rise in the incidence of perforated peptic ulcer in women over the age of 65 is related to the usage of NSAIDs. Collier and Pain in 1985 found that, among 269 patients with perforated peptic ulcer, NSAIDs were taken by 47% of 168 patients over the age of 65 years compared with 7% of 168 controls of the same age. In a more recent study of 80 patients, approximately half of all patients with a perforated peptic ulcer were taking NSAIDs (Horowitz *et al.*, 1989).

5.2.4 THE ULCERS

Perforated ulcers may be situated in the duodenum, pyloric or prepyloric area or elsewhere in the stomach. In most studies, patients with prepyloric and pyloric ulcers are included in the duodenal ulcer group because they tend to share many of the characteristics of duodenal ulcers (Horowitz *et al.*, 1989) whereas gastric ulcers are considered separately. The ratio of duodenal ulcer:gastric ulcer varies widely. Studies showed a ratio of 8.8:1 in Oxford

(Watkins *et al.*, 1984), 12:1 in Glasgow in 1978–1980 (McKay and McCardle, 1982) and 25:1 in Aberdeen (Hendry *et al.*, 1984).

The term 'acute ulcer' generally refers to patients with a history of less than 3 months and 'chronic ulcer' denotes patients with a significantly longer history before perforation. At operation acute ulcer perforations appear as a round hole in the duodenum with a pale, smooth, sharply defined margin but it should be noted that around 30% of patients who have a history of 'acute ulcer' will have scarring of the duodenum at operation.

The mean size of perforated duodenal ulcers in one report was 10 mm whereas the equivalent size for perforated gastric ulcers was 30 mm (Horowitz *et al.*, 1989). Perforated duodenal ulcers are most commonly seen in the anterior or antero-superior aspect of the first part of the duodenum whereas perforated gastric ulcers are usually situated on the lesser curve of the stomach. Most gastric ulcers perforate anteriorly with only 9% perforating posteriorly (Hodnett *et al.*, 1989). Perforated duodenal ulcers are never malignant whereas a varying proportion of perforated gastric ulcers eventually turn out to be cancerous. In a recent study of 202 patients with perforated gastric ulcer, 183 patients had biopsy material taken and of these ten were malignant (Hodnett *et al.*, 1989).

5.2.5　CLINICAL PRESENTATION

Most patients with perforated peptic ulcer will complain of the very sudden onset of severe pain in the upper abdomen. They can often remember just what they were doing at the time. The pain, which is constant and very severe, tends to be situated in the upper abdomen initially but quickly spreads to the whole abdomen. In addition, spread of gastrointestinal contents to the undersurface of the diaphragm produces referred pain to the shoulder area and the patient may have marked difficulty in breathing. Vomiting is also a frequent feature.

It is important to enquire about previous symptoms of indigestion and abdominal pain, particularly to ask if the diagnosis of peptic ulcer has ever been made, and to ask about the drug history, especially whether the patient has taken NSAIDs or corticosteroids. The surgeon should also enquire about previous medication for ulcer symptoms and in particular whether endoscopy has been performed and if so, whether *Helicobacter pylori* has been found and treated.

Patients with a perforated ulcer tend to lie still with a quick, shallow breathing pattern. Pallor is common and sweating is frequently evident. There may be signs of peripheral vasoconstriction, but these patients are not in surgical shock unless the perforation occurred many hours earlier, when they may show tachycardia and hypotension. In addition to the abdomen being tender in most cases there will be evidence of board-like rigidity due to spasm of the abdominal wall muscles. So tight is the abdomen that rebound tenderness is not obtainable. If the perforation is still localized to the upper abdomen, guarding and tenderness in the upper abdomen may be the only features. Liver dullness is usually replaced by a resonant note on percussion. Bowel sounds may or may not be audible.

The classical symptoms and signs are modified in some patients, particularly in the elderly and in those who are immunosuppressed or on corticosteroids. One of the most hazardous times for a patient to sustain a perforated ulcer is in the postoperative period after an entirely unrelated abdominal procedure, since abdominal pain and clinical signs will be interpreted in the light of the recent operation, rather than any new illness. Diagnosis is often delayed in patients who are in medical wards with other illnesses.

5.2.6 INVESTIGATIONS

The most useful radiological investigation in patients with suspected perforated peptic ulcer is the plain antero-posterior chest radiograph taken in the upright position to include the diaphragm and upper part of the abdomen. Because the patient is in pain, help is frequently required in the Radiology Department to keep the patient as upright as possible. Intraperitoneal gas may be visible under either diaphragm, around the stomach or below the liver. During the first 8 hours after perforation, around 50–60% of patients will have a positive chest radiograph, and after 8 hours intraperitoneal gas is seen in over 80% of patients (Lee *et al.*, 1977).

If the plain chest film is negative a water-soluble contrast study of the oesophagus, stomach and duodenum may be helpful. Fraser and Fraser (1974) studied 25 patients with perforated duodenal ulcer, using water-soluble contrast, and there was leakage of contrast material in 21. In a further three patients, although there was no leakage of contrast, there was free intraperitoneal gas on the plain film. The only patient who had no leakage of contrast or intraperitoneal gas proved to have a sealed ulcer at operation. If the water-soluble contrast study shows no evidence of leak it may be worthwhile obtaining an ultrasound examination of the abdomen to see if there is free fluid in the abdomen. The fluid can be aspirated to determine its nature.

Serum amylase estimation should be performed along with a full blood count and serum urea and electrolyte estimation. Although very high levels of serum amylase will point the diagnosis more towards pancreatitis, it should be realized that high levels may be seen in patients with perforated ulcer or intestinal ischaemia, and this is discussed on p. 383.

5.2.7 DIFFERENTIAL DIAGNOSIS

Although in a typical case there will be no major difficulty in making a diagnosis of perforated peptic ulcer, in other situations the diagnosis is elusive and valuable time elapses before the patient has appropriate treatment. Perforation of a duodenal ulcer occasionally produces mainly right-sided signs, and tenderness may be most marked in the RLQ. The sudden onset is unlike **acute appendicitis**, but this is a much commoner emergency than a perforation and sometimes a right gridiron incision can justifiably be made first in an obese patient when the diagnosis is in real doubt (p. 61).

Perforations of other parts of the gastrointestinal tract also lead to diagnostic confusion, particularly when the erect chest X-ray shows intraperitoneal gas. Although **perforated diverticulitis** will usually cause lower abdominal pain in the first instance, by the time many patients come to hospital there will be generalized abdominal tenderness and guarding; in both cases exploration is necessary.

Mesenteric vascular occlusion sometimes mimics the symptoms and signs of perforated peptic ulcer if the patient is seen more than 12–24 hours after the onset of symptoms. At an early stage, mesenteric vascular occlusion will present with very severe abdominal pain without dramatic abdominal signs but in the succeeding 12–24 hours abdominal signs similar to those of perforated peptic ulcer and hypovolaemic shock will be seen in both cases.

Although the pain of **ruptured abdominal aortic aneurysm** is sometimes felt in the upper abdomen, more commonly the patient also has backache and loin pain. Fainting and hypotension associated with the onset of abdominal pain are common associated features of ruptured abdominal aortic aneurysm.

Strangulating obstruction of the small bowel presents with severe onset of mid-abdominal pain rather than upper abdominal pain and abdominal signs may not be prominent initially. A plain radiograph of the abdomen will usually show dilated loops of small bowel, a feature not usually seen in patients with perforated peptic ulcer.

Intraperitoneal haemorrhage can present in the guise of a perforated peptic ulcer, as in the case of the woman described on p. 456. Ruptured tubal pregnancy can cause sudden generalized abdominal pain, with shoulder pain and diffuse tenderness and guarding. The early evidence of hypovolaemia, a history of menstrual irregularity, and the relative rarity of a perforated ulcer in a young woman should suggest the diagnosis.

Acute cholecystitis is another condition that produces features similar to perforated peptic ulcer. The patient with cholecystitis initially complains of severe midline upper abdominal pain and a few hours later the pain and tenderness tend to settle in the right upper quadrant. Unless the gallbladder has ruptured, the abdominal signs will tend to be more localized to the right upper quadrant and the rest of the abdomen is usually soft and less tender.

Acute pancreatitis can be a difficult differential diagnosis. In most cases of perforated ulcer the almost immediate onset of diffuse abdominal tenderness and rigidity is quite different to the severe pain but relatively moderate epigastric tenderness of pancreatitis. However, in a few patients with perforation the signs can be consistent with pancreatitis, the serum amylase can be raised and there may be no gas under the diaphragm (p. 383). Diagnostic peritoneal aspiration and a water-soluble contrast study can be very helpful.

Close attention to the history, particularly pain coming on after an episode of vomiting, sometimes points towards **Boerhaave's syndrome**. Boerhaave's syndrome is often diagnosed as perforated peptic ulcer and if the patient is operated on for suspected perforated peptic ulcer the diagnosis of ruptured oesophagus may be missed with disastrous consequences: in this event, with no perforation found, it is crucial that the surgeon examines the hiatus to look for extravasated gastrointestinal contents. It is essential to open the peritoneum overlying the abdominal oesophagus so that the lower oesophagus can be explored (see p. 159).

5.2.8   MANAGEMENT

After a diagnosis of perforated peptic ulcer is made time must be spent improving the patient's condition. With the rise in incidence of perforated peptic ulcer in the elderly female population, many patients will have coincidental medical problems that require attention.

Once a diagnosis is made there is no merit in withholding analgesia, and opiate drugs will usually be required to make the patient comfortable. A nasogastric tube should be inserted, the stomach should be aspirated and the tube should be placed on free drainage. Intravenous fluids will be necessary and the volume of crystalloid or colloid given will depend on the estimate of deficit of intravascular volume as well as overall fluid balance. In patients who have had the perforation for more than 24 hours who are hypotensive and dehydrated a urinary catheter should be inserted and hourly urine volume measurements made. Even if the patient has a history of only a few hours of abdominal pain at the time of admission it is reasonable to give broad-spectrum antibiotic therapy intravenously as soon as the diagnosis of perforation is made, although these need not be continued postoperatively in uncomplicated acute perforation with rapid treatment. Antibiotics become more important with increasing delay to diagnosis and treatment because bacterial overgrowth in the peritoneal cavity is inevitable.

Conservative management

By the time the operation is performed some perforated duodenal ulcers are sealed by a plug of omentum, and this has encouraged surgeons to capitalize on nature's way of dealing with a perforation and treat patients conservatively. The first major trial of conservative treatment was undertaken by Hermon Taylor at the King George Hospital, Ilford from 1944 onwards.

A protocol for management was devised and consisted of the following steps.

1. When the patient is admitted and the history and clinical findings are suggestive of perforated peptic ulcer, analgesia is given. A large orogastric tube is passed to empty the stomach and a nasogastric tube is then inserted.
2. An erect antero-posterior chest X-ray is taken to include the diaphragms and a further radiograph taken of the upper abdomen to demonstrate the position of the nasogastric tube. The diagnosis is critically reviewed if no gas is seen under the diaphragm.
3. The nasogastric tube is aspirated at 15-minute intervals and the result is recorded. Regular blood pressure and pulse rate recordings are taken and an intravenous infusion is set up.
4. If the treatment is successful the patient will begin to feel better and the pain tends to ease over the succeeding few hours.
5. A further erect chest radiograph is taken at 12 hours. If treatment is successful the amount of subdiaphragmatic gas should be less. If gas increases or pain is worse, operation is necessary.
6. Aspiration is continued until gastrointestinal function returns.

In 1957 Taylor reported 10 years experience of managing 256 patients with perforated ulcer, 208 of whom had been treated by the conservative method. Of the 79 patients with acute ulcer only two died. There were 177 patients who were considered to have chronic ulcer and of these 15% died. When followed up, only 14% were symptom-free and over half the patients had required surgery for their ulcer. Of 22 patients with gastric ulcer, seven died postoperatively.

There are two contraindications to conservative treatment.

*   It should not be attempted if there is reason to believe that the ulcer is **chronic or sited in the stomach**, because these ulcers rarely seal spontaneously.
*   It should not, in general, be applied to patients 'not fit for operation'. The reason for this is often the presence of a large volume of irritant gastric content in the peritoneal cavity. They need rapid resuscitation and, as soon as there is a reasonable response, laparotomy and thorough cleansing of the abdomen before closure of the perforation. This removal of the source of their severe illness offers these patients the only hope of recovery.

Because of the perception that the results of treatment were indifferent, conservative treatment of the perforated peptic ulcer never gained widespread acceptance. However a randomized trial was reported in 1989 from Hong Kong comparing conservative treatment with operative treatment for perforated peptic ulcer (Crofts *et al.*, 1989). Of 83 patients entered into the study, 40 were randomized to conservative treatment and 43 to surgical treatment. There was no clear advantage demonstrated for conservative management. It did not suit older patients, and four carcinomas (three gastric and one in the sigmoid colon) were found among the 83 patients. Eleven of the 40 patients treated conservatively had to be operated on after 12 hours observation. However, the authors concluded that in patients who are thought to have perforated peptic ulcer it is worthwhile considering an initial period of conservative treatment in those under 70 years of age.

It should be emphasized that conservative management is demanding, and judgement regarding when to operate in these patients is difficult. There is always the concern that a different condition needing urgent operative treatment is present. It is also clear that patients whom surgeons would like to treat conservatively, i.e. the unfit and the elderly, are those who do least well on conservative therapy. For these reasons, conservative treatment is still rightly not a popular option except in certain circumstances. These are:

- where there is clinical evidence that the perforation is already sealed; in a typical case the water-soluble contrast study suggests that the perforation has already sealed, or the symptoms and signs subside quickly after commencement of conservative treatment;
- in patients who are at exceptionally high risk from surgery, e.g. patients who have had recent myocardial infarction, or have other grave chronic diseases;
- in patients who are living in isolated places or at sea and are far from surgical help.

Operative treatment for perforated duodenal ulcer

There have been dramatic changes in both the elective and emergency management of peptic ulcer in the past few years. Since eradication of *Helicobacter pylori* from the stomach results in healing of duodenal ulcer in most patients, elective operations for chronic peptic ulcer are now rarely performed. This has resulted in problems of maintaining the skills of trained surgeons and catering for the needs of trainees, who rarely see and infrequently perform elective peptic ulcer surgery. More recently there has been a considerable overall reduction in the incidence of perforated peptic ulcer in the UK (Jibril *et al.*, 1994) so that surgeons have also become much less experienced in managing difficult cases of perforated peptic ulcer. At the same time there has been a concomitant increase in the proportion of patients with perforated peptic ulcer who are elderly women and are less fit for emergency operative procedures.

At laparotomy, most surgeons will use a midline incision. The size of the incision depends on many factors but it is important that it is long enough to allow the surgeon to visualize the perforation adequately and aspirate and lavage the whole peritoneal cavity. General anaesthesia will be used in the vast majority of patients but suture of a perforation is feasible under local anaesthetic in a patient who is unfit for general anaesthesia.

In some cases food debris and bile-stained fluid are spread throughout the peritoneal cavity; in others the perforation produces minimal contamination. As much fibrinous material as possible is removed from the peritoneal cavity and, if there is a fibrinous film overlying the diaphragmatic surface of the liver, this should be removed by careful mopping and irrigation. If the perforation occurred several days before operation and there are collections of infected material between loops of small bowel, the small bowel should be exteriorized and cleaned thoroughly. Lavage of the peritoneal cavity should be performed with several litres of physiological saline warmed to body temperature. Finally, a litre of 0.1% tetracycline solution in physiological saline is poured into the peritoneal cavity. After a few minutes most of this can be removed by suction. Attention is then turned to the perforated ulcer.

Simple suture

Most perforated duodenal ulcers will be suitable for simple closure. However, large perforated ulcers that involve a significant part of the circumference of the duodenum should not be sutured because (1) there is a significant risk of breakdown of the repair and (2) there is a risk of producing pyloric stenosis.

Closure of a small ulcer is straightforward (Figure 5.2). Three sutures are placed, one above the ulcer, one through the ulcer and the third below it. The middle suture should be placed at least 1 cm on either side of the perforation so that the tendency to cut out is reduced. Although chromic catgut has been used in the past for this purpose, a 3/0 polydioxanone or 3/0 polyglactin suture on a round-bodied half-circle 26 mm needle is now preferred. A tag of omentum is brought up to the perforation and the sutures are tied over it, closing the perforation.

Laparoscopic repair of perforated duodenal ulcer was first reported in 1990 by Mouret and colleagues. Since then a number of different techniques of closure of the perforation have been described, including both sutureless and sutured methods. It is evident from the surgical literature that adequate lavage of the peritoneal cavity can be achieved by the laparoscopic route. A recent randomized study (Lau *et al.*, 1996) designed to compare open techniques with laparoscopic repair of perforated duodenal ulcer concluded that the amount of analgesia required after a laparoscopic repair was less than after open surgery, but laparoscopic repair took significantly longer than open repair and there was no significant difference in hospital stay. The randomized trial also included a comparison of sutured with sutureless laparoscopic repair. Suture repair was done using an extracorporeal knotting technique. The sutureless

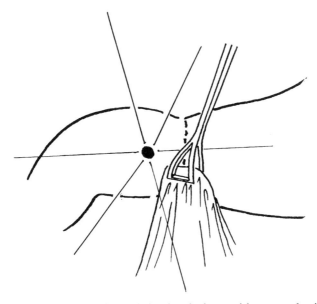

Figure 5.2 Suture closure of a perforated duodenal ulcer, with omental reinforcement.

method consisted of inserting a piece of gelatin sponge into the perforation and fibrin glue was used to fix the gelatin sponge in the perforation, the latter method proving to be significantly the quicker. A limiting factor of laparoscopic repair is that peptic ulcer perforations greater than 1 cm in diameter cannot be satisfactorily repaired, and a further problem is the difficulty in obtaining the experience required to acquire the necessary skills. Because of the small numbers of perforated ulcers seen in the UK and the fact that not all surgeons have the necessary training, it seems unlikely that laparoscopic repair of perforated ulcer will become the method of choice of repair of perforated duodenal ulcer in the foreseeable future.

The outcome of sutured closure of a pyloroduodenal ulcer is uncertain. For a truly acute ulcer the immediate outlook is good, and the likelihood of further ulceration fairly low: in 120 acute ulcers oversewn in Aberdeen, 24% later had recurrence of dyspepsia and 14% required surgery for a recurrent ulcer (Valerio *et al.*, 1985). Suture closure of chronic ulcers is more risky. Among 125 such patients, 14 bled after the operation, four had to return to theatre and seven died. Three re-perforated and eight developed outlet obstruction, of whom five required another operation. On follow-up 60% had a recurrent ulcer and 50% later required a definitive ulcer operation (Valerio *et al.*, 1985).

Some care is therefore needed in selecting patients for simple closure. Fortunately the older patients, who are most at risk, have a higher proportion of acute ulcers, so the shorter simpler operation is a reasonable choice in most of these patients, followed by *H. pylori* eradication therapy, if appropriate.

Definitive surgery
In the first half of this century, when duodenal ulcer was common, most elective surgical operating lists would contain at least one patient who needed a partial gastrectomy to terminate a long history of pain, often complicated by perforation or haemorrhage. In about 1933 Yudin in Moscow decided that when a patient with such a history perforated, it was sensible, provided the patient was fit, to perform the gastrectomy there and then, rather than close the perforation, wait for the probable recurrence of symptoms and then perform the gastrectomy electively. As vagotomy and a drainage operation was increasingly practised this operation supplanted gastrectomy (Boey *et al.*, 1982). In Aberdeen during 1972–1987 381 patients were treated for a pyloroduodenal perforation and 133, believed to have a chronic ulcer, had a definitive operation as emergency treatment for the perforation (128 vagotomy and drainage, five partial gastrectomy). There were three deaths (2.2%), all in patients over 70 years of age (Valerio *et al.*, 1985).

At the time the results suggested that this was a reasonable policy. However, with the introduction of H_2-receptor antagonists and *H. pylori* eradication therapy, and the sharp fall in the number of patients who require elective surgery for a chronic pyloroduodenal ulcer, there are now few indications for a definitive operation at the time of perforation.

This is now more or less limited to the patient with a large chronic duodenal ulcer which it is not possible to close safely – because of the rigidity of the ulcer edges – by sutures tied over omentum. Careful assessment may also show that suture closure is likely to precipitate pyloric obstruction.

In these circumstances on some occasions it is possible to carry out combined excision of the perforated ulcer and Finney pyloroplasty (Figure 5.3 and p. 29) with truncal vagotomy.

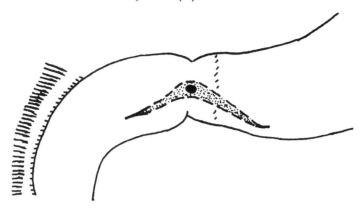

Figure 5.3 Excision of a perforated pyloroduodenal ulcer as part of a pyloroplasty incision. Peritoneum lateral to the second part of the duodenum has been divided to improve the mobility of the duodenal loop.

If the ulcer is too large and rigid to allow this then vagotomy and antrectomy or a Polya-type gastrectomy, with careful closure of the duodenum (p. 31), can be used. Now that few surgeons perform highly selective vagotomy it is rarely appropriate to use this demanding procedure in an emergency operation.

Operative treatment for perforated gastric ulcer

There is general agreement that perforated gastric ulcers are not suitable for laparoscopic management and should be treated at open operation. The treatment of choice will depend on the size of the ulcer, its position, the extent of contamination of the peritoneal cavity, the time lapse since the perforation occurred and the general condition of the patient. Small ulcers in the gastric antrum are best treated by simple excision and suture: the excised specimen is sent to the pathologist to confirm that the lesion is benign. Larger ulcers in the antrum may require to be managed by gastrectomy, particularly if a large portion of the circumference of the stomach is involved by the ulcer. When the perforation is situated high on the lesser curve and it is small (less than 1 cm in diameter) it will usually be possible to excise the ulcer and close the stomach. However if the ulcer is large and shows signs of chronicity with contraction of the lesser curve it will be necessary to excise the ulcer using a Pauchet manoeuvre (see Figure 8.6). If there is suspicion that the lesion may be a gastric carcinoma, after frozen section confirmation it is best to proceed with a gastrectomy with wide margins of clearance. There is recent evidence that simple closure using an omental patch for the treatment of perforated gastric ulcer is associated with a high mortality. In a study of 185 patients treated surgically for perforated gastric ulcer the mortality was 11.3% for those treated using definitive operative procedures whereas the mortality rate rose to 29% in patients treated by closure of the ulcer (Hodnett *et al.*, 1989).

Perforated gastric ulcers are more dangerous than pyloroduodenal ulcers. They have a considerably higher operative mortality and there is always the possibility of the ulcer being a carcinoma; in that event few patients survive more than a year. In patients over 70, Irvin (1989) found an operative mortality for duodenal ulcers of 26%, for gastric ulcers of 41%. In these patients the surgical procedure should be kept as simple as possible.

5.2.9   ERADICATION OF *HELICOBACTER PYLORI*

Since eradication of *H. pylori* has been shown to be associated with peptic ulcer healing in more than 90% of cases it is logical to give eradication therapy to all patients who have had perforated duodenal ulcer treated by simple closure who are HP-positive. Although supporting data are lacking it is probably also worthwhile treating all patients with *Helicobacter* infestation who have had perforated gastric ulcer treated by simple closure. The identification of HP-positive patients may be made by biopsy at the time of operation, e.g. in patients who have had perforated gastric ulcer. More commonly the issue will be addressed by the surgeon a few days after the operation for perforated ulcer when the patient is recovering from the operative procedure.

The HP status of the patient is best assessed by a $[^{13}C]$ or $[^{14}C]$urea breath test (UBT) or by serological tests. Sensitivity and specificity of UBT for *Helicobacter* infection is 98–99% (Rauws *et al.*, 1989). Enzyme-linked immunosorbent assay (ELISA) is a reliable serological test for *Helicobacter* infection with sensitivity and specificity of over 90%. If either test is positive the patient should be given a course of eradication therapy. In our own practice this is started before the patient goes home from hospital. Most recent evidence suggests that a 1-week 'triple therapy' course of a proton pump inhibitor, e.g. omeprazole, with clarithromycin and either metronidazole or amoxycillin will cure HP infection in around 90% of cases (Malfertheiner *et al.*, 1997). Although there is clear evidence that eradication therapy leads to cure of non-perforated duodenal ulcer, it should be pointed out that as yet there is almost no information in the surgical literature about the long-term follow up of patients who have had simple closure of perforated peptic ulcer followed by a course of HP eradication therapy. Although patients with perforated peptic ulcer who are on NSAIDs have a lower incidence of HP infection than those not on NSAIDs, it is still worthwhile checking the HP status of these patients postoperatively. The NSAID should be stopped if possible and eradication therapy given since there is some evidence that NSAIDs and HP may act synergistically in causing ulceration (Heresbach *et al.*, 1992).

5.2.10   PERFORATION INTO THE LESSER SAC

This is a diagnosis that is not infrequently raised in differential diagnosis but only rarely substantiated, occurring in about 1% of the perforations. It may occur in a penetrating ulcer of the lesser curvature of the stomach, or of the duodenum.

The clinical picture depends very much on whether there is leakage of the gastric contents through the foramen of Winslow, with general peritoneal contamination. If this happens the acute onset of pain and marked upper abdominal signs will usually lead to a diagnosis of perforation of a peptic ulcer. Feldman (1950) managed to collect 48 case histories of perforations into the lesser sac; 32 had been diagnosed as perforations but he gives no details of the other patients.

In our small experience the sudden onset of acute upper abdominal pain, sometimes also felt in the back, with variable signs of upper abdominal peritonism, rather suggests acute pancreatitis. Feldman (1950) found that half the patients had free subdiaphragmatic gas: shoulder pain and the serum amylase may also be helpful in differentiation. A water-soluble contrast study can be most useful.

5.2.11   INTRATHORACIC PERFORATION OF A PEPTIC ULCER IN A HIATUS HERNIA

This can produce a difficult clinical picture, and fortunately it is a rare event. An obese 70-year-old lady had acute severe continuous epigastric pain for 6 hours before admission. She had difficulty in breathing and was very tender in the epigastrium, but she was too obese for the surgeon to decide whether there was guarding. A plain X-ray showed no subdiaphragmatic gas but there was a gas shadow behind the heart. A gastrografin swallow showed an inverted stomach in a para-oesophageal hernia and when a later film was taken there was some gas under the left diaphragm and a suspicion of a leak of gastrografin behind the cardiac shadow. Laparotomy showed a perforated duodenal ulcer which lay within the para-oesophageal hernial sac (see Figure 5.5).

Some patients have severe retrosternal pain and shock and the clinical picture resembles a perforation of the oesophagus or a coronary thrombosis. Passage of a nasogastric tube and injection of gastrografin is again very helpful.

5.2.12   THE ASSOCIATION OF PERFORATION AND HAEMORRHAGE IN PEPTIC ULCERATION

This association, when it occurs, is likely to be fatal if not treated promptly and effectively. Perforation and haemorrhage in a peptic ulcer may be related in one of three ways.

Haemorrhage precedes perforation

This is a particularly dangerous sequence because the patient is likely to be admitted to a medical ward with the haematemesis. A patient with haematemesis or melaena is generally assumed to have a peptic ulcer, and such patients are expected to complain of abdominal pain. It is easy for the junior doctor to prescribe an antacid or analgesic rather than to examine the patient. When a patient complains of a new symptom it is crucial that he is examined as carefully as if he was being seen for the first time. In this way alone can the practitioner get away from the strong temptation to explain a new symptom in terms of the current diagnosis.

Once the patient is examined the diagnosis should be quite clear. Haemorrhage, followed by perforation, of an ulcer suggests an active, well-established lesion, so there are good grounds for performing definitive surgery.

Haemorrhage follows closure of a perforation

This is a well known complication of suture closure of a perforation of a chronic ulcer and has been considered (p. 172). This is a dangerous complication and is very likely to require surgical arrest, and this should not be delayed.

Simultaneous perforation and haemorrhage

This combination is unusual. If the perforation presents as a surgical emergency with the usual abdominal signs then the correct approach, surgical treatment, will be taken. If the patient presents with a haematemesis, however, he or she is likely to be thought 'medical' and the abdominal signs may not make a sufficient impression on the physician looking after him/her. A patient with ulcer haemorrhage who also has pain must always be very carefully observed because they tend, even if they do not perforate, to bleed particularly severely.

Perforation and haemorrhage is a certain indication for surgery and simple suture will not usually suffice. It should particularly be remembered that one ulcer may perforate and another may bleed: it is, for instance, important to look for a posterior duodenal ulcer when closing a perforation on the anterior duodenal wall.

REFERENCES

Bell, G. D. and Powell, K. U. (1993) Eradication of *Helicobacter pylori* and its effect in peptic ulcer disease. *Scand. J. Gastroenterol. Suppl.*, **28**, 7–11.

Boey, J., Lee, N. W., Koo, J. *et al.* (1982) Immediate definitive surgery for perforated duodenal ulcers. A prospective controlled trial. *Ann. Surg.*, **196**, 338–344.

Collier, D. St J. and Pain, J. A. (1985) Non-steroidal anti-inflammatory drugs and peptic ulcer perforation. *Gut*, **26**, 359–363.

Crofts, T. J., Park, K. G. M., Steel, R. J. C. *et al.* (1989) A randomised trial of nonoperative treatment for perforated peptic ulcer. *N. Engl. J. Med.*, **320**, 970–973.

Dean, P. (1894) Excision of perforated ulcer of the duodenum. *Lancet*, **i**, 1191.

Feldman, M. (1950) Peptic ulcer perforation into the lesser sac: study of 57 collected cases. *Annu. J. Dig. Dis.*, **17**, 333–334.

Fraser, G. M. and Fraser, I. D. (1974) Gastrografin in perforated duodenal ulcer and pancreatitis. *Clin. Radiol.*, **25**, 397–402.

Hendry, W. S., Valerio, D. and Kyle, J. (1984) Perforated peptic ulcer in North-East Scotland (1972–1981). Part I: Epidemiology. *J. R. Coll. Surg. Edin.*, **2**, 69–72.

Heresbach, D., Raoul, J. L., Bretagne, J. F. *et al.* (1992) *Helicobacter pylori*: a risk and severity factor of non-steroidal anti-inflammatory drug induced gastropathy. *Gut*, **33**, 1608–1611.

Hodnett, R. M., Gonzalez, F., Lee, W. C. *et al.* (1989) The need for definitive therapy in the management of perforated gastric ulcers. *Ann. Surg.*, **209**, 36–39.

Horowitz, J., Kukora, J. S. and Ritchie, W. P. (1989) All perforated ulcers are not alike. *Ann. Surg.*, **209**, 693–697.

Illingworth, C. F. W., Scott, L. D. W. and Jamieson, R. A. (1944) Acute perforated peptic ulcer. *BMJ*, **ii**, 655–658.

Irvin, T. T. (1989) Mortality and perforated peptic ulcer: a case for risk stratification in elderly patients. *Br. J. Surg.*, **76**, 215–218.

Jibril, J. A., Redpath, A. and MacIntyre, I. M. C. (1994) Changing pattern of admission and operation for duodenal ulcer in Scotland. *Br. J. Surg.*, **81**, 87–89.

Koo, J., Ngan, Y. K. and Lam, S. K. (1983) Trends in hospital admission, perforation and mortality of peptic ulcer in Hong Kong 1970–1980. *Gastroenterology*, **84**, 1558–1562.

Kriege, H. (1892) Ein Fall von einem frei in die Bauchhohle perforirten Magengeschwur. Laparotomie. Naht der Perforationsstelle. Heilung. *Berl. Klin. Wschr.*, **29**, 1244.

Lau, W. Y., Leung, K. L., Kwong, K. H. *et al.* (1996) A randomized study comparing laparoscopic versus open repair of perforated peptic ulcer using suture or sutureless technique. *Ann. Surg.*, **224**, 131–138.

Lee, P. W. R., Costen, P. D. M., Wilson, D. H. *et al.* (1977) Pneumoperitoneum in perforated duodenal ulcer disease – a further look. *Br. J. Clin. Pract.*, **31**, 108–110.

MacKay, C. (1966) Perforated peptic ulcer in the West of Scotland 1954–63. *BMJ*, **i**, 701–705.

MacKay, C. (1977) Prevalence of peptic ulcer and its complications. *Scot. Med. J.*, **22**, 288–289.

McKay, A. J. and McArdle, C. S. (1982) Cimetidine and perforated peptic ulcer. *Br. J. Surg.*, **69**, 319–320.

MacLaren, R. (1894) Discussion on operative treatment of perforative ulcer of the stomach and intestines. *BMJ*, **ii**, 863–864.

Malfertheiner, P., Megraud, F., O'Morain, C. *et al.* (1997) Current European concepts in the management of *Helicobacter pylori* infection – the Maastricht consensus report. 1997. *Eur. J. Gastroenterol. Hepatol.*, **9**, 1–2.

Marshall, B. J. and Warren, J. R. (1984) Unidentified curved bacilli in the stomach of patients with gastritis and peptic ulceration. *Lancet*, **i**, 1311–1314.

Morse, T. H. (1894) Ruptured gastric ulcer. *Lancet*, **i**, 671–673.

Mouret, P., Francois, Y., Vignal, J. *et al.* (1990) Laparoscopic treatment of perforated peptic ulcer. *Br. J. Surg.*, **77**, 1006.

Ng, E. K. W., Chung, S. C. S., Sung, J. J. Y. *et al.* (1996) High prevalence of *Helicobacter pylori* infection in duodenal ulcer perforations not caused by non-steroidal anti-inflammatory changes. *Br. J. Surg.*, **83**, 1779–1781.

Ng, K. W., Sung, J. Y. and Chung, S. C. S. (1997) Letter. *Br. J. Surg.*, **84**, 1030.

Rauws, E. A. J., Royen, E. A. U., Langenberg, W. *et al.* (1989) [14]C Urea Breath Test in *H. pylori* gastritis. *Gut*, **30**, 798–803.

Reinbach, D. H., Cruickshank, G. and McColl, K. E. L. (1993) Acute perforated duodenal ulcer is not associated with *Helicobacter pylori* infection. *Gut*, **34**, 1344–1347.

Taylor, H. (1957) Non-surgical treatment of perforated peptic ulcer. Gastroenterology, **33**, 353–368.

Valerio, D., Hendry, W. S. and Jones, P. F. (1985) Perforated peptic ulcer in North-East Scotland, 1972–81. Part 2: definitive treatment or oversew? *J. R. Coll. Surg. Edin.*, **30**, 364–368.

Walt, R., Katschinski, B., Logan, R. *et al.* (1986) Rising frequency of ulcer perforation in elderly people in the United Kingdom. *Lancet*, **i**, 489–492.

Watkins, R. M., Dennison, A. R. and Collin, J. (1984) What has happened to perforated peptic ulcer? *Br. J. Surg.*, **71**, 774–776.

5.3 DIAPHRAGMATIC HERNIA

Diaphragmatic hernia shares with the other internal abdominal hernias (Chapter 6) the fact that symptoms associated with the condition are acute, signs are few, and the penalties of delay in diagnosis are severe. Herniation through the diaphragm can occur in three distinct circumstances.

1. Traumatic rupture of the diaphragm may be immediately followed by herniation and strangulation (p. 471).
2. A diaphragmatic defect may be present but asymptomatic for months or years. It may be a congenital hernia, an undiagnosed traumatic rupture, or a silent disruption of a diaphragmatic suture line. Suddenly a viscus herniates through the defect and becomes trapped.
3. Hiatus hernia of the sliding or axial type rarely causes obstruction, but a para-oesophageal hernial sac is always open to receive a viscus, usually stomach, and produce an obstruction.

Not every obstructed diaphragmatic hernia is a strangulated hernia, but all are serious and share a similar presentation, in which it is easy to miss essential physical signs. Because they are uncommon they have to be actively considered in differential diagnosis.

Clinical features

There is often a history of recurrent dyspepsia, and there may be a past history of serious injury to the trunk, or of thoracotomy.

Because of the protective effect of the liver, 90% of diaphragmatic hernias are on the left side. The sudden migration of a viscus into the thorax, often after a heavy meal or strong exertion (there is a clear association with pregnancy and parturition), causes acute epigastric and substernal pain and breathlessness, with pain going through to the back, referred to the left shoulder and retching is common.

Patients with an acute herniation look ill, they are dyspnoeic and if strangulation supervenes they may become hypotensive. The mediastinum is shifted to the right, movement of the left chest is diminished, air entry is poor and often there is dullness at the bases. Sometimes bowel sounds are heard in the chest. Abdominal signs may be few, but in two of Hoffmann's (1968) four cases epigastric tenderness and guarding was marked.

An erect antero-posterior chest X-ray, including the diaphragms, is essential. Positive signs are shift of the mediastinum and an air bubble, and/or fluid levels, above the diaphragm. Care must be taken that the high arched shadow of the fundus of the herniated stomach is not mistaken for a high diaphragm. A barium swallow can give valuable information. If intestine is trapped there will be signs of intestinal obstruction in the abdominal X-ray.

There are four main types of diaphragmatic hernia: about 60% of strangulations occur in traumatic hernias, about 20% in hiatus hernias, 15% in congenital defects, and 5% in disrupted suture lines in the diaphragm (Carter and Giuseffi, 1948; Hoffmann, 1968).

5.3.1   TRAUMATIC RUPTURE OF THE DIAPHRAGM

The mechanism of closed and penetrating injuries of the diaphragm and their immediate consequences are considered in Chapter 10, p. 471.

Many of these tears go unnoticed (particularly when they are due to closed injuries) and they can remain silent for months and years, until some event causes a viscus to enter the thorax and become arrested in it. Hegarty *et al.* (1978) saw 25 patients who presented 5 or more months after the injury: 17 presented as an emergency, eight with signs of small-bowel obstruction, nine with epigastric pain and dyspnoea due to migration of stomach or colon. The onset of strangulation can be speedy, because many of these defects in the diaphragm are small, and, therefore, recognition and release of the viscus are urgently required.

'Spontaneous' rupture is also described (McIndoe and Hopkins, 1986).

5.3.2   INCISIONAL HERNIA OF THE DIAPHRAGM

Incisions are made in the diaphragm during many procedures, and in some silent disruption of the suture line occurs, producing a situation very similar to traumatic disruption. The presence of a thoracotomy scar can provide a hint of this possibility.

5.3.3   CONGENITAL DIAPHRAGMATIC HERNIA

Most babies born with a Bochdalek hernia in the left postero-lateral area of the diaphragm show immediate signs of respiratory difficulty due to hypoplasia of the lungs (Figure 5.4).

If the defect is not occupied by abdominal organs during intrauterine development the baby may develop normally, and then the patent defect may be the site of sudden herniation of viscera at any time. Occasionally, strangulation occurs as a result of herniation of bowel through a patent foramen of Morgagni, behind the xiphisternum (Gray, 1981).

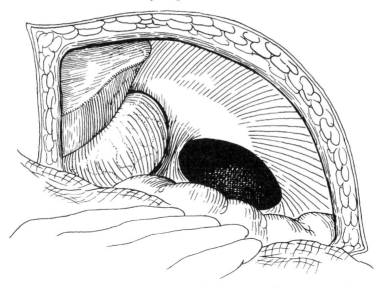

Figure 5.4 The typical deformity of a left Bochdalek hernia. The contents of the hernia have been withdrawn from the pleural cavity, and are held retracted under the assistant's hand.

5.3.4   DIAPHRAGMATIC HERNIA AND GASTRIC VOLVULUS

When a sizeable para-oesophageal hernia exists, the fundus of the stomach can roll up into it, and may or may not produce immediate symptoms. Para-oesophageal hernias are uncommon, constituting about 5% of all hiatus hernias. In the course of operating on 537 patients with a hiatus hernia Beardsley and Thomson (1964) encountered only 13 with acute gastric obstruction, of whom 12 had a gastric volvulus lying within a large para-oesophageal hernia. The stomach rolls upward, along its long axis (organo-axial) into the hernia sac (Figure 5.5).

The oesophagogastric junction is acutely angled and this causes dysphagia and usually prevents passage of a nasogastric tube. In some patients this is a relatively chronic condition, in others an acute strangulating obstruction occurs, with the symptoms of acute retrosternal and epigastric pain and retching, already described. A perforated ulcer in the inverted stomach gives a similar picture. Fluid accumulates in the obstructed stomach and it can become enormously distended (Hill, 1973). If a nasogastric tube can be passed through the obstruction 'a rush of gas and fluid, up to 3500 cc' can be withdrawn. If this is not possible, the situation is urgent, because the blood supply to the stomach may become impaired.

5.3.5   OPERATIVE TECHNIQUE

These patients need speedy preparation for emergency surgery. In all these patients with acute urgent symptoms, the likelihood is that the viscus will have migrated very recently into the chest, and so it will be relatively free of adhesions, and withdrawal through a high midline

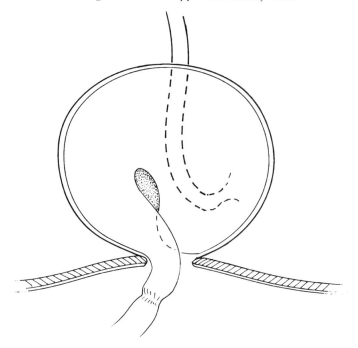

Figure 5.5 Diagram of a complete organo-axial volvulus of the stomach up into a paraoesophageal hernial sac. The acute bend in the oesophagogastric junction is shown.

abdominal incision will be feasible. However, conversion to a thoracolaparotomy incision is sometimes necessary.

The reason for difficulty in reduction may be tense dilatation of the stomach or colon with gas and fluid, and then it is useful to pass a wide catheter into the entering viscus, advance it through the tight diaphragmatic defect, and aspirate the distended herniated viscus (Gray, 1981). Great care must be taken in reducing the herniated viscera, especially the spleen and any organs with impaired circulation. The hernial sac is removed and then the defect requires closure with non-absorbable sutures. Assessment of viability of the reduced viscera follows.

When repairing a para-oesophageal hernia several sutures are placed behind the oesophagus and tied, and the same sutures are then used to attach the posterior wall of the oesophagus to the repair. The remainder are then placed in front of oesophagus. The defect may be large – up to 10 cm in diameter (Haas *et al.*, 1990) and sutures tend to cut out – so it can be helpful to use Teflon pledgets to support the sutures. A fundoplication may usefully be added, and finally the stomach is fixed by making a gastrostomy.

5.4 GASTRIC VOLVULUS

This is a rare condition when it occurs in the absence of a diaphragmatic abnormality. Wastell and Ellis (1971) and Carter *et al.* (1980) reviewed the condition and described a total of 33 cases – in only two of which was there no associated diaphragmatic defect. Spontaneous

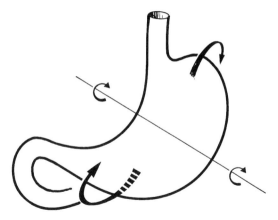

Figure 5.6 The axis of rotation of the mesenterio-axial variety of gastric volvulus.

volvulus is, therefore, rare because the stomach is usually well tethered by its oesophageal and duodenal attachments, by the left gastric artery and, to a lesser degree, by the great omentum. If the stomach folds on its long axis this is named **organo-axial volvulus** and if it rotates on a line from the middle of the lesser to the middle of the greater curvature this is termed **mesenterio-axial volvulus**: here the antrum moves forward and upwards over the fundus, which sinks downwards and backwards (Figure 5.6).

The symptoms and signs of this condition are very similar to those already described. A mass can sometimes be felt and an erect plain X-ray can show a double fluid-level in the left hypochondrium (Figure 5.7). Treatment comprises reduction, repair of the diaphragmatic defect if present, gastropexy and in those cases with gastric necrosis, gastric resection.

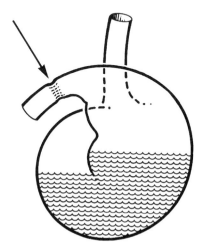

Figure 5.7 Appearance of a plain erect X-ray in mesenterio-axial volvulus of the stomach.

REFERENCES

Beardsley, J. M. and Thompson, W. R. (1964) Acutely obstructed hiatus hernia. *Ann. Surg.*, **159**, 49–62.

Carter, B. N. and Giuseffi, J. (1948) Strangulated diaphragmatic hernia. *Ann. Surg.*, **128**, 210–225.

Carter, R., Brewer, L. A. and Hinshaw, D. B. (1980) Acute gastric volvulus. *Am. J. Surg.*, **140**, 99–106.

Gray, F. J. (1981) Strangulated hernia of the foramen of Morgagni: introducing a principle for the reduction of obstructed intra-abdominal hernias. *Austr. N.Z. J. Surg.*, **51**, 314–317.

Haas, O., Rat, P. Christophe, M. *et al.* (1990) Surgical results of intrathoracic gastric volvulus complication hiatus hernia. *Br. J. Surg.*, **77**, 1379–1381.

Hegarty, M. M., Bryer, J. V., Angorn, I. B. *et al.* (1978) Delayed presentation of traumatic diaphragmatic hernia. *Ann. Surg.*, **188**, 229–233.

Hill, L. D. (1973) Incarcerated paraesophageal hernia: a surgical emergency. *Am. J. Surg.*, **126**, 286–291.

Hoffmann, E. (1968) Strangulated diaphragmatic hernia. *Thorax*, **23**, 541–549.

McIndoe, G. A. J. and Hopkins, N. F. G. (1986) 'Spontaneous' rupture of the diaphragm. *Postgrad. Med. J.*, **62**, 389–391.

Wastell, C. and Ellis, H. (1971) Volvulus of the stomach: a review with a report of eight cases. *Br. J. Surg.*, **58**, 558–562.

6

Small-bowel emergencies

6.1 INTESTINAL OBSTRUCTION

When Frederick Treves wrote his Jacksonian Prize essay on Intestinal Obstruction in 1884 he clearly distinguished the 'great variety of conditions which, although unlike in character, have yet the common property of bringing about, mechanically, an obstruction to the passage of matter along the intestine' (Treves, 1899). He described adhesive bands causing strangulation, annular carcinomas, volvulus, intussusception and gallstone ileus. Some could cause death within 48 hours while others developed over weeks and months. Treves advised surgeons to be much readier to open the abdomen, and in the previous year Henry Clark, Surgeon to Glasgow Royal Infirmary, had observed that 'it is too much the custom to wait till the patient is moribund and then very wisely decide that he is too far gone for operation'.

In 1885 Thomas Bryant, Surgeon to Guy's Hospital, established the fundamental differences between strangulating and non-strangulating obstructions, and in 1896 John B Murray in Chicago described the distinctive features of 'adynamic ileus' and contrasted it with mechanical obstruction. In spite of the clarity of these descriptions, mortality remained formidable, with ill and dehydrated patients being operated on while deeply anaesthetized with noxious agents.

In 1912 Hartwell and Hoguet made a key contribution when they demonstrated that dogs with complete obstruction of the duodenojejunal junction died, if untreated, in a few days but survived up to 3 weeks if given subcutaneous infusions of physiological saline. There was a major advance in the field of diagnosis when Schwarz (1911) described the patterns of fluid and gas distribution to be seen in plain X-rays of the obstructed abdomen.

6.1.1 THE EFFECTS OF INTESTINAL OBSTRUCTION

The results of extensive investigations can be summarized under four headings.

1. Obstruction of the small bowel leads to **loss of alimentary secretions**.
2. Increasing distension produces a **rise in intraluminal pressure**.

Emergency Abdominal Surgery. Edited by Peter F. Jones, Zygmunt H. Krukowski and George G. Youngson. Published in 1998 by Chapman & Hall, London. ISBN 0 412 81950 3.

3. **Bacterial multiplication** occurs in the retained secretions.
4. Intestinal strangulation involves **impairment or arrest of the blood supply** to the bowel.

1. Loss of alimentary secretions

In the normal adult some 7–9 litres of gastrointestinal juice is secreted each day, of which 98.8% is reabsorbed in the lower ileum and colon, leaving about 100 ml to be passed *per rectum*. In a **high jejunal obstruction** the secretions of the stomach, duodenum, pancreas and biliary tree continue to be produced, there is no reabsorption and the consequence is voluminous and effortless vomiting. There is minimal distension of bowel; a good estimate of the loss can be made and replaced, so the patient will soon be ready for operation.

Low small-bowel obstruction produces a more complex situation.

- Progressively higher levels of intestine above the obstruction become distended by the retained secretions and swallowed air. Vomiting may be delayed and by then there is considerable distension.
- Distended bowel becomes congested, reabsorption is impaired, and in fact the volume of secretion is increased (Shields, 1965). Johnson *et al.* (1978) found an increase in osmolality of the retained secretions due to enzyme activity, leading to an influx of fluid to restore osmotic balance.
- The clinical picture can be deceptive because vomiting is delayed, and it is easy to overlook the fact that as much as 2 litres of extracellular fluid is sequestrated in the obstructed bowel. Serum electrolytes may be unaltered but plasma volume is substantially reduced: this will be demonstrated by tachycardia, modest hypotension, pale cool extremities, and reduced urine output and a rise in serum creatinine.

  It is vital to remember this haemodynamic effect when the abdominal film shows multiple fluid levels in distended small bowel.

2. Distension and its effects

For a long time the source of the air above the fluid in obstructed small bowel was uncertain. Wangensteen and Rea (1939) showed conclusively that, if a dog with a low ileal obstruction also had a cervical oesophagostomy, so that no swallowed air could reach the abdomen, the small bowel did not become distended and, if given Ringer's solution intravenously the dog could survive for several weeks. Dogs who were given an ileal obstruction only quickly became distended and did not survive more than 5 days. They calculated that 72% of the gas in obstructed bowel was swallowed air.

In obstructed small bowel the intraluminal pressure rarely exceeds 8 cmH$_2$O (Sperling, 1938). However in the colon the ileocaecal valve is often competent, so the colon above the obstruction becomes a closed loop, and pressures above 25 cmH$_2$O are not uncommon. This can be harmful, especially in the thin-walled caecum (Saegesser and Sandblom, 1975) and perforation is not unusual (p. 266).

3. Bacterial growth

The bacterial flora of the upper small bowel is relatively scanty and limited to Gram-positive aerobes. In the distal ileum coliforms and anaerobic *Bacteroides* spp. are numerous; in obstruction the bacterial count rises sharply, coliforms and aerobic cocci predominating

(Sykes *et al.*, 1976). Beyond the ileocaecal valve anaerobes come to outnumber aerobes by a factor of 100–10 000:1, and nearly one third of faecal dry weight is composed of viable bacteria. The major anaerobic genus is *Bacteroides* (Simon and Gorback, 1984).

In small-bowel obstruction this highly infective fluid is confined to the bowel (except in strangulation) unless an intraoperative spill occurs. This must be avoided and one of the first steps should be to empty obstructed bowel content back into the stomach, whence it can be aspirated (p. 191).

4. Intestinal strangulation

The patient with a strangulated loop of bowel suffers all the effects just described, with the additional hazard of an impaired blood supply to the gut.

Most strangulations occur when a loop of bowel is caught under an adhesive band, or in the neck of a hernial sac. This tends to produce immediate occlusion of the mesenteric veins, but arterial input into the loop can, for a time, continue, so venous engorgement continues until there is interstitial haemorrhage into the bowel wall and some loss into the lumen. Eventually arterial circulation cannot continue and viability is lost: the aim of surgical treatment is to release the loop before this stage is reached. Bussemaker and Lindeman (1972) clamped the arteries and veins supplying a length of the distal ileum of dogs: after 4 hours the mucosa was necrotic but if the clamps were removed the bowel survived and the mucosa was normal 3 weeks later. With release after 6 hours the bowel survived but a late stricture developed. Release after 8 hours was followed by perforation of the non-viable bowel.

Bacterial multiplication
Bacterial multiplication in a strangulated loop is remarkable and within 24 hours Powley (1965) found 100 000 000 faecal organisms per millilitre of intestinal content. When the ileum of germ-free dogs was obstructed and the venous drainage interrupted, the bowel remained viable in 19 out of 21 dogs when explored at 100 hours. In a similar experiment in five control dogs all were dead within 37 hours, with perforation of a stinking, gangrenous loop of bowel (Thomas *et al.*, 1965). The effect of faecal organisms within a strangulated loop is to hasten proteolysis, and therefore expedite disruption of the bowel. During this process exudate leaks through the disintegrating wall, inoculating the peritoneum with a lethal mixture. This is so potent that even a strangulated knuckle of bowel a few centimetres long in a hernial sac offers a real threat, and it is essential to provide full systemic antibiotic cover and local antibiotic washout of the operation site.

Hypovolaemia and strangulation
When a long loop of small bowel becomes strangulated there is immediate occlusion of the venous drainage but for some time arterial perfusion continues, so a considerable volume of blood becomes isolated from the general circulation, within the hyperaemic loop. Holt (1934) found that, when the venous drainage of a 100 cm long loop of small bowel was obstructed for 4 hours, 50% of the dog's normal blood volume was trapped in the loop.

In clinical practice this does not often occur but if, as in malrotation (p. 209) a length of small bowel hangs on a narrow pedicle and undergoes volvulus then this picture can appear and the patient becomes dangerously hypovolaemic and hypotensive. The abdominal pain is severe but, at first, the abdominal signs are so few that dangerous delay in diagnosis can occur (p. 209).

6.1.2   THE CAUSES OF INTESTINAL OBSTRUCTION

When Treves was writing his essay in 1884 the major cause of obstruction was a strangulated hernia, and this was still true in 1932 when Vick reviewed the work of 19 British hospitals. Among some 6000 patients, 55% had an obstructed external hernia, 25% had an adhesive obstruction and in 17% the obstruction was due to malignant disease.

Since then, increasing numbers of patients have undergone a laparotomy and had elective repair of a hernia, and currently, in Western countries, about 40% of patients have an adhesive obstruction, in 20–25% the cause is a neoplasm (usually in the colon) and between 15% and 25% have an obstructed hernia (Bevan, 1984; McEntee *et al.*, 1987; Table 6.1).

In less developed countries, where there are few elective hernia repairs, and relatively few laparotomies to produce postoperative adhesions, these ratios are reversed. In Nigeria, 40–50% of obstructions are due to strangulated external hernia, 15–20% are due to intussusception in 5–15-year-olds, and adhesions and volvulus each account for some 10% (Cole, 1965; Chiedozi *et al.*, 1980). Neoplastic obstruction is unusual, although in Malaysia the Chinese show a relatively high incidence of neoplastic adhesive obstruction while Malaysian and Indian inhabitants rarely suffer in this way but have a high incidence of obstructed hernia (Ti and Yong, 1976). Volvulus of both small and large bowel is unusually common in Eastern Europe and the Middle East (p. 208). Obstruction by worms, especially *Ascaria* (p. 244), and tuberculous enteritis (p. 230) are other important causes of small-bowel obstruction in Third World countries.

The other major cause of intestinal obstruction is neurogenic, adynamic or paralytic ileus, most often seen in association with diffuse peritonitis (Chapter 4, p. 258).

Mortality

Intestinal obstruction has always carried a relatively high mortality, and until the 1930s this was partly due to the restricted use of intravenous fluid therapy and nasogastric suction, and the administration of relatively noxious anaesthetic agents. Since Vick's 1932 survey, when adhesive and neoplastic obstruction carried a mortality of 40%, there has been steady improvement. With wide recognition of the dangers of strangulating adhesive obstruction, and the challenge of large-bowel obstruction in the elderly, mortality percentages are now generally within single figures. However, this is only achieved with a high level of expertise in operative technique and, equally important, in pre- and postoperative care.

6.1.3   GENERAL PRINCIPLES OF DIAGNOSIS

History and clinical examination

Treves, in 1884, remarked on the diversity of the symptomatology, ranging from severe urgent colic to grumbling discomfort, occurring over a few hours to a few weeks.

It is worth re-emphasizing that a careful history can help as much as anything else in understanding the acute abdomen, and this is certainly true in intestinal obstruction. Severe central colicky abdominal pain, accompanied by vomiting and constipation, must be considered to arise from obstructed intestine until proved otherwise. A confusing history can be given by patients with incomplete small-bowel obstruction (p. 228), and the slow unimpressive history of neoplastic colonic obstruction (p. 267) must be remembered.

Table 6.1 Aetiology of small bowel obstruction in North America and the UK; percentages are based on the figures of Stewardson *et al.* (1978), Bizer *et al.* (1981) and McEntee *et al.* (1987)

Cause	%
Adhesions	40

- Postoperative (90%)
- Spontaneous (4%)
- Secondary to adjacent disease (3%)
- Meckel's diverticulum (2%)

Hernia	20

- External
  - Inguinal
  - Femoral
  - Incisional
  - Obturator
- Internal
  - Diaphragmatic
  - Paraduodenal etc
- Iatrogenic
  - Paracolostomy
  - Polya antecolic anastomosis

Neoplasms	20

- Carcinoma, primary and secondary
- Carcinoid
- Lymphoma
- Leiomyosarcoma
- Polyps (Peutz–Jeghers)

Inflammatory	6

- Crohn's disease
- Ileocaecal tuberculosis
- Endometriosis

Mesenteric vascular occlusion	6
Intraluminal obstructions	5

- Gallstones, food, worms
- Meconium ileus equivalent
- Foreign bodies

Iatrogenic	3

- Mechanical obstruction
  - Irradiation
  - Intramural haematoma (anticoagulants)
  - Potassium chloride and practolol
- Drug induced
- Functional obstruction

It is wise to spend time, both over the history and in sitting beside the patient, watching, palpating and listening to the abdomen. In this way the vital sign may be observed of the 30 seconds during which waves of peristalsis stand out in a ladder pattern on the abdominal wall and a rush of high-pitched tinkles and splashes can be heard. If, when listening to the history, the patient loses concentration and grimaces and grunts, bare the abdomen and watch and listen – this is the moment at which a confident diagnosis of intestinal obstruction can be made.

The **age of the patient** may be helpful in so far as, for example, intussusception is seen in infancy and neoplastic obstruction in later life.

Abdominal distension is a sign that is thought to accompany an obstruction, and it can be very impressive in large-bowel obstruction, especially volvulus of the sigmoid. However, the sign depends on a relatively slow development of distension in a fair length of bowel, so it is dangerously absent if a strangulation occurs in a loop of proximal jejunum or there is a volvulus of the small bowel in a patient with malrotation (p. 209).

The hernial orifices must be examined in every case of acute abdominal pain. **There are no exceptions to this important rule**. It is characteristic of strangulated femoral hernia that the patient complains only of central colicky abdominal pain: she may not know she has a hernia and often it is not painful (p. 216). If not purposefully sought, this relatively non-tender lump can be missed. A strangulated inguinal hernia is usually both painful and tender.

A **rectal examination** should be done, and if it is available a **specimen of vomit** must be examined: faeculent vomit is more or less certain to indicate an obstruction.

Radiography

In most cases of intestinal obstruction radiography has an important role to play in reaching a diagnosis. Schwarz in Vienna in 1911 was the first to describe the gas-distended loops seen in intestinal obstruction and the fluid levels visible in films taken with a horizontal tube. The appearances regarded as typical of small-bowel obstruction are best seen **when a simple adhesive obstruction affects the ileum**.

- **Upright film**.
  - A number of smooth and parallel-sided gas-distended loops are seen, scattered through the abdomen, each ending above a fluid-level.
  - The levels at the end of each loop lie at a different height, suggesting a positive pressure being exerted on the distal level.
  - Gas-distended jejunum shows a typical 'coiled-spring' appearance due to the volvulae conniventes: these are less conspicuous in gas-distended ileum.
  - In mechanical small-bowel obstruction gas is usually absent from the colon.
  - The number of distended loops provides a fair guide to the level of obstruction.
- If the patient cannot stand the exposure should be made with the patient in **lateral decubitus** and the tube horizontal.
- **Supine film**. The film should be large enough to include the diaphragms and the minor pelvis. This is the best position for showing the distribution of gas in the bowel, and radiologists tend to regard this view as more informative than the upright film.

Simple adhesive obstruction of the jejunum, especially when sited in its upper reaches, is less likely to produce these appearances because swallowed air tends to be returned to the stomach and is evacuated during vomiting. A gas pattern may not be seen, or these may be just one or two gas-filled loops with a fluid-level.

It is here that the virtues of water-soluble contrast radiography in the investigation of intestinal obstruction should be remembered. Epstein (1957) found that, if gastrografin, which contains 37% iodine, is injected down a nasogastric tube (100 ml for adults, 20–50 ml for children), the normal transit time to the colon is 30–90 minutes. The patient is asked to lie on the right side, semi-prone, to encourage passage through the pylorus, and supine films are exposed at 30 minutes and 2–4 hours. In simple high jejunal obstruction the 30-minute film will show contrast lying in one or two dilated jejunal loops only and this failure to progress will be confirmed in later films.

This useful investigation can be safely used in any doubtful case of small-bowel obstruction. Joyce *et al.* (1992) studied 127 patients between the ages of 11 months and 91 years who clinically and radiologically appeared to have an obstruction of small bowel. They found that, if contrast was arrested in the small bowel, with no passage into the colon, at 4 hours this indicated an organic obstruction. Assalia *et al.* (1994) emphasized that the osmolarity of gastrografin is six times that of extracellular fluid, so it is essential to rehydrate the patient before giving it, basing the requirement on the vital signs, urine output, correction of any serum electrolyte values, and occasionally central venous pressure readings. The stomach is then aspirated dry, the gastrografin injected, the tube spigoted for 2 hours and the patient postured to promote gastric emptying.

The osmotic effect of gastrografin can also be used as treatment in patients with partial obstruction (p. 198) and early postoperative intestinal obstruction (p. 196).

Strangulation of small bowel by a band is likely to occur when a loop of bowel with its mesentery becomes caught under a band or, occasionally, when the trapped loop undergoes volvulus. In this dangerous situation it is important to recognize that plain abdominal films are not always abnormal, and this can lead to a dangerous delay. Gough (1978) reported 71 patients who needed laparotomy for adhesive obstruction: 40 had strangulated bowel, but of these 40, 16 had a normal-looking or equivocal plain abdominal film on admission. The clear lesson from this analysis is that a strangulating obstruction continues to be suspected chiefly on clinical grounds. A patient is admitted with a short history of severe central abdominal pain, which is often more constant than colicky, accompanied by frequent vomiting. There is a scar of a previous laparotomy in nine out of ten patients. The temperature, pulse rate and white cell count can all be within normal limits but examination of the abdomen will arouse suspicion. In 22 of the 40 patients there was abdominal tenderness and guarding at the time of admission. By the time laparotomy was decided on 37 showed guarding and tenderness and in every case of gangrenous bowel there were signs of peritoneal irritation.

Vest (1962) made the useful observation that a strangulating obstruction induces marked inhibition of peristalsis, and objective evidence of this is obtained if the gastrografin contrast study is performed, because the contrast does not leave the stomach. Another sign of this is that the abdomen is silent, in contrast to the loud noises heard in non-strangulating obstructions.

Ultrasonography

Ultrasonography can provide information on fluid-filled dilated loops of small bowel, images of the contents being whirled about during hyperperistalsis, and evidence of oedema of the bowel wall. Ko *et al.* (1993) in South Korea performed a retrospective study on 54 patients with surgically proven small-bowel obstruction. They reviewed sonographic images and plain abdominal X-rays and considered that ultrasound was able to establish the presence of obstruction in 89% of the patients, compared to accuracy of 71% in the X-rays. Ultrasonography may be helpful in ill patients who can be examined at the bedside, and it would be particularly useful in pregnant patients. Its place may become clearer with increasing experience.

Computed tomography

Computed tomography is also undergoing assessment. Megibow (1994), in a review, considered that the role of CT should be restricted to patients in whom there is clinical suspicion of obstruction but in whom plain X-rays do not confirm this. It may be helpful in identifying strangulated bowel.

6.1.4 GENERAL PRINCIPLES OF TREATMENT

The treatment of intestinal obstruction is timely surgical relief of the cause: the exception is when the obstruction is functional, as in paralytic ileus (p. 258) and colonic pseudo-obstruction (p. 303).

Preoperative preparation

As soon as mechanical obstruction is diagnosed the surgeon should operate without delay, especially if there is any chance of strangulation. In every case, however, the question must be asked whether a period of preparation will improve the chances of survival. If the patient presents early and the diagnosis can be promptly reached, it is unlikely that the effects of starvation, vomiting and sequestration of fluid in the obstructed bowel will be great, and a short period of intravenous fluid infusion should render the patient fit for surgery.

The late case of small-bowel obstruction requires more thoughtful handling. For example, an elderly woman presents with gallstone obstruction of the low ileum, which can easily have been present for 3–4 days. Such a patient will be seriously dehydrated, may well be in low-output renal failure and will need judicious management.

If a patient has been obstructed for several days and there is no sign of peritonitis then it is reasonable to conclude that there is no strangulation, and then time can be given to careful preparation for operation. The distended small bowel can contain 2–3 litres of fluid, an unknown quantity will have been lost in vomit, and the patient will have drunk little or nothing. A total deficiency of 6–8 litres of water may exist, but great care must be exercised over speed of replacement, especially in an elderly patient with cardiorespiratory problems.

- A peripheral vein can be cannulated and blood withdrawn for haematological and biochemical analysis. Hartmann's solution can safely be given at a rate of 1 litre in $1-1\frac{1}{2}$ hours. In a hypotensive patient blood gases must be estimated and a plasma expander used. In the elderly patient in this delicate situation, placement of a central venous catheter will give much needed guidance on speed of infusion, and in a few seriously ill patients a Swan–Ganz catheter will be needed to measure central venous and pulmonary wedge pressure and cardiac output. If this level of attention is needed the patient should be nursed in an intensive care unit, or a least a high-dependency unit.

- Urinary output must be recorded by passing a catheter and measuring hourly urine volumes.
- Low ileal secretions can contain 40 mEq of potassium per litre, so substantial deficiencies can be present. Once the CVP returns to normal and hourly urine output comes up to 30 ml, potassium replacement should commence. Serum sodium and potassium levels should be carefully reviewed as rehydration proceeds.
- It is a mistake to wait until there is complete restoration of all theoretical deficiencies and a decision should be made in consultation with the anaesthetist on the timing of the operation. A nasogastric Anderson sump drain tube is inserted to make certain the stomach is empty. Anti-embolism stockings are fitted, and at induction of anaesthesia the patient is given 5000 units of heparin subcutaneously, and this will continue twice daily. The handling of obstructed bowel may cause bacteraemia and prophylactic antibiotics are started before the abdomen is opened.

The operation

It is accepted practice to place compressive leggings or boots on the patient. It is important to maintain body warmth by the use, where necessary, of a heating blanket or 'warm touch': this reduces the metabolic response to surgery and prevents clotting problems.

A vertical incision is preferred because the extent of the operation cannot be predicted and it is readily extended. When re-entering the abdomen, it is often right to re-open the previous incision but it is wise to extend it either upwards or downwards; this allows the first entry into the peritoneum to be made at a point at which bowel is unlikely to be adherent to the back of the scar. A midline incision is now generally used because it allows quick and accurate closure, with excellent long-term results (p. 20).

Intestinal decompression

In small-intestinal obstruction the surgeon always has to deal with loops of bowel distended with wind and intestinal secretions, and these produce several difficulties.

- In a low obstruction the numerous loops make exposure of the cause difficult, and if they are not emptied both surgeon and anaesthetist will have problems in securing closure of the incision.
- Rupture of tightly distended bowel during handling is a real risk.
- Distended bowel is likely to recover more slowly than bowel that has been decompressed.

The advantage to the surgeon of working on decompressed bowel has led to the design of various devices for aspirating the contents through suckers and trocars (Moynihan, 1926; Savage, 1960), but it is difficult to do this without some soiling with highly infective bowel content, and there is a real risk of later leakage from the puncture site. The authors have seen this cause fatal peritonitis after relief of a simple adhesive obstruction.

It is neater and easier to achieve decompression by gently milking the contents back, in stages, into the stomach, whence it is aspirated through a wide nasogastric tube (Jones and Matheson, 1968). It is best to start in the upper jejunum, squeezing the content upwards, hand over hand, into and through the duodenal loop and pylorus. The process is repeated at a lower level, advancing the fluid up again into the stomach, and this is continued until the whole bowel above the obstruction is empty, and a good view of the cause can be obtained. Obstructed small bowel becomes oedematous, and this manoeuvre must be done gently – particular care must be exercised over stripping bowel between the straight middle and index fingers.

Claims have been made that this cannot be done because the duodenum and pylorus oppose retrograde decompression, but we have disproved this over many years. However, a watch must be kept that the duodenum does not become over-distended. Another criticism is that this practice entails much handling of bowel, but this is not less than will occur in any attempt to aspirate the bowel, or in persuading dilated loops back into the abdomen before closing the incision. Shields and Dudley (1971) have shown that the natural oedema of obstructed bowel is accentuated after decompression but recovery of motility is not affected. However, the bowel is certainly more sensitive to any overload of intravenous fluid, and this is a reminder of the importance of attention to this aspect of postoperative care.

Once the bowel is decompressed the cause of the obstruction can be identified. Assessment of viability is considered on p. 199, and techniques of resection are described on p. 21.

Postoperative care

This follows standard lines. After the relief of a small-bowel obstruction the return of peristalsis and passage of flatus may seem to be delayed. A difficult differential diagnosis has sometimes to be made between a functional prolongation of ileus and an early adhesive obstruction and this is considered on p. 195.

REFERENCES

Assalia, A., Schein, M., Kopelman, D. *et al.* (1994) Therapeutic effect of oral gastrografin in adhesive, partial small bowel obstruction: a prospective randomised trial. *Surgery*, **115**, 433–437.

Bevan, P. G. (1984) Adhesive obstruction. *Ann. R. Coll. Surg. Engl.*, **66**, 164–169.

Bizer, L. S., Liebling, R. W., Delany, H. M. *et al.* (1981) Small bowel obstruction. *Surgery*, **89**, 407–413.

Bryant, T. (1885) *On the Mode of Death From Acute Intestinal Strangulation and Chronic Intestinal Obstruction*, J. A. Churchill, London.

Bussemaker, J. B. and Lindeman, J. (1972) Comparison of methods to determine viability of small intestine. *Ann. Surg.*, **176**, 97–101.

Chiedozi, L. C., Aboh, I. O. and Piserchia, N. E. (1980) Mechanical bowel obstruction: review of 316 cases in Benin City. *Am. J. Surg.*, **139**, 389–393.

Clark, H. E. (1883) On a case of obstruction of the bowels due to volvulus treated by abdominal section; recovery. *Lancet*, **ii**, 678–680.

Cole, G. J. (1965) A review of 436 cases of intestinal obstruction in Ibadan. *Gut*, **6**, 151–153.

Epstein, B. S. (1957) Non-absorbable water-soluble contrast mediums: their use in diagnosis of intestinal obstruction. *J.A.M.A.*, **165**, 44–46.

Gough, I. R. (1978) Strangulating adhesive small bowel obstruction with normal radiographs. *Br. J. Surg.*, **65**, 431–434.

Hartwell, J. A. and Hoguet, J. P. (1912) Experimental intestinal obstruction in dogs with special reference to the cause of death and the treatment by large amounts of normal saline solution. *J.A.M.A.*, **59**, 82–85.

Holt, R. L. (1934) The pathology of acute strangulation by the intestine. *Br. J. Surg.*, **21**, 582–603.

Johnson, L., Nordstrom, H. and Nylander, G. (1978) Experimental studies on fluid patho-physiology in small intestinal obstruction in the rat. 1. Effects of intraluminal hyperosmolality. *Scand. J. Gastroenterol.*, **13**, 49–56.

Jones, P. F. and Matheson, N. A. (1968) Operative decompression in intestinal obstruction. *Lancet*, **i**, 1197–1198.

Joyce, W. P., Delaney, P. V., Gorey, T. F. *et al.* (1992) The value of water-soluble contrast radiology in the management of acute small bowel obstruction. *Ann. R. Coll. Surg. Engl.*, **74**, 422–425.

Ko, Y., Lim, J., Lee, H. W. and Lim, J. W. (1993) Small bowel obstruction: sonographic evaluation. *Radiology*, **188**, 649–653.

McEntee, G., Pender, D., Mulvin, D. *et al.* (1987) Current spectrum of intestinal obstruction. *Br. J. Surg.*, **74**, 977–980.

Megibow, A. (1994) Bowel obstruction: evaluation with CT. *Radiol. Clin. North Am.*, **32**, 861–870.

Moynihan, B. G. A. (1926) *Abdominal Operations*, W. B. Saunders, Philadelphia, PA, vol. 1, p. 490.

Powley, J. M. (1965) Unexpected deaths from small bowel obstruction. *Proc. R. Soc. Med.*, **58**, 870–873.

Saegesser, F. and Sandblom, P. (1975) Ischaemic lesions of the distended colon: a complication of obstructive colorectal cancer. *Am. J. Surg.*, **129**, 309–315.

Savage, P. T. (1960) The management of acute intestinal obstruction. *Br. J. Surg.*, **47**, 643–654.

Schwarz, G. (1911) Die Erkennung der tieferen Dunndarmstenose mittels des Roentgenverfahrens. *Wien. Klin. Wschr.*, **24**, 1386–1394.

Shields, R. (1965) The absorption and secretion of fluid and electrolytes by the obstructed bowel. *Br. J. Surg.*, **52**, 774–779.

Shields, M. A. and Dudley, H. A. F. (1971) Effects of open and close decompression on the water content and motility of experimentally obstructed small bowel. *Br. J. Surg.*, **58**, 337–339.

Simon, G. L. and Gorback, S. L. (1984) Intestinal flora in health and disease. Gastroenterology, **86**, 174–194.

Sperling, L. (1938) Mechanics of simple intestinal obstruction. *Arch. Surg.*, **36**, 778–815.

Stewardson, R. H., Bombeck, C. T. and Nyhus, L. M. (1978) Critical operative management of small intestine. *Ann. Surg.*, **187**, 189–193.

Sykes, P. A., Boulter, K. H. and Schofield, P. F. (1976) The microflora of the obstructed bowel. *Br. J. Surg.*, **63**, 721.

Thomas, M. A., Heneghan, J. B., Mathieu *et al.* (1965) Strangulation obstruction in germ free dogs. *Surgery*, **58**, 37–46.

Ti, T. K. and Yong, N. K. (1976) The pattern of intestinal obstruction in Malaysia. *Br. J. Surg.*, **63**, 963–965.

Treves, F. (1899) *Intestinal Obstruction*, 2nd edn, Cassell, London.

Vest, B. (1962) Roentgenographic diagnosis of strangulated closed loop obstruction of the small intestine. *Surg. Gynecol. Obstet.*, **115**, 561–567.

Vick, R. M. (1932) Statistics of acute intestinal obstruction. *BMJ*, **ii**, 546–548.

Wangensteen, O. H. and Rea, C. E. (1939) The distension factor in simple intestinal obstruction. *Surgery*, **5**, 327–339.

6.2 ADHESIONS AND BANDS

Although patients with small-bowel obstruction are very familiar to surgeons, they contribute fewer than 5% of all urgent surgical admissions. Adhesions and obstructed hernias account for some two-thirds of all these cases, and are of particular importance because they are the two main causes of strangulation of bowel.

All modern surveys of adhesive small-bowel obstruction show that 80–90% of these patients have at some time had a laparotomy, and although it is often a simple operation appendicectomy has throughout the century been one of the principle sources of adhesion and bands that later cause obstruction. It is necessary to consider what is known about the formation of adhesions after laparotomy.

6.2.1 AETIOLOGY

Wherever the peritoneum is inflamed or injured there is a tendency for adhesions to form and, with time, they tend to disappear. When an appendix abscess is drained it is confined by some apparently strong adhesions, yet when interval appendicectomy is undertaken 2–3 months later, quite often little sign of adhesions around a fibrosed appendix can be found.

The first step in adhesion formulation is an inflammatory reaction in the peritoneum, which may be a reaction to the operation itself or to bacterial infection. This reaction can be minimized by good operating technique, including the avoidance of talc and starch powder in gloves, and by use of damp gauze swabs. Ellis (1962) demonstrated that ischaemia of the peritoneum due to suturing is a powerful cause of adhesion formation. The effects of infection can be reduced by antibiotics.

Histological study of experimental adhesion formation shows that the inflammatory reaction may be followed by fibrin deposition within an inflammatory exudate, fibroblast invasion and collagen formation, which in turn matures to form fibrous adhesions (Milligan and Raftery, 1974). However, this sequence is not inevitable because normal mesothelial cells produce fibrinolysins which, though at first depressed, regain their activity at 3–4 days and are most active at about 8 days, providing physiological prevention of adhesion formation (Thompson and Whawell, 1995). The degree to which this process operates determines whether fibrinous adhesions are lysed or go on to be invaded by fibroblasts and become organized.

Although it would appear to be desirable to prevent adhesion formation, it has to be remembered that sound healing of gastrointestinal and vascular anastomoses depends on deposition and organization of fibrin, and so does the limitation of infection. Both anti-inflammatory agents and anticoagulants (which limit fibrin production) will, in an adequate dose, limit adhesion formation, but their harmful effects on wound healing and haemostasis prevent their use. Experiments show that mesothelial cells naturally produce plasminogen activator activity (PAA) and this is the source of fibrinolysis – the lysis or persistence of fibrinous adhesions depends on the degree to which this natural process is active. The theory behind the use of viscous macromolecular solutions such as dextran to prevent adhesions around, for example, operations on the fallopian tube, is that these solutions entrap PAA and perpetuate its action in a localized area. With the manufacture of recombinant tissue plasminogen activator (rt-PA), which can replace absent PAA, a possible method of diminishing adhesion formation has been opened up. Animal experiments using a dose of 3 mg rt-PA in 3 g of sodium hyaluronate suggest that this can be used safely and that rt-PA does not weaken the healing of anastomoses or incisions (Menzies and Ellis, 1991).

Becker *et al.* (1996) report that a sodium hyaluronate-based bioresorbable membrane was placed beneath the abdominal incision in 175 patients having total colectomy and ileoanal pouch construction, with ileostomy. When the ileostomy was closed 6–8 weeks later, laparoscopy through the ileostomy incision showed there were adhesions to the back of the vertical incision in 85 of 90 control patients and 42 of 85 patients given the membrane. An alternative hyaluronate preparation applied as a thick solution to the exposed bowel throughout the laparotomy may also be effective but, although this is available in Europe it remained to be approved by the American FDA at the end of 1997.

'**Reperitonealization**' was long considered to be desirable after, for example, performing right hemicolectomy. Experiments have shown, however, that when areas of parietal peritoneum are removed and kept under observation, at 2 days the raw area is glistening and by 7 days it is covered by mesothelial cells and few adhesions form (Williams, 1955). Experience shows the truth of this work on the occasions when the abdomen has to be reopened after total colectomy.

When insertion of sutures produces avascularity of tissue and its overlying peritoneum, adhesions are very likely to form, and act as vascular grafts to support ischaemic tissue (Ellis, 1962).

In about 10% of adhesive obstructions there is **no history of laparotomy** and the bands may be **congenital**, as in some cases of Meckel's diverticulum, or **inflammatory**, such as may form after salpingitis.

6.2.2 OCCURRENCE

About nine out of every ten patients with adhesive intestinal obstruction will have had a previous laparotomy, and two-thirds of these will have been performed on the appendix, colon and rectum, or the pelvic organs. Krook (1947) calculated that 5% of the patients having an operation on these viscera would later suffer adhesive obstruction, but the incidence for operations on the colon can be as high as 20% (Lockhart-Mummery, 1967). Some 20% of these obstructions occur during the first postoperative year, and the majority arise during the first 4 weeks, and are considered separately as 'early postoperative obstructions'. Among the other 80%, about half present with an obstruction within 5 years of operation, but in 17% over 20 years passed before obstruction occurred (Raf, 1969).

6.2.3 EARLY POSTOPERATIVE OBSTRUCTION

This condition can be one of the more difficult conditions to manage in emergency abdominal surgery. As a starting point it is useful to consider the normal process of recovery from abdominal surgery.

If interference with the peritoneum has been minimal, as in inguinal hernia repair, there is little or no effect on the ability to drink and eat – a point repeatedly illustrated in day-surgery units. It is also now recognized that patients with non-perforated acute appendicitis can drink and take some light diet as soon as they recover from anaesthesia, and can leave hospital within 24 hours (Ramesh and Gallard, 1993).

The small bowel regains mobility and propulsion within a few hours of an abdominal operation but the colon reacts quite differently, and after colonic resection it can remain quiescent for 3–4 days. During that time small-bowel peristalsis propels swallowed air into the colon, which distends, but passage of flatus *per rectum* is delayed until colonic activity returns (Wilson, 1975).

Bowel sounds can, consequently, be misleading. They can return quite early with small-bowel activity, but this does not mean that the colon is active. If the patient looks well, and the abdomen is flat and relaxed, then it is reasonable to await events even if several days have passed since the operation.

On the other hand the surgeon is understandably worried if, after 4 or 5 days, the patient looks uncomfortable and anxious, there is some tachycardia, the abdomen is somewhat distended and resonant, bowel sounds are few and the X-rays show gas in dilated small bowel with little gas in the colon.

The question is whether this situation requires operative relief, or whether it is reasonable to await fibrinolysis and spontaneous separation of adhesions. Provided there is no serious colicky pain or other suggestions of strangulation it is reasonable to continue nasogastric suction for another 24 hours while giving careful attention to fluid and electrolyte balance. If there is still no progress there are two main possibilities to consider.

1. If there has been an operation for peritonitis, or if there has been a bowel resection and anastomosis (and the possibility of a leak from the suture line), there are reasons to suspect that **paralytic or neurogenic ileus** may be present. A rise of temperature and pulse, in an anxious, uncomfortable patient with a distended, tense, resonant and silent abdomen would support this suspicion. If an anastomotic leak is a possibility a water-soluble contrast study, either antegrade or by enema, is necessary. In some cases further active surgical intervention is needed, in others a conservative line of treatment is correct and these issues are considered on p. 259.

2. Most patients have a degree of **mechanical obstruction** and there are four possible causes for this.

    (a) The first priority is to decide whether a loop of bowel has become strangulated, either under a band or by slipping through a peritoneal defect, particularly if there has been an attempt to 'reperitonealize' after resection, e.g. closure of the pelvic peritoneum after rectal excision. The patient is likely to be restless and complaining of colic, and there may be abdominal tenderness.

    (b) In this situation the obstruction is usually due to adhesions and good judgement is needed to decide whether at this stage it is right to try the effect of a bolus of gastrografin: this contrast agent has an osmotic pressure six times greater than extracellular fluid and the additional fluid that this draws into the bowel can, in incomplete obstruction, lead to its resolution. This means that complete restoration of fluid balance is necessary before using this method, and considerable caution should be exercised in the presence of a newly made anastomosis. Joyce *et al.* (1992) injected 100 ml of gastrografin down the nasogastric tube of nine postoperative patients and exposed X-rays at 30 minutes and 4 hours: in eight they saw contrast in the colon at 4 hours and the obstruction resolved. Frager *et al.* (1995) examined 36 postoperative patients in this situation with CT scan 1–2 hours after giving 500 ml of gastrografin and they were able to distinguish mechanical obstruction in 31 patients from paralytic ileus in five: 20 of their 31 patients required laparotomy for release of the obstruction.

    (c) The small bowel is involved in a residual abscess, e.g. after an appendicectomy or beside an anastomosis.

    (d) The cause of the obstruction is not connected with the operation. This may be strangulation in a pre-existing hernia or, as in a recent patient, due to previous undiagnosed disease: a primigravida of 45 years required delivery by caesarean section. Three days later she vomited profusely and became distended: exploration revealed Crohn's disease in 45 cm of terminal ileum.

Sykes and Schofield (1974) remark that 'the diagnosis of intestinal obstruction depends upon being constantly alert to the possibility of its presence, and this is particularly apposite in the early postoperative period in view of the diagnostic difficulties'. A few of these patients need to be promptly identified and operated upon, while in most a careful examination by the same team at least twice in each 24 hours is essential.

Generally, if there has been no progress clinically and radiographically over 36–48 hours, then re-exploration would be indicated. By this time the commonest cause of obstruction, plastic fibrinous adhesions, are unlikely to resolve and require gentle separation. This is a good reason for being sceptical about the use of a Miller–Abbot or Cantor tube. They are difficult to pass successfully, but if this is achieved the decompression of the small bowel makes the patient feel better: this can make it all the more difficult to decide on the need for laparotomy. There are many references to the risks of unduly delayed laparotomy in the American literature (Bizer *et al.*, 1981; Brolin, 1984).

It is usual to reopen the previous vertical incision. A light, gentle touch is needed in these re-explorations because there are multiple fibrinous adhesions – some separate readily but others are tougher and it is easy to tear the oedematous wall of the obstructed bowel: the assistant has to be very careful as well as the surgeon. Sutures cut out of this friable bowel, so a fistula is a real possibility. Exceptional care is needed in the neighbourhood of abscesses, where the bowel is particularly friable.

The distended loops are lifted out and separated one by one, and then emptied back into the stomach. Eventually the point of obstruction is found and the kink straightened out. If need be the whole small bowel must be gently freed – this is much to be preferred to the misguided advice to leave matted loops in the pelvis alone and to anastomose mid-ileum to transverse colon.

The abdomen is thoroughly washed out with tetracycline solution and carefully closed after gently replacing the bowel back in the abdomen. A case may be made for placing a sheet of hyaluronate film between the bowel loops and the anterior abdominal wall to reduce the risk of adhesions at this point. The value of hyaluronate solution to coat the bowel throughout the procedure should be considered in cases of recurrent adhesive obstruction.

Parenteral nutrition has to be considered early as a prolonged convalescence is expected. It is probably better to insert the central venous feeding cannula at the time of laparotomy. A chest X-ray is taken to check the position of the cannula and for presence or absence of pneumothorax. Only when the doctor responsible for insertion of the line is happy on both points can fluid administration begin.

6.2.4   LATE ADHESIVE OBSTRUCTION

Symptoms and signs

Virtually every patient with this condition complains of acute abdominal pain of sudden onset. The obstruction inevitably involves the small bowel and is therefore centred on the umbilicus and is characteristically colicky. Silen *et al.* in 1962 pointed out that, although the pain of a strangulating obstruction is often said to be constant, 50% of patients have colicky pain. Almost all patients vomit, often repeatedly, and the vomit may be faeculent. Less than 50% complain of constipation because there is hardly time to appreciate this when patients present with severe symptoms (Gough, 1978).

On examination, the general condition of the patient is commonly satisfactory apart from dehydration due to vomiting and cessation of drinking. Strangulation does not necessarily alter the general state of the patient unless the affected loop is long: this leads to significant loss of blood into the loop, as already described (p. 185). Tachycardia and peripheral vasoconstriction are the early signs of this occurrence and should be taken seriously because, as noted earlier, abdominal signs may be few.

Abdominal examination is critical, but it has to be appreciated the signs are not always obvious and great care must be taken if they are to be elicited.

The **hernial sites** must always be examined. The scar of an **abdominal incision** will generally be present. Although abdominal distension is often present, it may not be in high jejunal obstruction and the speed with which strangulation can occur means that there can be little or no distension. It is critical to be aware of this. **Abdominal tenderness** is often present, but all studies comparing both single and strangulating obstructions show no differences in incidence, about two-thirds showing tenderness. However, all cases of patients with a gangrenous loop of bowel show localized tenderness, guarding and release pain. Auscultation may give the essential sign of obstructive intestinal sounds coinciding with the patient feeling colicky pain. It is no good expecting to hear this sign during a casual few seconds of auscultation. Take time and watch the patient's face: when the patient's expression changes, suggesting that a spasm of colic is starting, this is the time to start auscultation. In strangulating obstruction there are few bowel sounds because of the associated general ileus: only one patient in four will show hyperactivity (Silen *et al.*, 1962).

One important though unusual physical sign may occur when a number of loops of strangulated bowel caught under a band become palpable as a tender mass. This could be mistaken for a twisted ovarian cyst, but this is not serious if this sign makes the surgeon press on with surgery. Inspection of vomit is useful, because occasionally faeculent vomitus will suggest intestinal obstruction when it had not previously been considered.

There is no clear-cut difference to be drawn between simple and strangulating obstructions, and this topic has been discussed on p. 189, along with the radiographic signs of small-bowel obstruction.

Treatment

If a patient who has been well suddenly develops the symptoms and signs of small-bowel obstruction it is wise to assume that there is a mechanical cause for it. If the hernial sites are normal and there is a scar on the abdomen it is more than likely that the cause will be an adhesion or band. In the absence of a scar many other causes, to be considered in later sections, may be responsible.

Conservative treatment
Although there has been much enthusiasm for treating presumed adhesive obstruction by 'drip and suck', this approach carries two major disadvantages.

- If successful, it leaves the true cause in doubt.
- It is generally acknowledged that it is difficult to distinguish simple and strangulating adhesive obstructions, so great caution must be exercised over choosing conservative treatment. Obstruction that develops after an earlier appendicectomy, large bowel and pelvic surgery does not often resolve without an operation (Meagher *et al.*, 1993).

There are two situations in which it is reasonable to adopt it.

- When there are good grounds for believing the obstruction to be incomplete. The severity of the patient's complaints is beginning to ease, there are no signs of peritoneal irritation and the abdominal film shows not only dilated fluid-containing small-bowel loops, but also some gas in the colon. It is reasonable to treat these patients with 'drip and suck', keep a close watch on progress and test the osmotic effect of gastrografin. Assalia *et al.* (1994) treated 107 such patients and after careful rehydration therapy 59 received 100 ml of gastrografin down the nasogastric tube and 48 acted as controls. Overall, conservative treatment was successful in 85%, but the test group moved their bowels sooner and only

10% needed a laparotomy compared with 21% of the control patients. These patients need to be followed up in the outpatient clinic because the actual cause of the obstruction is not known. The patient may have Crohn's disease, a small-bowel neoplasm or slowly obstructing carcinoma in the proximal colon.

- The patient has had multiple previous operations for adhesive obstruction. This problem is considered on p. 200.

Operative technique

If there is a vertical scar from the previous operation, it is usually best to reopen this. Bowel may be adherent to the back of the scar so it is best to extend one end of the incision, deepen it down to the peritoneum and enter where the peritoneum is likely to be free of adhesions. A finger can then palpate the back of the scar and identify any adherent bowel. A wide exposure is likely to be needed.

Once the abdomen is opened it may be clear that there is strangulation present because there is a release of serosanguinous fluid. There may be extensive adhesions in cases of recurrent obstruction. Fortunately, in most patients the adhesions are confined to one point where a band is constricting the bowel. The distended bowel is gently delivered from the wound until the point of obstruction is reached. If possible, the bowel is decompressed by retrograde stripping as mentioned earlier.

Most often, the bowel is trapped by a fibrous band that is attached to either bowel or mesentery. The bowel is likely to show some degree of strangulation. This may vary from cyanosis to frank gangrene. It is not unusual for the band to 'give' when the bowel is being mobilized. If not, it may require division. It is now important to judge the viability of the bowel. This requires a degree of judgement and experience. A quick change of colour to a healthy pink resolves all the doubt about the viability in the loop but the question arises as to what to do with the constriction ring where the band held the loop. It is at this point that changes in colour are difficult to detect, as the area may be bruised. Palpation is always helpful. If the ring has the same consistency as the rest of the bowel then it is likely to be viable and safe. If it is grey and remains so and feels thin then it must be deemed non-viable. If this ring is very narrow it may be treated by unfolding it with a series of Lembert sutures, but resection may be needed.

If the strangulated loop does not speedily return to a normal colour, then tests of viability must be applied. It is worth remembering that strangulation by a band or by the neck of a hernial sac always means constriction of the mesentery and venous engorgement, while arterial inflow continues. This leads to severe congestion of the mesentery and bowel and local patches of haemorrhage develop. Only at a comparatively late stage do these changes lead to venous thrombosis and arterial obstruction.

Although experience is all-important, Bhajekar in 1947 suggested a useful classification of strangulation into three stages.

1. The bowel is deeply cyanosed but the serosa glistens, the consistency of the bowel is normal and there may be peristalsis. Following division of the band there is an immediate change of colour as venous drainage is resumed and well-oxygenated arterial blood perfuses the loop. There is no difficulty in deciding on viability.
2. The bowel is severely congested and dark blue in colour. Subserous haemorrhage is marked but patchy, and the test is to watch the colour change between the patches after division of the band. If these areas become pink and the wall of the bowel feels normally

thick this suggests viability: if mesenteric arterial pulsation is seen and there are some peristaltic movements, then these are useful confirmatory signs. It is useful to wrap bowel in a saline pack at 40°C and leave this for 5 minutes for a review of the rest of the abdominal organs, in particular eliminating any possibility of another distal obstruction. After 15 minutes it should be possible to reach a decision on viability, but this can be very difficult for a surgical trainee, who should have no hesitation in seeking the opinion of a senior colleague.

3.   The bowel looks black and green, and is inert and without mesenteric pulsation, and the bowel wall feels thin and fragile. This bowel requires resection.

Difficulties arise when the situation is on the borderline between stages 2 and 3. Generally, when there is a relatively short length of bowel of doubtful viability it is quicker and safer to resect. When longer loops of bowel are involved, which if resected may lead to the small-bowel syndrome, it is worthwhile considering reoperating on the patient after 24 hours to reassess the situation: the 'second look' operation.

Multiple adhesions
The division of a band is a simple matter and the problem is to decide whether the bowel trapped by it is viable. With multiple adhesions the problem is to disentangle the obstructed adherent loops and to find the point of obstruction. This can be a daunting and stressful task. The surgeon has to be patient and careful. It is useful to start at a point where it appears slightly easier to separate bowel. Once a difficult area is reached then move to another area until the situation clears. We prefer to use a sharp scalpel for this task, stroking the plane between the loops of adherent bowel, which are held under slight tension. Scissors can be used but only with great caution, because it is easy to cut too deeply and so enter the bowel. This is serious because, however carefully closed, this is a weak point during a period of ileus, and it can leak and cause a fistula. Because the bowel is matted together, strangulation is unlikely and the obstruction is usually due to kinking of the bowel: this point is indicated by the fact that the bowel below it is empty.

The tendency to circumvent these difficult situations by freeing a good length of upper small bowel and then perform a side-to-side anastomosis to bowel below the obstruction, thereby bypassing matted loops, should be avoided. This is bad practice because the defunctioned loops are still obstructed and have to empty in a retrograde fashion through the short circuit, often causing symptoms.

6.2.5   RECURRENT ADHESIVE OBSTRUCTION

This event is unusual. Most patients who suffer a band obstruction are not troubled in this way again. Krook (1947) followed up 309 patients after their first adhesiolysis and found that only 14% had required division of adhesions on a second occasion. Among this group 15% had required a third adhesiolysis. Fortunately this is a small group but they are particularly unfortunate because 'the results of these repeated operations (are) anything but encouraging – every fresh intervention gives a result inferior to the preceding one' (Krook, 1947). Some of these patients have a persistent low-grade obstruction and suffer recurrent colic and distension, and the need to exist on a sloppy, low-residue diet.

When operation has to be undertaken for an established obstruction the technical problems just described of separating multiple adhesions can be very considerable. For a long time ways were sought that would encourage the inevitable new adhesions, following the latest operation, to form in a favourable pattern, with the loops of small bowel adhering, and forming smooth rounded curves rather than kinks.

Noble (1937) thought this could be encouraged by stitching the small bowel in a ladder pattern, but this was not successful often enough to be taken up, and some patients had problems with fistulae.

In 1956 White suggested that a Miller–Abbott tube should be threaded down the whole length of the small bowel after all adhesions had been divided. The hope was that the intrinsic stiffness of the tube would hold the bowel in an orderly pattern, without kinks, as new adhesions formed in the weeks after the operation. Baker in 1968 introduced a long 16 FG Foley catheter, which was easier to introduce, and in 1974 we began to use a 300 cm 18 FG Foley catheter, introduced through a jejunostomy, and later reported our long-term results (Jones and Munro, 1985). In ten patients who had already had one laparotomy for adhesive obstruction, and in six who had had between two and four previous operations for adhesive obstruction, none had, over a period of 4–11 years, suffered any recurrence. The technique is fully described in that report and we believe that it is one worth considering when faced with one of the small but unfortunate group of patients who recurrently suffer complete adhesive obstruction and require a progressively more difficult operation for its relief.

REFERENCES

Assalia, A., Schein, M., Kopelman, D. *et al.* (1994) Therapeutic effect of oral gastrografin in adhesive partial small bowel obstruction: a prospective randomized trial. *Surgery*, **115**, 433–437.

Baker, J. W. (1968) Stitchless plication for recurring obstruction of the small bowel. *Am. J. Surg.*, **116**, 316–324.

Becker, J. M. M., Dayton, M. T., Fazio, V. W. *et al.* (1996) Prevention of postoperative abdominal adhesions by a sodium hyaluronate-based bioresorbable membrane: a prospective, randomised, double-blind multicentre study. *J. Am. Coll. Surg.*, **183**, 297–306.

Bhajekar, M. V. (1947) Strangulated inguinal hernia. *Arch. Surg.*, **54**, 41–57.

Bizer, L. S., Liebling, R. W., Delany, H. M. *et al.* (1981) Small bowel obstruction. *Surgery*, **89**, 407–413.

Brolin, R. E. (1984) Partial small bowel obstruction. *Surgery*, **95**, 145–149.

Ellis, H. (1962) The aetiology of postoperative adhesions. *Br. J. Surg.*, **50**, 10–16.

Frager, D. H., Baer, Rothpearl, A. *et al.* (1995) Distinction between postoperative ileus and mechanical small bowel obstruction: value of CT. *A.J.R.*, **164**, 891–894.

Gough, I. (1978) Strangulating adhesive small bowel obstruction with normal radiographs. *Br. J. Surg.*, **65**, 431–434.

Jones, P. F. and Munro A (1985) Recurrent adhesive small bowel obstruction. *World J. Surg.*, **9**, 868–875.

Joyce, W. P., Delaney, P. V., Goery, T. F. *et al.* (1992) The value of water soluble contrast radiology in the management of acute small bowel obstruction. *Ann. R. Coll. Surg. Engl.*, **74**, 422–425.

Krook, S. S. (1947) Obstruction of the small intestine due to adhesions and bands. *Acta Chir. Scand.*, **95**(Suppl. 125), 1–200.

Lockhart-Mummery, H. E. (1967) Intestinal polyposis: the present position. *Proc. R. Soc. Med.*, **60**, 381–384.

Meagher, A. P., Moller, C. and Hoffman, D. C. (1993) Non-operative treatment of small bowel obstruction following appendicectomy or operation on the ovary or tube. *Br. J. Surg.*, **80**, 1310–1311.

Menzies, D. and Ellis, H. (1991) The role of plasminogen activator in adhesion prevention. *Surg. Gynecol. Obstet.*, **172**, 362–366.

Milligan, D. W. and Raftery, A. T. (1974) Observations on the pathogenesis of peritoneal adhesions: a light and electron microscopic study. *Br. J. Surg.*, **61**, 274–280.

Noble, T. B. (1937) Plication of small intestine as prophylaxis against adhesions. *Am. J. Surg.*, **35**, 41–44.

Raf, L. E. (1969) Causes of abdominal adhesions in cases of intestinal obstruction. *Acta Chir. Scand.*, **135**, 73–76.

Ramesh, S. and Gallard, R. B. (1993) Early discharge from hospital after open appendicectomy. *Br. J. Surg.*, **80**, 1192–1193.

Silen, W., Hein, M. F. and Goldman, L. (1962) Strangulation obstruction of the small intestine. *Arch. Surg.*, **85**, 121–129.

Sykes, P. A. and Schofield, P. F. (1974) Early postoperative small bowel obstruction. *Br. J. Surg.*, **61**, 594–600.

Thompson, J. N. and Whawell, S. A. (1995) Pathogenesis and prevention of adhesive formation. *Br. J. Surg.*, **82**, 3–5.

White, R. R. (1956) Prevention of recurrent small bowel obstruction due to adhesions. *Ann. Surg.*, **143**, 714–719.

Williams, D. C. (1955) The peritoneum: a plea for a change in attitude towards this membrane. *Br. J. Surg.*, **42**, 401.

Wilson, J. P. (1975) Postoperative mobility of the large intestine in man. *Gut*, **16**, 689–692.

6.3   OBSTRUCTED INTERNAL HERNIAS

Intestinal obstruction due to bowel being trapped in one of the internal hernial sites is a rarity. However, these cases will present with symptoms and signs that are usually indistinguishable from band obstruction, so they must be considered alongside this much commoner cause. Internal hernias are those that occur entirely within the peritoneal cavity: strictly they do not include hernias (such as those through the diaphragm) that occur through the abdominal wall but produce no external swelling.

The sites at which internal hernias occur are:

1.   around the duodenojejunal flexure (paraduodenal);
2.   in the sigmoid mesocolon;
3.   through the foramen of Winslow;
4.   through the gaps in the mesenteries or the broad ligament;
5.   alongside the bladder;
6.   spigelian hernia.

Zimmermann and Laufman (1953) found only 12 cases in 10 years work in Cook County Hospital, Chicago, which has 3500 beds and a heavy emergency load, so the chances of an individual surgeon seeing such a hernia area are small, and the likelihood of making a preoperative diagnosis is slim. Among every ten such hernias, about half are paraduodenal, with single examples of the other five varieties.

Rare as they are, these hernias are important to understand because it is unlikely that the surgeon will be expecting to find one, and it will be discovered at exploratory laparotomy for intestinal obstruction. A paraduodenal hernia can appear to be exceptionally complex if it is encountered without prior knowledge of its anatomy.

6.3.1   PARADUODENAL HERNIA

This type accounts for about 50% of all internal hernias. It is fairly easy to recognize and to treat if the anatomy is appreciated. Andrews (basing his text on an idea of Herzler's) gave the first clear description of this hernia in 1923, and his explanation has become the accepted one. The hernia is well described by Bartlett *et al.* (1968).

Embryology

The rotation of the midgut occurs during the eighth to 11th weeks of fetal life and during this time both the pre- and postarterial loops normally rotate anticlockwise through 270° to take up their adult positions. In **right paraduodenal hernia** the prearterial loops rotate through only 90° and, as a consequence, the duodenum passes straight down into the jejunum and the small intestine occupies the right half of the abdomen. The postarterial loop, however, continues to rotate and so comes round and covers up the small bowel with the expanded ascending mesocolon (Figure 6.1).

As a consequence only the terminal ileum is truly intraperitoneal, with the rest of the small gut lying behind, and covered over by, the proximal colon and its mesocolon. The foramen through which the terminal ileum emerges from the retroperitoneal cavity is the point at which a loop of small gut can prolapse and become strangulated, kinked or twisted. In the anterior edge of this foramen will run the ileocolic artery and vein.

A **left paraduodenal hernia** seems to form after normal rotation of both pre- and postarterial loops has gone through 270°. The prearterial loop then invaginates into the descending mesocolon, behind the inferior mesenteric vein and is covered by the mesocolon (Figure 6.2).

Once again, it is only the terminal ileum that is intraperitoneal. It is helpful to term this type a 'hernia beneath the descending colon' and the right paraduodenal type a 'hernia beneath the ascending mesocolon'.

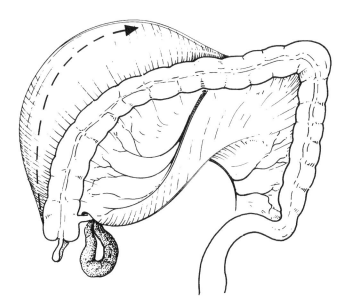

Figure 6.1 Right paraduodenal hernia. The postarterial loop of the midgut advances over the prearterial loop and covers it, leaving only the terminal ileum within the peritoneal cavity. A loop of small bowel has prolapsed through the foramen through which terminal ileum emerges. The dotted line indicates the incision that mobilizes the colon and releases the small bowel.

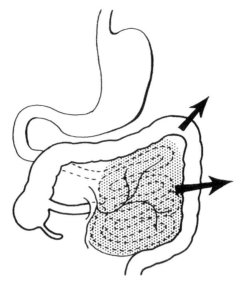

Figure 6.2 Left paraduodenal hernia. The arrows indicate the manner in which, in the process of rotation and fixation of the colon, the left mesocolon comes to cover the small bowel.

Clinical picture

The existence of these hernias is quite consistent with a normal existence and some individuals presumably never know that they have such an anomaly. Most cases come to light when a loop of bowel prolapses through the foramen, or torsion within the sac occurs. Occasionally a patient will have recurrent abdominal pain and the mass of the bowel within the sac becomes palpable. Cases of acute intestinal obstruction due to this cause can be seen from the neonatal period up to old age, and a high proportion of them involve strangulation of the obstructed loop. The characteristic emergency presentation is with colicky pain of sudden onset and of increasing severity, with vomiting and constipation. In these conditions the mass produced by the hernia is not likely to be felt. The plain abdominal X-ray may show coils of small bowel crowded into one side of the abdomen or the other.

Nevertheless, the condition is so uncommon that an accurate preoperative diagnosis is unlikely and the patient will come to operation as a case of acute small-bowel obstruction, most probably due to adhesions or bands.

Treatment

On opening the abdomen little or no small bowel will be visible and collapsed colon will be seen, either lying over or displaced by a tense peritoneum-covered mass containing small intestine: usually a discoloured strangulating loop will be seen emerging from the foramen of the hernia.

The right paraduodenal hernia is the easier to release. An incision is made parallel to and lateral to the ascending colon and caecum, through the peritoneal sac. This allows the right half of the colon to move to the left and releases the small bowel in the sac. The peritoneal division can be carried under the lower pole of the caecum to the foramen, and this line of incision is quite safe because it lies behind the ileocolic vessels, which run in the anterior edge of the foramen. Once this incision is completed small bowel is completely freed and it can be placed on the right side of the abdomen, with the colon on the left. The strangulated loop is examined and dealt with appropriately (p. 199).

A left paraduodenal hernia is not so easy to deal with. If a loop of small gut is strangulated in the foramen, it will be too tight to allow manual withdrawal of the remainder of the bowel into the abdomen: gentle digital dilatation may allow reduction of the strangulated loop, followed by withdrawal of the rest of the small bowel. If adhesions prevent this then it would be reasonable to mobilize the descending colon along its lateral aspect, if necessary with the splenic flexure, and turn the descending mesocolon medially to reveal the small bowel held confined within it. If it is really necessary, the neck of the foramen can be divided anteriorly but this means ligation and division of the inferior mesenteric vein and the left colic artery, and circulation in the colon must be carefully checked.

Paracaecal hernia also appears to be caused by an error in the rotation process, although it is much less pronounced than in paraduodenal hernias. When the caecum descends into the right iliac fossa it normally becomes completely attached to the posterior abdominal wall. This process of attachment may fail to some extent, leaving a retrocaecal cavity in communication with the peritoneal cavity. A loop of small bowel can become incarcerated in such a cavity and so produce intestinal obstruction.

6.3.2   HERNIA INTO THE SIGMOID MESOCOLON

The fossa sigmoidalis occurs in most people. The sigmoid mesocolon lies in front with the parietal peritoneum covering the bifurcation of the left common iliac artery, which is in turn crossed by the left ureter. In some the fossa is just a pyramid with its apex at the point where the two limbs of the sigmoid mesocolon meet, but in many people the fossa continues upwards rather in the shape of a finger of a glove.

Although the presence of such a fossa is frequent it is very rare to see an intersigmoid hernia. Clemenz and Kemmerer (1967) found only 34 cases in the literature in the 80 years up to 1964.

Diagnosis is usually made at laparotomy for intestinal obstruction. The distended loop of small bowel can be traced into the fossa, from where the obstructed segment can be teased out and dealt with accordingly. The opening into the fossa is closed by a non-absorbable suture.

6.3.3   HERNIA THROUGH THE FORAMEN OF WINSLOW

This is a rare form of hernia and Kiviniemi *et al.* (1984) found that only 115 cases had been described up to 1977.

Most people will have a small patent foramen of Winslow so it must be abnormally wide before such a rare hernia will occur. .

In a series of 90 cases the hernia contained small bowel in 57 cases, ileum and caecum in 27 and transverse colon in six: the age range was from 20–60 years (Erskine, 1967).

In common with other unusual hernias, the diagnosis is often made at laparotomy. However, some unusual features have been described. As well as having classical signs of acute small-bowel obstruction, the patient may note that the pain is eased by sitting up in bed with the knees drawn up to the chin or hunched in a chair. This observation was made as far back as 1888 by Treves, who also noted that pain may also be felt in the back.

A suggestive sign, if it is noticed, is a palpable epigastric mass consisting of herniated bowel in the lesser sac. It is easily missed because it is fairly soft and the patient finds it difficult to relax when lying flat. The mass is usually tender, but even if it is not felt then epigastric tenderness can be elicited. Distension is not a prominent sign and bowel sounds may be obstructive or totally absent. Obstructive jaundice due to pressure on the bile duct in the anterior wall of the foramen has been reported.

Successful radiological diagnosis is again unusual and depends on a loop caught in the lesser sac being outlined by gas- and fluid-levels. These appearances will be similar to a high small-bowel loop lying in front of the stomach. Contrast radiology is unlikely to be used in the emergency setting, although in the subacute situation a gastrografin meal may be helpful.

Treatment

At laparotomy the distended lesser sac is filled with bowel, but its significance may only be appreciated when the distended bowel is followed distally. Usually, gentle traction will reduce the hernia, but the duodenum may need to be mobilized by Kocher's manoeuvre to enlarge the foramen. If this fails because the bowel in the hernia is grossly distended the best method of decompression is to insert a 20 FG whistle-tip catheter, through a purse-string suture, into healthy bowel close to the foramen, pass it up the lumen into the distended bowel and apply gentle suction. By careful manipulation of the bowel the distension can be relieved and the bowel carefully withdrawn from the lesser sac. This technique is safer than direct puncture of the obstructed bowel, with the inherent risk of contamination.

Still and Scott in 1967 reported the only case of this type of hernia occurring during pregnancy. Intermittent pain was present for 40 hours before it became severe and laparotomy was decided upon. At the 36th week the uterus prevented access to the site of obstruction so a caesarean section was performed. This resulted in the delivery of a live child and provided access to the hernia, which was reduced.

The reported results of these operations have been good.

6.3.4   TRANSMESENTERIC HERNIA

This is the one type of hernia that does not have a true sac. The small bowel passes through a solitary hole, usually with smooth edges and of obscure origin, within the mesentery of the small intestine, transverse or sigmoid mesocolon, and becomes entrapped.

There are about 130 examples recorded in the literature. The consensus as to the origin is that they are congenital and this theory receives some support from the number of cases reported in young children. A defect may arise after a resection of bowel, with dehiscence of the closure of the mesentery.

Transomental hernia is a similar type of hernia in which bowel passes through a defect in the greater omentum. Defects in this structure are quite often seen at laparotomy and it is surprising that this type of hernia does not occur more often. Such defects can be produced at the time of operation and it is the author's practice to close these with an absorbable suture.

Hernia through the broad ligament has also been described; there is no embryological explanation for this and herniation is rare.

There are no special features in the presentation and management is immediate surgery. Some thought is needed to be given to preservation of the mesenteric circulation. The subject is extensively reviewed by Janin *et al.* (1980).

6.3.5 SUPRAVESICAL HERNIA

A supravesical hernia is one that commences its course by passing through one of the two supravesical fossae, i.e. the two triangles bounded in the midline by the medial umbilical ligaments (obliterated umbilical artery), and below by the transverse fold of the peritoneum where the fundus of the bladder meets the anterior abdominal wall. Supravesical hernia can be divided into two types.

- **External supravesical hernia**. These will appear as an ordinary direct hernia. It has been estimated that about 50% of all direct hernias are also supravesical: i.e. the neck lies medial to the obliterated umbilical artery. This does not modify the clinical appearance or operative treatment in any way.
- **Internal supravesical hernia**. Here the neck of the sac is the peritoneum of the supravesical fossa, usually 2–3 cm in diameter, and the fundus of the sac lies in the prevesical space (Figure 6.3).

  This is one of the rarest hernias, only 40–50 examples having been described. Nearly all were revealed by a loop of bowel becoming trapped and obstructed in the hernial sac. There is a strong tendency for these hernias to be associated with an inguinal hernia.

A majority of patients will be elderly men and they are likely to present with the symptoms of an internal small-bowel obstruction. At laparotomy, the small bowel will be trapped in the hernia and reduction can be achieved by carefully incising the neck of the

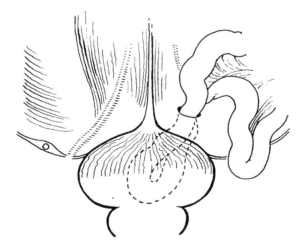

Figure 6.3 Internal supravesical hernia.

sac away from the bladder. If there is a reflex retention of urine it may be necessary to break off the operation and catheterize the bladder in order to improve the exposure. The hernia defect is simply repaired by sewing up the neck of the hernial sac with a non-absorbable suture.

6.3.6 SPIGELIAN HERNIA

This is a hernia through the semilunar line, at the lateral edge of the rectus abdominis, where the posterior rectus sheath is deficient, below the arcuate fold. The hernial ring is a defect in transversus abdominis and the hernial sac is often interparietal, covered by external oblique aponeurosis; consequently it may not be palpable when the patient is lying down. A strangulated spigelian hernia will present as a tender area, which may be mistaken for a haematoma of the rectus sheath but ultrasound can give a picture of the hernial ring.

External oblique has to be split to achieve access to the sac, and the opening in internal oblique and transversus is closed with non-absorbable sutures (Spangen, 1984).

REFERENCES

Andrews, E. (1923) Duodenal hernia – a misnomer. *Surg. Gynecol. Obstet.*, **37**, 740–750.
Bartlett, M. K., Wang, C. and Williams, W. H. (1968) Paraduodenal hernia. *Ann. Surg.*, **168**, 249–254.
Clemenz, F. W. and Kemmerer, W. T. (1967) Intersigmoid hernia. *Arch. Surg.*, **94**, 22–24.
Erskine, J. M. (1967) Hernia through the foramen of Winslow. *Surg. Gynecol. Obstet.*, **125**, 1098–1109.
Janin, Y., Stone, A. M. and Wise, L. (1980) Mesenteric hernia. *Surg. Gynecol. Obstet.*, **150**, 747–754.
Kiviniemi, H., Ramo, J., Pokela, R. *et al.* (1984) Herniation through the foramen of Winslow. *Acta Chir. Scand.*, **150**, 501–502.
Spangen, L. (1984) Spigelian hernia. *Surg. Clin. North Am.*, **64**, 351–366.
Still, R. M. and Scott, R. (1967) Hernia through the foramen of Winslow in pregnancy. *J. Obstet. Gynaecol. Br. Cwlth*, **74**, 939–940.
Treves, F. (1888) A clinical lecture on the hernia into the foramen of Winslow. *Lancet*, **ii**, 701–703.
Zimmermann, L. M. and Laufmen, H. (1953) Intra-abdominal hernias due to developmental and rotational anomalies. *Ann. Surg.*, **138**, 82–91.

6.4 VOLVULUS OF THE SMALL BOWEL

All forms of intestinal volvulus, affecting small as well as large bowel, are relatively common in some countries with a largely rural population. Small-bowel volvulus, which is a rare cause of obstruction in Western Europe, North America and Australasia, accounts for 15% in Northern India (Agrawal and Misra, 1970), 20% in Iran (Saidi, 1909) and 30% in Kenya (Kerr and Kirkaldy-Wallis, 1946). In some of these volvuli of the small-bowel adhesions or a Meckel's diverticulum form the axis of rotation, but the majority of cases reported from these countries follow a uniform pattern. The volvulus occurs almost exclusively in wiry, healthy farmers and seems commonest in the summer when they work all day in the fields and return home in the evening to a large meal. An interesting variety of this is seen in Moslem countries, when annual observance of Ramadan leads to a particularly large amount of food and drink being taken after a day-long fast. In Afghanistan incidence is always much higher during Ramadan (Duke and Yar, 1977) and is believed to be due to a large and relatively indigestible meal based on wholegrain flour arriving quickly in an empty small bowel. At laparotomy the twisted loops of small bowel tend to be loaded with 1–2 litres of thick, undigested food, often suspended on an unusually long mesentery. Perry (1983) demonstrated experimentally that the sudden distension of small bowel imparts a rotational driving force, because the antimesenteric aspect can elongate while the shorter mesenteric side of the bowel is relatively inelastic.

In the relatively few reports of apparently spontaneous small-bowel volvulus occurring in Western Europe, it is of interest that in several cases they had imbibed or eaten unusually freely shortly before the onset. Spontaneous small-bowel volvulus accounted for only 0.5% of a series of 2295 patients with small-bowel obstruction studied in Stockholm (Raf, 1969). In a few patients congenital malrotation or non-rotation of the midgut has resulted in the bowel hanging on a relatively unattached mesentery liable to volvulus at any time (see Figure 3.10). Characteristically, this complication occurs during the first week or two of life but occasionally volvulus of the malrotated midgut can present in children and adults (Devlin, 1971). In acute attacks the patient complains of pain and vomiting with upper gastric distension and the X-ray may show a characteristic gas distension of the duodenal loop, suggesting occlusion of duodenojejunal flexure by volvulus. In older patients there may be a history of recurring attacks of upper abdominal colic, followed several hours later by diarrhoea, which may be blood-stained. Some attacks of midgut volvulus are due to an adhesion or a Meckel's diverticulum suspending a narrow-based loop of bowel, while in others a mesenteric cyst has been responsible. Many, however, appear to be idiopathic.

Clinical picture

All attacks of small-bowel volvulus follow a similar pattern. It is quite important to be aware of this uncommon entity because the patients can present in a very serious condition.

There is an acute onset of severe central abdominal pain, which may be colicky and constant. This is followed by vomiting but this tends not to be copious, although it may be blood-stained. It is quickly apparent that the patient is greatly distressed by the severity of the pain, tends to lie or kneel in one position that gives relief and is most reluctant to move from that position (Tagart, 1950). The other striking feature is the speed at which patients show signs of hypovolaemic shock, due to sequestration of blood in the obstructed loop, consequent on obstruction of the venous drainage (p. 185). Webber (1945) described a 9-year-old boy who became profoundly shocked within 10 hours of the onset of abdominal pain, and was dead within 16 hours: the autopsy showed a volvulus of the whole small bowel. It has to be remembered that as much as 50% of the total circulating blood volume can be accommodated in a volvulus of the whole small bowel.

The other striking feature of these patients is that the congested bowel does not at first produce much peritoneal irritation (like other causes of mesenteric ischaemia) so although the patient is in great pain, and is clearly acutely ill, the abdominal signs are few – moderate tenderness and no more than a suggestion of guarding. Bowel sounds are few or absent. The abdominal X-ray may or may not show distended bowel and fluid levels. Talbot (1960) saw five such patients in two years and emphasized the mildness of the abdominal signs. These patients are not often seen, so this clinical picture needs to be remembered, because the most energetic resuscitation must go hand-in-hand with laparotomy, when untwisting of the bowel

– if it is viable – will restore a considerable volume of blood to the circulation. It is important to lift out the whole of the small bowel so that the volvulus can be recognized and reduced by counterclockwise rotation. In assessing viability, resuscitation and oxygenation need to be well advanced, so that mesenteric perfusion is optimal. Sight and smell may indicate that the bowel is no longer viable, and some extensive resections have to be performed. The value of 'second-look' laparotomy in 24–48 hours must be remembered. When resection is required, special attention must be paid to visible arterial pulsation at the suture line.

Goodwin (1968) reports the remarkable history of a 38-year-old woman at term in her fourth pregnancy. She complained of severe **upper** abdominal pain when admitted with poor labour pains, and began to vomit bile. There were few abdominal signs, but after 12 hours the abdomen was tender, blood pressure 90/60, pulse 140. At laparotomy there was a volvulus of most of the small bowel. Caesarean section delivered a stillborn baby, and after resection 45 cm of jejunum was anastomosed to 30 cm of ileum. On the fourth day the anastomosis had to be revised and an ischaemic patch excised, yet 3 years later she was well, with one stool a day.

Before closing the abdomen attention should be directed to the base of the mesentery because in some cases malrotation will have resulted in the upper jejunum and the lower ileum lying close together, and instead of the usual long insertion of the base of the small-bowel mesentery, the base is very short. A Ladd's band may require division, and the duodenojejunal junction may need to be freed. In these patients the small bowel should be laid in the right half of the abdomen, the colon in the left. Appendicectomy should be performed (p. 81).

REFERENCES

Aggrawal, R. L. and Misra, M. K. (1970) Volvulus of the small intestine in Northern India. *Am. J. Surg.*, **120**, 366–370.

Devlin, H. B. (1971) Midgut malrotation causing intestinal obstruction in adult patients. *Ann. R. Coll. Surg. Engl.*, **48**, 277–237.

Duke, J. H. and Yar, M. S. (1977) Primary small bowel volvulus. *Arch. Surg.*, **112**, 685–688.

Goodwin, D. P. (1968) Volvulus of the small intestine in labour. *Br. J. Surg.*, **55**, 469–470.

Kerr, W. G. and Kirkaldy-Wallis, W. H. (1946) Volvulus of the small intestine. *BMJ*, **i**, 799–801.

Perry, E. G. (1983) Intestinal volvulus: a new concept. *Austr. N.Z. J. Surg.*, **53**, 483–486.

Raf, L. E. (1969) Causes of small intestinal obstruction: a study covering the Stockholm area. *Acta Chir. Scand.*, **135**, 67–72.

Saidi, F. (1969) The high incidence of intestinal volvulus in Iran. *Gut*, **10**, 838–841.

Tagart, R. E. B. (1950) Volvulus of the small intestine: the position of relief. *Lancet*, **i**, 71–73.

Talbot, C. H. (1960) Volvulus of the small intestine in adults. *Gut*, **1**, 76–80.

Webber, B. (1945) Volvulus of the small intestine. *BMJ*, **ii**, 863–864.

6.5 IATROGENIC INTERNAL HERNIAS AND OBSTRUCTIONS

6.5.1 PARASTOMAL HERNIAS

Among patients with a permanent left iliac terminal colostomy, herniation alongside the stoma occurs in 5–10% (Devlin, 1988). The hernial sac may be interstitial (within the layers of the abdominal wall) or subcutaneous. It is rare for strangulation to occur, but if this is suspected it is wise to perform a laparotomy, extract the strangulated bowel and treat it appropriately. If gangrene is present and a resection is needed, the risk of postoperative sepsis is high, in spite of local and systemic application of antibiotics; it may then be wise to defer specific repair of the hernia. Devlin (1988) describes methods of repair.

Herniation alongside or within the everted bowel of a spout ileostomy is unusual, particularly when the ileum is brought along an extraperitoneal channel and the size of the trephine of the skin and abdominal wall is carefully tailored. Leong *et al.* (1994) followed up 150 patients who had an ileostomy fashioned at St Mark's Hospital and, after 20 years, 16% showed some herniation and 27 (18%) had experienced an episode of intestinal obstruction. Of these, 13 required laparotomy but only three were for impaction of small bowel in a parastomal hernia, nine others being for adhesions and one for recurrent Crohn's disease. These patients show signs of small-bowel obstruction and a mass beside the ileostomy which may or may not be tender. Cuthbertson and Collins (1977) had two patients with a 2–3-day history, and both required 2–4 feet (60–120 cm) of gangrenous bowel to be removed and the ileostomy to be resited.

With increasing use of loop ileostomies to protect low rectal anastomoses, a number of cases of volvulus immediately beneath the stoma have been seen. The insertion of a Foley catheter down the proximal limb often relieves the obstruction, only for it to recur when the catheter is removed. At laparotomy the volvulus is untwisted and the antimesenteric aspect of the ileum sutured to the peritoneum of the anterior abdominal wall over several centimetres (Anderson *et al.*, 1994). The authors have also seen volvulus occur in the ileum just proximal to the point at which it enters the abdominal wall to form a permanent end ileostomy.

Foley catheterization may also relieve this obstruction, and if it is retained for a day or two the obstruction may not recur.

6.5.2 HERNIAS DUE TO AMBULATORY PERITONEAL DIALYSIS

Since the introduction of continuous ambulatory peritoneal dialysis (CAPD) in 1976, it has become widely used, and two complications involve the appearance of hernias.

Any pre-existing but asymptomatic hernial sac is likely to be revealed by the introduction of CAPD. The patient complains of a painless swelling in the groin or scrotum, which with pressure can be emptied into the peritoneal cavity. If peritonitis should supervene the swelling may become painful.

The more important hernias are those that arise as a direct consequence of CAPD. The Tenckhoff catheter is inserted at laparotomy and, because wounds in uraemic patients do not heal normally, special care has to be taken with closure. However, incisional hernias occur, and there are a number of examples of strangulation of small bowel in hernias beside the catheter exit site, several of Richter-type (Engeset and Youngson, 1984). It is necessary for all who care for CAPD patients to be aware of this and, if pain and vomiting occur, to examine closely the possible hernial sites, because the lump can be small, difficult to palpate, with the added problem of diagnosis of a Richter hernia (p. 216).

6.5.3 HERNIAS SECONDARY TO LAPAROSCOPY

Intestinal complications secondary to the widespread use of laparoscopy have been relatively few. However, some examples of diathermy injury to bowel occurred after the introduction of laparoscopic interruption of the Fallopian tubes, and it must always be remembered that diagnosis of injury to small intestine can be particularly difficult, in part because of the slow onset of symptoms (p. 436).

The small defect left after removal of the laparoscope can develop into a hernial sac, and into it small bowel can enter and strangulate, with particular dangers attached to a Richter's hernia. This can occur at any time. We have seen three examples in the weeks after laparoscopy, one as recently as the second postoperative day, when an elderly woman vomited repeatedly: at laparotomy a knuckle of upper jejunum was completely obstructed within a left port site incision. The other two patients had Richter hernias. Incidence of port site hernias in 3000 laparoscopic procedures performed by one surgeon in Aberdeen is 0.1%. Patterson *et al.* (1993) review the subject and comment on the need for care in closure of port sites.

6.5.4   RETRO-ANASTOMOTIC HERNIAS AFTER PARTIAL GASTRECTOMY

This is now an unusual operation, but there are still patients who had this operation in the 1950s and 1960s when it was the standard procedure for chronic duodenal ulcer. When a Polya gastrectomy is concluded by forming an anterior gastrojejunostomy, a hiatus is formed between the transverse colon and the afferent and efferent loops. Herniation of a loop of bowel through this hiatus was known early in the century but was only described in detail in the 1950s by Stammers, who, in 1954, collected 16 examples. In eight a loop of jejunum had become caught in the hiatus, in five the afferent loop had doubled back on itself behind the efferent loop (Figure 6.4), and these were especially prone to the development of gangrene. In some cases omentum moved into the gap.

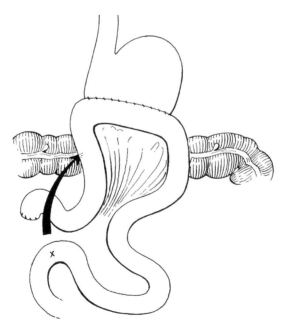

Figure 6.4 Following antecolic gastrojejunostomy the afferent loop can pass through the space behind the efferent loop and become obstructed.

Most patients presented in the postoperative period, about the fifth day, with pain and vomiting, and an opaque swallow was a key to the diagnosis. Nowadays, examples are more or less limited to late-onset cases, when the patient presents with the signs of a high intestinal obstruction, and this leads to early laparotomy. As Stammers remarked, half the secret in dealing with this unusual problem is to know that it occurs. Reduction of the loop and assessment of viability may be all that is required, although an unduly long afferent loop may need shortening.

6.5.5 RETROGRADE JEJUNOGASTRIC INTUSSUSCEPTION

This has always been an unusual complication of gastrojejunostomy and now that this is an uncommon operation, it is rarely seen.

It can occur days after the completion of the operation, with colicky upper abdominal pain and vomiting. If an opaque meal is given a filling defect may be seen in the stomach. Delayed intussusception can occur months or years after the operation, with the patient smitten with acute epigastric pain and vomiting: at first food and bile are vomited but later blood is brought up. In about 50% of patients an epigastric mass is palpable.

An opaque meal shows a typical rounded filling defect, or the intussusception might be seen at endoscopy for haematemesis. In 94 collected cases it was the efferent loop that entered the stomach in 73, and in 14 distal efferent loop intussuscepted into proximal efferent loop (Conklin and Markowitz, 1965). Ready *et al.* (1984) emphasize the importance of prompt diagnosis and operation in these patients, and they report an important case.

A 56-year-old man had had a Polya gastrectomy, with enteroanastomosis, 35 years before he presented with upper abdominal pain and vomiting. There was a tender mass in the left side of the epigastrium and the serum amylase was 2400 u/l. He had a haematemesis but gastroscopy showed no abnormality. After observation for $2\frac{1}{2}$ days, and a further haematemesis, his condition deteriorated and he came to laparotomy. A retrograde intussusception of the efferent loop had passed across the enteroanastomosis, up the afferent loop into the stomach. The pancreas was normal; 30 cm of gangrenous jejunum had to be resected and the Polya anastomosis reconstructed. This report is an important reminder of the truth of the aphorism (p. 384) that a gastrectomized patient with acute abdominal pain and a raised serum amylase is likely to have an obstruction of the afferent loop rather than acute pancreatitis (Everett and Sampson, 1969).

6.5.6 INTESTINAL OBSTRUCTION AFTER ABDOMINOPERINEAL EXCISION

The obstruction classically associated with this operation was herniation of small bowel through the space lateral to the left iliac colostomy, but this has been overcome by the technique of extraperitoneal colostomy. Johnson *et al.* (1981) reported 396 combined excisions without such a hernia being seen. Most obstructions are due to adhesions, and the majority arise during the patient's stay in hospital, so they present all the problems of the early differential diagnosis of postoperative ileus and mechanical obstruction (p. 195). An important variety is strangulation of a loop of small bowel in a defect in the pelvic peritoneal suture line.

REFERENCES

Anderson, D. N., Driver, C. P., Park, K. G. M. *et al.* (1994) Loop ileostomy fixation: a simple technique to minimise the risk of stomal volvulus. *Int. J. Colorect. Dis.*, **9**, 138.

Conklin. E. F. and Markowitz, A. M. (1965) Intussusception: a complication of gastric surgery. *Surgery*, **57**, 480–488.

Cuthbertson, A. M. and Collins, J. P. (1977) Strangulated para-ileostomy hernia. *Austr. N.Z. J. Surg.*, **47**, 86–87.

Devlin, H. B. (1988) *Management of Abdominal Hernias*, Butterworths, London, pp. 177–186.

Engeset, J. and Youngson, G. G. (1984) Ambulatory peritoneal dialysis and hernial complications. *Surg. Clin. North Am.*, **64**, 385–392.

Everett, W. G. and Sampson, D. (1969) Afferent loop obstruction mimicking acute pancreatitis. *Br. J. Surg.*, **56**, 843–844.

Johnson, W. R., McDermott, F. T., Pih, C. E. *et al.* (1981) Small intestinal obstruction following resection for carcinoma of the rectum. *Austr. N.Z. J. Surg.*, **51**, 34–36.

Leong, A. P. K., Londono-Schimmer, E. E. and Phillips, R. K. S. (1994) Life-table analysis of stomal complications following ileostomy. *Br. J. Surg.*, **81**, 727–729.

Patterson, M., Walters, D. and Browder. W (1993) Postoperative bowel obstruction following laparoscopic surgery. *Am. Surgeon*, **59**, 656–657.

Ready, A. R., Downing, R. and Black, J. (1984) Elevated serum amylase in association with jejuno-gastric intussusception. *Br. J. Surg.*, **71**, 844.

6.6   STRANGULATED EXTERNAL HERNIAS

6.6.1   INTRODUCTION

A strangulated hernia was for centuries the commonest cause of bowel obstruction, and this pre-eminence has only disappeared in countries with comprehensive health services, where many laparotomies are performed and so adhesive obstructions are often seen.

In Uganda 77% of all obstructions were due to hernias (Hall-Craggs, 1960) and in northern Nigeria the proportion was 65% (Chiedozi *et al.*, 1980). In Westernized countries strangulated hernias now account for 15–20% of bowel obstructions (Stewardson *et al.*, 1978; McEntee *et al.*, 1987), a substantial fall from Vick's large survey in England in 1932, when external hernias caused 55% of obstructions. The only comparable recent figure was found in Bournemouth, in a restricted group of 218 patients over 75 years of age with intestinal obstruction, of whom 115 (53%) had a strangulated external hernia (Blake and Lynn, 1976).

6.6.2   INCIDENCE, AGE AND MORTALITY

Inguinal hernias are about eight times more common than femoral hernias, but although they only constitute about 10% of all external hernia, 40% of femoral hernias are admitted as an emergency, compared to 5–10% of inguinal hernias (Nicholson *et al.*, 1990). Inguinal hernias are seen about six times more often in men than women, but for femoral hernias this ratio is about 5:1 in favour of women. Umbilical hernias are seen in equal numbers, but incisional hernias are about three times more frequent in women.

Strangulation of an external hernia is seen throughout life. It is a common event in inguinal hernias in the first months of life (p. 126), but it then becomes an unusual event until about the age of 40 years: incidence then rises steeply, reaching a maximum between 70 and 80 years of age (Andrews, 1981). Age is closely related to postoperative mortality, with an average age at death of 76 years. The other major factor affecting mortality is delay. Andrews (1981) found that among patients who arrived within 24 hours the mortality rate was 1.4%, but for those who came after 48 hours it was 21%.

There are two factors at work here. Patients who have been starved and have been vomiting for 2 or more days are likely to be seriously dehydrated, and need careful assessment and judicious resuscitation before surgery. Even so, this alone make recovery more difficult in the elderly.

Bowel that has been strangulated for more than 48 hours is very likely to need resection. This adds a major immediate risk in the shape of infection from gangrenous bowel and surrounding fluid, and a later one from the risks of resection and anastomosis.

6.6.3 PATHOLOGY

Any acute episode of intestinal obstruction which is associated with sudden pain or swelling in an external hernia must be termed a strangulated hernia, because there is no way in which external examination can determine whether the blood supply of the trapped bowel is or is not imperilled. 'Incarceration' is too benign a term to apply to a condition that can be so dangerous. 'Irreducibility' is applicable to many cold hernias (especially femoral, umbilical and incisional) found in patients who are well and with no acute symptoms: it should be applied only to this group.

The constricting ring that causes the strangulation is usually the neck of the sac, but in inguinal hernia the external abdominal ring may play this role, and is the reason why sedation of the infant with a strangulated hernia may result in relaxation of the abdominal muscles, with reduction of the hernia.

About a quarter of strangulated hernias contain omentum only, but in the other 75% containing bowel circulation is to some extent compromised. In patients admitted within 24 hours the bowel resection rate is 7%, but among those who wait more than 48 hours resection is needed in 27% (Andrews, 1981).

6.6.4 FEMORAL HERNIA

Delay before admission is characteristic of patients with a strangulated femoral hernia. A total of 100 patients seen by Thomas (1968) had had symptoms for 2.8 days compared with 45 patients with an obstructed inguinal hernia who had waited only 27 hours. The reasons for this are very important. Dunphy in 1940 pointed out that only one quarter of his patients had felt any pain in their femoral hernia, and only 42% knew they had a hernia. Nicholson *et al.* (1990) found that only 35% of their patients were referred to hospital with a correct diagnosis, and Hjaltason (1981) reported that in six of 46 patients the hernia was not palpated in the ward, the true diagnosis only being made at laparotomy.

Most of these patients, who are often well-covered, do not complain of their hernia, hence the reiterated advice to **make a thorough examination of the hernial sites in every patient, of all ages, who complains of acute abdominal pain**.

Clinical picture

Some 80% of patients are between 50 and 80 years of age, five out of six are women and 30% have significant cardiorespiratory disease (Chamary, 1993). Most patients complain of acute central colicky abdominal pain, consequent on the obstruction of the trapped small bowel. In a minority the hernial content is omentum with only vague abdominal discomfort, although the hernia may be painful.

A lump will be found in the groin, provided it is carefully sought, in the classic position, but it will **not** always be tender. In 51 patients Dunphy (1940) found no tenderness in 22, some tenderness in 10, and it was marked in 19. This absence of tenderness, compared to a strangulated inguinal hernia, can be most disquieting but it must not exclude the diagnosis.

The abdominal signs will be those of small-bowel obstruction, which in an obese patient may be hard to decide on. Auscultation over 2–3 minutes may yield the diagnostic build-up of obstructive sounds.

Richter's hernia

Well over 50% of Richter's hernias occur in a femoral hernia, most others in incisional or umbilical hernias and about 15% in inguinal hernias. It is a hernia – usually affecting terminal ileum – in which a portion of the circumference of the bowel wall is imprisoned, thus narrowing but not obliterating the lumen (Treves, 1887).

A lump is not always palpable but Gillespie *et al.* (1956) found that in 20 patients 18 had **tenderness** over the hernial site (11 were femoral, five incisional or umbilical, and four inguinal hernias). All complained of abdominal pain or discomfort, 14 had nausea and vomiting, eight showed abdominal distension and two-thirds of the 17 who had an abdominal X-ray showed signs of obstruction. In patients without clear signs of obstruction suspicion must be high if there is nausea and discomfort and tenderness over a hernial site.

The bowel released from a Richter's hernia must be assessed and treated accordingly. If there is a small patch of ischaemia, it may be possible to excise it and close the defect transversely, after the style of a Mickulicz pyloroplasty.

Littré's hernia

Littré's hernia is generally taken to be any hernia containing incarcerated Meckel's diverticulum. About one-half occur in inguinal and one-quarter in femoral hernias (Perlman *et al.*, 1980).

Treatment

There is no place for postural treatment in strangulated femoral hernia. The method of repair described by McEvedy (1950), based on Henry's (1936) extraperitoneal approach, is superior to any other, although a transverse muscle-splitting incision is much to be preferred to a vertical incision.

The skin incision runs in a skin crease, from a point medial to the anterior superior iliac spine to a point short of the midline (see Figure 3.12); it is centred on the lateral edge of the rectus sheath. External oblique is split in the line of its fibres to reveal the linea semilunaris. This is incised horizontally with a knife and the anterior rectus sheath is opened medially with scissors: this split is extended laterally by incising the muscular internal oblique and transversus abdominis and then the two index fingers are used to widen this muscle-splitting incision.

Retractors are inserted, and transversalis fascia is opened to reveal the surface of the peritoneum. The rectus is now retracted medially (taking care to avoid damaging the inferior epigastric vessels) and the lower lip of the incision is retracted downwards. Blunt dissection outside the peritoneum will lead down to the neck of the femoral hernia as it enters the femoral canal. If bowel is involved in the hernia then it is wise at this stage to open the peritoneum near the neck of the hernia and secure one of the intestinal loops with a Babcock's forceps, to avoid the possibility of the bowel escaping after release (Figure 6.5).

The bowel must now be eased out of the hernia, and this usually entails dilatation of the fibrous neck of the sac, which is the actual cause of the strangulation. If a pair of Moynihan cholecystectomy forceps is introduced into the neck of the sac and gently opened up, the neck will be dilated from within and this usually allows the strangulated bowel to be withdrawn. This is wrapped in a warm saline towel while the sac is withdrawn through the femoral canal.

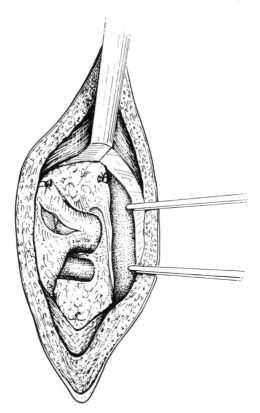

Figure 6.5 Preperitoneal approach to a right femoral hernia. The surgeon's view, looking down under the lower flap of the incision, with the inferior epigastric vessels divided and rectus abdominis retracted medially. The neck of the sac is passing into the femoral canal, medial to the femoral vein, and behind the inguinal ligament. An incision to the neck of the sac allows strangulated bowel to be secured.

If the fundus of the femoral hernia feels bulky then it is worth modifying this procedure. Dissect down in the subcutaneous plane of the lower skin flap until the sac is reached and clean and isolate it. This is easily done. Now cut gently through the layers, which are numerous, until peritoneum is reached. It is worth taking some trouble, by packing off with swabs and by having the sucker working, to avoid spillage of the dangerous and very infective fluid that could be spilt when the sac is opened. A bacteriological swab must be taken. Having done this, withdraw the loop of bowel in the manner already described and then amputate the sac at the level of the fossa ovalis. Doing this avoids having to pull the bulky fundus of the femoral hernial sac through the femoral canal.

Now return to the abdomen, draw the neck of the sac out of the femoral canal and turn attention to the strangulated bowel, which is assessed by the methods already described (p. 199). If the bowel is viable it is returned to the abdomen. The whole of the sac is removed. The gap in the peritoneum that is left by doing this, and the incision already made to secure the bowel, are closed with a running suture of 3/0 Prolene.

If the viability of bowel remains in doubt then it should be wrapped in a warm saline towel while the repair is completed. This is done by placing one or two unabsorbable sutures to bring the inguinal ligament down to its pectineal part, thus occluding the entrance to the femoral canal. Avoid compression of the femoral vein by careful placement of the sutures – one of the hazards of the low approach is that these sutures cannot be accurately sited and there is a risk of causing deep vein thrombosis. Alternatively, the femoral canal can be closed by inserting into it a cone of rolled-up Prolene/Marlex mesh.

If resection of bowel proves necessary it is easy to draw out the intestines through the peritoneal incision: this also is awkward if the low approach is used.

The incision is closed, after thorough antibiotic washout, with interrupted 3/0 Prolene, and a running suture of 2/0 polydioxanone to external oblique.

Results
These are directly related to the length of time which elapses before the patient is admitted. Those who arrive after 48 hours are likely be dehydrated and exhausted, and much more likely to require a bowel resection. They require high-quality preoperative preparation and careful surgery to avoid contamination from ischaemic bowel. With 30% of patients having established cardiovascular disease, and the high average age of these patients, expert postoperative care is needed. Recent reports show a mortality rate of 4% (Chamary, 1993) to 8% (Nicholson *et al.*, 1990).

6.6.5 INGUINAL HERNIA

This common emergency should not present any major difficulty in diagnosis.

The patient is usually a man and is most likely to be between 40 and 70 years of age, though the condition is not rare both above and below these ages. Almost all patients know that they had a hernia before and they recognize that it has suddenly become tense and painful. In only 10% of Frankau's (1931) 650 patients was strangulation the first sign of the presence of a hernia, and in only 2% of his series was the lump not painful. The major hazard of strangulated femoral hernia (the patient's ignorance of the presence of a strangulated hernia) is therefore not a problem with inguinal hernia.

Usually the lump is obvious and on inspection, very tense and tender on palpation, with no cough impulse, and there are signs of intestinal obstruction on abdominal examination.

Some 97% of strangulated inguinal hernias are oblique, and about 60% are right-sided. The sac will contain small intestine in about 80% of patients, quite often with some omentum being trapped as well. The appendix was found in the sac in three of Frankau's (1931) patients, and a Meckel's diverticulum in four. Large intestine is found in only about 5% of strangulated inguinal hernias, in contrast to the frequency with which sigmoid colon in a sliding left inguinal hernia becomes irreducible. If omentum only is strangulated there is a painful lump but no abdominal signs or symptoms. This is seen in about 10% of patients.

The major differential diagnosis is to recognize when an inguinal hernia is irreducible but not strangulated. This may be seen in a long-standing scrotal hernia as a result of adhesions, but the most likely emergency presentation is when an elderly patient has a left sliding inguinal hernia within which hard faecal masses can slip into the herniated sigmoid colon and prove very difficult to reduce. The hernia is irreducible and may be a little tender but there are no signs of obstruction and the scybala in the loop are usually easily recognizable.

The other major diagnostic problem is torsion of an ectopic testicle: examination of the scrotum should immediately make clear what has happened. Occasionally a retroperitoneal haemorrhage can present as a swelling in the inguinal canal, and postoperative peritonitis can occasionally cause confusion when pus collects in a pre-existing inguinal sac (Cronin and Ellis, 1959; p. 153). This produces a tender tense swelling that closely resembles a strangulated hernia.

Treatment by posture

The use of posture should not be forgotten in adults because it can so easily be practised while the preparations for operation are going on.

Bowesman (1951) has argued most cogently for this method, based on his experience in the Gold Coast. Over a 12-year period during which he used immediate operation, Bowesman noted that he did not see gangrenous bowel if the duration of strangulation did not exceed 24 hours. He found that he had a high mortality with this universal policy of early operation, so he decided to try postural treatment if it was certain that the hernia had been present for less than 24 hours. (He continued to operate forthwith on those whose hernias had been strangulated some 24 or more hours or in whom he thought a Richter's hernia was present.)

The regime was:

- 2 foot (60 cm) blocks at the foot of the bed;
- morphine 30 mg; (20 mg is the usual dose);
- warm blankets around the patient;
- flexion of hips and knees.

He found a reduction rate of 72%, which occurred on average some 4 hours after the start of postural treatment and was not likely to happen after 6 hours. In 10 out of 47 patients the hernia did not reduce and it had to be operated on. None of these 47 patients died. Three who had strangulated hernias of more than 24 hours duration needed a resection and of these one died.

This is an impressive record and shows the safety of postural treatment when its application is strictly controlled. All the 34 patients who were treated by posture subsequently had an elective repair without mishap.

Operation

This is indicated in any patient in whom postural treatment has been tried for a few hours, and anyone unsuited to it.

Local anaesthesia may be the best choice, either by reason of local circumstances or because the patient is deemed unfit for general anaesthesia. Lignocaine 0.5% with 1 in 200 000 adrenaline can be used up to a total of 50 ml. Starting 2.5 cm medial to the anterior superior iliac spine the subcutaneous tissues are infiltrated along the line of the incision, over the external ring and down on to the sac. The incision is made down to external oblique and then the tissues deep to it are infiltrated, working from the external ring laterally. The neck of the sac may need careful infiltration.

Sometimes the additional relaxation of the external ring induced by the anaesthetic is followed by reduction of the hernia. In that case repair should proceed in the normal way.

If the hernia remains strangulated a generous incision is needed, made in the long axis of the sac, and it is deepened down to the external oblique: this is opened, lateral to the external ring, in the line of its fibres, first being split laterally, then down to and through the external ring, and onward, opening external spermatic fascia. It may now be possible to tease the sac out of its coverings, dissect the spermatic cord away from it and bring the sac out on to the surface, where the discoloured bowel and bloodstained fluid content can be seen. The sac is very carefully opened and as soon as fluid runs out, a bacteriological swab is taken and the fluid is mopped up while the sac is split towards the fundus. Sometimes opening up external oblique releases the strangulation, but the tight neck of the sac may have to be sought, and the conjoint tendon will need firm retraction upwards while the neck is sought at the internal ring. Haemostats should be placed on each side of the incised edges of the sac. Once the neck of the sac has been incised it should then be possible to draw out some normal bowel and commence assessment of the viability of the strangulated bowel (p. 199). Occasionally, in a large hernia, colon is trapped in an inguinal hernia, and this is usually a **sliding hernia** of caecum and the appendix on the right, or the sigmoid colon on the left. A sliding hernia is usually only covered by peritoneum on its medial aspect (Figure 6.6), and the strangulation may affect small bowel, which slips into this narrow finger of peritoneum.

The appearance and feel of the contents may raise a suspicion that colon is present, with no true peritoneal sac, and this lateral extraperitoneal aspect of the colon should be left severely alone. The medial side of the region of the internal ring should be explored to see if peritoneum can be identified; any small bowel should be assessed and the peritoneal defect closed with a purse-string suture. Colon is then returned to the abdomen and a careful repair of the inguinal canal is performed.

If there is ever a serious doubt about the viability of colon involved in a hernia then the only safe course is to perform a laparotomy and make a complete mobilization and inspection of the suspect area. This is considered in the next section.

Usually, repair of the breach in the peritoneum at the neck of the sac is easily dealt with by twisting the sac and ligating the neck in the usual manner. However, in large hernias in which the division of a large sac has had to be carried up to the deep inguinal ring, repair can call for some care, and it is here that it is important to have the edges of the defect controlled in haemostats, while the defect is closed with a running suture of 2/0 or 3/0 Prolene.

The use of a non-absorbable mesh now plays a major part in elective inguinal hernia repair. A sheet of Prolene or Marlex mesh, 11×6 cm, is shaped and sutured to the conjoint tendon

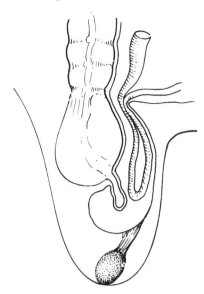

Figure 6.6 Sliding hernia. The diagram shows how the sigmoid colon on the left or the caecum on the right slide down the inguinal canal only covered medially and anteriorly by peritoneum. These hernias usually have a long history and should be suspected in an elderly man with a big hernia; peritoneum should be sought at the internal ring, on the medial aspect of the colon.

and the inguinal ligament, and laterally split into two tails, encircling the spermatic cord at the internal ring. This acts as a reinforcement to the posterior wall of the inguinal canal.

The authors have used this on 12 occasions for a strangulated hernia, a single injection of prophylactic antibiotic being given as the mesh is inserted. Some doubt must be expressed over whether this is a wise step when gangrenous bowel has been delivered and resected.

Reduction en masse

This is the classic complication of an attempt to reduce a strangulated hernia – almost always inguinal – by taxis. It requires some force to achieve this and it happened more often when surgeons were unwilling to operate. It is now a rarity, but needs to be understood in the event of it happening.

Mass reduction means that a strangulated hernia is reduced by pressure to lie deep to the abdominal wall, where it cannot be seen and rarely felt, while obstructive symptoms and signs continue. In the presence of a lax internal ring the inguinal hernial sac and its contents (still held and obstructed by the tight neck of the sac) can be displaced to lie deep to the abdominal muscles, in a properitoneal position (Figure 6.7). (The suggestion that a pre-existing properitoneal sac has to be present before this can happen is now discounted as unlikely.)

The patient is usually an elderly man who has controlled an inguinal hernia with a truss. The hernia often comes down and is replaced by the patient. On this occasion this has proved to be painful and difficult, and a few hours later abdominal colic and vomiting commence.

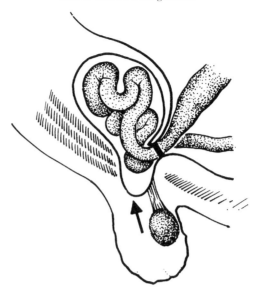

Figure 6.7 Reduction *en masse*. Massive reduction of a scrotal hernia and its contents through the internal ring into a properitoneal position. The testis is drawn upwards through traction on the spermatic cord.

There are likely to be signs of small-bowel obstruction, with some tenderness over the inguinal area, and perhaps the impression of a deep mass. The inguinal canal may feel boggy. Barker and Smiddy (1970) have described a useful additional sign in two patients – the testis is drawn up near the external ring, and traction upon it produces pain in the iliac fossa. This is due to the traction on the spermatic cord produced by the mass reduction of the hernial sac, to which the spermatic cord is adherent.

Treatment requires good access to the inner aspect of the abdominal wall and is best obtained through a generous vertical laparotomy incision. The neck of the sac should be sought, and the contained bowel released, withdrawn and assessed in the usual way. The sac is removed and the opening in the peritoneum at the neck of the sac is opened up to provide access to the inner aspect of the internal ring. This needs to be repaired and use of a sheet of Prolene or Marlex mesh may provide useful reinforcement.

6.6.6   UMBILICAL HERNIA

Among 100 patients with a strangulated hernia, about 10 will occur in a paraumbilical hernial sac (Hjaltason, 1981). Although relatively few are seen, they carry a particularly high risk to the patient. This is partly because a resection of damaged bowel is required in 25% (Andrews, 1981) and partly because almost all the patients are elderly, they are usually obese and 85% have a serious associated problem such as cardiovascular disease or diabetes (Gibson and Gaspar, 1959).

There is another important feature of umbilical hernia contributing to the high mortality, and that is the difficulty of deciding whether strangulation has occurred in a hernia that has for long been known to be irreducible. This can be difficult both for patient and doctor and often leads to delay in admission. The majority of patients have had a paraumbilical hernia for a long time. This they have come to tolerate, and they are used to episodes of discomfort associated with it. The usual signal that the hernia has strangulated is onset of nausea and vomiting associated with cramping or steady abdominal pain, and tenderness of the hernia. One reason for delay is that colon may be involved in the hernia, and obstruction of colon does not cause such acute pain and vomiting as occurs with small-bowel obstruction. These factors may combine to make the patient procrastinate, so that, by the time of admission, there is discoloration of skin over the hernia, and a serious degree of water and electrolyte depletion. Even then, vigorous replacement therapy and good surgery can save the day.

Experience teaches that, though there is no doubt that a patient has an irreducible umbilical hernia, it can be difficult to be sure whether strangulation is certain: in these circumstances it is much wiser to carry out an emergency repair as soon as the patient has been made as fit as is possible for the operation. Delay in recognizing strangulation after admission occurred in one-third of the 171 patients reviewed by Gibson and Gaspar (1959).

Operation

This can be a difficult procedure and should not normally be tackled without at least experienced guidance. This is because these hernias are often large, and contain both small and large intestine and omentum, which are adherent to each other.

The best approach is to make two long transverse incisions above and below the neck of the hernia. If the neck is wide the incision climbs on to the sac in order to provide enough skin to allow the skin edges to come together at the end of the operation. The two skin flaps are dissected up so as to expose the normal anterior rectus sheath on each side and define accurately the neck of the sac.

These landmarks having been made clear, the sac is opened at a convenient point and the task of sorting out the contents begun. Generally, the contents are more adherent at the fundus than at the neck, so it pays to open the sac 1–2 cm up from the neck and work round. Sometimes it is helpful to split the sac up towards the fundus, open it out and see what it contains. Omentum is often widely adherent to the sac and usually the best course is to amputate this omentum by multiple ligatures of bunches of tissue at the level of the neck of the hernia. By now the neck should be clearer and any bowel going up into the sac can be identified and followed up and released. This can involve a good deal of patient work with fine dissecting scissors and the scalpel.

Strangulated small bowel is likely to be free because it will only recently have entered the sac. It can be released by making horizontal incisions out into the anterior and posterior rectus sheaths, at 3 and 9 o'clock on the circumference of the neck of the hernia. Viability is assessed in the usual way. Exceptional care must be taken over assessing any strangulated colon. When there is doubt it is much wiser to resect, because the penalties of retaining non-viable colon are so severe. Immediate anastomosis may be appropriate but it may be wiser to exteriorize the two ends of bowel as faecal and mucous fistulae rather than attempt anastomosis. Thorough antibiotic lavage of peritoneum and wound is important before attempting closure. When a considerable length of small bowel has been involved in a large strangulated umbilical or incisional hernia, and is of doubtful viability, it can be very helpful to employ the 'second look' procedure (p. 200). This may allow the conservation of significant lengths of small bowel which at first sight appeared not to be viable.

When all bowel has been reduced into the abdomen, and omentum has been either reduced or excised, the neck of the sac should be clear and ready for repair. It is rarely possible to suture a separate peritoneal layer and reliance must be placed on the suture of the upper and lower edges of the defect. A Mayo type of repair is usually possible and gives two suture lines instead of the single one when the edges are only apposed. This involves cleaning the upper and lower flaps and then inserting interrupted silk sutures to bring the lower flap up behind the upper flap. The edge of the upper flap is then sutured to the front of the lower flap. An overlap of 1.5–2.0 cm should be obtained. If the tissues do not allow a tension-free overlap, a piece of Marlex or Prolene mesh, soaked in antibiotic solution, can be cut to size and sutured into position to repair the defect.

In these poor-risk patients, close collaboration between surgeon and anaesthetist both before and after operation is of particular importance, and a number will require intensive therapy facilities.

6.6.7   INCISIONAL HERNIA

Incisional hernias have become progressively less common, as has burst abdomen, with the general acceptance among surgeons that abdominal incisions cannot safely be closed with catgut. Jenkins (1976) emphasized the importance of the large-bite, slack-suture technique, in which the length of the suture was some four times the length of the incision. With this technique, using continuous non-absorbable sutures, he closed 1505 incisions with only one evisceration. Those who have followed his methods have experienced rates of wound dehiscence of much less than 1%.

When incisions sutured in various ways are followed up over 10 years, Mudge *et al.* (1986) found that wounds sutured with catgut only have a 14% incidence of incisional hernia; in those closed with nylon only it is 7.7%. They found that only 4.3% of hernias appeared during the first year after operation. Advanced age, obesity, postoperative distension and, most of all, wound infection are the important factors favouring subsequent herniation (Bucknall *et al.*, 1982).

Most incisional hernias are diffuse bulges and are unlikely to strangulate. The smaller local breakdowns, with a sharp edge to the linea alba defect, are those most likely to harbour a strangulation. Even gridiron incisions can cause trouble and in Aberdeen, where some 650 appendicectomies were performed annually, ten incisional hernias were seen during 1971–1974 and five contained strangulated bowel (Pollet, 1977).

The onset of pain and vomiting, with a tense tender area in the hernia, and signs of intestinal obstruction, will leave no room for doubt about the diagnosis and the need for exploration.

Repair

As in dealing with paraumbilical hernia, the first step is to expose normal tissues and this usually means obtaining a clear view of the anterior rectus sheaths up to the point of disruption in the midline. Once all sides of the hernia are clearly isolated it is then best to open up one of the side walls of the sac, find an area free of adhesions and then work up towards the fundus. The method of dealing with the contents follows the same lines as in umbilical hernia.

Once the contents have been reduced and the sac has been excised an attempt should be made to bring the edges of the linea alba together. If this is not possible it is well worth making a vertical relieving incision down the lateral one-third of one anterior rectus sheath. This immediately relaxes the tissues in the midline but preserves the abdominal wall because the rectus abdominis remains covering the posterior rectus sheath. By using this relaxing incision at one or both sides the peritoneum and the linea alba should come together without undue tension and the repair can commence. The flap of medial rectus sheath obtained from the relaxing incision in one (or both) rectus sheaths is brought across and sewn to the opposite rectus sheath. If this does not repair the defect a mesh repair can be performed. As always, if strangulated bowel has been released a thorough antibiotic lavage of the whole wound must be carried out.

6.6.8   OBTURATOR HERNIA

This hernia is better known than might be expected in view of its rarity and infrequent diagnosis before operation. Rogers (1959) found 12 cases among 3000 small-bowel obstructions seen over 22 years in Los Angeles, but Archampong (1968) had the extraordinary experience of treating 6 patients in 8 months in one surgical unit in Welwyn, Hertfordshire, and all survived.

Anatomy

The obturator foramen is almost closed by the obturator membrane. Where the obturator artery and nerve slip out of the pelvis, under the pubic bone, in the subpubic groove, they leave a gap in the membrane. This passage is called the obturator canal and it is 2–3 cm long. The membrane itself is strong so the gap has tough edges and is very liable to cause strangulation of small bowel, which is the usual structure to become incarcerated.

Clinical picture

About 90% of patients are elderly women, who are notably thin: 20 adult patients seen over 10 years in Thailand (Martin and Welch, 1974) only weighed between 26 and 35 kg! The history of abdominal colic and vomiting often extends over several days, so dehydration is marked. Diagnosis of an obturator hernia depends on a complaint of pain in the distribution of the obturator nerve, i.e. the antero-medial aspect of the thigh from the perineum to the knee. This was pointed out by Howship in 1840. Close questioning is needed to check the exact distribution of the pain, which can easily be confused with rheumatism. The sensation may be one of pricking, tingling or sharp pain, intermittent or continuous. It is usually eased by moving the leg to a new position and especially by flexing the hip. In view of the advanced age of many patients and their general condition, which is often poor, it is not surprising that this symptom is only elicited from 50% of patients who prove to have an obturator hernia.

A thin elderly woman shows signs of established small-bowel obstruction, usually without any abdominal scar or palpable hernia. It is rarely possible to feel a mass, or tenderness, below the inguinal ligament, although sometimes the mass can be felt *per vaginam*: often no lump is felt.

In these circumstances diagnosis depends on recognizing Howship's symptom, and this is clear-cut in less than half of patients, so most come to laparotomy for a small-bowel obstruction.

Treatment

It is clear from what has been said that a few hours spent in preparing the patient for operation will be repaid.

If it is strongly suspected that there is an obturator hernia then it will probably be best to make a low paramedian incision. This will give excellent access if the diagnosis is correct and still allow abdominal exploration if it is incorrect. If the diagnosis can be confidently made then McEvedy's approach would give good access.

Reduction of the strangulated bowel has usually been a simple matter, dilatation of the neck of the sac only being needed to release the bowel. Viability will be judged on the usual criteria. Although several complex methods of repair are described, there does not seem to be any need to go beyond inversion of the sac and ligation of the base. If the defect in the obturator membrane seems to be particularly large then a mesh repair would probably be appropriate.

6.6.9   LUMBAR HERNIA

This unusual hernia is rarely the site of a strangulation. It occurs through the triangle of Petit, bounded in front by external oblique, behind by latissimus dorsi and below by the iliac crest. The peritoneal sac needs to be opened, emptied and tied off at its neck. A mesh repair may be needed to cover the defect.

6.6.10   INTESTINAL STENOSIS AFTER RELEASE OF STRANGULATED HERNIA

When a loop of strangulated small intestine is released the surgeon studies it and decides whether it is viable or non-viable. It may be easy to decide that the bowel falls into one or other category. Bowel that is doubtfully viable will from time to time be returned to the abdomen when it is partially ischaemic. This does not affect all coats sufficiently to allow perforation but some part of the wall undergoes necrosis and is replaced by fibrous tissue. This must happen fairly often to some degree but it is rare for the fibrosis to produce intestinal stenosis.

Cherney examined the literature in 1958 and could only find 82 examples. This is not a good indication of incidence because most surgeons have probably seen one or more examples of this change. Cherney (1958) found that many of these patients had seen rectal bleeding during their convalescence. One-third of the patients developed diarrhoea within days or weeks of the operation. Signs of slowly increasing small-bowel obstruction develop some 3–4 weeks after the release of the bowel. Cherney found that the strangulated hernia responsible had been inguinal in 39, femoral in 31, umbilical in three and ventral in four. Resection of the affected segment will be required. The same changes can be seen in bowel released from strangulation under a band.

REFERENCES

Andrews, N. J. (1981) Presentation and outcome of strangulated external hernia in a district general hospital. *Br. J. Surg.*, **68**, 329–332.

Archampong, E. Q. (1968) Preoperative diagnosis of a strangulated obturator hernia. *Postgrad. Med. J.*, **44**, 140–143.

Barker, K. and Smiddy, P. G. (1970) Mass reduction of inguinal hernia. *Br. J. Surg.*, **57**, 264–266.

Blake, R. and Lynn, J. (1976) Emergency abdominal surgery in the aged. *Br. J. Surg.*, **63**, 956–960.

Bowesman, C. (1951) Reduction of strangulated inguinal hernia. *Lancet*, **i**, 1396–1397.

Bucknall, T. E., Cox, P. J. and Ellis, H. (1982) Burst abdomen and incisional hernia: a prospective study of 1129 major laparotomies. *BMJ*, **284**, 931–933.

Chamary, V. L. (1993) Femoral hernia: intestinal obstruction is an unrecognized source of morbidity and mortality. *Br. J. Surg.*, **80**, 230–232.

Cherney, L. S. (1958) Intestinal stenosis following strangulated hernia. *Ann. Surg.*, **148**, 991–994.

Chiedozi, L. C., Aboh, I. O. and Piserchia, N. E. (1980) Mechanical bowel obstruction: review of 316 cases in Benin City. *Am. J. Surg.*, **139**, 389.

Cronin, K. and Ellis, H. (1959) Pus collections in hernial sacs. *Br. J. Surg.*, **46**, 364–367.

Dunphy, J. E. (1940) The diagnosis and surgical management of strangulated femoral hernia. *J.A.M.A.*, **114**, 394–396.

Frankau, C. (1931) Strangulated hernia: a review of 1487 cases. *Br. J. Surg.*, **19**, 176–191.

Gibson, L. D. and Gaspar, M. R. (1959) A review of 606 cases with umbilical hernia. *Int. Abs. Surg.*, **109**, 313–322.

Gillespie, R. W., Glas, W. W., Mertz, G. H. and Musselman, M. M. (1956) Richter's hernia. *Arch. Surg.*, **73**, 590–594.

Hall-Craggs, E. C. B. (1960) Sigmoid volvulus in an African population. *BMJ*, **i**, 1015–1017.

Henry, A. K. (1936) Operation for femoral hernia by a midline extraperitoneal approach. *Lancet*, **i**, 531–533.

Hjaltason, E. (1981) Incarcerated hernia. *Acta Chir. Scand.*, **147**, 263–267.

Howship, J. (1840) *Practical Remarks on the Discrimination and Appearances of Surgical Disease*, J. A. Churchill, London.

Jenkins, T. P. N. (1976) The burst abdominal wound: a mechanical approach. *Br. J. Surg.*, **63**, 873–876.

McEntee, G., Pender, D., Mulvin, D. *et al.* (1987) Current spectrum of intestinal obstruction. *Br. J. Surg.*, **74**, 977–980.

McEvedy, P. G. (1950) Femoral hernia. *Ann. R. Coll. Surg. Engl.*, **7**, 484–496.

Martin, N. C. and Welch, T. P. (1974) Obturator hernia. *Br. J. Surg.*, **61**, 547–548.

Mudge, M., Harding, K. E. and Hughes, L. E. (1986) Incisional hernia. *Br. J. Surg.*, **73**, 82.

Nicholson, S., Keane, T. E. and Devlin, H. B. (1990) Femoral hernia: an avoidable source of surgical mortality. *Br. J. Surg.*, **77**, 307–308.

Perlman, J. A., Hoover, H. C. and Safer, P. K. (1980) Femoral hernia with strangulated Meckel's diverticulum (Littré's hernia). *Am. J. Surg.*, **139**, 286–289.

Pollet, J. (1977) Appendectomy wounds do herniate. *J. R. Coll. Surg. Edin.*, **22**, 274–276.

Rogers, F. A. (1960) Strangulated obturator hernia. *Surgery*, **48**, 394–403.

Stewardson, R. H., Bombeck, C. T. and Nyhus, J. M. (1978) Critical operative management of small bowel obstruction. *Ann. Surg.*, **187**, 189–193.

Thomas, D. (1968) Acute small bowel obstruction. *Austr. N.Z. J. Surg.*, **37**, 302–306.

Treves, F. (1887) Richter's hernia, or partial enterocoele. *Medico-Chir. Trans.*, **52**, 149.

Vick, R. M. (1932) Statistics of acute intestinal obstruction. *BMJ*, **ii**, 546–548.

6.7　STENOSIS OF THE SMALL BOWEL

About 15% of obstructions of the small intestine are due to narrowing of the lumen due to intramural disease, which may be inflammatory, neoplastic or iatrogenic in origin (Table 6.1). It is useful to bring these stenoses together because they all present in similar ways, and may even prove difficult to differentiate at laparotomy.

Presentation may be as a typical acute small-bowel obstruction, with sudden onset of pain and vomiting, and signs suggesting a non-strangulating obstruction. This acute onset is usually due to impaction of food at the point of narrowing and with conservative management the impaction may disintegrate. Another most important mode of presentation is a gradual development of epigastric and umbilical pain, nausea, anorexia and occasional vomiting. These symptoms can be unimpressive and unless the examiner is fortunate enough to be watching the abdomen as a wave of peristalsis passes through a small-bowel loop, causing it to become visible and palpable, it is easy to miss the fact that the patient is obstructed. If suspicion is aroused in outpatients it is always worth having immediate erect and supine plain X-ray of the abdomen.

However, the symptoms are likely to suggest one of the infinitely commoner gastroduodenal disorders so, unless the request for a barium meal specifically requests a follow-through examination, the meal report is likely to show no abnormality. The most accurate examination is a small-bowel enema: when Maglinte *et al.* (1984) examined 56 patients suspected of a partial obstruction, a hold-up was demonstrated in 37, and of these 24 had an immediate laparotomy with confirmation of the presence of obstruction. In 13 conservative management led to resolution of the obstruction, and they were investigated further, revealing Crohn's disease (CD) and other small-bowel disorders. The 19 patients with a normal result all settled.

That this presentation is not uncommon is shown by the fact that, during a 15-month period, we treated 11 such patients, and in the first patient it took 2 months to reach a correct diagnosis. These subacute obstructions were due in three instances to primary carcinoma of the ileum, in one to direct invasion of ileum by a rectal carcinoma, in three there was Crohn's enteritis, two were due to irradiation stenosis of ileum, in one there was a lymphoma of jejunum, and in another gradual stenosis had occurred beneath a thick band. Other recent examples have included endometriosis involving ileum, and potassium-induced strictures.

6.7.1   INFLAMMATORY CAUSES

Crohn's disease

The most common cause of stenosis in Western countries is Crohn's disease of the small bowel and ileocaecal angle. There are regional variations in the segments of the intestine most affected: in the Grampian region of Scotland in 445 patients seen over a 25-year period, we found that small bowel was primarily involved in 30%, the colorectum in 41% and in the remaining 29% lesions were distributed over the whole length of the alimentary tract.

With many patients having small-bowel involvement a degree of obstruction is common, mostly causing some pain after meals, with anorexia, nausea and some distension of the abdomen. A few patients present with an established subacute obstruction, with loops of distended bowel showing visible peristalsis and audible peristaltic sounds. Table 6.2 lists the main indications for the 625 operations that were required in 445 patients: in 186 patients with obstructive symptoms, 67 presented with a major obstructive episode requiring urgent surgery.

Many of these obstructed patients settle if they are starved and given intravenous fluids, blood as required and intravenous vitamins. If obstruction is due to active oedematous disease steroids may be helpful, but they are not useful if stenosis is due to fibrosis. If malnutrition is evident hyperalimentation may be very helpful in preparing the patient for

Table 6.2 Indications for surgery in 445 patients
undergoing 625 operations for Crohn's disease in the
Grampian region, 1975–1992 (N.B. Patients have more
than one indication)

Indications	No. of patients	%
Obstructive symptoms	186	29
Diarrhoea	184	29
Chronic ill health	180	29
Pain	131	21
Fistula – abdominal	79	13
Mass	77	12
Acute obstruction	67	11
Toxic/fulminant colitis	46	8
Weight loss	45	7
Abscess – abdominal	44	7

operation. This need not necessarily be by the intravenous route, because drip-feeding *via* a fine nasogastric tube can be very useful. Investigations can proceed and an operation take place at the best time.

However, in a number of patients the obstruction does not relent. In 431 patients who needed ileocaecal resection in Stockholm, Hellers (1979) found that 87 (20%) required urgent surgery, 36 (8%) for small-bowel obstruction. (Another seven had diffuse peritonitis and 44 were thought to have acute appendicitis – p. 249.) Among 344 elective resections, 77 were done for continuing incomplete obstruction.

In these patients whose obstruction shows no sign of abatement the laparotomy most often reveals typical ileocaecal CD. However, some show a localized lesion in the small bowel and it can then be difficult, in a new patient, to know whether the lesion is due to CD, or a neoplasm, or rarely tuberculosis or endometriosis: this difficult differential diagnosis is further considered on p. 233.

Before embarkation on any resection it is important to make a close examination of the whole small bowel for signs of a skip lesion. These are short patches of paler, thicker bowel with fatty thickening of the adjacent mesentery. Palpation of the normally supple mesentery is one of the best ways of picking up these lesions. Resection of the lesion causing obstruction is necessary, both as treatment and for histological diagnosis.

There is now sufficient evidence to show that taking an extra length of normal-looking bowel above the macroscopic upper limit of abnormality is a mistake. This does not guard against recurrence and tends to sacrifice bowel that can be of great value if there is recurrence. Pennington *et al.* (1980) looked at this topic in detail by recording the histology of both ends of 103 resection specimens, and following the progress of patients for 3 or more years. The suture line recurrence rate was much the same whether there was no sign of Crohn's changes at the suture line (35% recurrence rate) or obvious, even naked eye, changes of CD (41% recurrence).

The obstructing segment is resected, dividing bowel about 5 cm above visible and palpable disease: close naked-eye inspection of the mucosa of both open ends is made, and sometimes there is visible mucosal ulceration that cannot be detected from outside, so a further 2–3 cm is resected and the inspection is repeated. A similar process takes place at the distal resection line, which is frequently in the ascending colon. There is no need to remove hepatic flexure, as in formal right hemicolectomy, if there is no pathological reason to do so. The whole emphasis is on resecting as short a length of small and large bowel as will best serve the later interests of the patient.

The reason for this is that the risk of recurrent disease is high. Some suggest that this is very common, but Shivananda *et al.* (1989) made a close study of the community in Leiden, with full follow-up. Among 210 patients with CD, 118 (56%) needed a resection: after 10 years 25% had required a further resection (17% for recurrence, 8% for persisting symptoms) and after 20 years 50% had evidence of recurrent disease.

So, conservation of bowel is of the first importance in prevention of the 'short bowel syndrome' and this had led to the important development of 'strictureplasty' and of very limited resection, originated by Lee and Papaioannou (1982). To overcome localized strictures they found it was safe to divide them longitudinally and close them transversely, like a Mickulicz pyloroplasty. Interrupted Gambee sutures of fine non-absorbable material are used. Sometimes, with a longer stricture, it is better to perform a Finney-type strictureplasty. Fazio *et al.* (1993) reviewed 116 patients with obstructed small-bowel CD, who had 452 strictureplasties, some having one, some as many as 15 of these procedures. Relief was obtained in 99% and only two patients required reoperation for postoperative sepsis. We have often been glad to make use of this procedure, which has contributed to only four of our patients requiring home parenteral nutrition. The subject is well reviewed by Alexander-Williams (1994).

Tuberculosis

Intestinal tuberculosis (TB) is not often seen in Western countries, although immigration can result in relatively high incidence in some localities. In India, Vaidya and Sodhi (1978) calculated that TB was responsible for 10% of small-bowel obstructions. In north-west London Palmer *et al.* (1985) saw 90 patients with abdominal TB during 1978–1983: 74 (82%) were Asians, 20 were from India and 45 were Indians who had lived in Africa. Only three of these patients were British natives. During the same period, 102 patients with Crohn's disease were seen, so TB must count as an important differential diagnosis among Asian citizens with abdominal symptoms.

Of the 90 patients, 39 had TB of the ileocaecal angle, and half of these patients presented as an emergency – ten with small-bowel obstruction, two had perforation with peritonitis and the remainder showed signs suggesting acute appendicitis. At laparotomy the naked-eye appearances of ileocaecal TB are very similar to ileocaecal CD, but fortunately the correct treatment for both is limited ileocaecal resection. Even under the microscope the differentiation can be difficult. Surgeons in the Indian subcontinent with a wide experience of TB are strong advocates of limited ileocaecal resection and of 'strictureplasty' – they value the speed with which ileoplasty can be performed in emaciated subjects (Pujari, 1979).

In Bradford, Addison (1983) found that tuberculous peritonitis in children and adolescents presented as an acute abdomen, with signs suggesting acute appendicitis. Palmer *et al.* (1985) practised observation in 16 patients with an acute abdomen and started treatment with ionized rifampicin and pyrazinamide: if the diagnosis of TB is confirmed chemotherapy must be maintained for 9–12 months.

Endometriosis

This is another unusual cause of small-bowel obstruction, causing a localized fibrotic kink that is difficult to distinguish from a neoplasm; this differential diagnosis is considered on pp. 233 and 514.

REFERENCES

Addison, N. V. (1983) Abdominal tuberculosis – a disease revived. *Ann. R. Coll. Surg. Engl.*, **65**, 105–111.
Alexander-Williams, J. (1994) Surgical management of small intestinal Crohn's disease: resection or strictureplasty? *Semin. Colon Rect. Surg.*, **5**, 193–198.
Fazio, V. W., Tjandra, J. J., Lavery, I. C. *et al.* (1993) Long-term follow up of strictureplasty in Crohn's disease. *Dis. Colon Rectum*, **36**, 355–361.
Hellers, G. (1979) Crohn's disease in Stockholm county 1955–1974. *Acta Chir. Scand. Suppl.*, **490**, 5–84.
Lee, E. C. G. and Papaioannou, N. (1982) Minimal surgery for chronic obstruction in patients with extensive or universal Crohn's disease. *Ann. R. Coll. Surg. Engl.*, **64**, 228–233.
Maglinte, D. D. T., Peterson, L. A., Vahey, T. N. I. (1984) Enteroclysis in partial small bowel obstruction. *Am. J. Surg.*, **147**, 325–328.
Palmer, K. R., Patil, D. H., Basran, D. H. *et al.* (1985) Abdominal tuberculosis in urban Britain – a common disease. *Gut*, **26**, 1296–1305.
Pennington, L., Hamilton, S. R., Bayless, T. H. and Cameron, J. L. (1980) Surgical management of Crohn's disease: influence of disease at margin of resection. *Ann. Surg.*, **192**, 311–318.
Pujari, B. D. (1979) Modified surgical procedures in intestinal tuberculosis. *Br. J. Surg.*, **66**, 180–181.
Shivananda, S., Hordijk, M. L., Pena, A. S. *et al.* (1989) Crohn's disease: risk of recurrence and reoperation in a defined population. *Gut*, **30**, 990–995.
Vaidya, M. G. and Sodhi, J. S. (1978) Gastrointestinal tract tuberculosis: a study of 102 cases including 55 hemicolectomies. *Clin. Radiol.*, **29**, 189–195.

6.7.2 NEOPLASMS

These tumours are unusual. In the Aberdeen hospitals some 350 new cases of colorectal cancer are seen each year. In contrast, seven primary small-bowel neoplasms presented during 1995 and most surveys show that they contribute 1–4% of all gastrointestinal neoplasms. The majority present as surgical emergencies so the emergency surgeon must know something of their behaviour and treatment.

Over 20 years 43 patients with a primary neoplasm presented to a district hospital in the south of England (Baillie and Williams, 1994). In 36 their symptoms were directly due to the neoplasms, and 31 were admitted as emergencies: of these ten had a small-bowel obstruction, ten an abdominal mass, seven had perforated, three were bleeding into the intestine and two had caused an intussusception. Of the 43 neoplasms seen at laparotomy, 38 were malignant and five benign. This low proportion of **benign neoplasms** is characteristic and these tumours (leiomyoma, lipoma, adenoma) present either as an intussusception (p. 246) or with melaena consequent on ulceration (p. 375). The congenital Peutz–Jeghers syndrome of multiple small-bowel polyps (due to a tree-like overgrowth of the muscularis mucosae) is well known, and they also cause intussusception and melaena.

The **malignant neoplasms** display quite a different incidence to those in the large intestine. Roughly equal numbers are seen of primary adenocarcinoma (30%), carcinoids (30%) and lymphomas (30%), with a few leio- or fibrosarcomata (10%). If the duodenum (where presentation is different) is excluded these neoplasms are fairly evenly divided between jejunum and ileum, except for carcinoids, of which 90% are in the ileum. Peak incidence is in the sixth and seventh decades. Although these patients generally come in as emergencies, they have often a history of recurrent abdominal pain, accentuated by food, and show the sign of visible peristalsis, characteristic of a slowly-increasing small-bowel obstruction.

Adenocarcinoma

Primary carcinomas of the small bowel generally present with symptoms of partial or complete obstruction. Although most can be resected about one-half already have metastases at the time of operation and not more than 25% survive 5 years (Barclay and Schapira, 1983).

Involvement of small bowel by blood-borne metastases from a distant primary is not unusual, for example from carcinoma of bronchus or breast, and these are not likely to be distinguished from primary tumours when seen as a single lesion at operation, so histological examination is important. Direct involvement of small bowel by colorectal or pelvic carcinomas is well recognized (p. 233).

Carcinoid tumours or argentaffinomas

This interesting group of tumours was described 100 years ago and became generally recognized when, in 1907, Obernsdorfer tried, by devising the term *Karzenoide*, to indicate that the histology of the tumour was at variance with the relatively favourable prognosis. Shortly after, Masson showed that the tumour cells had argentaffin characters and were neoplasms of the enterochromaffin cells of the small gut, which secrete 5-hydroxy tryptamine (5-HT). 5-HT was isolated in 1948 and in 1952 Biorck demonstrated that patients with a carcinoid tumour can produce excessive 5-HT which will cause flushing, colicky abdominal pain, diarrhoea and damage to the right heart valves (the carcinoid syndrome). Woods *et al.* (1985) give a useful review of this tumour.

About 45% of carcinoids occur in the vermiform appendix (p. 77), where they are generally only recognized when routine histological examination follows incidental appendicectomy or when carcinoid happens to be associated with acute appendicitis. The fact that these tumours are usually symptomless, and sometimes not visible on external inspection, underlines the importance of having a firm rule that all excised appendices are examined histologically. Carcinoid of the appendix is most often seen in the third decade.

About 30% of carcinoids arise in small bowel, mostly in ileum, and contrast in many ways with those in the appendix. The average age of occurrence is later, around 55 years. Whereas only one appendicular carcinoid in 20 is found to have metastasized, this will have occurred in about 50% of intestinal carcinoids (Welch and Malt, 1977). However, if the primary is below 1 cm in diameter prognosis is good (Barclay and Schapira, 1983). About 25% of patients present with intestinal obstruction, the others complaining of recurrent pain and bowel disturbance, with a few showing signs of carcinoid syndrome. Typically, the primary lies in the submucous layer, producing a small firm, pale, yellow, circumscribed tumour that tends to spread into the muscle and then out into the mesentery and the nodes. Endarteritis and fibrosis are prominent and produce the narrowing of the lumen that eventually leads to intestinal obstruction. In some there is a mass adherent to adjacent loops of small bowel.

Spread to the liver and other distant sites is found is about one-third of laparotomies. It is well worthwhile to resect accessible hepatic metastases (Woods *et al.*, 1985).

Generally, it is advisable to carry out a radical resection of a carcinoid, because even tumours more than 2 cm in diameter show 20% survival at 5 years, and only a few are as large as that.

Regular examination of urine for the oxidation product of 5-HT – 5-HIAA – is a way of detecting recurrence, but recently estimation of platelet serotonin levels has been found to be more sensitive and accurate (Kema *et al.*, 1992).

There are considerable problems in managing the carcinoid syndrome, and these have been reviewed by Basson *et al.* (1993).

Lymphomas

Nearly half the non-Hodgkin's lymphomas that principally affect the alimentary tract present as emergencies. In Aberdeen 45 such patients were seen over 5 years, arising in a population of 450 000 (Green *et al.*, 1979), and small bowel was involved in 15. Of these nine were operated on as an emergency, in six for perforation with peritonitis and in three for obstruction.

At operation a length of pale, thickened intestine is seen, with considerable mesenteric thickening and lymphadenopathy. In some perforation has occurred through the base of a penetrating ulcer, in others the mural thickening has produced obstruction. Non-traumatic perforation of small bowel is always unusual, and because these appearances are difficult to distinguish from CD and treatment is so different there is a strong case for an immediate histological report: either frozen section can be done or the tumour can be opened, its surface imprinted on a slide and the Romanowsky-stained film examined by the pathologist. If the appearances are those of lymphoma, Talamonti *et al.* (1990) have provided powerful evidence of the superior results of immediate radical resection.

The prognosis in small-bowel lymphoma depends very much on the stage of the disease, and on skilful coordination of chemo- and radiotherapy with the oncologists. We found 60% survival at 3 years, falling to 20% at 5 years (Green *et al.*, 1979).

Treatment

The emphasis already laid on histological diagnosis bears repetition because a localized lesion in the small bowel may be due to CD, to a neoplasm, to endometriosis or to radiation. They all look rather similar yet require, literally, radically different treatment.

Limited resection is vital in CD, and all that is needed in endometriosis. For the neoplasms a well-planned radical resection of the primary and associated mesenteric and para-aortic lymph nodes is the key to sound treatment, but this can involve ligation of mesenteric vessels that deprives a substantial length of bowel of its blood supply. This is correct in treating malignant disease, but clearly inappropriate in other situations.

Secondary carcinoma

When small-bowel obstruction is found to be due to direct invasion of its wall by another neoplasm, usually a colorectal carcinoma, it can be difficult in the emergency to know what to do. With a patient in good condition and an experienced surgeon it may be practical to combine resection of the affected loop with a radical large-bowel resection (p. 280). However, if this seems unwise, a side-to-side enteroenterostomy will overcome the small-bowel obstruction and plans can be made for an early return for radical removal of all neoplastic tissue.

Walsh and Schofield (1984) raise the important issue of the patient who, having already had treatment for malignant disease, later develops small-bowel obstruction. This may be due to a blood-borne metastasis from, for example carcinoma of the breast, or to direct invasion from recurrent carcinoma of bowel or ovary. On the other hand it may be due to a benign condition such as adhesions, or to a treatable problem such as postirradiation stenosis (p. 234). In fact, Walsh and Schofield found that 15 of their 53 patients had a correctable non-malignant condition, and it was possible to carry out a useful resection in 40. It is very clear therefore that the bias in these patients should be towards exploration; only in a small minority will it be clear that it is kinder not to re-explore.

REFERENCES

Baillie, C. T. and Williams, A. (1994) Small bowel tumours: a diagnostic challenge. *J. R. Coll. Surg. Edin.*, **39**, 9–12.

Barclay, T. H. C. and Schapira, D. V. (1983) Malignant tumours of small intestine. *Cancer*, **51**, 878–881.

Basson, M. D., Ahlman, H., Wangberg, B. *et al.* (1993) Biology and management of the midgut carcinoid. *Am. J. Surg.*, **165**, 288–297.

Green, J. A., Dawson, A. A., Jones, P. F. and Brunt, P. W. (1979) The presentation of gastrointestinal lymphoma: study of a population. *Br. J. Surg.*, **66**, 798–801.

Kema, I. P., de Vries, E. G. E., Scheilings, A. M. J. *et al.* (1992) Improved diagnosis of carcinoid tumours by measurement of platelet serotonin. *Clin. Chem.*, **38**, 534–540.

Talamonti, M. S., Dawes, L. G., Joeh, L. R. J. *et al.* (1990) Gastrointestinal lymphoma: a case for primary surgical resection. *Arch. Surg.*, **125**, 972–977.

Walsh, H. J. P. and Schofield, P. F. (1984) Is laparotomy for small bowel obstruction justified in patients with previously treated malignancy? *Br. J. Surg.*, **71**, 933–935.

Welch, J. P. and Malt, R. A. (1977) Management of carcinoid tumours of the gastrointestinal tract. *Surg. Gynecol. Obstet.*, **145**, 223–227.

Woods, H. F., Bax, N. D. S. and Smith, J. A. R. (1985) Small bowel carcinoid tumours. *World J. Surg.*, **9**, 921–929.

6.7.3   IATROGENIC STENOSES

Radiation injury

Radiation plays a major role in the management of some abdominal malignancies, such as carcinoma of the uterine cervix, ovary and urinary bladder, and increasingly it has a role in the treatment of carcinoma of the rectum. The distal small bowel, caecum, sigmoid colon and rectum all lie within the fields of pelvic radiotherapy and are affected by it.

Acute epithelial injury occurs to the intestinal mucosa after each treatment, and most patients experience some nausea and diarrhoea during treatment. Some 3 weeks after completion of treatment the mucosa returns to apparent normality, and there may be no more trouble. However, anyone receiving a total dose of 5000–6000 rad can have more severe effects, and radiation proctitis can last for some time: in 10–20% of these patients some later effects will be noticeable (Berthrong, 1986). These chiefly affect the submucosa, where vasculitis is followed by fibrosis. Between 6 months and 25 years later these changes may lead to sufficient stenosis to produce obstruction, or ulceration and adhesion to adjacent viscera may lead to fistula formation.

Among 93 patients referred to the Mayo Clinic, 76 had intestinal obstruction, 11 a fistula, four presented with melaena and two had a free perforation with a pelvic abscess: in 84% the ileum was principally affected (Schmitt and Symmonds, 1981). A majority of patients present in the 5 years after treatment, but when the interval is much longer it is easy for a patient to forget about the treatment – not realizing its significance.

When a patient who has had irradiation presents with intestinal obstruction it is most important not to assume that there is a recurrence of the malignancy. Walsh and Schofield (1984) saw 20 patients who had pelvic radiotherapy and later obstructed and in six this was due to recurrent carcinoma. However, in 12 the cause was radiation damage, of whom nine did well after resection, and this has been our experience.

The ideal treatment is to resect the affected segment, which looks pale and thick, and is nearly always in the terminal ileum. However, it is essential to include all irradiated bowel and this can be a difficult decision, although it is rare for jejunum, and relatively rare for proximal ileum, to be affected. The site of division must look and feel normal and the cut end must bleed freely with a good visible arterial pulse in the mesentery. On the distal side it is likely that caecum will be affected and generally it is wise to make an end-to-end ileocolic anastomosis near the hepatic flexure. Adhesions are nearly always numerous and these operations can take some time. With care over resection lines and the technique of anastomosis (p. 21) these patients should make a good recovery. However, this will also depend on the general nutritional state of the patient, and if this is seriously depleted then a period of intravenous feeding before operation, continued for a short time after, may be important.

Occasionally, laparotomy will reveal a true frozen pelvis: with patience these matted loops can generally be unravelled but rarely a side-to-side anastomosis to short-circuit the area may be best. If perforation occurs fairly soon after irradiation and there is a severe peritonitis, it may be much wiser to perform a quick resection and bring out the ileum as a terminal ileostomy, returning after some months for a carefully considered anastomosis.

To prevent some of these problems the author has lifted small bowel out of the pelvis in the course of performing pelvic exenteration for gynaecological disease. Six patients needed postoperative radiotherapy so the small bowel was held in the upper abdomen by using a sling of absorbable mesh, which was sutured posteriorly to the pelvic brim, running the suture laterally and anteriorly to end at the level of the umbilicus. These patients proceeded to radiotherapy and experienced no problems from the mesh, which would have dissolved over the space of a few weeks.

REFERENCES

Berthrong, M. (1986) Pathologic changes secondary to radiation. *World J. Surg.*, **10**, 155–170.

Schmitt, E. H. and Symmonds, R. E. (1981) Surgical treatment of radiation induced injuries of the intestine. *Surg. Gynecol. Obstet.*, **153**, 896–900.

Walsh, H. J. P. and Schofield, P. F. (1984) Is laparotomy for small bowel obstruction justified in patients with previously treated malignancy? *Br. J. Surg.*, **71**, 933–935.

Potassium-induced stenosis of the small intestine

During April and May 1964, four patients were admitted to St Erik's Hospital, Stockholm, with intestinal obstruction due to a short non-specific stricture of the small bowel (Lindholmer *et al.*, 1964). These patients were so similar that further enquiry was made and revealed that all were taking thiazide and potassium chloride orally. A wider search revealed that 20 patients had been treated over seven years for the same condition and 17 had received thiazide and potassium chloride. In each case there was a narrow circumferential ulcer of the terminal ileum, which had produced marked stenosis of the lumen.

This seems to be the first description of what is now a well-known condition. A few months later, Baker *et al.* (1964) reported 12 similar patients in Minneapolis and showed good grounds for believing that enteric-coated potassium chloride tablets were the responsible agent.

Experimental work by Lawrason *et al.* (1965) in monkeys showed that oral administration of potassium chloride caused ulceration of small intestine but this did not happen if thiazide only, or the enteric-coating alone, were given. Some have suggested that potassium chloride will only induce ulceration and subsequent fibrosis of the small intestine if there is already vascular insufficiency in the bowel. The major factor is probably slow intestinal transit, which allows prolonged contact.

It soon became clear that enteric-coated potassium chloride tablets broke down in about 15 minutes in the small bowel, allowing a high local concentration of potassium chloride to produce necrosis of the mucosa and submucosa, which was followed by fibrosis and stenosis. By 1965 over 300 such cases had been reported (Boley et al., 1965); the enteric-coated tablets were withdrawn and slow-release tablets were substituted in which the salt was embedded in a wax matrix from which it was released over about 4 hours.

Leizonmark and Raf (1985) have studied this topic in detail and calculate that the enteric-coated tablet caused 20 times as many complications as the slow-release tablets. They were only able to find 22 cases of ulceration in Stockholm County during 1970–1983. Of these, 17 had a stenotic obstruction and there were five perforations. All the ulcers occurred in the ileum, mostly near to the ileocaecal valve, and all showed an ulcer with sharp edges and very marked fibrosis in the submucosa. In the 17 stenoses the ulcer was circumferential and 1–2 cm wide, so the stenotic segment was very short. All needed resection and anastomosis and the patients made a good recovery.

It appears that potassium-induced strictures may not be so rare because eight were reported early in 1976 in *The Lancet*, four having been seen within 2 years in the small population of the Isle of Skye (Ball, 1976). These reports suggest that in some well known formulations of thiazide diuretics with potassium chloride the expected slow-release of potassium can in some individuals be quick, or the tablet be held up so that its contents are released at one spot. Tresadern *et al.* (1977) reported four progressive small-bowel strictures in a child who accidentally swallowed an overdose of thiazide potassium chloride slow-release tablets.

The answer seems to be to prescribe the necessary potassium chloride supplement as an effervescent draught, although newer micro-encapsulated formulations are said to be safer.

The non-steroidal anti-inflammatory drugs, such as diclofenac, naproxen, tolmetin, flurbiprofen, sulindac and piroxicam, and the little-used phenylbutazone, all have a mild inflammatory effect on the intestinal mucosa, and occasionally have been associated with diaphragm-like strictures (Colin, 1991).

REFERENCES

Baker, D. R., Schroder, W. H. and Hitchcock, C. R. (1964) Small bowel ulceration apparently associated with thiazide. *J.A.M.A.*, **190**, 586–588.

Ball, J. R. (1976) Potassium strictures of the upper alimentary tract. *Lancet*, **i**, 495–496.

Boley, S. J., Allen, A. C., Schultz, L. and Schwartz, S. (1965) Potassium-induced lesions of the small bowel. I Clinical Aspects. *J.A.M.A.*, **193**, 997–1000.

Colin, R. (1991) Les complications digestives des anti-inflammatoires non-steroidiens. *Schweiz. Med. Wschr.*, **121**, 716–721.

Lawrason, F. D., Alpert, E., Mohr, F. L. and McMahon, P. G. (1965) Ulcerative-obstructive lesions of the small intestine. *J.A.M.A.*, **191**, 105–107.

Leizonmark, C. E. and Raf, L. (1985) Ulceration of the small intestine due to slow-release potassium chloride tablets. *Acta Chir. Scand.*, **151**, 273–278.

Lindholmer, B., Nyman, E. and Raf, L. (1964) Non-specific stenosing ulceration of the small bowel: a preliminary report. *Acta Chir. Scand.*, **128**, 310–312.

Tresadern, J., Rickwood, A. M. K. and Spitz, L. (1977) Multiple small bowel strictures in a child with accidental potassium chloride ingestion. *BMJ*, **ii**, 1124–1125.

Other mechanical obstructions

A remarkable example of this was the **sclerosing peritonitis due to practolol** that caused considerable problems in 1974–1976. The entire small intestine was covered in a membrane, which acted as a cocoon around the bowel and mesentery, causing shortening and angulation, and consequent obstruction. Fortunately, there was a good plane of cleavage between the membrane and the serosa of the bowel and mesentery, and with patience the whole bowel could be freed, and there was no recurrence. Practolol was withdrawn in 1976, and no other beta-blocker has shown this serious side-effect (Jackson, 1977).

However, a more serious form of sclerosing peritonitis has appeared in patients on **continuous ambulatory peritoneal dialysis** (CAPD). This treatment, introduced in 1976, has proved to be of great value, but from 1983 reports began to appear of a serious form of peritonitis in some patients. At the Western Infirmary in Glasgow, during 1982–1987, 14 patients on CAPD presented with attacks of colicky abdominal pain and a loss of the efficacy of dialysis. They showed signs of small-bowel obstruction. At operation a thick fibrous membrane was found covering the bowel and mesentery, which had contracted and drawn the bowel up, out of the pelvis, and encapsulated it. In this case there was no sign of the plane of cleavage found in practolol peritonitis, and it was very difficult to provide any useful surgical relief. Ten of the 14 patients died after the operation, some from cachexia following extensive resection, which had seemed the only course open to the surgeon.

The cause of this very worrying condition remains obscure, although contamination of the perfusate with chlorhexidine, used in the disinfecting of tubing, appeared to be a factor. Fortunately this grave complication has a low incidence, but its occurrence is quite unpredictable (Hollman *et al.*, 1991).

The use of an **oral contraceptive** with a relatively high oestrogen content has been occasionally associated with mesenteric venous thrombosis. This grave emergency (p. 529) doe not usually present until severe ischaemic changes have occurred, and in a recent experience complete midgut ischaemia necessitated so wide a resection that the patient only survives on home parenteral nutrition (Rose, 1972).

Patients on long-term **anticoagulant therapy** with warfarin occasionally present with **intramural intestinal haematoma** (Herbert, 1968). This event, which is rare, is not necessarily related to overdose, but it is a reminder of the importance of including current medication when taking the patient's history.

The combination of long-term taking of an anticoagulant with acute abdominal pain, vomiting and constipation should raise this condition as a possibility. The INR is likely to be significantly over 2.5, with signs of small-bowel obstruction. An opaque meal and follow-through is likely to show – usually in the jejunum – a rigid narrowed segment with a coarse mucosal pattern, with spike-like projections of barium lying between the mucosal folds.

When a laparotomy has been performed, a haemoperitoneum is usually found, with a distended glistening segment of bowel, purple-black in colour causing the obstruction. Similar segments are often seen further down the small bowel. The distinctive feature is that the mesenteric pulsation and circulation is obviously normal, and in fact these changes are reversible. If the diagnosis can be made on the basis of the history and radiological findings, conservative treatment can reasonably be pursued, and resolution of the haematomas awaited. Histological examination of resection specimens show submucosal haemorrhage, with patent vessels and a viable intestinal wall. Herbert (1968) reviewed 88 patients, and all 47 treated conservatively survived. If laparotomy is undertaken and the characteristic appearances are found it is reasonable to withhold resection and await resolution.

Drug-induced functional obstruction

This can occur with a number of different pharmaceuticals (George, 1980). All opiate-type narcotics reduce peristaltic activity by reducing smooth muscle tone. When methadone is given in doses of 60–100 mg daily in the substitution treatment of heroin addiction all patients suffer from severe constipation and sometimes become so obstructed that laparotomy has been required for a picture of severe paralytic ileus.

Similar effects may occur with the tricyclic antidepressants: amitriptyline and nortriptyline have atropine-like effects and Milner and Hills (1966) saw three patients on standard dosage who presented with a picture of advanced paralytic ileus, one requiring a laparotomy. They considered imipramine to be the safest of these drugs.

Anticholinergic drugs such as orphenadrine used in the treatment of parkinsonism can have a similar effect. Daggett and Ibrahim (1976) described such a patient who appeared to have an obstructed carcinoma of the colon.

In view of the wide use of these drugs it is wise to make particular enquiry about medication when faced with a patient who appears to have unexplained paralytic ileus (p. 258).

REFERENCES

Daggett, P. and Ibrahim, S. Z. (1976) Intestinal obstruction complicating orphenadrine treatment. *BMJ*, **i**, 21–22.

George, C. F. (1980) Drugs causing intestinal obstruction. *J. R. Soc. Med.*, **73**, 200–204.

Herbert, D. C. (1968) Anticoagulant therapy and the acute abdomen. *Br. J. Surg.*, **55**, 353–357.

Hollman, A. S., McMillan, M. A., Briggs, J. D. *et al.* (1991) Ultrasound changes in sclerosing peritonitis following CAPD. *Clin. Radiol.*, **43**, 176–179.

Jackson, B. T. (1977) Surgical treatment of sclerosing peritonitis cause by practolol. *Br. J. Surg.*, **64**, 255–257.

Milner, G. and Hills, N. F. (1966) Adynamic ileus and nortriptyline. *BMJ*, **i**, 841–843.

Rose, M. B. (1972) Superior mesenteric vein thrombosis and oral contraceptives. *Postgrad. Med. J.*, **48**, 430–433.

6.8   OBTURATION OF SMALL BOWEL

6.8.1   GALLSTONE OBSTRUCTION

This is the classical cause of intestinal obstruction by obturation of the lumen and has been recognized since 1654 when the first example, confirmed by autopsy, was described by Bartholin.

In spite of this, gallstone obturation of the intestines has always been a diagnosis more missed than made preoperatively. It is not common (1–2% of all cases of intestinal obstruction are due to a gallstone) and it occurs in the elderly, who are often tolerant of pain, and in the obese, who can hide considerable pathology. About 85% of patients are women. The mortality is still high (15–20%) so there is every reason, with an increasingly aged population, to be on the watch for gallstone ileus.

Pathology

It has been calculated that 5% of gallstones migrate into the intestinal tract and that 0.5% cause intestinal obstruction (Raiford, 1962). Almost all of the migratory 5% pass through a cholecystoduodenal fistula. It is a fairly common experience when operating on a gallbladder to find that Hartmann's pouch is adherent to the junction of the first and second parts of the duodenum. If, in these circumstances, the gallbladder becomes both obstructed and inflamed then the formation of a cholecystoduodenal fistula is not surprising. This is followed by the passage of one or more stones into the duodenum. The majority of stones that pass into the intestine in this way will not be large enough to cause any trouble, and the patient is often unaware of anything amiss. Day and Marks (1975) found that most of the stones causing obstruction are more than 3 cm in diameter, with a range of 1.5–5.5 cm. Gallstone obstruction may occur after ERCP for stones retained in the bile ducts (Taylor *et al.*, 1984).

It is interesting to speculate on whether gallstones can enter the duodenum through the bile duct and the ampulla of Vater, and then grow by accretion to a size that is likely to cause an obstruction. We have dealt with a very large gallstone in the duodenum which caused pyloric obstruction: the findings at operation made it clear that this 4 cm stone could not recently have passed from the gallbladder into the duodenum and must have been growing within the duodenum for, at least, many months. It is noticeable that less than half the patients give a history of gallbladder disease and this suggests either that transit of a gallstone through a cholecystoduodenal fistula is often a silent process or that it can happen a long time before the stone causes intestinal obstruction. In the 37 patients seen by Clavien *et al.* (1990), 25 had a cholecystoduodenal fistula, in four the gallbladder communicated with the colon, and in eight the path of the fistula was uncertain.

The terminal ileum is the site of the great majority of gallstone impactions. Collected statistics suggest that 75% occur in this region, 10–15% occur in the jejunum. Arrest at other sites is rare: duodenum (3%), colon (4–5%), stomach (1–2%).

Clinical picture

This is, characteristically, an elusive diagnosis. An elderly obese woman complains of rather vague abdominal pain and vomiting, which comes and goes. The pain is usually central and colicky, but it may localize in the right lower abdomen and this will naturally suggest appendicitis. There is usually constipation, and the vomiting is repeated and troublesome. This disease progresses in a notably inconstant fashion. After a time the pain eases and the patient does not complain for hours or days until the next episode of impaction occurs. In this inconclusive way the stone travels down the small intestine, sometimes being held up with consequent colic, and then travelling on further with relief of pain and vomiting, and passage of flatus *per rectum*. A sense of urgency is readily dissipated in the face of these characteristic fluctuations of the symptoms and signs.

Although Hesselfeldt and Jess (1982) found that patients took, on average, 5 days to reach hospital, the delay ranged between a few hours and 120 days! In hospital some delays extended up to 14 days before laparotomy was undertaken.

Nevertheless, this clinical picture is most characteristic of gallstone obstruction of the small intestine, and it should not be considered unlikely just because there is no clear history of chronic gallbladder disease: this is absent in about half the patients. Generally, the signs suggest a small-bowel obstruction. If auscultation of the abdomen is practised during an episode of colic obstructive sounds are likely to be heard and small-bowel loops may be felt to harden, a sign characteristic of an obstruction that has been present for some days.

Plain radiography of the abdomen will nearly always show dilated small-bowel loops, usually with fluid levels. Rigler *et al.* (1941) described three specific signs in plain X-rays.

- the presence of gas in the biliary tree – this is seen in 50–60% of most reports;
- signs of intestinal obstruction;
- aberrant site of a radio-opaque gallstone – most often in the right lower quadrant – seen in about 30% of patients.

The presence of two of these three signs is generally considered to be diagnostic of gallstone ileus. Occasionally, when the signs suggest a high obstruction, an opaque meal will show a large stone obstructing the duodenum.

Diagnosis

Most of these patients will have a diagnosis of small-bowel obstruction made, but Clavien *et al.* (1990) found that a gallstone impaction was only suspected in 17% at admission. This rose to 70% by the time operation was undertaken, after a delay varying between 5 hours and 14 days. Precision in diagnosis can be difficult in a well-covered elderly patient: in some the picture will suggest the obstructive presentation of acute appendicitis in the elderly, and in nine of Clavien's patients an arteriogram had been done on suspicion of mesenteric ischaemia. However, in a typical case the long and variable history is very suggestive in itself.

Treatment

These patients are generally poor operative risks. Among 45 patients treated by Kurtz *et al.* (1985) 21 had significant respiratory disease, 16 had cardiac disease and 18 were diabetics: most will have been starving and will be dehydrated. Much care is therefore needed over preoperative preparation.

The operation will often be done without certain knowledge of the cause of the obstruction and the incision will therefore be an exploratory one in the midline. The diagnosis is immediately obvious when the dilated bowel is traced down to the site of the obstruction.

When the stone is stuck in the terminal ileum it may be worth trying gently to milk it through the ileocaecal valve into the caecum. If this succeeds enterotomy is avoided and the risk of septic complications much diminished. However, Andersson and Zederfeldt (1969) had one patient whose ileum was split open by the manipulations and one in whom the stone impacted in the sigmoid, which was narrowed by diverticular disease: the second laparotomy proved fatal. This experience suggests that it is wise to have a bias towards enterotomy but before doing this the bowel should be emptied retrogradely into the stomach (p. 191). This serves two useful purposes.

- It makes closure of the abdomen less difficult, which is a great help in the obese.
- Emptying the bowel upwards from the point of obstruction automatically means that every part of the bowel is surveyed and that a second stone, if present, will be found.

This is a matter of real practical importance because recurrent gallstone obstruction is well recognized. Buetow *et al.* (1963) found 44 examples in the literature and added two of their own. Both of these patients recovered but it is most undesirable to expose elderly patients to a condition which is both dangerous and preventable.

The search for a further stone must be carried to the gallbladder itself. There is often a cholecystoduodenal fistula and many surgeons believe that this is best **not** disturbed at the time of the obstruction. A stone that will cause obstruction is, however, quite large (most are more than 3 cm and all more than 2 cm in diameter) so it is not difficult to feel a stone of this size through the wall of the gallbladder. If found the wise thing is to perform a cholecystotomy to remove the stone, and to tie a Malecot catheter into the gallbladder and bring it out through a stab subcostal incision.

The search for a second stone must be particularly careful if the obstructing stone is found to be faceted, or if preoperative ultrasonography has shown multiple stones. Stones found in the course of the search through the small bowel can usually be brought down to the level of the obstructing stone and removed through the same enterotomy.

Occasionally, perforation or pressure gangrene will dictate making a short resection, but generally it is best to gently milk the stone up into normal bowel and remove it through a longitudinal incision. If it is not movable it must be removed through an incision over it and then it is important to check the viability of this segment of bowel before closing it. A transverse closure with interrupted serosubmucosal sutures of 2/0 or 3/0 braided nylon or polydioxanone is recommended.

It remains to decide whether immediate or elective surgery is indicated for the gallbladder. The repair of a cholecystoduodenal fistula is rarely a simple matter. The experience of Andersson and Zederfeldt (1969) is cautionary. They had five patients who were subjected to cholecystectomy and fistula closure at the time of operation for gallstone obstruction, and three died, two with peritonitis secondary to failure of healing of the duodenal closure.

Clavien *et al.* (1990) argue that one-stage removal of the impacted stone, fistula repair and cholecystectomy is a reasonable course when the patient is fit for the operation and the surgeon experienced. They did this in eight patients with two deaths. In 23 patients the stone only was removed, with five deaths, and four patients suffered recurrent obstruction from residual stones.

On balance, we believe it is wiser to restrict the operation to removal of the obstruction, combined with a most thorough search for other stones, including removal of a stone from the gallbladder.

The decision on later exploration of the biliary tree will generally hinge on whether the patient experiences further trouble. We have had a patient develop severe biliary pain due to stones in the common bile duct after a gallstone obstruction and here the indication to operate on the biliary tract was clear. Among the 27 patients followed up by Hesselfeldt and Jess (1982) five complained of biliary dyspepsia and three required cholecystectomy.

The **mortality** of gallstone ileus remains around 18% in the three latest reports totalling 121 laparotomies (Hesselfeldt and Jess, 1982; Kurtz *et al.*, 1985; Clavien *et al.*, 1990). These patients are poor risks but there is certainly room for improvement by way of speedier diagnosis, both before and after admission to hospital.

REFERENCES

Andersson, A. and Zederfeldt, B. (1969) Gallstone ileus. *Acta Chir. Scand.*, **135**, 713.

Buetow, G. W., Glaubitz, J. P. and Crampton, R. S. (1963) Recurrent gallstone ileus. *Surgery*, **54**, 716–724.

Clavien, P. A., Richon, J., Burgan, S. *et al.* (1990) Gallstone ileus. *Br. J. Surg.*, **77**, 737–742.

Day, E. A. and Marks, C. (1975) Gallstone ileus. *Am. J. Surg.*, **129**, 552–558.

Hesselfeldt, P. and Jess, P. (1982) Gallstone ileus. *Acta Chir. Scand.*, **148**, 431–433.

Kurtz, R. J., Hermann, T. M., Beck, A. R. and Kurtz, A. B. (1985) Patterns of treatment of gallstone ileus over a 45-year period. *Am. J. Gastroenterol.*, **80**, 95–98.

Raiford, T. S. (1962) Intestinal obstruction caused by gallstones. *Am. J. Surg.*, **104**, 383–394.

Rigler, L. G., Bormann, C. N. and Noble, J. F. (1941) Gallstone obstruction: pathogenesis and roentgen manifestations. *J.A.M.A.*, **117**, 1753–1759.

Taylor, J. D., Zaman, K., Fossard, D. P. and Carr-Locke, D. (1984) Gallstone ileus: a 12-year review, with special reference to ERCP and endoscopic sphincterotomy. *Br. J. Surg.*, **71**, 992.

6.8.2   OBSTRUCTION DUE TO FOOD

Turtle eggs and grasshoppers eaten whole are two of the unlikely foods that have caused bolus obstruction of the intestines: they figure among 61 other foods that Stephens (1966) found to be a cause of this form of intestinal obstruction. It is not rare and most busy units will see one or two cases each year. Elliott (1932) brought the condition to general notice and Ward-McQuaid made an excellent review in 1950.

Poorly chewed oranges, dried fruit eaten uncooked which then swells as it absorbs water in the gut, and masses of gobbled peanuts are the commonest agents. Local customs operate, such as eating the persimmon or date-fruit in North America and Israel (Kaplan *et al.*, 1985): this fruit contains a tannin which produces a sticky coagulum in contact with gastric acid and this traps pulp and seeds into a bezoar (Goldstein *et al.*, 1984). In Hong Kong preserved ginger root, which is a favourite among the young, is eaten quickly and is liable to swell as it passes down the intestine (Liu and Ho, 1983). Meat is rarely a problem, presumably because it is more likely to be digested than cellulose. 'Fruit stone ileus' has been described (Weaver and Trapnell, 1973) where a swallowed stone remains in a narrowed segment of gut for a long time, gradually increasing in size through accretion, until it causes an obstruction. Excessive intake of unprocessed bran can also produce large-bowel obstruction through impaction in the distal colon and rectum (Kang and Doe, 1979).

A bolus that would pass down the normal small bowel is likely to obstruct at an adhesive kink and it is our impression that this causes a number of early readmissions after laparotomy. The patient is pleased to satisfy a returning appetite, and eats quickly, with inadequate mastication. These episodes of partial obstruction generally settle with 24 hours of starvation.

Robles *et al.* (1994), working in Murcia in a fruit-growing area of Spain, saw 117 admissions of 99 patients with gastrointestinal bezoars, mostly of persimmons, vegetables and oranges. In 30 the stomach was affected, causing dyspepsia, and only two required an urgent operation for pressure necrosis of the gastric wall. In 86 episodes the small bowel was obstructed, completely in 78, and all required a laparotomy: in 69 of these cases the patient had required gastric surgery in the past, mostly truncal vagotomy and pyloroplasty.

Clinical picture

These patients frequently do not connect their symptoms with the food responsible for them. They present with the acute onset of severe abdominal colic and vomiting, with constipation. The severe pain and repeated vomiting can rapidly result in an ill-looking patient with signs of hypovolaemia.

The abdomen is more or less distended, according to the level of obstruction and the time it has been present, and is usually markedly tender. Bowel sounds are loud and obstructive and occasionally the impacted bolus can be palpated. Plain abdominal films show the usual signs of a small-bowel obstruction.

Diagnosis

This is one of the less common obstructions and it has to be thought of if it is to be diagnosed. Everything depends on obtaining a positive dietary history. However, some care must be exercised in its interpretation, especially in a gastrectomized patient who may very well have an adhesive obstruction.

Treatment

In the presence of a suggestive history conservative measures are justified provided the progress of the patient is most carefully watched.

If there is any misgiving then laparotomy must be undertaken because the diagnosis of bolus obstruction may be wrong, or the bolus may not move without operative help. There is usually no difficulty in making the diagnosis once dilated bowel has been traced to the site of impaction. The decision to be made is whether to gently break up the bolus and squeeze it into the caecum, or whether to extract it by enterotomy. Only a careful assessment of this situation and a trial of milking can decide this. It is certainly far safer to perform enterotomy than to persist in milking to the extent that the bowel wall is damaged. Pressure ischaemia of the bowel seems to be more or less unknown. If an enterotomy is made it seems wise to incise the bowel longitudinally over the bolus, and, after evacuation, to sew it up in the transverse axis with interrupted serosubmucosal sutures of 3/0 braided nylon or poly-dioxanone. Before closing, it is essential to check the bowel proximal to the obstruction, and the stomach, for other bezoars (Kaplan *et al.*, 1985).

Wound infection is a particular hazard so protection of wound edges and antibiotic lavage are important precautions.

REFERENCES

Elliott, A. H. (1932) Intestinal obstruction caused by food. *Am. J. Med. Sci.*, **184**, 85–94.

Goldstein, S. S., Lewis, J. H. and Rothstein, R. (1984) Intestinal obstruction due to bezoars. *Am. J. Gastroenterol.*, **79**, 313–318.

Kang, J. Y. and Doe, W. F. (1979) Unprocessed bran causing intestinal obstruction. *BMJ*, **i**, 1249–1250.

Kaplan, O., Klausner, J. M., Lelcuk, S. *et al.* (1985) Persimmon bezoars as a cause of intestinal obstruction: pitfalls in their surgical management. *Br. J. Surg.*, **72**, 242–243.

Liu, P. H. W. and Ho, H. L. (1983) Ginger and drug bezoar induced small bowel obstruction. *J. R. Coll. Surg. Edin.*, **28**, 397–398.

Robles, R., Parrilla, P., Escamilla, C. *et al.* (1994) Gastrointestinal bezoars. *Br. J. Surg.*, **81**, 1000–1001.

Stephens, F. O. (1966) Intestinal colic caused by food. *Gut*, **7**, 581–584.

Ward-McQuaid, N. (1950) Intestinal obstruction due to food. *BMJ*, **i**, 1106–1109.

Weaver, P. C. and Trapnell, D. H. (1973) Fruit stone ileus. *Br. J. Surg.*, **60**, 237–239.

6.8.3 OBSTRUCTION DUE TO WORMS

Although almost unknown in Western countries, obturation of the small bowel by masses of *Ascaris lumbricoides* is common throughout Africa and the East. In Cape Town Louw (1966) found that ascariasis accounted for 12.8% of admissions of 730 African children with acute abdominal pain, and it was only exceeded in frequency by acute appendicitis. Children from families living in poor hygienic conditions, aged 3–5 years, are the most often affected, and they may also suffer from penetration of the worms into ducts, causing acute pancreatitis and cholecystitis. The commonest event is obstruction of the small bowel by an impacted mass of worms, which may be incomplete or complete. The weight of a mass of worms can cause intestinal volvulus, and this can go on to ischaemic necrosis of the bowel (Cole, 1965).

Wasadikar and Kulkarni (1997) in India saw 92 patients (76 were children) with roundworm obstruction. In 68 the obstruction was not complete and after 2–3 days of intravenous fluids and nasogastric suction they passed a bolus of 25 to several hundred worms. They were then treated with mebendazole. The 24 patients with a complete obstruction were in a much more serious state, and five died during resuscitation from gangrene due to small-bowel volvulus and intussusception. In 18 the abdomen was tender and in 15 there were signs of peritonitis and roundworm toxaemia (delirium and muscular twitching). Many were malnourished. Ultrasonography in seven patients showed a 'railway track' appearance in a longitudinal scan and a 'bull's eye' sign in the transverse scan, and an akinetic dilated loop of bowel signified strangulation in two. At laparotomy the worms may be squeezed through terminal ileum into the caecum, but this could only be done in two patients: 11 required enterotomy and extraction of worms and six resections were done for gangrene. The combination of long-standing malnutrition and the severity of the bowel changes mean that ascariasis is a serious condition, and seven of the 19 patients died postoperatively.

REFERENCES

Cole, G. J. (1965) Surgical manifestations of *Ascaris lumbricoides* in the intestine. *Br. J. Surg.*, **52**, 444–447.

Louw, J. H. (1966) Abdominal complications of *Ascaris lumbricoides* infestation in children. *Br. J. Surg.*, **53**, 510–521.

Wasadikar, P. P. and Kulkarni, A. B. (1997) Intestinal obstruction due to ascariasis. *Br. J. Surg.*, **84**, 410–412.

6.8.4 MECONIUM ILEUS EQUIVALENT

It is well recognized that a proportion of new-born babies with cystic fibrosis suffer from meconium ileus. The occurrence of some degree of intestinal hold-up in children and young adults with cystic fibrosis is less well known. It has, understandably, been termed meconium ileus equivalent (MIE) but Park and Grand (1981) suggest that 'distal intestinal obstruction syndrome' would be a better term. They argue that, although the most severe cases of distal ileal obstruction are due to putty-like faecal material stuck in the lumen, many more minor episodes are due to poorly digested food, impaired intestinal motility and dehydration. This certainly corresponds with the clinical picture, which may be one of abdominal colic and distension that settles quickly, or may sometimes be a full obstructive episode with a palpable mass of partly digested food impacted in terminal ileum, due to a combination of thick intestinal mucus, water-insoluble mucoprotein and insufficiency of pancreatic enzymes. Hunton *et al.* gave a full review in 1966.

Eight of 53 patients, aged between 2 and 17 years, attending a cystic fibrosis clinic in Dublin (Hanly and Fitzgerald, 1983), were found to suffer from MIE. The diagnosis should be considered when a cystic fibrosis patient complains of abdominal colic. In about half there will be a palpable mass in the right lower quadrant, and the abdominal X-ray may show signs of obstruction and a bubbly appearance of air mixed with faecal accumulations. It is important for the surgeon to recognize this condition because it usually responds well to medical treatment, and the main problem is whether the obstruction is due to MIE or to a cause that requires surgical relief.

A boy of 6 years with cystic fibrosis gave a history of several recent attacks of abdominal pain. On New Year's Day he was admitted with severe intestinal colic and vomiting. There was no evidence of intestinal obstruction on clinical or radiographic examination. A mass palpable just above the umbilicus was taken to be inspissated material in the bowel. Next day, after gastrografin had passed through normal-looking small bowel he was comfortable and we could feel no mass. He went home on acetyl cysteine but continued to experience colic from time to time. He was re-admitted on 14 January with a recurrence of severe intestinal colic and a palpable elongated lump, this time in the left iliac fossa. Once again there was no evidence of obstruction but rectal examination showed a little blood on the finger stall. A diagnosis of intussusception was made and a caecocolic intussusception was reduced: the apex was normal caput caeci.

Intussusception is a well recognized complication of cystic fibrosis, although a large clinic in Boston saw only 22 episodes in 19 patients over 17 years, during which they cared for over 1000 patients (Holsclaw *et al.*, 1971). A correct diagnosis was made on the clinical picture in 18: only two required resection among 19 patients operated on, the remainder being easily reduced. Holsclaw *et al.* suggest that a barium enema is therefore likely to achieve both diagnosis and full reduction, and should be tried. It is certainly desirable to avoid operation in patients with intestinal complications of cystic fibrosis because these patients so easily run into respiratory difficulties after laparotomy, and the majority respond to medical treatment.

The object is to dislodge the semi-solid tenacious material that is stuck in terminal ileum and caecum. N-acetyl cysteine by mouth or enema does this by reducing the viscosity of the mucoproteins that glue the faecal mass to the mucosa: sodium diatrizoate (gastrografin) acts partly as a wetting agent and mainly because it is hyperosmolar, so the outpouring of intestinal secretion that it stimulates helps to wash out the impacted faeces. Copeland *et al.*

(1984) successfully used 150 ml of 2% N-acetyl cysteine six times a day, given through a tube into the stomach: alternatively it can be given as an enema. Gastrografin can similarly be used either by mouth or as an enema.

The effect of these measures will be closely watched. Generally they are effective over 24–48 hours, but it will be remembered that when a faecal mass is not palpable it may not be MIE causing the obstruction, and there may be a surgical cause requiring laparotomy.

REFERENCES

Copeland, G., Waldron, R. and Wilson, W. A. (1984) Meconium ileus equivalent. *J. R. Coll. Surg. Edin.*, **29**, 325–326.

Hanly, J. G. and Fitzgerald, M. X. (1983) Meconium ileus equivalent in older patients with cystic fibrosis. *BMJ*, **286**, 1411–1413.

Holsclaw, D. S., Rocmans, C. and Swachman, H. (1971) Intussusception in patients with cystic fibrosis. *Pediatrics*, **48**, 51–58.

Hunton, D. B., Long, W. K. and Tsumagari, H. Y. (1966) Meconium ileus equivalent: an adult complication of fibrocystic disease. *Gastroenterology*, **50**, 99–102.

Park, R. W. and Grand, R. J. (1981) Gastrointestinal manifestations of cystic fibrosis: a review. *Gastroenterology*, **81**, 1143–1161.

6.9   INTUSSUSCEPTION IN THE ADULT

This is a relatively unfamiliar occurrence compared to the well-known intussusceptions of infancy, and only 5–10% of intussusceptions occur after the age of 12. Only 50 examples were found in the five Glasgow teaching hospitals over the 20 years 1954–1974 (Murdoch and Wallace, 1977), so each hospital saw only one case every 2 years.

In contrast to the situation in infancy, the assumption must be that the intussusception has been initiated by a pre-existing abnormality in the wall of the bowel that will require resection. In the small bowel these tend to be benign neoplasms or a Meckel's diverticulum, but in the colon a carcinoma is the most likely leading point. Numbers of intussusceptions in the small and large intestines are roughly equal. Roper (1956) analysed the literature and found that the major causes of intussusception in 133 patients over 10 years of age were: benign neoplasms, 42; malignant neoplasms, 49; Meckel's diverticulum, 7; other causes, 18. In 18 no cause could be found.

Neoplasms
In the small bowel lipomas, adenomas, haemangiomas and leiomyomas, generally polypoid in shape, make up about 75% of the neoplasms, and the other 25% are carcinomas, carcinoids, lymphomas or metastatic melanoma (Azar and Berger, 1997). Once over the age of 5 years, lymphoma is an important cause of small-bowel intussusception (p. 233), which may cause attacks of pain and vomiting over days or weeks (Youngson and Scotland, 1981).

In the large bowel, the majority of the neoplasms causing an intussusception are polypoid adenocarcinomas: they may arise in any part of the large bowel, although those we have seen have been either caecal or rectal: one presented as a bleeding mass at the anus. An occasional colonic adenoma or leiomyoma will act as leading point.

In the small intestine it is important to remember that a Peutz–Jeghers hamartoma is likely to cause an intussusception and then it is necessary to hunt for others. Eosinophilic granuloma has been found as a leading point (Antrum *et al.*, 1983).

Meckel's diverticulum

This can cause an intussusception at any age, although most occur before 10 years of age. About 20% occur after the age of 20. Only about 5% of the complications of Meckel's diverticulum are intussusceptions, and small-bowel obstruction is more often due to a mesodiverticular band (Diamond and Russell, 1985). Presentation may resemble a small-bowel neoplasm (Williamson *et al.*, 1984).

The vermiform appendix

This may initiate an intussusception, either because there is a neoplasm in it (Langsam *et al.*, 1984) or because the appendix stump, after appendicectomy, acts as a leading point (Wolfson *et al.*, 1984 and p. 67). Danielson (1969) reported 12 such cases: onset of crampy abdominal pain occurs some days after appendicectomy, there may be bloody stools, and a mass may be felt in the right abdomen. A barium enema should give a characteristic 'coiled spring' appearance, and should be obtained whenever there is doubt. Right hemicolectomy is usually needed.

Other causes

A few cases have been due to ectopic pancreatic tissue in the wall of the small bowel and a few have been initiated by foreign bodies in the lumen, such as bezoars. Inflammatory disease of the small bowel is a well-described though rare cause: Goodall (1963) has analysed this subject in detail and has found examples of intussusception secondary to typhoid fever, amoebic and bacillary dysentery and tuberculous enteritis.

Idiopathic group

The size of this group varies considerably among reports. In Glasgow (Murdoch and Wallace, 1977) 24 of 50 patients over the age of 21 had no demonstrable cause for their intussusception. Other papers report a much lower percentage. The apex of an intussusception in an adult requires very careful inspection before it is accepted that there is no definable leading point.

Clinical features

Apart from the clinical picture normally associated with obstruction of the small or large intestine, there are some special features that may suggest that intussusception has occurred. However, most cases are diagnosed at laparotomy.

History

It is characteristic in the benign neoplastic group for there to be a history of recurrent episodes of abdominal pain and vomiting that have resolved, and in our experience this also occurs in intussuscepting carcinomata in the caecum. A history of rectal bleeding is not common unless the causative neoplasm lies low in the colon. A young patient who gives a history of recurrent episodes of colic and vomiting and who has a palpable abdominal mass might reasonably be suspected of having an intussusception secondary to Meckel's diverticulum.

Signs

A palpable mass is present in many intussusceptions and one of the features of these masses, among those that resolve spontaneously, are that they may be present one day and absent on the next. This is highly suggestive of recurrent intussusception. On the whole, the general picture of intussusception in the adult is not so acute and distressing as it is in the child, although a proportion certainly require emergency surgery. Auscultation of the abdomen can sometimes reveal obstructive sounds when nothing else definite had been found on routine abdominal and rectal examination.

An urgent barium enema can be of great help in establishing a diagnosis, as in infancy. The signs are quite characteristic, with the intussusception forming a rounded filling defect with the column of barium dividing around it and thinning out at the edges. Sometimes the mucosal pattern of the intussusception is very well shown and demonstrates the 'coiled spring' sign. In small-bowel intussusception, a micro-opaque meal may delineate distended small bowel and demonstrate that an obstruction is present.

Treatment

This will depend on the findings at operation. When the intussusception is irreducible, or a sizeable mass is palpable in the bowel, suggesting a neoplasm, then resection is needed. When a carcinoma is suspected then a full radical resection is needed and in six intussusceptions of colorectal carcinomas it has been possible to perform a standard resection with restorative anastomosis, and these patients have had good immediate and long-term results. Polyps may be removable by enterotomy and local removal. Lipomata and leiomyomata are intramural and need resection.

The site where problems will arise is the ileocaecal valve. Every operator who deals with childhood intussusception will know the remarkable swelling of the valve that can sometimes be felt after successful reduction and how, even in infants, there can be doubt about the possible presence of tumour. In these circumstances caecotomy may be helpful and biopsy of doubtful areas may be needed.

REFERENCES

Antrum, R. M., Craven, J. L. and Hall, R. (1983) Polypoid eosinophilic granulomas of the terminal ileum presenting with intussusception. *J. R. Coll. Surg. Edin.*, **28**, 337–339.

Azar, T. and Berger, D. L. (1997) Adult intussusception. *Ann. Surg.*, **226**, 134–138.

Danielson, K. S. (1969) Ceco-colic intussusception – a post-operative complication of appendicectomy. *N. Engl. J. Med.*, **280**, 35–37.

Diamond, T. and Russell, C. F. J. (1985) Meckel's diverticulum in the adult. *Br. J. Surg.*, **72**, 480–482.

Goodall, P. (1963) Intussusception in adults complicating specific inflammatory diseases of the intestine. *Gut*, **4**, 132–135.

Langsam, L. B., Raj, P. K. and Galang, C. F. (1984) Intussusception of the appendix. *Dis. Colon Rectum*, **27**, 387–392.

Murdoch, R. W. G. and Wallace, J. R. (1977) Adult intussusception in Glasgow 1968–74. *Br. J. Surg.*, **64**, 679–680.

Roper, A. (1956) Intussusception in adults. *Surg. Gynecol. Obstet.*, **103**, 267–270.

Williamson, R. C. N., Cooper, M. J. and Thomas, W. E. G. (1984) Intussusception of invaginated Meckel's diverticulum. *J. R. Soc. Med.*, **77**, 652–655.

Wolfson, S., Shachor, D. and Freund, U. (1984) Ileocolic intussusception in an adult – a post-operative complication of appendicectomy. *Dis. Colon Rectum*, **27**, 265–266.

Youngson, G. G. and Scotland AD (1981) Small bowel lymphoma presenting as chronic adult intussusception. *Scot. Med. J.*, **26**, 260–261.

6.10 OTHER SMALL BOWEL EMERGENCIES

6.10.1 ACUTE CROHN'S DISEASE

Among the 445 patients with proven Crohn's disease (CD) treated in Aberdeen during 1975–1992, 9.4% were operated on as an emergency and 19% required an urgent operation. These patients presented in a number of guises, and many came to operation with a provisional diagnosis of acute appendicitis, so it is important to recognize these various presentations. Prognosis can materially depend upon taking the correct steps at emergency laparotomy.

(a) Crohn's ileocolitis that presents as acute appendicitis

In the Aberdeen study of 445 patients with Crohn's disease (CD) who required an operation during a 27-year period, there were six who appeared to have acute appendicitis. They had marked tenderness and guarding over the right lower quadrant, and under the anaesthetic a mass was palpable. At operation there was a segment of terminal ileum, 30–60 cm in length, covered in fibrin and pus, the ileal wall was thickened with the fat-wrapping typical of CD. The mesentery contained enlarged, juicy lymph nodes. There could be no doubt that these patients had CD and a limited ileocaecal resection was performed with a good recovery.

Weston *et al.* (1996) have reviewed this subject. Among 1421 patients with CD, 36 presented in this way, and 10 had an ileocolic resection, 23 an appendicectomy and in three the abdomen was closed. They were followed for a mean of 14 years. Five of the 10 resected patients were well, but five had required further resections. Of the 23 having an appendicectomy, 20 had undergone later resection, over one-third during the first year. Clearly it is correct to proceed to emergency resection, bearing in mind the strict principles of resection for CD (p. 229).

The rare occurrence of CD being confined to the appendix, only recognized when an inflamed appendix is submitted to histological examination, is considered on page p. 78.

(b) Acute appendicitis complicating Crohn's ileitis

Again, this is a rare event. Rawlinson and Hughes (1985) treated a 25-year-old man with symptoms and signs of acute appendicitis who was on 2.5 mg of prednisolone daily for proven Crohn's ileitis. Twelve hours after commencing intravenous fluids and hydrocortisone there was no improvement and laparotomy was undertaken. They found typical acute appendicitis unconnected with well-marked changes of CD in 30 cm of terminal ileum. Ileocolectomy was performed and the patient went on to make a good recovery. Histology confirmed the two independent diagnoses.

We have operated on a woman with a slightly different problem. She presented with severe right iliac fossa pain and a tender mass. Under anaesthesia a slightly mobile mass was felt. On opening the abdomen she had CD of the terminal ileum and a mucocele of the appendix. Limited right hemicolectomy removed both problems.

(c) Acute terminal ileitis

Whereas the above conditions can reasonably be resolved at operation, acute terminal ileitis can present quite a problem. Many a surgeon has operated on a patient who is usually aged between 16 and 40 and presents with a short history of abdominal pain suggestive of acute appendicitis. At operation the appendix appears normal, but the terminal 20–30 cm of ileum is beefy and red with pus and fibrin on its surface. There is marked lymphadenitis with thickening of the mesentery. There is no fat wrapping, as seen in Crohn's disease, but there is a great similarity. A young inexperienced surgeon would be advised to call on a senior colleague. Once the difference in appearance between ileitis and CD is appreciated it is important to know what the surgical approach should be. An understanding of the natural history is essential.

Kewenter *et al.* (1974) in Gothenberg made a thorough study of 72 such patients who had been treated between 1951 and 1965 in the course of performing 10 625 operations for suspected acute appendicitis. All had an appendicectomy, except for one who had an immediate hemicolectomy, and all recovered. Between 5 and 20 years later Kewenter *et al.* managed to recall 68 of the 72: one was the patient who had the immediate resection. Among the 67 appendicectomies one had formed a fistula and subsequently had a hemicolectomy. Seven others required right hemicolectomy between 1 and 15 years after their appendicectomy for histologically proven CD. Among the 59 remaining patients 38 were well and 21 had some abdominal pain: all these had a small-bowel enema, barium enema and sigmoidoscopy and all were found to be normal except for one patient who had typical terminal ileum CD. Therefore, of the 68 patients followed up over at least 5 years, 10 had CD but 58 (85%) showed no signs of developing it.

Yersinia enterocolitica or *Y. pseudotuberculosis* can produce acute terminal ileitis with considerable mesenteric adenitis. The diagnosis can be confirmed by culturing the organism from the lumen of the appendix or the stools and by finding raised antibody titres (Mair, 1977). These infections usually resolve spontaneously, but the organism is sensitive to tetracycline so this may speed recovery (Morain, 1981). It is clearly helpful to prove the diagnosis of yersiniasis in these patients, if possible, because the prognosis is so different from CD. However, it is clear that there is no way in which by inspection at operation the majority of patients (whose terminal ileitis is due to yersiniasis) can be distinguished from the 10–15% in whom the ileitis is the fist sign that they have CD. The operative procedure should therefore be to remove the appendix, take a culture from its lumen and submit it for histological examination. The remainder of the small bowel is examined for evidence of CD. Antibody titres are estimated at the time of operation and 7–10 days later. Provided the caecum looks normal there is no risk of fistula formation in removing the appendix. If the caecum is abnormal this strongly suggests the diagnosis of CD.

Postoperatively, it is important to continue to monitor the patient's progress. The author has seen two patients who did not improve. One developed generalized peritonitis within 4 days of the laparotomy at which terminal ileitis had been diagnosed and the abdomen closed. At the second laparotomy there was a free perforation and the patient underwent a resection of the ileum with ileostomy and a mucous fistula. Histology confirmed CD. The patient required a prolonged period of intensive care. The second patient continued to complain of localized pain with increasing toxicity following a laparotomy for 'ileitis'. A further laparotomy was undertaken and a limited right hemicolectomy was performed. Histology again confirmed CD.

(d) *Intra-abdominal sepsis – free perforation*

In 1957 B. B. Crohn wrote 'free perforation of ileitis into the peritoneal cavity never occurs, or at least I have never seen it'. However, in 1952 in Liverpool, Gow and Walsh had described two cases, both of which caused diffuse and fatal peritonitis; they also mentioned an example in 1937. By 1965 Crohn reported seven perforations in 'acute regional ileitis', but remained sceptical about perforation occurring in established granulomatous ileitis; however, this does occur. Steinberg *et al.* (1973) reported seven perforations among 360 patients with proven CD, six in ileum and one in sigmoid colon: these had occurred proximal to a stricture that had caused obstruction. Makowiec *et al.* (1993) reviewed their experience in 384 patients and concluded that obstruction due to CD did not increase the risk of perforation. Bundred *et al.* (1985) in Edinburgh confirmed the rarity of perforation. Among 612 patients with CD, four of 414 patients with small-bowel disease and six of 198 patients with colonic CD had suffered a free perforation. Four of these patients were on corticosteroid treatment and diagnosis was delayed until gas was seen under the diaphragm.

In the Grampian series of 445 patients, eight had a free perforation, six in small bowel and two in the sigmoid colon. Six patients were known to have CD. In two the diagnosis was made on the histology of the resected specimen.

Simple suture is quite inappropriate, and carries a high mortality. Resection is necessary, but primary end-to-end anastomosis should be restricted to patients in good condition, without gross peritoneal soiling. This is often present, and time must be given to a thorough peritoneal toilet and debridement (p. 145) with antibiotic lavage, and careful consideration of the appropriate choice of stoma. It may be best to form a double-barrelled ileocolostomy. For a colonic perforation, after resection, an ileostomy will be needed, and a distal mucous fistula. Greenstein *et al.* (1987) used enterostomies in their 30 patients and there were no deaths.

(e) Intra-abdominal sepsis – abscess formation and rupture

Very few abscesses present as an emergency. Among 415 patients with CD, Greenstein *et al.* (1987) had only nine who presented with spontaneous perforation of an abscess into the peritoneal cavity. In CD abscesses form between bowel loops, between the leaves of the mesentery, between bowel and the abdominal wall, especially in the pelvis, and into the psoas sheath. Should one rupture the situation will be dealt with according to basic principles of management of CD and peritonitis.

(f) Massive haemorrhage

In Aberdeen, 10 patients among 510 with a confirmed diagnosis of CD presented with severe haemorrhage (Driver *et al.*, 1996). In five the haemorrhage was the first sign of the disease and the average transfusion required was 11 units.

In spite of attempts to localize the source of bleeding by colonoscopy and angiography (p. 000) this was successful in only one patient, who was bleeding from an ulcer just proximal to an ileorectal anastomosis: total colectomy had been performed 10 years previously. Seven of the other nine had a colonic site of bleeding and all required colectomy and ileostomy to achieve haemostasis. Two patients bled from the ileum: one had four separate areas of CD and all four were removed by limited resection. The last specimen contained fresh clot.

These histories show that this can be a serious complication and localization of the bleeding point difficult. The rules for investigating severe rectal haemorrhage must be remembered, including the importance of gastroduodenal endoscopy (p. 377).

Haemorrhage may also occur from the site of an anastomosis or a strictureplasty. Gardiner *et al.* (1996) saw four cases of severe haemorrhage in 52 patients who required 241 strictureplasties in the course of 76 operations. Three patients settled with conservative care but one required two laparotomies before the bleeding was arrested. On-table endoscopy and enteroscopy may be needed (Ozuno and Fazio, 1995).

REFERENCES

Bundred, N. J., Dixon, J. M., Lumsden, A. B. *et al.* (1985) Free perforation in Crohn's colitis: a 10 year review. *Dis. Colon Rectum*, **28**, 35–37.

Crohn, B. B. (1957) Indications for surgical intervention in regional ileitis. *Arch. Surg.*, **74**, 305–311.

Crohn, B. B. (1965) The pathology of acute regional ileitis. *Am. J. Dig. Dis.*, **10**, 565–572.

Driver, C. P., Anderson, D. M. and Keenan, R. A. (1996) Massive intestinal bleeding in association with Crohn's disease. *J. R. Coll. Surg. Edin.*, **41**, 152–154.

Gardiner, K. R., Kettlewell, M. G. W. and Mortensen, N. J. M. (1996) Intestinal haemorrhage after strictureplasty for Crohn's disease. *Int. J. Colorect. Dis.*, **11**, 180–182.

Gow, J. G. and Walsh, A. (1952) Acute perforation in regional enteritis. *Br. J. Surg.*, **39**, 445–447.

Greenstein, A. J., Scahar, D. B., Main, D. *et al.* (1987) Spontaneous free perforation and perforated abscess in 30 patients with Crohn's disease. *Ann. Surg.*, **205**, 72–76.

Kewenter, J., Hulten, L., Kock, N. G. (1974) Relationship and epidemiology of acute terminal ileitis and Crohn's disease. *Gut*, **15**, 801–804.

Mair, N. S. (1977) Yersinia infections, in *Topics in Gastroenterology 5*, (eds S. C. Truelove and E. Lee), Blackwell Scientific Publications, Oxford, p. 325.

Makowiec, E. C., Jehle, E. C., Koveker, G. *et al.* (1993) Intestinal stenosis and perforating complications in Crohn's disease. *Int. J. Colorect. Dis.*, **8**, 197–200.

Morain, C. O. (1981) Acute ileitis. *BMJ*, **283**, 1075–1076.

Ozuno, G. and Fazio, V. W. (1995) Management of gastrointestinal bleeding after strictureplasty for Crohn's disease. *Dis. Colon Rectum*, **38**, 297–300.

Rawlinson, J. and Hughes, R. G. (1985) Acute suppurative appendicitis: a rare associate of Crohn's disease. *Dis. Colon Rectum*, **28**, 608–609.

Steinberg, D. M., Cook, W. T. and Alexander-Williams, J. (1973) Free perforation in Crohn's disease. *Gut*, **14**, 187–190.

Weston, L. A., Roberts, P. L., Schoetz, D. J. *et al.* (1996) Ileocolic resection for acute presentation of Crohn's disease of ileum. *Dis. Colon Rectum.*, **39**, 841–846.

6.10.2 NON-TRAUMATIC PERFORATION OF SMALL BOWEL

In most Western countries this is an unusual cause of peritonitis, although more often seen in tropical countries due to typhoid fever (p. 254) and enteritis necroticans. These patients will present with the signs of peritonitis, and are almost certain to be suspected of perforated appendicitis or a perforated peptic ulcer. Leizonmark *et al.* (1984) describe 112 patients seen in Stockholm, and review the subject.

Among the serious causes of perforation are **small-bowel lymphomas** (p. 233), **Crohn's ileitis** (p. 250), **tuberculous enteritis** (p. 230) and the **late effects of radiation** (p. 234). These can be difficult to distinguish on naked-eye inspection, but require a different range of treatment and this is considered on pp. 233 and p. 235.

Conditions as various as **Meckel's diverticulum** (p. 101), **diverticulosis of small bowel** (p. 256), **polyarteritis nodosa** (p. 543) and **yersiniosis** (p. 250) can be complicated by perforation. Enteritis due to *Yersinia enterocolitica* usually produces a febrile illness with vomiting and diarrhoea but can go on to a serious illness with perforating ulcers in jejunum or ileum. Cultures of faeces seem unreliable and a rising serum antibody titre seems the most reliable method of diagnosis (Browning and Weir, 1985). They had to perform two resections for multiple perforations and maintain high dosages of chloramphenicol over many days in a gravely ill patient.

One of the commoner causes of perforation is penetration of the bowel wall by a **swallowed foreign body**. Of these, fish bones and toothpick splinters are most often seen – and felt: a sharp prick on the finger as the small bowel is reviewed has several times drawn our attention to the cause of peritonitis. The mentally retarded may eat dangerous objects that can cause perforation (Harrison, 1980).

Enteritis necroticans or acute gangrenous enteritis is rare in temperate climates but is familiar in South-east Asia, Papua New Guinea and some parts of Africa. The subjects are usually poorly nourished children, eating a largely vegetable diet, who partake of poorly cooked pig meat. This is heavily contaminated with *Clostridium welchii* C and B toxin elaborated by the bacteria (Lawrence and Walker, 1976). Because the subjects are vegetarians, proteolytic enzymes are low so the toxin is not destroyed and can invade the mucosa of the jejunum, with consequent necrosis and shedding of considerable areas of mucosa. This causes abdominal colic, vomiting and diarrhoea. In some there is gas formation in the submucosa and if inflammation penetrates the muscularis perforation is likely: patients are then admitted gravely ill with general peritonitis. A number of similar cases were recorded in Germany in 1944–1948, when malnourished individuals were suddenly offered meat. Urgent operation, peritoneal cleansing and resection of the oedematous and congested small bowel back to healthy tissue, with anastomosis or stoma formation, are required (Archampong, 1985).

Patients who recover without perforation may present later with a fibrous stricture where granulation tissue has covered denuded muscularis.

Ingested potassium chloride was an important cause of small-bowel injury (p. 236), but with the development of slow-release preparations this is now unusual. Farquharson-Roberts *et al.* (1975) describe a case of perforation probably due to slowed intestinal transit time. Leizonmark and Raf (1985) collected 22 patients who sustained small-bowel damage from slow-release tablets and nine of them had perforated.

Tablet containing **ferrous sulphate** can also cause focal necrosis and perforation if held up undissolved in, for instance, a jejunal diverticulum (Ingoldby, 1977). Slow-release **indomethacin** can have a similar effect (Day, 1983).

All reports mention a number of patients in whom no cause for a perforation can be found. Cronin (1959) reviewed this subject and suggested that some were due to a sudden rise of pressure within bowel while it lies against a hernial orifice, with a blow-out occurring in the unsupported wall.

The important topic of the occurrence of perforation of small and large bowel in patients who are on **high dosage of corticosteroids** must be remembered and is particularly relevant in the management of inflammatory bowel disease. The effect of this medication is to modify very considerably the reaction of the parietal peritoneum – and so guarding and tenderness – to perforation.

In many of these situations it is likely that there will be doubt, at the time of operation, about the cause of the perforation, so it will be important to obtain histological material. This may be easy because it is necessary to resect in order to deal properly with the situation, e.g. in Crohn's disease. However, if simple suture seems to be appropriate then it is wise to carry out a limited excision around the perforation before inserting Gambee sutures: the tissue so obtained must be submitted to histological examination.

REFERENCES

Archampong, E. Q. (1985) Tropical diseases of the small bowel. *World J. Surg.*, **9**, 887–896.

Browning, G. G. P. and Weir, W. R. C. (1985) Intestinal perforation associated with *Yersinia enterocolitica* infection. *BMJ*, **290**, 1872.

Cronin, K. (1959) The problem of spontaneous rupture of the normal alimentary canal. *Br. J. Surg.*, **47**, 43–50.

Day, T. K. (1983) Intestinal perforation associated with osmotic slow release indomethacin capsules. *BMJ*, **287**, 1671–1672.

Farquharson-Roberts, M. A., Giddings, A. E. B. and Nunn, A. J. (1975) Perforation of small bowel due to slow release potassium chloride (slow-K). *BMJ*, **iii**, 206.

Harrison, R. A. (1980) Pica: an unusual cause of intestinal perforation. *Br. J. Clin. Pract.*, **34**, 155–156.

Ingoldby, C. J. H. (1977) Perforated jejunal diverticulum due to local iron toxicity. *BMJ*, **i**, 949–950.

Lawrence, G. and Walker, P. D. (1976) Pathogenesis of enteritis necroticans in Papua New Guinea. *Lancet*, **i**, 125–126.

Leizonmark, C. E. and Raf, L. (1985) Ulceration of the small intestine due to slow-release potassium chloride tablets. *Acta Chir. Scand.*, **151**, 273–278.

Leizonmark, C. E., Fenyo, G. and Raf, L. (1984) Non-traumatic perforation of the small intestine. *Acta Chir. Scand.*, **150**, 405–411.

6.10.3   TYPHOID FEVER AND THE ACUTE ABDOMEN

If this seems an unlikely subject for concern to most readers of this book, it is worth remembering that this is still a very common disease. Holidaymakers in Spain and Italy should remember that 15 000–20 000 cases are notified yearly in each of these countries while it is exceedingly common in South America, Africa and the East. The surgeon in a tropical country is very much aware of the enteric fevers and their ability to mimic or produce surgical emergencies, while the surgeon in Western Europe cannot afford to forget it, especially among those who have recently travelled abroad: it is worth remembering that TAB inoculation has not been a wholly reliable preventive among Service personnel in the Middle East.

The enteric fevers can only be contracted by drinking or eating food contaminated by a human carrier. In the small bowel, the organisms penetrate the Peyer's patches, where they multiply and spread through the blood stream to liver and spleen. After some 10–14 days the organisms re-emerge into the blood and heavily recolonize the gut *via* the bile. It is then that deep ulceration of Peyer's patches in distal ileum may cause perforation, or loss of blood *per rectum*.

The patient complains of malaise, headache, anorexia, cough and fever. There is usually constipation at this stage, though thin, green stools may be passed later. During this first week the blood culture is usually positive. If untreated, the patient is gravely ill by the end of the first week, confused and restless, with a doughy somewhat distended abdomen. The rose macules may be seen at this stage and the spleen becomes palpable. The Widal test is not much help at first but a rising titre of O antigen from 1:80 to over 1:200 is very suggestive.

Perforation

The surgeon's main task is to identify those who have perforated. Incidence varies, from as much as 15–30% in West Africa down to 1–2% in South Africa, Papua New Guinea and India (Richens, 1991). The perforations occur characteristically on the antimesenteric aspect of terminal ileum, in ulcerated Peyer's patches, and are longitudinal in shape and sometimes multiple. There is little tendency to fibrinous sealing or localization, so peritoneal contamination is widespread.

Patients have usually been feverish and ill for a week or more. Archampong (1985) in 315 patients in Ghana, found abdominal tenderness (100%), guarding (79%), rigidity (33%), distension (82%) and fever over 38°C in 54%. About 80% show free gas under the diaphragm. Sometimes the picture suggests intestinal obstruction.

Management

There is now a consensus that operative treatment gives the best results. Preoperative preparation is very necessary, because these patients are seriously dehydrated (4–5 litres deficit), acidotic and anaemic (mean Hb = 7.5 g/dl). Parenteral treatment is commenced with chloramphenicol and metronidazole. A urine output of 30–50 ml/h should be achieved. Then, excision and suture of the perforation(s) and thorough peritoneal toilet with antibiotic lavage are performed.

A mortality rate of about 15% is widely reported, depending very much on the stage at which patients reach hospital. In Nigeria, Badezo and Arigbabu (1980) treated 110 patients with suture repair, and 55 with resection and anastomosis for multiple perforations. They introduced a catheter into the upper abdomen and a drain into the pelvis and irrigated the abdomen for 5 days with chloramphenicol and trasylol in dextran, and recorded only five deaths.

Haemorrhage may occur in the third week and is best treated by transfusion and skilful medical management.

In the Aberdeen outbreak of typhoid fever in 1964 several patients were treated for advanced appendicitis, because their complaints had been attributed to typhoid fever, which they did not have. It is wise to remember that there are many causes of peritonitis, and this is another reason for preferring laparotomy to conservative treatment.

REFERENCES

Archampong, E. Q. (1985) Tropical diseases of the small bowel. *World J. Surg.*, **9**, 887–896.

Badezo, O. A. and Arigbabu, A. O. (1980) Operative treatment of typhoid perforation with peritoneal irrigation: a comparative study. *Gut*, **21**, 141–145.

Richens, J. (1991) Management of bowel perforation in typhoid fever. *Trop. Doctor*, **21**, 149–152.

6.10.4 DIVERTICULOSIS OF THE SMALL INTESTINE

Diverticula of the duodenum are sometimes seen in barium meals and at laparotomy surgeons are familiar with the incidental finding of multiple jejunal diverticula. The great majority of these diverticula cause little or no trouble. A few patients suffer chronic dyspepsia, and Phillips (1953) gave an excellent description of the chronic functional obstruction that is now well recognized as a complication of jejunal diverticulosis (Krishnamurthy *et al.*, 1983). Bacterial colonization occasionally causes megaloblastic anaemia.

Acute diverticulitis, perforation, haemorrhage and acute intestinal obstruction are all recognized complications of diverticulosis and generally, because of their rarity, are only diagnosed when revealed at laparotomy. The subject is well reviewed by Walker (1945).

It is generally agreed that jejunal diverticula are acquired and, in common with colonic diverticula, they show an increasing incidence with increasing age. They arise at the point in the jejunal wall where the vasa recta pierce the muscular wall. They are usually multiple, do not have a muscular covering and are often initially intramesenteric and not easy to see unless the jejunum is deliberately distended. Diverticula are commoner in the upper than the lower jejunum and are only rarely seen in the ileum (Cocks and Zino, 1968).

Petrie *et al.* (1972) examined all barium studies made in the north-east of Scotland during 1967–1970. In a total of 29 512 examinations, 1935 small intestinal studies were made and diverticula were found in seven men and 12 women. This compared with the finding of colonic diverticula in 635 men and 932 women, which gives a useful indication of the rarity of diverticula in the small bowel and also confirms the known tendency for alimentary diverticula to occur more frequently in women.

Perforation and acute jejunal diverticulitis

These two complications are not easy to separate because a number of patients who present with suppurative peritonitis do not have a demonstrable perforation, although one or more diverticula are acutely inflamed and may be surrounded by a local abscess. Phillips (1953) saw a rolled-up tomato skin projecting from a diverticulum.

These patients present in a variety of ways. Most are likely to be considered to have acute appendicitis or acute colonic diverticulitis. The oedema produced by the local inflammation may cause acute intestinal obstruction (Walker, 1945). It is important to remember, therefore, that jejunum as well as ileum is one of the areas that must be examined when, at laparotomy for suspected appendicitis, the appendix looks normal.

Most reports (Roses *et al.*, 1976) emphasize that, because of the intramesenteric situation of these diverticula, there is an inflammatory mass, often covered by fibrin or pus, within the mesentery. The correct treatment is to resect the affected segment of jejunum. There are usually a number of diverticula, and a judgement has to be made whether removal of all diverticula, along with the affected segment, is reasonable, or whether this would mean removal of too much small bowel.

Duodenal diverticula

Duodenal diverticula rarely become inflamed but Donald (1979) reports two patients who developed acute pain and tenderness in the right upper quadrant and were thought to have acute cholecystitis. Both had a retroperitoneal inflammatory mass, lateral to and behind the second part of the duodenum, due to a perforated diverticulum. For the first patient Donald excised the diverticulum and sutured the inflamed duodenal wall, and this was followed by a temporary duodenal fistula. In the second patient he thought it safer to add a vagotomy, antrectomy and gastrojejunal anastomosis, because of uncertainty over the security of the duodenal closure.

Acute diverticulitis in the terminal ileum

This is very unusual. It is particularly likely to present as acute appendicitis, but does not look much like acute Meckel's diverticulitis because it lies principally in mesentery. Limited enterectomy or ileocolectomy will probably be the correct operation (Cocks and Zino, 1968).

Acute haemorrhage

The reports of this unusual source of severe alimentary tract haemorrhage all emphasize the large volumes of blood lost. Taylor (1969) reviewed the literature and found that 25 out of 35 patients required transfusion of more than 5 litres of blood, and 30 needed a laparotomy to secure haemostasis. In most patients there is no haematemesis, but this can occur if the diverticulum is in duodenum, or high in jejunum.

Spiegel *et al.* (1982) report three elderly patients with severe rectal haemorrhage, who each needed 10–13 units of blood, in whom a superior mesenteric angiogram clearly demonstrated the bleeding point. Between 20 and 90 cm of jejunum was resected and the bleeding point was demonstrated in two. In these patients gastroduodenoscopy is likely to show fresh blood entering duodenum from below, so attention will be focused on the small bowel at laparotomy.

The duodenal loop must also be closely examined. In Donald's (1979) patient the second part contained a diverticulum but it did not appear to be bleeding. The hepatic flexure was fully mobilized and then a large diverticulum was found in the third part with an active bleeding point. A total of 3.5 litres of blood had to be given intraoperatively in addition to 4 litres in the 8 hours before operation. The diverticulum was excised and vagotomy, antrectomy and gastrojejunostomy performed.

If the stomach and duodenum, and remainder of the gut are normal, and the jejunum is tense with blood and contains many diverticula, it is reasonable to assume that one or more of these are the source of bleeding, and to resect. If this specimen is opened along its antimesenteric aspect, blood cleared out and then the mesentery massaged, one diverticulum may fill with blood.

Acute intestinal obstruction

This can occur in several ways. An inflamed jejunal diverticulum may become adherent to another structure and thereby kink the bowel, or form the apex of a volvulus (Donald, 1979). Some diverticula become filled with inspissated food residue, and this may form into a faecolith, migrate into the lumen and cause bolus obstruction (Bewes, 1967).

REFERENCES

Bewes, P. C. (1967) Surgical complications of jejunal diverticulosis. *Proc. R. Soc. Med.*, **60**, 225–227.

Cocks, J. R. and Zino, F. J. (1968) Acute diverticulitis of the terminal ileum. *Br. J. Surg.*, **55**, 45–49.

Donald, J. W. (1979) Major complications of small bowel diverticula. *Ann. Surg.*, **190**, 183–188.

Krishnamurthy, S., Kelly, M. M., Rohrmann, C. A. and Schuffler, M. D. (1983) Jejunal diverticulosis. *Gastroenterology*, **85**, 538–547.

Petri, J. C., Needham, C. D. and Gillanders, L. A. (1972) Survey of alimentary radiology findings in North-East of Scotland Region (1967–70). *BMJ*, **ii**, 78–81.

Phillips, J. H. C. (1953) Jejunal diverticulosis. *Br. J. Surg.*, **40**, 350–354.

Roses, D. F., Gouge, T. H., Scher, K. S. and Ranson, J. H. C. (1976) Perforated diverticula of the jejunum and ileum. *Am. J. Surg.*, **132**, 649–652.

Spiegel, Schultz, R. W., Casarella, W. J. and Wolff, M. (1982) Massive haemorrhage from jejunal diverticula. *Radiology*, **143**, 367–371.

Taylor, M. T. (1969) Massive haemorrhage from jejunal diverticulosis. *Am. J. Surg.*, **118**, 117–120.

Walker, R. M. (1945) The complications of acquired diverticulosis of the jejunum and ileum. *Br. J. Surg.*, **32**, 457–459.

6.11   INTESTINAL OBSTRUCTION IN OLDER PATIENTS

With advancing age the incidence of appendicitis falls away, intestinal obstruction becomes the commonest abdominal emergency (Irvin, 1989) and beyond 75 years of age nearly 60% of abdominal emergencies involve obstruction (Blake and Lynn, 1975). Strangulated hernia (30%) and adhesions and carcinoma of the colon (20%) are the main causes, so adhesive obstruction is no longer, as in the younger age groups, the principal source of obstruction. Over the age of 60 the mortality rate rises from around 1% to about 12% in the 60-year-olds and to 20% in patients over 80: much of this is due to intercurrent disease, and the inability of older patients to contend with postoperative complications.

REFERENCES

Blake, R. and Lynn, J. (1976) Emergency abdominal surgery in the aged. *Br. J. Surg.*, **63**, 956–960.
Irvin, T. T. (1989) Abdominal pain: a surgical audit of 1190 emergency admissions. *Br. J. Surg.*, **76**, 1121–1125.

6.12   NEUROGENIC, ADYNAMIC OR PARALYTIC ILEUS

Throughout ancient and medieval times the term 'ileus' was applied to all forms of intestinal obstruction and it was not until the late 19th century that Treves in 1884 (Treves, 1899) clearly separated the mechanical obstructions from the ileus that is due to loss of the propulsive power of the intestine. As a consequence, swallowed air and water and the alimentary secretions accumulate, the bowels progressively distend and there is total constipation. There is no point of mechanical obstruction so this state cannot be directly treated by surgical intervention.

Much experimental work has been done, because in the first 50 years of the development of abdominal surgery this worrying postoperative complication was relatively common, and not infrequently fatal.

Peritonitis is the classic cause of adynamic ileus, and it was regularly seen in the days before antibiotics, when many patients had diffuse peritonitis due to perforations of the alimentary tract. Arai in 1922 performed the crucial experiments, which showed that, if the splanchnic nerves of a cat were divided and then peritonitis was induced, the passage of barium through the inflamed bowel still proceeded normally. This showed that peritonitis did not produce its effect directly on the bowel musculature but induced an inhibitory effect on the bowel by stimulating the function of the splanchnic nerves (Neely and Catchpole, 1971).

This theory also explained other causes of ileus. **Disturbance of the retroperitoneal area** through which the splanchnic nerves run, is a well-recognized cause of ileus. Fractures of the spine, retroperitoneal haemorrhage, a difficult nephrectomy, immobilization of a patient on a plaster bed, and acute pancreatitis are among recognized precipitating factors.

Metabolic disorders, especially cellular potassium deficiency, is at least a contributory factor in the occurrence of adynamic ileus (Streeten and Ward-McQuaid, 1952).

A number of **drugs**, such as the phenothiazines and tricyclic antidepressants, and anticholinergics such as propantheline, produce inhibition of intestinal function (p. 238).

It is also worth considering what can be done at the time of abdominal operation to prevent the onset of ileus. Efficient treatment of peritonitis, as detailed in Chapter 4, good, gentle surgical technique, nasogastric suction where indicated, combined with a cautious start to postoperative fluid intake and careful accounting of fluid and electrolyte intake and output, with special reference to potassium metabolism, are all contributions to prevention of ileus.

Adynamic ileus is now an unusual condition, but it will be suspected when one of the possible causes is operative. Most often a patient who has had an operation for diffuse peritonitis remains unwell. On the second or third day there is frequent vomiting, or aspiration through the nasogastric tube of dirty brown fluid, in quantity. The patient is anxious and uncomfortable, the pulse fast, the abdomen considerably distended, tense, resonant and silent. Neither flatus nor faeces is passing. Review of fluid and electrolyte balance may show that it has fallen behind the losses. A plain abdominal film shows gas-distended small **and** large bowel, with fluid levels. This presence of gas in the colon suggests that there is no mechanical obstruction in the small bowel, but it is still very important to consider whether an organic condition is present. This possibility must be regularly reviewed.

Treatment

The first task is to make the anxious patient more comfortable and morphine should be used effectively. It is important to review the biochemical status of the patient because losses of extracellular fluid can be large, both in vomit and aspirate and in fluid loss into the distended bowel. Blood transfusion may be indicated. Some have found it helpful, after full restoration of normovolaemia, to inject 30–40 ml of gastrografin down the nasogastric tube and expose X-rays at 30 minutes and 3–4 hours later. This may confirm patency of the small bowel and the osmotic effect of gastrografin may promote bowel movement (Zer *et al.*, 1977).

It should be remembered that the reason for the ileus may be concealed. The first warning of an anastomotic leak after colorectal surgery may be that, at about the sixth day, the picture of adynamic ileus develops, and then the correct reaction would be to check the state of the anastomosis with a water-soluble contrast enema.

As a general principle, great caution would have to be exercised over using gastrografin in the presence of fresh bowel anastomosis.

Pharmacological treatment

If ileus persists then a change to a more active regime must be considered. The case for this has been well argued by Neely and Catchpole (1971). They base their case on the work that suggests that persistent ileus is due to sympathetic overactivity mediated through the splanchnic nerves: the argument is, therefore, that pharmacological blockade of the sympathetic nervous system should remove the inhibitory effect of this overaction and therefore promote recovery from ileus.

On the practical side, Neely and Catchpole emphasize the importance of the patient being in water and electrolyte balance, and being normovolaemic. It must also be emphasized that the surgeon should be as certain as possible that there is no mechanical element in the obstruction. If these conditions are met then the effect of guanethidine can be tried. The patient should lie flat and the blood pressure should be frequently checked. There is likely to be a 10–20 mmHg fall, but this should not be exceeded.

Add 20 mg of guanethidine to 200 ml of physiological saline and this mixture is run into a vein over 30 minutes. The blood pressure is measured every 5 minutes and auscultation of the abdomen is maintained. When bowel sounds become established it is recommended that the effect of the guanethidine should be potentiated by injecting small doses of a parasympathomimetic drug. The authors use either one subcutaneous injection of bethanechol chloride 2.5 mg or repeated intravenous injections of neostigmine to a total of 0.5 mg. (The simplest method is to add 0.5 mg neostigmine to 20 ml of water in a syringe. Then 2 ml of this solution will contain 0.05 mg prostigmine and 2 ml can be given through the infusion every 3–4 minutes.) As a result of this treatment flatus is likely to be passed before all the neostigmine has been given and no more should be used once this has happened. If abdominal colic is produced no more neostigmine should be given.

Neely and Catchpole record that they have found this treatment effective and have not had any ill-effects in more than 30 patients, and our experience confirms these claims. This concept has a sound basis and gets away from the idea that ileus is a mysterious condition. After ensuring that any precipitating factor has been effectively treated, the surgeon can apply a logical treatment.

REFERENCES

Arai, K. (1922) Experimentelle Untersuchung über die Magen-Darmbewegungen bei akuter Peritonitis. *Arch. Exp. Pathol. Pharmakol.*, **94**, 149.

Neely, J. and Catchpole, B. (1971) Ileus: the restoration of alimentary tract motility by pharmacological means. *Br. J. Surg.*, **58**, 21–27.

Streeten, D. H. P. and Ward-McQuaid, J. N. (1952) Relation of electrolyte changes and adrenocortical activity to paralytic ileus. *BMJ*, **ii**, 587–592.

Treves, F. (1899) *Intestinal Obstruction*, 2nd edn, Cassell, London.

Zer, M., Kaznelson, D., Feigenberg, Z. *et al.* (1977) The value of gastrografin in the differential diagnosis of paralytic ileus versus mechanical intestinal obstruction. *Dis. Colon Rectum*, **20**, 573–579.

6.13   ACUTE DILATATION OF THE STOMACH

This is another unusual disturbance of alimentary tract function. During the first 40 years of this century surgeons were unhappily familiar with patients who, following major abdominal surgery, became anxious and pale after about 48 hours, hypotensive, and began to vomit dark brown or black vomit: if a stomach tube was passed litres of this fluid was aspirated. Acute dilatation had a sinister reputation, and carried a mortality of 30–40%.

With widespread adoption of postoperative nasogastric suction and better understanding of fluid and electrolyte balance during and after the Second World War, this condition has become a rarity, but its effects are serious and recognition is important. The large amounts of fluid in the stomach are due to gastric hypersecretion, with some mucosal bleeding: this outpouring occurs very rapidly and the loss of extracellular fluid is reflected in the hypotension, which can be severe, and calls for very urgent intravenous infusion of electrolyte and colloid solutions. It should be remembered that the potassium content of the aspirated juice is about 15 mEq/l (Starr, 1953). With energetic treatment acute dilatation generally disappears as quickly as it came, but introduction of oral feeding clearly should be most carefully watched.

Acute gastric dilatation has been known for a long time as a complication of placing a patient flat on his/her back in a plaster bed or a hip spica, and is known as 'the body cast syndrome' (Dorph, 1950). If the patient is kept recumbent there is a strong tendency to recurrence. It may also complicate blunt abdominal trauma and Kasenally *et al.* (1976) were particularly impressed with the improvement in the cardiorespiratory state of their two patients after the aspiration of large volumes of fluid and gas from the stomach.

Acute dilatation is seen from time to time after a patient with anorexia nervosa suddenly eats a large meal (Brook, 1977) and Saul *et al.* (1981) saw a patient in whom this led to fatal perforation. Similar problems arose in 1945 when released prisoners of war understandably ate a normal-sized meal, which was more than they could accommodate (Markowski, 1947).

REFERENCES

Brook, G. K. (1977) Acute gastric dilatation in anorexia nervosa. *BMJ*, **ii**, 499–500.

Dorph, M. H. (1950) The cast syndrome. *N. Engl. J. Med.*, **243**, 440–442.

Kasenally, A. T., Felice, A. G. and Logie, J. R. C. (1976) Acute gastric dilatation after trauma. *BMJ*, **ii**, 21.

Markowski, B. (1947) Acute dilatation of the stomach. *BMJ*, **ii**, 128–130.

Saul, S. H., Dekker, A. and Watson, C. G. (1981) Acute gastric dilatation with infarction and perforation. *Gut*, **22**, 978–983.

Starr, K. W. (1953) Acute postoperative dilatation of the stomach. *Ann. R. Coll. Surg. Engl.*, **12**, 71–87.

7

Large-bowel emergencies

7.1 INTRODUCTION

Until the 1950s the surgery of colonic and rectal emergencies had remained virtually unchanged for half a century. Laparotomy, identification and perhaps drainage of the lesion, with formation of a proximal colostomy, was the recognized treatment for obstructions and perforations. A majority of the patients were elderly, many with medical problems, and the general experience was that about 30% or more of these patients died after operation. Those who survived required a second operation to resect the lesion, and a third to close the colostomy. Many patients did not undergo the second or third operations because they died, were found unfit for further surgery or the progression of the original disease precluded further surgical intervention.

This resolve to do the minimum of surgery at the first operation was based on a well-founded concern for the dangers faced by these patients. The obstructed colon is fragile and loaded with highly infective fluid faeces. In perforations, the dangers of causing or spreading faecal peritonitis are great. Thus in past decades, the surgeon's instinct suggested that the patient was so ill that only limited surgery could be sustained. Anaesthesia was primitive; there were no antibiotics or intensive therapy. Intravenous fluid replacement was a relatively new concept and, consequently, relative inaction by the surgeon was a reasonable judgement.

The evidence that initiated a changing attitude started when it was appreciated that the only method by which a patient with fulminating ulcerative colitis could be consistently rescued (which at the time carried a mortality of about 50%) was to perform an emergency colectomy and ileostomy before perforation took place (Brooke, 1954). At about the same time, it was recognized that it was safer and technically little different to carry out immediate resection and anastomosis for an obstruction of the proximal colon than it was to perform an ileotransverse colonic anastomosis (Baranofsky, 1950). It then became clear that among patients with perforated sigmoid diverticular disease, the results were better if immediate resection by the Hartmann's operation were performed (Boyden and Neilson, 1960), instead of draining the perforation and making a proximal transverse colostomy. As experience has increased, with the evolution of intensive therapy units, an understanding of sepsis prevention and treatment, as well as the management of sick patients during complex surgery

Emergency Abdominal Surgery. Edited by Peter F. Jones, Zygmunt H. Krukowski and George G. Youngson. Published in 1998 by Chapman & Hall, London. ISBN 0 412 81950 3.

Table 7.1 197 consecutive colorectal emergencies

Carcinoma	No 83	Died 5
Obstructed	73	4
Perforated	9	1
Haemorrhage	1	
Immediate resection (12% mortality)	74	5

Diverticular disease	No 43	Died 6
Perforated	29	
Purulent	20	3
Faecal	9	
Obstructed	3	3
Haemorrhage	5	
Non-perforated	6	
(3 with small bowel obstruction)		
Immediate resection	37	6

'Colitis'	No 28	Died 5
Crohn's	12	
Ulcerative	16	3
Perforated	8	
Fulminant	8	2
Megacolon	6	
Ileocaecal mass/abscess	3	
Haemorrhage	3	
Immediate resection	28	5

Miscellaneous	No 43	Died 4
Volvulus	10	
Injuries	10	
SMA occlusion	4	
Strangulation	4	
Pseudo-obstruction	4	
Angiodysplasia	2	
Intussusception		
Pancreatic pseudocyst		
Pseudomembranous colitis		
Ischaemic colitis	1 each	
Faecal impaction		
Polyarteritis		
Radiotherapy		
Torsion appendix epip		
Immediate resection	25	4

by modern anaesthetic techniques, the majority of patients with a major large-bowel emergency can be treated by immediate resection.

The place of immediate resection is illustrated in Table 7.1 which summarizes all the large-bowel emergency operations performed over a 10-year period in a general surgical unit receiving all emergency admissions, on every fourth day, from a population of 400 000.

Among the 197 operations, which illustrates the range of emergency large-bowel surgery, 164 (83%) involved resection of the lesion. The mortality rate of 12% could be improved on, but only four of the 20 patients who died were under 68 years of age and these four all had perforated inflammatory bowel disease – a reminder of the serious consequence of leakage from the large intestine.

There may be a temptation for the less experienced surgeon to attempt local repair of a perforation, on the grounds that the defect is small and to resect might seem an over-reaction: however, experience teaches that suture of large-bowel perforations in the presence of established peritonitis is not safe, and resection of the perforated lesion is required, with an end stoma and end mucous fistula, or a Hartmann's operation.

An important corollary of this move towards immediate resection is that the surgeon performing the emergency operation must have acquired considerable personal experience in the performance of major elective large-bowel operations. These procedures require considerable clinical judgments for all phases of patient management (resuscitation, intra- and postoperative care), and in addition, the procedures themselves are technically demanding. Only in this way can the best results be obtained by safe and expeditious surgery (Phillips *et al.*, 1985).

REFERENCES

Baronofsky, I. D. (1950) Primary resection and aseptic end-to-end anastomosis for acute or subacute large bowel obstruction. *Surgery*, **27**, 664–672.

Boyden, A. M. and Neilson, R. O. (1960) Reappraisal of the surgical treatment of diverticulitis of the sigmoid colon. *Am. J. Surg.*, **100**, 206–209.

Brooke, B. N. (1954) *Ulcerative Colitis and its Surgical Management*, E. & S. Livingstone, Edinburgh.

Phillips, R. K., Hittinger, R., Fry, J. S. *et al.* (1985) Malignant large bowel obstruction. *Br. J. Surg.*, **72**, 296–302.

7.2   OBSTRUCTIONS OF THE LARGE INTESTINE

There are considerable differences between the obstructions of the large and small intestine. The small bowel obstructs between two and three times more frequently than the large gut, and from a wide variety of causes. In the large bowel there are only two major causes of obstruction, namely carcinoma and volvulus. Bowel strangulation, which is a constant concern in small-bowel obstruction, is unusual in this part of the gut.

More than 50% of all large-bowel emergencies are caused by obstruction, of which 70% are secondary to carcinoma (Table 7.2).

Table 7.2 Causes of obstruction of colon in 103
consecutive patients

Cause		No.
Carcinoma		73 (70%)
Volvulus		10
• Sigmoid colon	6	
• Caecum	2	
• Transverse colon	1	
• Splenic flexure	1	
Megacolon complicating inflammatory bowel disease		6
Strangulation of colon		4
• External hernia	3	
• Band	1	
Pseudo-obstruction		4
Diverticular disease*		3
Intussusception		1
Faecal impaction		1
Pancreatic pseudocyst obstructing colon		1
		103
		(53% of all colorectal emergencies)

* There were also four cases of small-bowel obstruction due to adhesions to
sigmoid diverticulitis

This pattern is seen in Western Europe, the UK, North America and Australasia (Campbell *et al.*, 1956; Carden, 1966). In Africa and Asia the picture is quite different, with volvulus of various types being the commonest cause (Sinha, 1969; Odonga, 1982).

Intramural obstruction by carcinoma, and occasionally by diverticular disease, present in a similar manner and may be managed in similar ways (pp. 266 and p. 301). Colonic volvulus is a distinctive group (p. 289). Pseudo-obstruction of the colon is an important differential diagnosis and remains a therapeutic problem (p. 303). Unusual causes of large-bowel obstruction are described on page p. 301. Megacolon (p. 321), strangulated hernia (p. 214) and intussusception (p. 246) are considered elsewhere.

REFERENCES

Campbell, J. A., Gunn, A. A. and McLaren, I. F. (1956) Acute obstruction of the colon. *J. R. Coll. Surg. Edin.*, **1**, 231–239.

Carden, A. B. G. (1966) Acute large bowel obstruction: aetiology and mortality. *Med. J. Austral.*, **1**, 662–663.

Odonga, A. M. (1982) Variety of volvuli of intestine seen at Mulago Hospital, Kampala, 1966–75. *E. Afr. Med. J.*, **59**, 711–714.

Sinha, R. S. (1969) A clinical appraisal of volvulus of the pelvic colon. *Br. J. Surg.*, **56**, 838–840.

Table 7.3 Site of carcinoma in 70 patients presenting with large bowel obstruction compared to 433 consecutive patients presenting in NE Scotland with colorectal cancer

Site of cancer	70 obstructed patients		433 consecutive patients (%)
	No.	%	
Caecum and ascending colon	17	24	27
Transverse colon	7	10	8
Splenic flexure	15	21	4
Descending colon	4	6	3
Sigmoid colon	19	27	19
Rectosigmoid junction and rectum	8	11	39

7.2.1 NEOPLASTIC OBSTRUCTION

Obstruction of the large bowel by a carcinoma is generally due to annular neoplasm producing gradual narrowing of the lumen with a few proliferative neoplasms causing obstruction, particularly in the caecum. Rarely obstruction is due to invasion by direct infiltration from an adjacent neoplasm (e.g. ovary), or by a blood born metastasis (e.g. carcinoma of the breast) developing in the wall of the colon.

Between 15% and 20% of patients with colorectal carcinoma first present to the hospital only when they have obstructed, and among those over 70 years of age the proportion who arrive obstructed is 30% (Phillips *et al.*, 1985; Waldron *et al.*, 1986). About one-third of obstructed carcinomas lie proximal to the splenic flexure, two-thirds at and beyond this point. An unusually high proportion of carcinomas at the splenic flexure obstruct (50%), but among rectal carcinomas this proportion is very low, about 5% (Phillips *et al.*, 1985; Table 7.3).

7.2.1.1 Pathology

The colon proximal to the obstruction compensates by work hypertrophy of the muscularis, and so for a time powerful peristalsis overcomes the effect of the narrowing. Gradually the rise of intraluminal pressure is transmitted along the lumen of the colon, which progressively distends. This effect is maximal in the thin-walled caecum, where the lips of the ileocaecal valve tend to occlude, often preventing decompression of the caecum into the ileum. At worst, the colon between the ileocaecal valve and the carcinoma becomes a 'closed loop', while the ileum continues to propel gas and faeces into this segment of the bowel. By the action of Laplace's law, the caecum dilates more easily than elsewhere because of its greater original diameter and thin wall.

In the initial phases of bowel obstruction, which is of gradual onset, blood flow to the obstructed segment has been shown to increase in several different animal models (Papanicolaou *et al.*, 1989).

However, as the process progresses, intraluminal pressure rises, blood flow diminishes (Coxon *et al.*, 1984) and makes the caecum especially liable to 'ulcero-haemorrhagic ischaemic colitis' (Saegesser and Sandblom, 1975). This process may proceed to full-thickness necrosis and perforation, which was first described by Heschl in 1880 and is a very important reason for taking special note of the caecal diameter on plain abdominal radiographs in the management of large-bowel obstruction, and anticipating the danger of caecal perforation by early surgery. (The same danger arises in some patients with pseudomechanical obstruction; p. 303.) As many as 15% of patients with neoplastic colonic obstruction can present with a perforation (Umpleby and Williamson, 1984), although this figure has now fallen. In some patients this perforation occurs at or near the carcinoma, but in most in the distended caecum. Therefore, it is unsound and unacceptable to suture the perforation even after decompression of the colon (Saegesser and Sandblom, 1975). The safe treatment for pressure perforation of the caecum is resection of all colon proximal to the obstruction (p. 271).

Another harmful effect of large-bowel obstruction is the great multiplication of microorganisms that occurs in the stagnant pool of faeces proximal to the site of obstruction. These microorganisms and their products become translocated into the draining vessels of the obstructed bowel segment. The bacteria can then be found inhabiting draining lymph nodes and 'toxins' are found in the portal system. This breakdown of the mucosal barrier is another reason to support the notion that resection of the obstructed bowel in a sick patient will assist other resuscitative measures.

Obstructive colorectal carcinomata tend to be more advanced than the non-obstructed case: although patients in Dukes stage B and C are approximately equal, there are fewer stage A patients and between 30% (Phillips *et al.*, 1985) and 40% (Umpleby and Williamson, 1984) have distant metastases at the time of presentation (stage D).

7.2.1.2 Clinical picture

It is typical of a neoplastic obstruction that the patient cannot give an exact time of symptom onset. Most patients have noticed some disturbance of bowel function over the preceding weeks or months, until this culminates in absolute constipation. Almost all experience some colicky lower abdominal pain and some notice distension with audible peristalsis. Vomiting only affects about half of patients because there is relatively little involvement of the small bowel. Most have lost some body weight.

Because vomiting is neither so frequent nor so productive as in small-bowel obstruction, the general condition of the patient may be relatively good, and this contrasts with the marked abdominal distension. Sometimes the distended caecum can be seen if light falls obliquely on the abdomen, and quite often it can be felt. A palpable carcinoma is unusual because it is generally quite small, and the tense colon prevents deep abdominal palpation. Percussion gives a hyper-resonant note, and tinkling obstructive bowel sounds can be heard sometimes without the help of the stethoscope. It is unusual to feel a rectal neoplasm, but blood may be seen on the examining finger. Sometimes a sigmoid carcinoma has prolapsed into the rectovaginal/vesical pouch and can be felt through the anterior wall of the rectum. Occasionally, a colonic carcinoma intussuscepts and can then be palpated *per rectum*. A gentle sigmoidoscopy may reveal a carcinoma at the level of the rectosigmoid junction.

In 10–15% of patients with a perforation there will be signs of peritoneal irritation, localized over the caecum, but sometimes it may be generalized. Among the 20% of patients with a carcinoma of the caecum or ascending colon, there is more likely to be a picture of small-bowel obstruction, and it may be possible to see peristalsis of these loops through the abdominal wall. This important sign is frequently associated with dangerously high intracolonic pressure and indicates gradually increasing small-bowel obstruction requiring urgent laparotomy after initial resuscitation and stabilization. These patients are usually elderly and are likely to be malnourished and anaemic with other medical problems; thus careful general assessment with a few hours spent to correct major problems, such as arrhythmias, dehydration and serious anaemia, is usually essential before surgery.

7.2.1.3   Radiography

The distribution and shape of the gas and fluid trapped in the obstructed bowel is just as helpful in the diagnosis of obstructions in the colon as it is in those of the small intestine.

- There is usually great gaseous distension of the colon down to the point of obstruction, and this can be seen in both the erect and supine films. It is characteristic for the distension to be most marked in the caecum and ascending colon because most obstructions are in the distal colon, where muscular hypertrophy is maximal just above the obstruction, while the wall of the proximal colon is far more distensible. A very large fluid level can usually be seen in the caecum and, if the patient lies in the left lateral position, a horizontal film may show this fluid level to be up to 30 cm in length. In distal obstruction fluid levels may also be seen in the transverse and descending colon.
- The distended proximal colon is often smooth-sided, but in the transverse colon it is usually possible to see haustrations, which clearly identify the distended viscus as colon.
- There will be no gaseous distension in the colon and rectum distal to the obstruction, which is usually 'empty' save for a small amount of residual gas.
- There are usually only a few small-bowel loops visible, although this depends on the competence of the ileocaecal valve. In obstructions sited in the caecum or ascending colon, there is often a typical small-bowel obstruction picture.
- It is important to remember that the distribution of gas in the colon can be misleading because the gas shadows may terminate far short of the obstructing lesion. This is caused by the lumen immediately proximal to the obstruction being filled with fluid or semi-solid faeces. McIver and Don (1965) have drawn particular attention to this column of faecal matter because it can often be seen as a soft tissue shadow outlining the descending colon (Figure 7.1), giving a strong hint that the site of the obstruction is in the sigmoid area. An emergency opaque enema should clarify this matter.
- It is necessary to remember how closely some cases of 'pseudomechanical obstruction' can mimic a neoplastic large-bowel obstruction, especially when idiopathic in origin (p. 303). This has led us and many others to use an emergency opaque enema as a method of identifying these patients, and it has proved to be safe and helpful. Stewart *et al.* (1984) report a trial in which all patients with suspected large-bowel obstruction had an emergency water-soluble contrast enema using 25% diodone. In 98 patients believed to have a mechanical obstruction on the basis of clinical examination and plain abdominal radiographs, this diagnosis was confirmed in 60 patients. However, in 38 patients the contrast flowed freely to the caecum, thus excluding a diagnosis of mechanical obstruction in the large bowel. Of this group of 38 patients, the final diagnosis included 11 patients with 'pseudo-obstruction'; three had small-bowel obstructions; and a mixed collection of inflammatory and neoplastic conditions producing large-bowel distension explained the remainder.

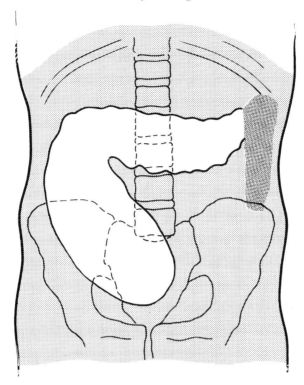

Figure 7.1 Possible appearance of a plain abdominal X-ray in obstruction of the sigmoid colon. The gas shadow stops at the splenic flexure because the descending colon is filled with faeces; this column may be seen as a faint shadow.

In a second group of 17 patients, Stewart *et al.* believed that the plain films suggested a diagnosis of pseudo-obstruction, and this diagnosis was confirmed in 15, but in two patients the emergency enema revealed an obstructing carcinoma.

A series of 91 emergency opaque enemas performed in Aberdeen (Koruth *et al.*, 1985a) produced a very similar result. Other similar studies have been reported more recently (Chapman *et al.*, 1992).

Consequently, we recommend the use of an emergency contrast enema and would now not be happy to explore a patient without the guidance of this examination except where signs clearly indicated perforation. Some use dilute barium, or gastrografin: the osmotic effect of gastrografin is sometimes helpful to relieve a pseudo-obstruction (p. 303).

7.2.1.4 Differential diagnosis

Most patients with neoplastic obstruction of the distal colon present in a typical manner, and the diagnosis is confirmed by sigmoidoscopy or opaque enema. Volvulus of the colon (p. 289) has a different but generally typical presentation. Many patients with pseudomechanical obstruction of the colon are already seriously ill, or have just given birth, often by caesarean section, so the clinical picture is different. However, in the idiopathic cases the differential diagnosis can be difficult and emergency contrast enema and colonoscopy can be vital to establish the diagnosis.

7.2.1.5   Treatment

The treatment of neoplastic obstruction of the large bowel remained largely static throughout the first half of this century. For obstruction in the proximal colon an ileotransverse anastomosis was the procedure of choice, and transverse colostomy was the treatment for obstructing carcinomas much beyond the midpoint of the transverse colon. Although these were relatively minor procedures Goligher and Smiddy (1957) in Leeds found that the mortality was about 30%, while the survivors had to face a resection and, for many, later closure of the colostomy.

FT Paul (1895) of Liverpool made a remarkable contribution with his concept of resecting an obstructing carcinoma and fashioning a double-barrelled colostomy at the first operation, and von Mickulicz (1903) independently devised a similar operation. However, this was really only applicable in the left colon and the sigmoid, and was not much used. Then Baronofsky (1950) and Gregg (1955) made the challenging suggestion that in selected patients it was possible not only to carry out a radical resection of an obstructed colonic carcinoma but also to perform an immediate anastomosis. Together they reported eight such patients, with no deaths.

Following this lead a number of surgeons practised primary resection and anastomosis when it was feasible (Hughes, 1966; Herrington *et al.*, 1967; Valerio and Jones, 1978) and recorded mortality rates around 10%. Considering the age, and often the infirmity, of many of these patients, a mortality rate much below 8–10% is difficult to achieve. An operation that can overcome obstruction in one stage, rather than in two or three, and with a lower mortality, has particular value for older patients.

This approach has now been widely adopted but its continued success will depend on careful patient selection, choice of method, and careful operative technique by surgeons with considerable experience of elective colorectal surgery.

It remains to be seen whether the introduction of the expanding metal stent will allow a lumen to be opened up within a distal colonic carcinoma so that the bowel can be decompressed and prepared for later elective resection.

General considerations

All these patients require the most careful assessment, because the first impression can be misleading. Nearly all suffer some degree of dehydration and consequent impairment of renal function depending on the extent of vomiting, starvation and sequestration of fluid in the large and small bowel. Occult loss of blood and restricted eating has often resulted in an iron-deficiency anaemia. The very marked dilatation which occurs in distal colonic obstruction may restrict diaphragmatic movement, resulting in respiratory complications. The enormous bacterial population of the obstructed colon greatly increases the risk of bacteraemia and multiple organ failure.

These effects will operate in varying degree so that some patients will only be slightly affected, while others will be gravely ill, requiring all the resources of an intensive therapy unit to prepare them for surgery. In all patients a complete physical examination must be followed by a full blood count, blood biochemistry, blood type and antibody screen, ECG, chest X-ray, erect and supine abdominal films and, frequently, blood gases. Central venous pressure measurements and hourly urinary output will be essential in some patients with dehydration and cardiac failure to assist in fluid and electrolyte management. Systemic antibiotics should be commenced (p. 143).

Most patients can be prepared for surgery in 3–6 hours. The degree of colonic distension, with its attendant risk of bowel perforation, makes it important to keep this time as short as possible.

A carefully thought-out plan with modern-day supportive care must be based on an assessment of the objectives of alternative treatment regimens in the context of the individual patient. What was the patient's life expectancy before the emergency occurred? Is there evidence of metastasis? What is the operative risk for a full laparotomy with resection? Could the patient be treated by the newer stenting method? What is known of this patient's wishes concerning mechanical life-sustaining measures?

As discussed later, we recommend that for those patients deemed fit enough for a laparotomy, then a bowel resection should be performed when technically possible. However, there are a small group of patients who are elderly, who are very sick because of cardiopulmonary compromise, with possible major fluid and electrolyte imbalance, with or without diabetes, but who do not exhibit signs of bowel perforation. In this small, select group of patients, the stenting method should be used. If this technique is not available, then a 'trephine' caecostomy should be considered to relieve the obstruction and provide a longer 'window of opportunity' to carry out intensive medical management, having decompressed the large gut. The latter group of patients will be small, but this procedure, which can be conducted under local anaesthesia, might, under very carefully defined circumstances, be life-saving when it is clear that general anaesthesia and a laparotomy would carry a prohibitive risk.

The proximal obstructed colonic segment

Until about 1950 it was customary to treat obstruction of the caecum and the ascending and proximal transverse colon by emergency ileotransverse colostomy, proceeding at a later date to resection. Goligher and Smiddy (1957) showed that this latter resection was only undertaken in seven of 28 such patients, whereas if an immediate right hemicolectomy was carried, 14 of 15 patients survived the one-stage operation. It soon became clear that this was much the better procedure (Samenius, 1962). There is now virtual unanimity among surgeons on this matter, and unless there is particularly heavy contamination due to caecal rupture, the hemicolectomy is concluded by making an ileotransverse anastomosis. However, ileotransverse reconstruction is not free from anastomotic leakage and Phillips *et al.* (1985) recorded in their prospective large-bowel cancer project a 12% anastomotic leakage in these patients. It may be that the safer procedure would be an ileostomy and mucous fistula, if the operation were being carried out by a somewhat less experienced surgeon or if there continued to be a high risk of cardiopulmonary compromise. It is clear that this form of anastomosis should be regarded as high-risk and that special attention to detail is mandatory (see below).

The use of extended right hemicolectomy in the treatment of carcinomas of the left half of the transverse colon and the splenic flexure continues to be controversial. The advantage of this procedure is that it removes all the obstructed colon and allows an anastomosis between relatively normal ileum and unobstructed distal colon. There can be no doubt about the value of this operation when the viability of the caecal area is in question. Saegesser and Sandblom (1975) treated 24 patients with 'diastatic' rupture of the colon proximal to the obstruction. In 11 patients the perforation was either sutured or exteriorized and the colon decompressed by transverse colostomy. All these patients died. Sandblom and Saegesser attributed this outcome to the generalized ischaemic damage of the colon in which suture repair of the perforation could not be expected to heal. They contrast this disastrous outcome with the results in 13 other patients, all of whom had the colon proximal to obstruction removed by subtotal colectomy followed by ileocolic anastomosis; there was only one death. Histological examination of the specimens showed widespread ischaemic lesions of the mucosa and submucosa, despite the generally normal outward appearance of the bowel. This process can proceed to 'acute necrotizing colitis', in which the tense colon shows patches of gangrene with offensive free fluid. This clearly needs complete resection down to and including the obstructing lesion (Teasdale and Mortensen, 1983).

Extended right hemicolectomy can be a safe operation. Koruth *et al.* (1985b) reported its use in 31 patients up to and including splenic flexure. There were two deaths, both in patients with hepatic metastasis. Morgan *et al.* (1985) also performed an emergency extended right hemicolectomy in 16 patients with obstructed carcinomas at and beyond the splenic flexure, with two deaths from myocardial infarction, but with no anastomotic leaks. Although this may be seen to be a major undertaking, we have found extended right hemicolectomy to be a relatively simple and safe procedure for obstructed carcinomas at, and just beyond, the splenic flexure (Koruth *et al.*, 1985b). When the caecum is tensely distended with a commencing split in the taenia, and whenever it has perforated, the safest treatment is resection. This operation deals definitively with the problem of faecal loading, and it will occasionally remove an unsuspected second carcinoma; Morgan *et al.* (1985) had two such cases. Some have criticized this operation on the grounds that it leads to postoperative diarrhoea, but in fact this resolves over a few weeks and patients settle to having one to three bowel movements per day with full control.

Technique
1. The incision needs to be generous because the caecum is so often tense and fragile. Generally, a vertical incision is best, but if the position of the carcinoma is known, and lies proximal to the hepatic flexure, then excellent exposure is obtained through a transverse muscle-cutting incision commencing in the right flank and ending near the midline. This incision heals strongly and is substantially more comfortable for the patient than a vertical incision.

2. Decompress the caecum if it is tense, blue and thin. It is much safer to aspirate the contents before mobilizing it. This can be done with the minimum of handling by the technique described on p. 281. However, incompetence of the ileocaecal valve in these proximal obstructions usually means that the tension in the caecum does not exceed a dangerous level.

3. Reduce the contents of the small bowel, because it is often distended, and it helps exposure and later abdominal closure to empty the small-bowel contents back into the stomach (p. 191).

4. A general examination of the abdomen includes examination of the liver for metastases and the remainder of the colon for a possible second neoplasm or other major disease. The presence of hepatic or other metastasis should not prevent excision of the primary neoplasm provided it is resectable.

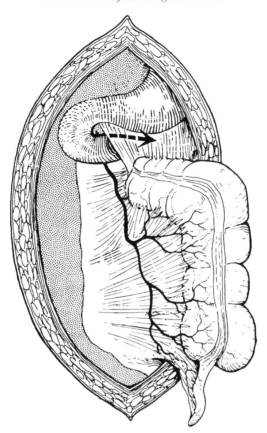

Figure 7.2 Right hemicolectomy. The right colon has been mobilized by dividing the peritoneum of the right paracolic gutter, revealing the right ureter. The arrow shows the plane in which the left index finger dissects behind the greater omentum.

5. The mobilization of the colon can now commence. The peritoneum of the lateral pericolic gutter is divided starting below, lateral to the appendix and working up to the hepatic flexure. It is important to take away a wide circle of peritoneum lateral to a carcinoma. Occasionally the tumour has become attached to the transversus abdominis and then a disc of this muscle should also be removed in continuity with the tumour.

The bloodless plane behind the caecum and ascending colon can now be opened and the proximal colon lifted out of the abdomen, being hinged on the mesocolon. The appendix and terminal ileum also needs to be freed by carrying the peritoneal incision around the caput caeci. The right ureter can be identified at this stage (Figure 7.2).

6. Transillumination of the ileal mesentery is helpful at this time. Select a suitable point for division of the ileum, ligate the marginal vessels and clear the ileum ready for division (Figure 7.3).

7. Mobilization of the hepatic flexure is the next step. Using the left index finger as a blunt dissector to identify the lateral edge of the greater omentum, open up a plane above the hepatic flexure, between the omentum in front and the duodenum behind (arrow in Figure

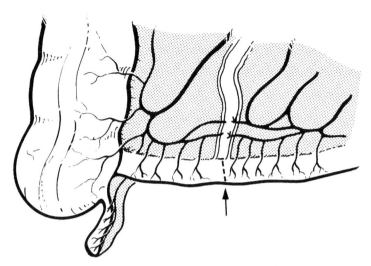

Figure 7.3 There are usually two parallel arcades to be divided in the terminal ileal mesentery. The arrow indicates the site of division of the ileum, the line slightly angled towards the bowel to be retained.

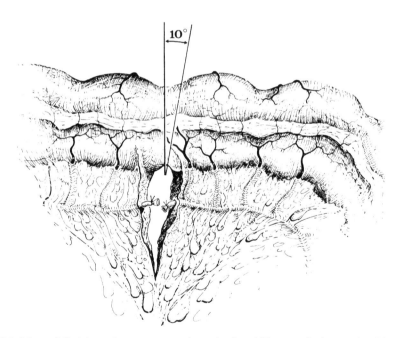

Figure 7.4 Line of division of transverse colon, sloping 10° towards the retained bowel. The marginal artery is just proximal to a vasa recta, to ensure the blood supply to the anastomosis.

7.2). The omentum can then be subdivided, tied and divided in bunches, preserving the gastroepiploic vessels. This reveals the loop of the duodenum and the head of the pancreas behind, which are gently separated from the colon and mesocolon, as the freed hepatic flexure is drawn up and out of the abdomen. This allows the ileocolic mesentery to be transilluminated and the ileocolic artery and vein can be isolated and tied just lateral to their origin from the superior mesenteric vessels. All the lymph nodes around the ileocolic vessels should be included in the specimen. When the ileocolic artery and vein have been divided, a specimen is held only by the ileum and the transverse colon and mesocolon. Usually there is a main branch of the middle colic artery to be divided, followed by the marginal artery, while leaving intact the arterial supply to the colon at the site of the anastomosis (Figure 7.4).

8. Division of the bowel is now undertaken. This is carried out between clamps (Schoemaker clamp to the ileum and a Parker–Kerr clamp to the colon). Bowel division must slope towards the retained bowel by approximately 10° to protect the blood supply to the antimesenteric border (Figures 7.3 and 7.4). The small bowel has already been emptied back into the stomach, and the colon beyond the obstruction should be empty so both can be divided and then the specimen is removed. There should be visible bleeding from both cut ends. If a sutured anastomosis is being constructed, the disparity between the circumference of the ileum and the colon can be overcome by a Cheatle cut-back in the ileum (Figure 7.5). We prefer a one-layer serosubmucosal suture to fashion the anastomosis (p. 24).

9. After thorough lavage of the anastomosis and peritoneal cavity with tetracycline solution (p. 145), the anastomosis can be laid back on the posterior abdominal wall. Although it is not necessary to close the mesentery gap, many surgeons carry out this procedure. However, this should be omitted if it is likely to give rise to tension in the mesentery.

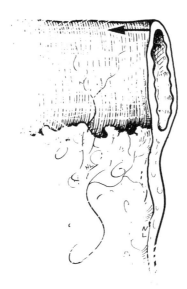

Figure 7.5 Cheatle cut-back. The length is adjusted so that the circumference of ileum equals the circumference of colon.

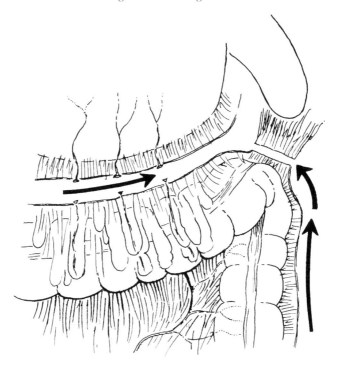

Figure 7.6 Mobilization of the splenic flexure. The arrows show the manner in which it is freed from both sides.

10. If extended right hemicolectomy is performed, the mobilization of the transverse colon proceeds distally. The first step is to separate the transverse colon from the stomach. When operating for a carcinoma of the colon, there is good reason to remove the great omentum with the transverse colon, just as it is removed in continuity with the stomach in gastric carcinoma. If division of the omentum branches of the gastroepiploic arch is performed 1–2 cm below the arch, the omentum will be divided transversely and the lesser sac will be opened up, allowing a clear view of the upper aspect of the transverse mesocolon. The branches of the middle colic artery can then be seen and divided. When the carcinoma lies in the transverse colon, it is important to secure these branches as deeply towards the posterior abdominal wall as possible, as they emerge from beneath the pancreas, so that all available lymph nodes are excised.

If the neoplasm is at the splenic flexure, the first step is to establish that the carcinoma is mobile. The spleen, stomach and diaphragm are all in close relationship to the splenic flexure of the colon and sometimes need to be removed in continuity with the carcinoma (Jones and Siwek, 1986). Usually, the splenic flexure can be freed from these structures, but if there is any difficulty, it is often easier to stand to the right of the patient while the assistant retracts the left costal margin. The other helpful step is to mobilize the splenic flexure from both sides. When the transverse colon has been mobilized as far as is convenient, the descending colon is then mobilized by incising the peritoneum on its lateral aspect, opening up the space behind the colon and working up in this plane towards the splenic flexure (Figure 7.6).

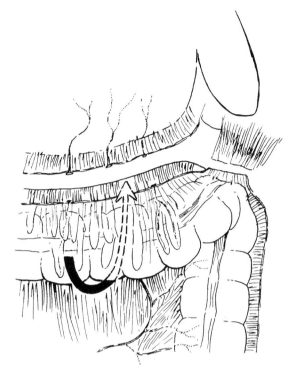

Figure 7.7 Mobilization of the splenic flexure – the arrow indicates the 'tenting' of the transverse mesocolon, which must be remembered when ligating the mesocolic vessels.

The transverse and the descending colon can then be drawn together towards the right iliac fossa, thus displaying more clearly the attachment of the splenic flexure and its mesocolon. It is wise to remember that the mesocolon is tented upwards at the splenic flexure and needs careful mobilization (Figure 7.7).

At this point, adhesions between the capsule of the spleen and surrounding structures are at greatest risk of being avulsed and causing splenic damage. Gentle dissection under direct vision is absolutely necessary, taking the dissection towards the spleen rather than the spleen towards the incision. If this dissection is difficult it is wise to move back to the transverse colon attachment and then return to the descending colon attachment, and if necessary to lengthen the incision. Every effort is needed to prevent splenic damage. Time, blood and immune functions are all lost if splenic bleeding requires its eventual removal.

Once the splenic flexure has been mobilized, it can be drawn out of the abdomen and the mesocolic vessels can be seen. These are the final branches of the middle colic artery and the left colic branch of the inferior mesenteric artery. If the duodenojejunal flexure is mobilized medially, the origin of the left colic artery can be found and ligated. In this way, the maximum number of potentially invaded lymph nodes can be removed. Finally, a suitable place for division of the descending colon is identified and cleared. There should be ample blood supply through the marginal arcade perfused by the sigmoid branches of the inferior mesenteric artery. Ileocolic anastomosis can then be performed by the surgeon's preferred method.

The distal obstructed colonic segment

Since Baronofsky and Gregg demonstrated in the 1950s the possibility of resecting obstructing carcinomas lying beyond the splenic flexure, and of performing immediate colonic anastomosis, this form of management has been widely adopted and its results reported. The advantage to the patient of all treatment being completed in one stage, without a stoma, are evident.

There are now three possible approaches.

Hartmann's resection must not be forgotten, because it will be the best solution for a patient who is very ill with spreading peritonitis due to perforation of the obstructing carcinoma itself, or for the patient who, with chronic medical disease, requires a swift and effective operation. It remains a safe operation for the general surgeon who does not often make large-bowel anastomoses. It has the important advantage that the carcinoma is removed at once: reconnection of colon to rectum can wait until the patient is fully fit.

However, the merits of a one-stage resection have been increasingly recognized (Phillips *et al.*, 1985; Koruth *et al.*, 1985b). Two methods are available, and both are directed to the management of the faecal overloading that occurs above the obstruction. This is a hazard during mobilization of the colon, with the wall – especially of the caecum – being tense and fragile. Baronofsky in 1950 solved this by resecting the whole of the distended colon, as well as the carcinoma, and anastomosing ileum to the rectosigmoid junction. This extension of extended right hemicolectomy into the left colon has now been extensively tested. It deals at a stroke with faecal loading. Quite often the caecum is in a dangerously fragile state, there may be a small perforation, and resection is much the safest solution. The operation also deals radically with those patients who have a silent second carcinoma – or adenomata – in the proximal colon. The major disadvantage of the operation is that when the ileum has to be jointed to the top of the rectum some patients suffer troublesome diarrhoea; they are a minority but this complication is unpredictable (Scotia Study Group, 1995; Deans *et al.*, 1994).

The alternative technique for dealing with faecal loading is to evacuate the loaded colon on the table. To avoid evacuating open bowel, Muir (1968) tied in a wide glass cannula attached to Paul's tubing above the obstruction but it was difficult to manipulate faeces through the tubing. In 1980 Dudley *et al.* substituted rigid anaesthetic scavenging tubing for the Paul's tube, and then irrigated the colon with saline running through a catheter tied into the caecum (see Figure 7.10). This was much more effective in thoroughly cleansing the colon, and an improved plastic cannula tubing and bag for collecting the effluent was introduced by Munro *et al.* (1987). This allowed clean prepared proximal colon to be used for the anastomosis, following radical segmental resection of the carcinoma.

These two methods had an extensive prospective randomized trial (Scotia Study Group, 1995). The conclusion was that hospital mortality and morbidity were not significantly different – the overall mortality rate was 12% and anastomotic leakage rate was 7% in 91 patients with a median age of 70 years, treated in 12 hospitals by 18 participating surgeons. On follow-up it was concluded that subtotal colectomy is a good operation for obstruction up to the level of the splenic flexure (and when there is caecal damage or perforation in more distal obstructions), but that the unpredictable effect of low ileocolonic anastomosis on bowel action makes wash-out and segmental resection preferable for obstructing tumours beyond the splenic flexure.

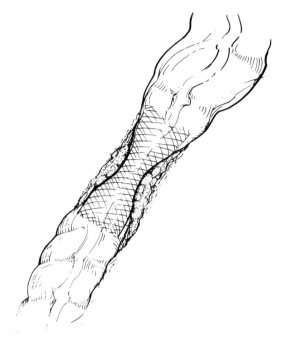

Figure 7.8 Diagram of an expandable metal stent, located within, and dilating up, an obstructing colonic neoplasm.

An essential feature of these one-stage operations is that success depends on careful patient selection and treatment by surgeons with considerable experience of elective colorectal surgery.

The role that expanding metal stents will play in the initial relief of left-sided colonic obstruction, by creating a lumen through the obstruction, remains to be seen. A guide wire is introduced under radiographic or colonoscopic control and passed through the obstruction. The stent is then passed along the wire, and placed within the carcinoma where it expands sufficiently to allow obstructed gas and faeces to pass, and for the bowel to be prepared for elective resection in the usual way (Figure 7.8). Canon *et al.* (1997) describe the technique and the problems which arise during trials of the method.

Finally a transverse colostomy can be established as the first step in treatment. This requires a laparotomy for its safe performance and is now more or less confined to situations in which the surgeon is not in a position to undertake resection.

Technique
There are four operations to be considered. If immediate resection is proposed, the choice lies between:

1. Hartmann's resection; and
2. resection and anastomosis.

The choice then lies between subtotal colectomy and segmental resection after colonic wash-out.

3. If protection of an anastomosis is needed, a **loop ileostomy** can be made.
4. Alternatively, a **transverse loop colostomy** can be used; this is also available as the emergency operation for relief of distal obstruction.

1. Hartmann's resection   Henri Hartmann devised his operation as a safe way to perform elective excision of low sigmoid and high rectal carcinomas, but as far as we know he did not use the procedure for emergencies (Sanderson, 1980). The principles of the operation are the same as those for elective resection, and the method can be adopted if, after resection, it is felt to be unwise to attempt an anastomosis. It is particularly suited to the distal obstructive neoplasm that is complicated by perforation and established peritonitis.

The operation proceeds as for a radical resection to the point when a right-angle clamp is applied at a suitable point below the carcinoma – usually at or a little below the rectosigmoid junction. The rectum is then thoroughly washed out and the bowel is divided immediately below the clamp. The rectum should be seen to bleed from the cut edge, and is then closed with one or two layers of 2/0 polydioxanone. The rectum should not be mobilized, and some sutures should be inserted to secure the closed end to the sacral promontory: this should help with access to it when the reconnection operation is performed (p. 30).

Before the specimen is removed the descending colon (but not the splenic flexure) should be mobilized enough to allow the divided end of the colon to lie without tension at skin level. A de Martel clamp is applied, the specimen is removed and the colostomy is formed, with mucocutaneous sutures, at a suitable site in the left lower quadrant.

Koruth *et al.* (1985b) used a Hartmann resection in 16 obstructive patients with one death.

The reported disadvantage of this procedure is that the subsequent restoration of bowel continuity can be a 'major undertaking'. This operation can be difficult on account of adhesions but, if several months are allowed to elapse before bowel restoration is attempted, the peritoneal cavity will have restored itself and the degree of adhesion is substantially reduced. It can be a very straightforward procedure.

2. Resection and anastomosis   When the surgical team has a bias towards performing immediate resection in suitable patients with colonic obstruction beyond the splenic flexure, experience shows that a high proportion prove to be suitable for this approach.

The technique of the operation generally follows standard practice. Patients are placed in the lithotomy–Trendelenburg position (Lloyd-Davies, 1939) because it is so valuable to have free access to the rectum; the second assistant can be much more helpful standing between the patient's legs, and the surgeon can also stand in this position to great advantage when dissecting the splenic flexure. The choice of operation depends on the circumstances. Generally, Hartmann's resection will be chosen if the obstruction has been complicated by perforation and there is an established peritonitis. The stoma should be created in a carefully chosen site marked on the abdominal wall preoperatively, to lie clear of the incision and of the anterior superior iliac spine, remembering that circumstances may require the patient to keep the stoma permanently.

If the peritoneum is clean and the patient is in good condition, then it is reasonable to consider colonic lavage, resection and anastomosis. If this choice is made, it is useful first to

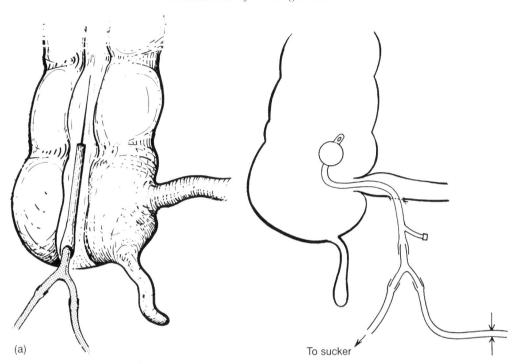

(a)

To sucker

Figure 7.9 A method of decompressing obstructed colon. **(a)** The gaseous content of the colon can be aspirated by connecting the sucker unit to a needle which is passed obliquely through a taenia. **(b)** Following insertion of the Foley catheter. The two arrows indicate where pressure is applied for aspiration and is released to allow movement of the catheter.

decompress the colon. First, gas should be aspirated by passing a 16 FG hypodermic needle attached to a sucker unit obliquely into the colon (Figure 7.9(a)).

Then the small-bowel contents are gently emptied back into the stomach (p. 191). The terminal ileum is then steadied and a purse-string suture is inserted into its antimesenteric border a few centimetres proximal to the ileocaecal valve, or the side of the appendix can be used. Antiseptic-soaked packs are then placed around the ileum. The suction unit is prepared by attaching a Y connection to a Foley catheter of 28 FG or 30 FG (Figure 7.9(b)). To one arm attach a piece of flexible tubing and attach the other to suction. Through an incision within the purse-string the lubricated catheter is passed through the ileocaecal valve into the caecum, and the balloon is inflated with approximately 25 ml of water. If the flexible tubing is now occluded, gas and faeces will begin to pass into the sucker tubing and the caecum will begin to deflate. By using such a wide catheter, much of the liquid faeces can be sucked out of the caecum, and then the contents of the transverse colon can also be gently milked back into the proximal colon. In this way the calibre of the colon is markedly reduced, allowing it to be easily manipulated.

It is very much easier and safer to perform the colonic irrigation if the distal colon has been mobilized, otherwise considerable difficulty can be met in easing the solid content around the splenic flexure, and Munro *et al.* (1995) find that mobilizing the proximal colon as well

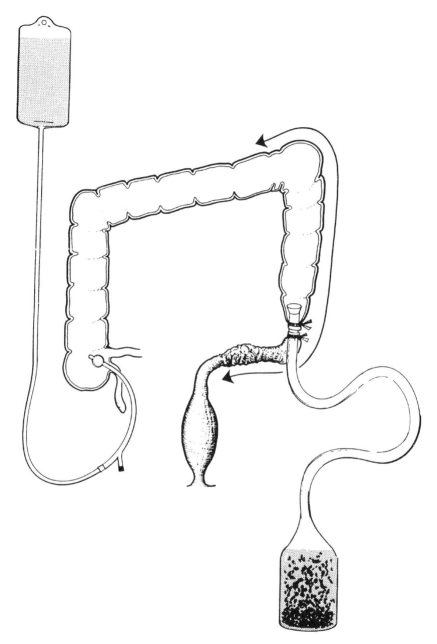

Figure 7.10 Intraoperative colonic lavage. The arrow indicates that the colon has to be mobilized and brought out of the abdomen before the cannula can be introduced. This is done when the carcinoma and the mesentery are ready for resection. A disposable irrigation collection system and bag is shown.

makes for a quicker and easier irrigation. A standard operation for resection of a distal colonic or rectosigmoidal carcinoma is therefore carried out with high ligation of the inferior mesenteric vessels and full mobilization of the splenic flexure. The point of distal division is cleared, a right angle clamp applied and the rectum washed out with a cytotoxic agent. The rectum is then divided below the clamp and the specimen is brought through the incision on to the abdominal surface, which is covered in towels. This provides very easy access to the sigmoid and descending colon.

The irrigation can now be started, using either disposable anaesthetic scavenging tubing sterilized in chlorhexidine in spirit or, if available, a disposable cannula, tubing and bag (Figure 7.10).

Faeces are stripped back from the bowel above the carcinoma, and a transverse incision is made through half the circumference of the colon into which the cannula is introduced. Two strong tape ligatures are now passed through the mesentery and tied very tightly around the cannula and the colon to make an absolutely watertight seal. The tubing hangs over the side of the table, and discharges into a receptacle resting on the floor.

The catheter in the caecum is then connected by sterile tubing to a 3 litre cystoscopy irrigation bag containing warmed tap water which is allowed to flow into the colon. It must be noted that the water should be as near body heat as possible in order not to reduce body temperature by heat exchange. Water and faeces are manually mixed to give a consistency that can gently be massaged along the colon and out through the cannula. A few solid blocks of faeces usually need breaking up. Soon fluid faeces are flowing easily out of the colon, into the tubing and bag and gradually, after 3–5 litres of water have been used, the colon is deflated and the effluent is clean. As much of the irrigating water as possible is drained out of the colon and then the colon is divided just above the cannula in the standard manner. The specimen and the tubing are discarded and the restorative anastomosis is carried out in a manner favoured by the surgeon.

A protective loop ileostomy (or for some surgeons transverse loop colostomy) is not generally necessary. If the irrigation is successful, the anastomosis has been made on bowel that is decompressed, clean and with a good blood supply. The work of Coxon *et al.* (1984) and Papanicolaou *et al.* (1989) has shown that mucosal blood flow in the left colon is increased in obstruction, and these circumstances are comparable to those found in elective restorative anastomosis.

The choice between subtotal colectomy and colonic washout, as the method of removing the gaseous and faecal load in the obstructed colon, has been discussed and will be decided by the circumstances. Both methods involve considerable manipulation of the colon proximal to the obstruction. Subtotal colectomy is safer if there are doubts about caecal viability, but is an extensive operation that leaves the patient with some increased stool frequency. Colonic wash-out may leave an unnoticed adenoma, or even a small carcinoma-*in-situ* in the retained colon, but if circumstances permit colonoscopy round to the caecum, on the table, can be done before making the anastomosis.

In practice (Koruth *et al.*, 1985c) we only made a protective transverse colostomy in five out of 61 immediate resections with anastomosis. There were four clinical anastomotic leaks, of which three healed spontaneously, but one patient died from continued sepsis. There were five deaths in all (8.4%), the other being due to medical complications.

3. Protective loop ileostomy This method can be used when the surgeon, at the end of carrying out a primary anastomosis, becomes concerned about the absolute proficiency with

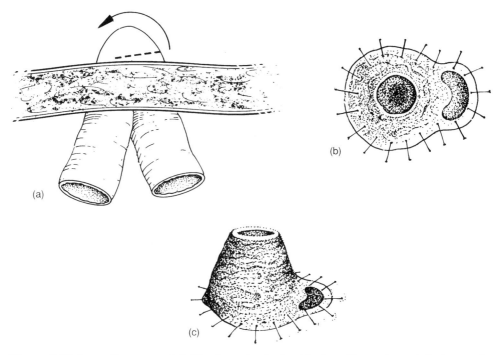

Figure 7.11 Loop ileostomy. **(a)** The loop is sited with the afferent loop inferior to the efferent loop. **(b)** Site of incision, carried round two-thirds of the efferent side of the loop. **(c)** The loop is supported by a short rod. The incised ileum is folded down to form a spout below the half-closed efferent side of the loop. Mucocutaneous sutures are inserted.

which the anastomosis is being created. If this concern exists, a loop stoma (preferably a loop ileostomy) should be constructed (Figure 7.11).

In anticipation, a site should be selected preoperatively to the right of the umbilicus, taking into account the position of the umbilicus, the anterior superior iliac spine, previous surgical incisions and the degree of obesity. A small disc of skin 1.5 cm in diameter is excised; a cruciate incision is made through the rectus sheath (anterior and posterior), being careful not to injure the epigastic vessels. The opening should admit two fingers very snugly. A loop of small bowel near the terminal ileum is identified, and a simple marker suture is placed in the antimesenteric border distal to the site for stoma formation. A small opening in the mesentery at the mesenteric border of the bowel is fashioned, preferably without dividing tissues. A catheter is looped through this orifice and brought out through the abdominal opening to facilitate the passage of the ileum through the abdominal wall. The bowel is gently eased through the abdominal wall, making sure that the proximal bowel is inferior and the distal bowel is superior in the opening.

A semi-lunar superficial excoriation of the serosa with diathermy is then carried out on the upper limb of the bowel. The stoma is not opened until the main incision has been closed and covered. The semi-lunar marking on the serosa is then deepened to open the bowel. The bowel wall is then folded back to form the loop ileostomy, and the distal component of the stoma can be sutured to the skin and subcutaneous tissue flush with the skin. Four to six sutures are placed above and below the catheter that was used to help bring the small bowel through the abdominal wall. The catheter is removed and may be replaced with a small glass or plastic rod, and a snugly-fitting stoma appliance is fixed to the skin.

The advantages of loop ileostomy over loop colostomy are that the stoma is smaller, easier to manage by the patient, has less odour and requires a simpler procedure to reduce it into the abdomen once the patient has recovered.

4. Transverse loop colostomy   This operation should not be performed 'blind' through a small incision. As early as 1894, Bland-Sutton pointed out that, if this incision is used, it is very difficult to bring out the tense loop of transverse colon, and furthermore, nothing is learned about the operability of the neoplasm and about its potential spread.

1. If the operation is purely to decompress the colon then a left paramedian incision is preferred, leaving the right upper quadrant free for the loop colostomy, with adequate room for the colostomy bag to adhere to intact skin. The paramedian incision can then be reopened when resection takes place. A midline incision usually comes too close to the transverse colostomy and will frequently get infected and may become disrupted.

2. The caecum is likely to be tense and blue, possibly with a split in the taenia. This gives warning of the tension within the colon, and it is much safer to decompress before attempting any exploration. It also makes delivery of the transverse colon much easier.

3. Palpation of the liver and the remainder of the large bowel and other viscera is now safer and operability of the primary tumour can be assessed. If the tumour appears to be inoperable, then a transverse loop colostomy is a reasonable approach to palliate the patient's symptoms.

4. The incision for the colostomy should be tailor-made, running transversely across the right upper rectus and the linea semilunaris, 2.5–3.0 cm long. The fingers of the left hand can be used to push forward the abdominal wall from within the abdomen, and the incision can be quickly made using cutting diathermy, the incision running transversely through the anterior rectus sheath, the rectus abdominis and the posterior rectus sheath into the peritoneum. The index and middle finger should just fit this wound.

5. The next step is to select the stoma site well into the right half of the transverse colon, so that when the loop of the colon is drawn out there is no danger of kinking the main branches of the middle colic artery which would supply the distal colon (*via* the marginal arcade) if a second-stage resection is to be carried out (Figure 7.12). The omentum is detached from the colon for 7–8 cm on either side of the selected point for the stoma. A 16 FG whistle-tip catheter is now drawn through the opening made in the mesocolon and used as a sling to draw the loop of colon through the colostomy incision (Figure 7.13); it should fit snugly in the incision.

6. Two subcutaneous tunnels some 4 cm long are now made for this catheter above and below the colostomy by passing forceps through short incisions and drawing the two ends of the catheter through them in each direction (Figure 7.14). Both ends are secured to the skin incision and the remainder of the catheter is discarded from both ends.

7. The suction catheter in the ileum is now carefully extracted (and subsequently discarded) making sure that faecal spillage is minimal. The incision and surrounding bowel is washed with tetracycline solution and it is repaired by tying the purse-string suture and oversewing it with a few Lembert sutures.

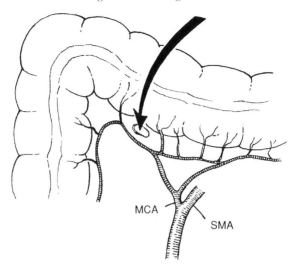

Figure 7.12 Diagram showing the site in the right colon for construction of loop colostomy.

8. After tetracycline lavage of the abdomen, the paramedian incision is closed.
9. The colostomy can then be opened by making a diathermy incision 2.0–2.5 cm long in the taenia coli. The interior is cleaned with mops and then the whole circumference of the colonic incision can be secured. Altogether, 12–14 interrupted sutures are placed; 3/0 chromic catgut on a curved cutting needle is very suitable for the purpose. Each stitch must be passed from skin into the full thickness of colon: this avoids islands of mucosa being transplanted into the skin, giving rise to a mucosal rosette and making it more difficult to manage the colostomy.

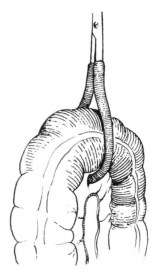

Figure 7.13 A catheter is passed through the mesentery and is used to draw the colon through the incision.

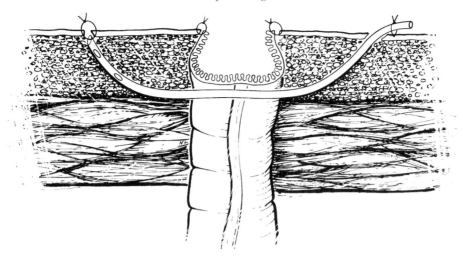

Figure 7.14 The subcutaneous path of the catheter that supports the loop. Rectus abdominis is shown in the longitudinal section. The clear area of the skin around the stoma allows efficient adhesion of the colostomy bag.

7.2.1.6 Late prognosis after tumour resection

All reports show that the outlook of patients with obstruction is poorer than that for patients with colorectal cancer presenting for elective resection. Five-year survival figures for patients having potentially curative surgery are 40% among the obstructed and 60% for the non-obstructed (Phillips *et al.*, 1985). Although immediate postoperative mortality is high in the former group, after 3 years the slopes of the survival curves are similar. The reasons for this differential death rate are not known.

7.2.1.7 The patient treated for malignant disease who develops late intestinal obstruction

This is a small but important group. The later occurrence of obstruction, usually in small bowel, may be due to recurrence of the primary (either by direct invasion in the abdomen, or by blood stream spread from, for instance, carcinoma of the breast). However, this must not be assumed. The obstruction may be due to adhesions or postirradiation stenosis (p. 234). Walsh and Schofield (1984) found that, among 53 patients previously treated for malignant disease who later obstructed, 15 had a correctable non-malignant cause and a useful resection to overcome the obstruction was done in 40. There should, if the conditions allow it, be a bias toward exploration.

REFERENCES

Baronofsky, I. D. (1950) Primary resection and aseptic end to end anastomosis for acute or subacute large bowel obstructions. *Surgery*, **27**, 664–666.

Canon, C. L., Baron, T. H. and Morgan, D. E. (1997) Treatment of colonic obstruction with expandable metal stents: radiologic features. *A.J.R.*, **168**, 199–205.

Chapman, A. H., McNamara, M. and Porter, G. (1992) The acute contrast enema in suspected large bowel obstruction: value and technique. *Clin. Radiol.*, **46**, 273–278.

Coxon, J. E., Dickson, C. and Taylor, I. (1984) Changes in intestinal blood flow during the development of chronic large bowel obstruction. *Br. J. Surg.*, **71**, 795–798.

Deans, G. T., Krukowski, Z. H. and Irwin, S. T. (1994) Malignant obstruction of the left colon. *Br. J. Surg.*, **81**, 1270–1276.

Dudley, H. A. F., Radcliffe, A. G. and McGeehan, D. (1980) Intraoperative irrigation of colon to permit primary anastomosis. *Br. J. Surg.*, **67**, 80–81.

Goligher, J. C. and Smiddy, F. G. (1957) The treatment of acute obstruction or perforation with carcinoma of the colon and rectum. *Br. J. Surg.*, **45**, 270–274.

Gregg, R. O. (1955) The place of emergency resection in the management of obstructing and perforating lesions of the colon. *Surgery*, **37**, 754–761.

Herrington, J. L., Lawler, M., Thomas, T. V. *et al.* (1967) Colon resection with primary anastomosis performed as an emergency and as non-planned operation. *Ann. Surg.*, **165**, 709–720.

Hughes, E. S. R. (1966) Mortality of acute large-bowel obstruction. *Br. J. Surg.*, **53**, 593–594.

Jones, P. F. and Siwek, R. (1986) *A Colour Atlas of Colorectal Surgery*, Wolfe Medical, London.

Koruth, N. M., Koruth, A. and Matheson, N. A. (1985a) The place of contrast enema in the management of large bowel obstruction. *J. R. Coll. Surg. Edin.*, **30**, 258–260.

Koruth, N. M., Hunter, D. C., Krukowski, Z. H. *et al.* (1985b) Immediate resection in emergency large bowel: a 7 year audit. *Br. J. Surg.*, **72**, 703–707.

Koruth, N. M., Krukowski, Z. H., Youngson, G. G. *et al.* (1985c) Intraoperative colonic irrigation in the management of left-sided large bowel emergencies. *Br. J. Surg.*, **72**, 708–711.

Lloyd-Davies, O. V. (1939) Lithotomy–Trendelenburg position for resection of rectum and pelvic colon. *Lancet*, **ii**, 74–76.

McIver, J. R. and Don, C. (1965) The fluid-filled colon in acute large-bowel obstruction. *AJR*, **94**, 410–415.

Mikulicz, J. von (1903) Small contributions to the surgery of the intestinal tract. *Boston Med. Surg.*, **148**, 608.

Morgan, W. P., Jenkins, N., Lewis, P. *et al.* (1985) Management of obstructing carcinoma of the left colon by extended right hemicolectomy. *Am. J. Surg.*, **49**, 327–329.

Muir, E. G. (1968) Safety in colonic resection. *Proc. R. Soc. Med.*, **61**, 401–408.

Munro, A., Steele, R. J. C. and Logie, J. R. C. (1987) Technique for intraoperative colonic irrigation. *Br. J. Surg.* **74**, 1039–1040.

Munro, A., Sulaiman, M. N., Borgstein, E. *et al.* (1995) Total colonic mobilization and exteriorization facilitates intraoperative colonic irrigation. *J. R. Coll. Surg. Edin.*, **40**, 171–172.

Papanicolaou, G., Ahn, Y. K., Nikas, D. J. *et al.* (1989) Effect of large-bowel obstruction on colonic blood flow. An experimental study. *Dis. Colon Rectum*, **32**, 673–679.

Paul, F. T. (1895) Colectomy. *BMJ*, **i**, 1136–1139.

Phillips, R. K. S., Hittinger, R., Fry, J. S. *et al.* (1985) Malignant large bowel obstruction. *Br. J. Surg.*, **72**, 296–302.

Saegesser, F. and Sandblom, P. (1975) Ischemic lesions of the distended colon: a complication of obstructive colorectal cancer. *Am. J. Surg.*, **129**, 309–315.

Samenius, B. (1962) Treatment of acute obstruction due to carcinoma of right half of colon with special reference to primary hemicolectomy. *Acta Chir. Scand.*, **123**, 415–421.

Sanderson, E. R. (1980) Henri Hartmann and the Hartmann operation. *Arch. Surg.*, **115**, 792–793.

Scotia Study Group (1995) Single-stage treatment for malignant left-sided colonic obstruction: a prospective randomized clinical trial comparing subtotal colectomy with segmental resection following intraoperative irrigation. *Br. J. Surg.*, **82**, 1622–1627.

Stewart, J., Finan, P. J., Courtney, D. F. *et al.* (1984) Does a water soluble contrast enema assist in the management of acute large bowel obstruction: a prospective study of 117 cases. *Br. J. Surg.*, **71**, 799–801.

Teasdale, C., Mortensen, N. J. McC. (1983) Acute necrotising colitis and obstruction. *Br. J. Surg.*, **70**, 44–47.

Umpleby, H. C. and Williamson, R. C. N. (1984) Survival in acute obstructing colorectal carcinoma. *Dis. Colon Rectum*, **27**, 299–304.

Valerio, D., Jones, P. F. (1978) Immediate resection in the treatment of large bowel emergencies. *Br. J. Surg.*, **65**, 712–716.

Waldron, P. P., Donovan, I. A., Drumm, J. *et al.* (1986) Emergency presentation and mortality from colorectal cancer in the elderly. *Br. J. Surg.*, **73**, 214–216.

Walsh, H. J. P. and Schofield, P. F. (1984) Is laparotomy for small bowel obstruction justified in patients with previously treated malignancy? *Br. J. Surg.*, **71**, 933–935.

7.2.2 VOLVULUS OF THE COLON

The sigmoid is the segment of the large gut that most often undergoes rotation, but volvulus of the caecum is well recognized, and the transverse colon may occasionally rotate.

7.2.2.1 Sigmoid colon

Although not frequently seen in Western Europe, North America and Australasia, a sigmoid volvulus is the second most common cause of large-bowel obstruction in other parts of the world and carries a high mortality if incorrectly treated. Perlmann (1925) in Minsk found sigmoid volvulus in 55% of 200 obstructed patients. Boulvin (1966), working in Iran, treated 1000 mechanical bowel obstructions over 8 years and 33% of these patients had volvuli, 282 of the sigmoid, 46 of the small bowel and 12 of the caecum. Sinha (1969) in North India also found that 30% of all obstructions were due to sigmoid volvulus. In Kampala, Uganda (Odonga, 1982), 3334 patients were treated for intestinal obstruction of whom 43% had an obstructed external hernia; sigmoid volvulus was the next most common cause (20%). It is believed that sigmoid volvulus in Brazil is associated with the megacolon due to trypanosomiasis (Chagas' disease), (Gama *et al.*, 1976).

In the UK the position is quite different. Anderson and Lee (1981) reported that of 3380 patients who were treated for intestinal obstruction, only 193 (5.7%) had a colonic volvulus. We saw a similar proportion (4.9%) among 122 obstructed patients in Aberdeen (Valerio and Jones, 1978).

It is noticeable that in countries where intestinal volvulus is common it is the custom to eat bulky vegetable diets.

Sigmoid volvulus is sometimes associated with megacolon, and Ryan (1982) noticed that these patients had a long past history of constipation, and generally continued to be constipated despite having a sigmoid resection to treat the volvulus.

Age

Sigmoid volvulus is regarded as a disorder of the elderly, but only half the patients present over the age of 60 years. Smith *et al.* (1977) have drawn attention to a group of young patients who suffer intermittent sigmoid volvulus. In India (Sinha, 1969) and Iran (Scott, 1965), the average age of patients is about 40 years. Generally, more men than women suffer from this diagnosis.

Pathology

In many patients, especially in the tropics, it is clear that the sigmoid loop has been undergoing self-limiting episodes of volvulus for some time. The base of the sigmoid loop is usually very narrow, thus providing a pedicle for the rotation. This can occur in a clockwise or anticlockwise direction through 180°–720°. The mesentery is often thickened with large vessels and the wall of the sigmoid is thick as a result of musculohypertrophy. These changes may help to protect the bowel against gangrene caused by venous occlusion at the point of the twist in the sigmoid mesentery.

Fortunately, the sigmoid loop is gangrenous in only 10% of these patients (although this proportion is much higher in ileosigmoid knot; p. 295). Nevertheless, it is very important to remember that this change can extend, because of retrograde venous thrombosis, beyond the actual area of the volvulus, and when resection is performed viability of the descending colon and of the rectum must be carefully established (Neely, 1970).

There is an association with pregnancy and the puerperium (p. 503), but the precise factors for the establishment of a persisting symptomatic volvulus are not known.

Recurrence

Once a patient has suffered a symptomatic sigmoid volvulus, there is a strong tendency for it to recur. However, on a temporizing basis, some may untwist as a result of the patient adopting the knee–elbow position, and others can be treated by large rectal tube intubation with or without the help of a sigmoidoscope. The threat and rate of recurrence is in no way diminished by simple operative untwisting. Shepherd (1968) found that, among 37 patients having sigmoidoscopic deflation, 15 recurred and, when operative detorsion was performed in 30 patients, 12 recurred. Thus, the recurrence rate was 40% in both groups.

Clinical pictures

Two major symptoms of sigmoid volvulus are abdominal pain and progressive abdominal distension. These may have been noted for hours only, or may have been developing over several days. In this connection, Hinshaw and Carter (1957) have made the useful point that 75–85% of their patients presented with a subacute progressive type of attack but that an important minority show an acute fulminating type of onset, which carries a high risk of strangulation. Arigbabu *et al.* (1985) provide strong evidence for making this clinical distinction in a study of 92 consecutive patients.

Subacute progressive type
It is common for the patient to recall previous attacks. The present episode may have lasted for 1–7 days. The onset is usually definite in time, with total constipation, lower abdominal colicky pain and rapidly progressive abdominal distension. The colicky pain lasts for approximately a minute, and the interval between spasms is very variable but may be as long as half an hour. Nausea and vomiting are common but the volume of vomitus is usually small. The occasional patient complains of intermittent diarrhoea, probably caused by the intermittent untwisting of the volvulus, allowing contents to proceed to the rectum.

On examination, the general state of the patient may show little change from that normal for the individual, but after 3–4 days of illness he or she is likely to be dehydrated. Gaseous abdominal distension is a striking finding, and wide loops of colon may be seen through the abdominal wall; these may become palpable when a spasm of colic is felt, and at that time high-pitched obstructive bowel sounds can be heard. On the other hand, gross general distension may be seen, maximal in the right upper quadrant. Abdominal tenderness is present but not marked. However, although this type of volvulus is not usually associated with gangrene, this complication can supervene if the volvulus continues over several days.

Acute fulminating type
Hinshaw and Carter (1957) found this syndrome in 13 of their 55 patients with sigmoid volvulus. In contrast to the subacute type, it occurred in younger patients and showed a shorter and more severe picture: the pain was more severe and colicky and vomiting occurred more frequently, while general malaise, hypotension and tachypnoea were noticeable. The very marked abdominal distension so characteristic of sigmoid volvulus may not be seen, because moderate distension is more likely in these patients. There will be signs characteristic of an internal strangulation of the gut: tenderness, muscle guarding, release pain and absent bowel sounds. The absence of bowel sounds was noted in 15 of the 134 patients recorded by Anderson and Lee (1981), and there was gangrene of the sigmoid in 13 of these 15 patients.

This picture is not so suggestive of sigmoid volvulus as the subacute type, although the plain abdominal radiographs may show characteristic changes. The important matter is to recognize the need for urgent laparotomy.

Radiology

Plain abdominal films are invaluable to confirm the diagnosis because the findings are usually quite characteristic. Rigler and Lipschultz (1940) seem to have been the first to describe them. In six patients they found:

- great gaseous distension of the sigmoid loop, which extends from the pelvis to below the left diaphragm. The loop is so tense that the outline is smooth, not haustrated, and it seems to originate from the left side of the pelvis. 'The bent inner tube of a tyre' is a useful simile.
- Erect views show wide fluid levels in both limbs of the closed loop. The air:fluid ratio is characteristically more than 2:1.

However, about one-third of patients do not show typical appearances. Young *et al.* (1978) found this in 14 of 40 patients with a proven sigmoid volvulus. The main difficulty arose from the very marked gaseous distension of the proximal colon, which obscured the outline of the sigmoid loop. They found the 'liver overlap sign' helpful. In this, the shadow of the volvulus can be seen to extend above the gas shadow of the hepatic flexure. None of their patients showed any small-bowel distension.

Agrez and Cameron (1981) have warned that the long dilated transverse colon in dilated obstruction makes a U-shaped gas-filled shadow in the mid-abdomen that can look very like a sigmoid volvulus. When there is doubt, it is worth carrying out an emergency contrast enema (p. 268). In sigmoid volvulus, the barium column narrows to a curving point 'like the beak of a bird of prey'.

It is reasonable to wonder how such large volumes of gas accumulate so quickly. Most of the gas is swallowed air which must be able to enter but not leave the loop. Similar tense wide distension of the colon is seen in distal carcinomatous obstruction, but this builds up over a number of days.

Differential diagnosis

The acute fulminating type does not, for reasons already given, offer much difficulty. The more common subacute type may provide some difficulty, although with experience the picture is characteristic. The contrast between the satisfactory general state of the patient and the abdominal distension is striking.

The major differential diagnosis has to be made from neoplastic obstruction of the left colon. The history is likely to be similar, although the change from normal bowel habit to constipation is likely to be much sharper and more recent in a patient with volvulus. The abdominal distension seen in both obstructions is very marked, but in neoplastic obstruction there is general smooth distension, whereas in volvulus it is rather characteristic for the individual loops of the colon to stand out under the abdominal wall. Plain radiography usually produces a characteristic picture of a sigmoid volvulus, and it is notable that caecal distension, which is characteristic of neoplastic obstruction, is absent.

Treatment

Volvulus of the sigmoid colon was first described in 1836 by von Rokitansky. The first successful surgical case was recorded by Waldenstrom in Sweden in 1878 although Erichsen had performed a laparotomy and emptied the colon through a rectal tube for this diagnosis in 1849.

Clark reported the first successful operative untwisting in Great Britain in February 1883, and the patient recovered even though he had been ill for over 3 weeks before laparotomy. These and other descriptions helped recognition of the condition and operative untwisting of the bowel became the standard treatment. However, it carried a high mortality and other methods have since been developed. It soon became clear that prognosis was much affected by the presence or absence of gangrene: ischaemic change carried a mortality of about two patients in every three treated by simple untwisting. The choice of treatment hinges on whether gangrene is suspected, so management is considered for two different clinical situations: (a) when gangrenous changes are not suspected and the diagnosis is certain, and (b) when gangrenous changes are suspected or proven.

(a) Gangrenous changes are not suspected and the diagnosis is reasonably certain
If no suspicion of gangrene is aroused by the clinical examination, it is likely that the sigmoid loop will be viable. When this is the case (and resection is, therefore, not mandatory), there is a choice of available treatments. The immediate aim is to deal safely with the emergency and the long-term aim is to prevent recurrence of torsion. The three main methods of treatment do not offer equally effective answers to these two problems.

Operative untwisting of the loop   This is simple and effective, in the short term, and allows confirmation of the diagnosis but it subjects elderly patients to all the stresses of a laparotomy and does nothing to prevent recurrence. The method used remains identical with that reported by Erichsen (1850): laparotomy, guiding a tube up the rectum through the twist into the loop, deflation and restoration of the normal lie of the colon. Today, there seems to be little support to favour this procedure. If the patient can be deflated by non-operative means then there is no immediate need for surgery. If sigmoidoscopic deflation fails and operation is necessary then there is much to be said for primary resection, because the mortality is not affected appreciably by the additional procedure and it eliminates later recurrence of the volvulus.

Endoscopic deflation   Non-operative treatment for sigmoid volvulus has been practised for a long time, and there are many records of a flatus tube entering the loop and allowing deflation. However, it is an uncertain approach to push a tube blindly through 10–15 cm of rectum and expect it to pass through the twisted area of the loop into the dilated colon without causing injury. It was Bruusgaard (1947) who established sigmoidoscopic deflation as a good emergency treatment.

The patient is placed in the knee–elbow position and the sigmoidoscope is passed. It travels usually some 15–25 cm before reaching the point of bowel twist, although occasionally a 30 cm sigmoidoscope is needed. When the twist is reached, a very careful examination of the mucosa is mandatory. If there are any signs of discoloration, or if blood-stained fluid is seen coming through the lumen of the bowel, then strangulation must be suspected and the procedure should be abandoned and immediate laparotomy performed (see below).

If the mucosa looks normal, the distal end of the sigmoidoscope is held firmly so that it lies immediately below the point of torsion. Then, a well-lubricated rectal tube of 1 cm internal bore is passed through the sigmoidoscope and eased by gentle pressure into the twisted colon to enter the dilated sigmoid. It is wise for the operator to be suitably clothed and shod because there is a massive and satisfactory discharge of flatus and liquid faeces when the tube negotiates the torsion and enters the fluid- and gas-filled sigmoid. It should be a rule that, if the fluid that is withdrawn is blood-stained, it must be assumed that there is at least an element of strangulation in the loop and operation is then immediately undertaken, even though the mucosa at the site of torsion looks normal. It is wise to leave the tube *in situ* in the loop to drain, and most surgeons recommend passing a stitch through the perianal skin (under local anaesthesia) to secure the rectal tube for 24–48 hours for further drainage.

Bruusgaard's (1947) collected results were impressive. A total of 123 patients had a sigmoidoscopic deflation and of these only nine were not successful and required immediate operation. In one case the tube perforated gangrenous bowel and, although immediate laparotomy was done, the patient died. The disadvantage of the method is seen when it is remembered that 31 were re-admitted with recurrence. It is this marked tendency towards recurrence of the volvulus after simple deflation that provides the evidence to support an elective resection of the affected loop after a few days of preparation.

In a few patients, the twist lies so high that the sigmoidoscope cannot reach. It is then that the colonoscope offers the chance of deflation when otherwise it would be necessary to proceed to emergency laparotomy. In these patients, the twist lies 35–40 cm from the anus (Starling, 1979). With gentle air insufflation the colonoscope may be passed through the torsion, and gas and liquid faeces aspirated. Arigbabu *et al.* (1985) successfully decompressed 83 patients through a flexible sigmoidoscope and went on to elective resection after 5 days: all patients recovered. It seems likely that this method will replace intubation through a rigid sigmoidoscope because it allows safe negotiation of the point of torsion but under direct vision.

Resection of sigmoid colon   This is done in two different circumstances.

1. **As an emergency**. Resection is essential if gangrene is present. Emergency resection of viable bowel will be indicated in the 7–10% of patients in whom sigmoidoscopic deflation fails and then it seems reasonable to resect, rather than just untwist the volvulus and wait for the next recurrence. Sinha (1969) performed 149 primary resections with anastomosis (but he does not report how many were for gangrene). There were nine anastomotic leaks so the method is not without its complications. Anderson and Lee

(1981) reported 70 emergency resections. There were nine deaths after 30 Paul–Mikulicz resections, and seven deaths after 37 resections with primary anastomosis, which were associated with five anastomotic leaks. It is much safer to perform an emergency Hartmann's resection and return to restore continuity when the patient is fit. Jones and Fazio (1989) argue for this method. (See below for the management of the volvulus when vascular compromise is present.)

2. **Elective resection**. There is much support for achieving immediate sigmoidoscopic or colonoscopic deflation and then proceeding 3–5 days later to elective resection. If precautions are taken it is very unlikely that gangrene from the sigmoid will be overlooked, and time is allowed for general assessment of the patient and for preparation of the bowel. Recurrence of the volvulus is unlikely within these few days.

Shepherd (1968) followed this plan and performed 74 early elective resections with two deaths. Using the same regimen, Boulvin (1966) operated on 21 patients without mortality. Both these experienced surgeons advised against open detorsion and support immediate deflation followed by early resection (Gibney, 1991).

(b) Gangrenous change is suspected or proven

Shepherd (1968) concluded that gangrene is unlikely to be missed provided that emergency laparotomy is always undertaken when: (1) the clinical picture suggests gangrene, or (2) sigmoidoscopy shows discoloured mucosa or yields blood-stained fluid, or (3) decompression by intubation or colonoscopy cannot be achieved.

In these situations there is no alternative to immediate laparotomy, and, if gangrene of the sigmoid is found, there is then no alternative to some form of resection.

The twist should not be reversed. In the presence of compromise of blood flow to the volvulus, the 'twist' should not be derotated when the abdomen is open. Rather, the volvulus should be maintained. Clamps should be applied to the bowel above and below the twist, and then the mesentery supplying the volvulus should be clamped. The purpose of this approach is to prevent sudden revascularization of the gangrenous (or compromised) segment. If this is allowed to occur, then there will be a sudden infusion of blood from the compromised volvulus into the portal circulation, which may have dramatic effect on cardiac functions. Furthermore, it may also explain some of the late deaths from sepsis seen if the volvulus is untwisted before vascular and luminal control has been achieved.

Hartmann's resection for gangrenous sigmoid volvulus   The patient should be set up in Lloyd-Davies's lithotomy–Trendelenburg position. A Foley catheter should be passed into the urinary bladder and attached to a sterile drainage bag. The advantage of this position is that it allows for better access for the preliminary sigmoidoscopy and passage of the rectal tube and, in addition, allows for greater access for abdominal surgery and the possible usage of an end-to-end stapling machine.

A wide-bore sigmoidoscope is passed gently through the rectum until the lower edge of the twist is reached. If gangrenous changes are only suspected on clinical grounds (and this is usually the case because pneumoperitoneum is rare) then it is helpful to know the appearance of the mucosa before laparotomy. Discoloration of the mucosa indicates a high likelihood of gangrene in the loop and is a useful warning sign of what the surgeon should expect.

A generous left paramedian or midline incision will give the necessary access.

The enormously distended and discoloured colon will immediately present and care must be taken when entering the abdomen through the peritoneum in order not to damage and enter the volvulus. It is wise to assume that the area of the twist is likely to be more unhealthy than the loop itself and any attempt to untwist the loop at this stage must be resisted. This is all too likely to result in a tear of the bowel with catastrophic faecal soiling of the abdomen. Any handling of the loop at this stage is liable to be difficult, so it is safer to perform a needle decompression to remove the contained gas. A large hypodermic needle is attached to the sucker system and then very gently passed into the sigmoid colon making sure only to enter the air component and keep the tip of the needle away from liquid faeces. If liquid faeces is touched by the needle, it will become blocked. Several litres of gas may be readily aspirated by this method, allowing safer access to the abdomen. At this point it may be worth a further attempt to pass a rectal tube through a sigmoidoscope as previously described in order to drain out the liquid component in the volvulus. If it is clear that the twist is very tight, then this further attempt at intubation can be omitted.

For reasons given above, proximal and distal luminal control and a clamp across the vascular supply to the mesentery should then be achieved.

Resection of the loop can proceed with division of the peritoneum lateral to the sigmoid colon and mesocolon. The whole sigmoid loop can then be drawn out of the abdomen so that in some cases the mesocolon can be transilluminated to identify the feeding vessels. Shepherd (1968) warns that the superior rectal vessels often take a looping course some distance into the sigmoid mesocolon in patients with volvulus, so that these vessels might be at risk. The sigmoid vessels need to be identified, tied and divided and the dissection taken back to points where the descending colon and the rectum are clearly viable. The proximal and distal bowel can be divided between clamps. The rectum must be divided where it is clearly viable, and it may be necessary to go down to mid-rectum to achieve this outcome. The rectal stump should be washed out with a cleansing solution through the rectal catheter, after which it is divided and, if bleeding is seen from the cut edge, closed by suture with one or two layers of 2/0 polydioxanone.

In the majority of cases an anastomosis will not be contemplated at this stage. The distal rectal stump should be sutured to the sacral promontory or presacral fascia to keep the remaining rectum straight and prevent its apex rotating forward to lie in the depth of the pelvis. This will assist reconstruction at a later date. The proximal colon is brought out as a colostomy to complete the Hartmann's procedure.

In an otherwise fit patient an experienced surgeon might decide on anastomosis and then on-table bowel irrigation should be undertaken to clear the proximal bowel.

Outcome

In the West the mortality rate among a generally elderly population is appreciable – between 17% and 30% – often as a result of intercurrent disease. In the Third World the patients are generally relatively young and fit (Baker *et al.*, 1994).

Ileosigmoid knot

This is a particularly dangerous form of volvulus which seems to be largely localized to Africa, although some cases have been reported from Scandinavia, Russia and India (Puthu, 1991). Shepherd (1967) has given the most detailed description, based on 92 cases seen in Uganda. There is a very acute onset of agonizing generalized abdominal pain and frequent vomiting. Hypovolaemic shock occurs early and distension is not usually so marked as in

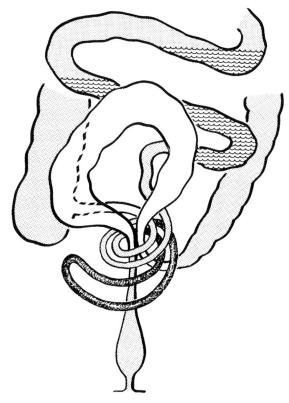

Figure 7.15 Ileosigmoid knot. The ileum wrapped around the sigmoid loop is usually gangrenous, and there are signs of a small-bowel obstruction above it.

sigmoid volvulus. There are often signs of peritonitis. The plain abdominal film shows a wide, dilated sigmoid colon and fluid levels in the small bowel.

The pathology is illustrated in Figure 7.15, which shows that the ileum is always ischaemic and the sigmoid often strangulated, hence the severe loss of blood into the mesenteries of the affected bowel.

This condition seems to be initiated by the ileum wrapping itself around a long sigmoid loop, but what causes it to have such strict geographical limits is not known. Ver Steeg and Whitehead (1980) give a good description of a single case seen in North America.

Speedy resuscitation is vital. The abdomen contains 1–2 litres of blood-stained fluid and the bowel and its lumen are full of blood, hence the hypovolaemia. It helps to mobilize the descending colon, sigmoid and upper rectum, first from the lateral side, identifying and protecting the left ureter. The whole sigmoid plus the knot can then be lifted out of the abdomen and properly visualized. The ischaemic ileum at the neck of the twist should be doubly clamped. The two ends of healthy ileum are laid aside while the ischaemic ileum is unwound and then discarded. The sigmoid is often ischaemic and a Hartmann's resection is required. Finally, an end-to-end anastomosis of ileum is needed, or the end of the ileum is implanted into the caecum. Often the greater part of the ileum needs removal.

REFERENCES

Agrez, M. and Cameron, D. (1981) Radiology of sigmoid volvulus. *Dis. Colon Rectum*, **24**, 510–514.

Anderson, J. R. and Lee, D. (1981) The management of acute sigmoid volvulus. *Br. J. Surg.*, **68**, 117–120.

Arigbabu, A. O., Badejo, O. A. Y. and Akinola, D. O. (1985) Colonoscopy in the emergency treatment of colonic volvulus in Nigeria. *Dis. Colon Rectum*, **28**, 795–798.

Baker, D. M., Wardrop, P. J., Burell, H. *et al.* (1994) The management of acute sigmoid volvulus in Nottingham. *J. R. Coll. Surg. Edin.*, **39**, 304–305.

Boulvin, R. (1966) L'intubation recto-sigmoidienne sous controle rectoscopique dans le volvulus aigu du sigmoide. *Lyon Chir.*, **62**, 19–23.

Bruusgaard, C. (1947) Volvulus of the sigmoid colon and its treatment. *Surgery*, **22**, 466–478.

Clark, H. E. (1883) Obstruction of the bowels due to volvulus, treated by abdominal section: recovery. *Lancet*, **ii**, 678–680.

Erichsen, J. (1850) Cases of intestinal obstruction, with remarks. *Lancet*, **i**, 108–109.

Gama, A. H., Haddad, J., Simonsen, O. *et al.* (1976) Volvulus of the sigmoid colon in Brazil. *Dis. Colon Rectum*, **19**, 314–320.

Gibney, E. J. (1991) Volvulus of the sigmoid colon. *Surg. Gynecol. Obstet.*, **173**, 243–255.

Hinshaw, D. R. and Carter, R. (1957) Surgical management of acute volvulus of the sigmoid volvulus. *Ann. Surg.*, **146**, 52–60.

Jones, I. T. and Fazio, V. W. (1989) Colonic volvulus. Etiology and management. *Dig. Dis.*, **7**, 203–207.

Neely, J. (1970) The management of gangrenous sigmoid volvulus. *Br. J. Surg.*, **57**, 670–672.

Odonga, A. M. (1982) Variety of volvuli of intestine seen at Mulago Hospital, Kampala 1966–1975. *E. Afr. Med. J.*, **59**, 711–717.

Perlmann, J. (1925) Klinische Beitrage zur Pathologie und chirurgischen Behandlung des Darmverschlusses. *Arch. Klin. Chir.*, **137**, 245–264.

Puthu, D., Rajan, N., Shenoy, G. M. *et al.* (1991) The ileosigmoid knot. *Dis. Colon Rectum*, **34**, 161–166.

Rigler, L. G. and Lipschultz, O. (1940) Roentgenology findings in acute obstruction of colon with special reference to acute volvulus of sigmoid. *Radiology*, **35**, 534–543.

Ryan, P. (1982) Sigmoid volvulus with and without megacolon. *Dis. Colon Rectum*, **25**, 673–679.

Scott, G. W. (1965) Volvulus of the sigmoid flexure. *Dis. Colon Rectum*, **8**, 30–34.

Shepherd, J. J. (1967) Ninety-two cases of ileo-sigmoid knotting in Uganda. *Br. J. Surg.*, **54**, 561–566.

Shepherd, J. J. (1968) Treatment of volvulus of the sigmoid colon: a review of 425 cases. *BMJ*, **i**, 280–283.

Sinha, R. S. (1969) A clinical appraisal of volvulus of the pelvic colon. *Br. J. Surg.*, **56**, 838–840.

Smith, R. B., Kettlewell, M. G. and Gough, M. H. (1977) Intermittent sigmoid volvulus in the younger age groups. *Br. J. Surg.*, **64**, 406–409.

Starling, J. R. (1979) Initial treatment of sigmoid volvulus by colonoscopy. *Ann. Surg.*, **190**, 36–39.

Valerio, D. and Jones, P. F. (1978) Immediate resection in the treatment of large bowel emergencies. *Br. J. Surg.*, **65**, 712–716.

Ver Steeg, K. R. and Whitehead, W. A. (1980) Ileo-sigmoid knot. *Arch. Surg.*, **115**, 761–763.

Young, W. S., Engelbrecht, H. E. and Stoker, A. (1978) Plain film analysis in sigmoid volvulus. *Clin. Radiol.*, **29**, 553–560.

7.2.2.2 Volvulus of the caecum and right colon

This is an unusual cause of intestinal obstruction: 41 of 193 colonic volvuli seen in Edinburgh over 13 years occurred in the caecum (Anderson and Lee, 1980).

Aetiology

Caecal volvulus is a misnomer in that most cases also involve the ascending colon and the ileum. Indeed, the condition cannot occur unless all these components are free to rotate. This usually depends on them hanging from a common ileocaecal mesentery and this, in turn, means that the normal fixation of the caecum and ascending colon to the posterior abdominal wall has not occurred. Wolfer *et al.* (1942) studied this matter in 125 cadavers in Chicago and found that in 11% the caecum was mobile enough to allow the development of a volvulus. If this proportion of people have a congenital abnormality allowing volvulus, then some special circumstances must determine the very small proportion who actually suffer from the diagnosis.

- There seems no doubt that an undue proportion of patients are pregnant (10% in the 100 patients studied by Donhauser and Atwell, 1949), and the difficulties of diagnosis if volvulus occurs at the time of delivery (Simons, 1950) or puerperium (Rose, 1941) are very great. It seems that the changes in the size of the uterus can produce conditions in which volvulus can occur (p. 503).
- There may be a history of a recent abdominal operation. Jordon and Beahrs (1953) found six examples in a 13-year period at the Mayo Clinic, five occurring within 11 days of major abdominal surgery.
- There is an important association between caecal volvulus and an obstructing lesion in the left side of the colon (Wilson *et al.*, 1954). They report eight patients with volvulus of the caecum, in four of whom there was a neoplasm in the left colon. They suggest that obstructive distension of the caecum may have predisposed to the volvulus. This suggests the importance of examining the whole length of the colon when operating on a patient with a volvulus of caecum.
- Among 50 patients, six were already in hospital for treatment of a medical disease (O'Mara *et al.*, 1979).

Pathology

The torsion usually takes place around the ascending colon (Figure 7.16).

This is followed by remarkable distension of the closed loop of bowel, usually at the site away from the right iliac fossa. Although only some 20% of caecal volvuli are gangrenous by the time of laparotomy (O'Mara *et al.*, 1979; Anderson and Lee, 1980), this is not a potential threat in all volvuli and signs may not indicate this. In a few patients (10%, O'Mara *et al.*, 1979) the caecum simply folds upwards, through 180°, at the junction with ascending colon, producing an acute kink (the 'caecal bascule') with the blood supply unaffected. Both forms of rotation create a closed loop.

Clinical picture

Females outnumber males by about 2:1. Caecal volvulus occurs at all ages, though more frequently over the age of 60.

Nearly all patients present with central abdominal pain, generally colicky in character. Most have vomited and are constipated (though a few complain of diarrhoea) but are in good general condition, apart from the minority with established gangrene. There is usually considerable distension, which may be asymmetrical, and in about 20% there is a palpable tympanitic mass, which may be tender. Bowel sounds, if heard, are obstructed.

Plain abdominal X-rays can be helpful. Anderson and Mills (1984) reviewed films from 45 proven cases and considered that a diagnosis of caecal volvulus could have been made in 40 patients. This is mainly based on the 'comma-shaped' caecal shadow lying away from the

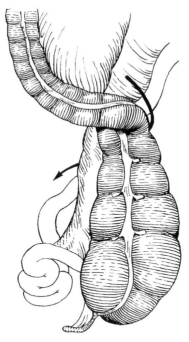

Figure 7.16 Caecal volvulus. The first stage of torsion of the ileocaecal mesentery.

right iliac fossa, usually in mid-abdomen or left upper quadrant with its concavity facing the right iliac fossa. A single long fluid level is seen in the erect film. Sometimes the distended caecum lies under the left diaphragm and resembles a dilated stomach; mottled faeces may be visible, but the issue can be settled by passing a nasogastric tube. Small-bowel shadows may be seen to the right of the distended caecum. If there is doubt about the interpretation, an emergency opaque enema will show a spiral pattern in the ascending colon, ending in a characteristic 'beak' (Dowling and Gunning, 1969).

Treatment

Although there are a few claims for reduction by colonoscopy, the great majority of these patients will require laparotomy as soon as preoperative treatment is complete. O'Mara *et al.* (1979) found that only two of nine patients with gangrenous bowel showed evidence of peritoneal irritation, indicating that early surgery is necessary in these patients.

When the abdomen is open through a vertical incision, the tense blue dilated volvulus will present. It is safer to decompress this bowel by the 'needle-suction' method described above. Once the tension in the area has been relieved, proximal, distal and mesenteric control can be secured as already described. Decompression through a trocar and cannula introduced through a purse-string can then be undertaken to further evacuate the volvulus. The site of aspiration is best oversewn and the soiled instruments discarded.

The dilated bowel can then be identified as caecum and ascending colon. If the volvulus is frankly gangrenous, it must be resected and the only reasonable way to do this is to perform a right hemicolectomy. A speedy resection and immediate end-to-end anastomosis can be accomplished quickly and is preferable. The essentials are that good bleeding must be seen from both ends of the bowel before they are joined, that the small intestine should be completely decompressed by retrograde emptying of contents into the stomach (p. 191) and a thorough antibiotic lavage of the peritoneal cavity should be performed. The technique of right hemicolectomy is discussed on page p. 272.

If the bowel proves to be viable after the volvulus has been untwisted, it is necessary to decide whether to resect or whether to perform a caecopexy to prevent recurrence of the volvulus. Some surgeons report favourably on caecopexy with tube caecostomy as a safe and effective way of fixing the caecum, but others have had problems with this approach. A neater solution is suggested by El-Katib (1973), in which a strip of polyvinyl alcohol sponge (4 cm × 15 cm) is fixed to the posterior abdominal wall behind the area over which the caecum would normally adhere. Fine, interrupted, non-absorbable sutures are then inserted to fix the back of the caecum to the sponge. The parietal peritoneum lateral to the strip is dissected up and sutured over the front of the caecum. El-Katib reports using this ingenious method in five patients with uneventful recoveries and periods of 6 months to 8 years without recurrence. However, the manner in which these sutures are placed into the bowel wall is critical and local faecal fistula into a sponge would be a very grave complication. We believe that right hemicolectomy offers the highest likelihood of uncomplicated recovery.

Postoperative deaths are now unusual, although Anderson and Lee (1980) saw three deaths among eight patients having a right hemicolectomy for gangrenous volvulus; all were due to septicaemia secondary to anastomotic leak. This is a serious reminder that the precautions advised are of particular importance and, if doubt exists concerning the security of an anastomosis, an end ileostomy and mucous fistula is a safer alternative that should readily be adopted in uncertain circumstances or if there is relative lack of experience by the surgeon to judge the issues.

REFERENCES

Anderson, J. R. and Lee D (1980) Acute caecal volvulus. *Br. J. Surg.*, **67**, 39–41.

Anderson, J. R. and Mills, J. O. M. (1984) Caecal volvulus: a frequently missed diagnosis? *Clin. Radiol.*, **35**, 65–69.

Donhauser, J. L. and Atwell, S. (1949) Volvulus of the caecum. *Arch. Surg.*, **58**, 129–148.

Dowling, B. L. and Gunning, A. J. (1969) Caecal volvulus. *Br. J. Surg.*, **56**, 124–128.

El-Katib, Y. (1973) Volvulus of the caecum: caecopexy by polyvinyl alcohol sponge. *Br. J. Surg.*, **60**, 475–478.

Jordan, G. L. Y. and Beahrs, O. H. (1953) Volvulus of the caecum as a post-operative complication. *Ann. Surg.*, **137**, 245–249.

O'Mara, C., Wilson, T. H., Stonesifer, G. L. *et al.* (1979) Cecal volvulus: analysis of 50 patients with long term follow up. *Ann. Surg.*, **189**, 724–731.

Rabinovici, R., Simansky, D. A., Kaplan, O. *et al.* (1990) Cecal volvulus. *Dis. Colon Rectum*, **33**, 765–769.

Rose, I. (1941) Volvulus of caecum. *BMJ*, **ii**, 577–578.

Simons, P. (1950) Volvulus of the caecum and pre-eclampsia complicating labour. *J. Obstet. Gynaecol. Br. Emp.*, **57**, 445–449.

Wilson, H. E., Desforges, G., Dunphy, H. G. *et al.* (1954) Volvulus of the caecum: possible predisposing lesions in the left colon. *Arch. Surg.*, **68**, 593–604.

Wolfer, J. A., Beaton, L. E. and Anson, B. J. (1942) Volvulus of the caecum: anatomical factors in its aetiology. *Surg. Gynecol. Obstet.*, **74**, 882–894.

7.2.2.3   Transverse colon

This is the most unusual form of colonic volvulus and fewer than 100 cases have been reported. Patients present with the symptoms of acute intestinal obstruction and usually have a marked degree of tympanitic abdominal distension, with obstructive bowel sounds. The X-ray picture shows very large gas-distended loops of colon, which is often interpreted as the much commoner sigmoid volvulus. The erect film shows wide large-bowel fluid levels (Anderson *et al.*, 1981).

If, at the time of laparotomy no vascular compromise is seen, the torsion should be unwound and a possible cause for the volvulus sought. In some reported cases there was distal obstruction by, for example, a sigmoid carcinoma and, consequently, it is important to make a thorough examination of the whole bowel under the circumstances. Associated defects of absence of hepatic and splenic flexures, attachment of the apex of the volvulus with adhesions and organo-axial rotation of the stomach have all been reported.

After simple detorsion the incidence of recurrence is high, so there is a good case for advising resection. Extended right hemicolectomy (p. 276) is likely to be the most appropriate procedure. If there is peritonitis with gangrene of the loop, it may be wiser to resect back to healthy bowel and fashion a proximal colostomy or ileostomy and a distal mucous fistula, and allow the patient to recover before restoring continuity.

Reference

Anderson, J. R., Lee, D., Taylor, T. V. *et al.* (1981) Volvulus of the transverse colon. *Br. J. Surg.*, **68**, 179–181.

7.2.3   UNUSUAL CAUSES OF LARGE-BOWEL OBSTRUCTION

Reports show that only 3–5% of all large-bowel obstructions are caused by diverticular disease and its complications (Campbell *et al.*, 1956; Koruth *et al.*, 1985; Table 7.2). It can, however, be surprisingly difficult to distinguish between an obstructing annular carcinoma in the sigmoid colon, and a short segment of narrowing caused either by the exceptional muscular thickening seen in diverticular disease (p. 308) or by the effects of a pericolic abscess. The distinction can be difficult to make in an opaque enema (although biopsy *via* a colonoscope can sometimes be helpful), but it can be just as difficult at the time of laparotomy. Under these circumstances clinical management should follow the lines already detailed for obstructing carcinomas.

The only additional point to be made is the need to be particularly careful if an anastomosis is to be performed on colon containing diverticula. Experience shows that, in dealing with a diseased sigmoid, it is not necessary to extend the resection proximally to include every diverticulum in the descending colon. The aim should be to find a segment of descending colon that is free of diverticular thickening and inflammation so that when the bowel is divided, the 2 cm of colon immediately proximal to the point of anastomosis is healthy, enabling a safe anastomosis to be performed.

By contrast, all the distal sigmoid colon involved with the diverticular process should be resected down to the uppermost portion of the rectum, where the taenia coli fan out to form the complete layer of longitudinal fibres seen in the rectum. Failure to carry out this more distal dissection has been associated with recurrence of the diverticulitis process in this segment and, because of the musculohypertrophy, has been associated with anastomotic leakage.

An important variety of intestinal obstruction occurs when a loop of small bowel becomes adherent to, and consequently kinked by, an area of diverticulitis. The patient presents with the picture of small-bowel obstruction. Experience shows that the kinked small bowel may be mobilized and straightened by separating the inflammatory adhesions to the sigmoid colon, without the surgeon realizing that the sigmoid pathology must also be considered for further treatment. These circumstances can also occur in Crohn's colitis. If the colonic pathology fails to resolve then re-exploration may be needed. Thus, careful assessment of the colon is needed by an experienced surgeon to decide whether the diverticulitis (or Crohn's disease) is likely to resolve with conservative management or whether resection is required.

Adhesions

In contrast to small-bowel obstruction, which is frequently caused by intraperitoneal adhesions, obstruction of the colon is rarely attributable to this cause (Campbell *et al.*, 1956; Agrawal *et al.*, 1984).

Radiation therapy

One of the long-term consequences of radiation is endarteritis obliterans resulting in fibrotic stricture of bowel adjacent to the treatment area. Although this usually affects the small bowel, strictures of the pelvic colon may produce large-bowel obstruction. This is treated in the same manner as outlined for the small intestine (p. 234). The need to perform wide resection of the irradiated rectosigmoid may mean that reconstruction will involve an endoanal anastomosis. Clearly, this procedure would be inappropriate in an emergency operation and is one of the situations better treated by diverting colostomy to alleviate the emergency and to allow full evaluation before elective surgery.

Acute pancreatitis

Acute obstruction of the transverse colon can occasionally be generated by acute pancreatitis: a pseudocyst can generate sufficient fibrosis just proximal to the splenic flexure to cause obstruction. Frisell *et al.* (1981) found 34 cases and reported two of their own. They recommended treatment by *en bloc* resection of the mass with the tail of the pancreas and the splenic flexure. However, some patients suffer a stenosis of the colon caused by the adjacent inflammatory process, which resolves as the cyst settles (Mair *et al.*, 1976; Russell *et al.*, 1983).

Endometriosis

Endometriosis occasionally causes sufficient narrowing to produce large-bowel obstruction (p. 513).

Intraluminal obstruction

Gallstone obstruction would appear an unlikely condition in the wide colon, but if a large stone enters the colon directly through a cholecystocolic fistula, then the stone may impact in a narrowed area due, for example, to sigmoid diverticular disease (Anseline, 1981).

Faecal impaction of unusual material that has been eaten can occasionally cause intraluminal obstruction. Large impacted faecoliths containing numerous matchsticks, perverse eating of large amounts of unprocessed bran and excess usage of hydrophilic colloid laxatives (such as Isogel and methyl cellulose) have all been reported, usually situated in the rectum (Kang and Doe, 1979).

REFERENCES

Agrawal, N. W., Akdamar, K. and Litwin, M. S. (1984) Post-operative adhesions causing colon obstruction. *Am. Surgeon*, **50**, 479–481.

Anseline, P. (1981) Colonic gallstone ileus. *Postgrad. Med. J.*, **57**, 62–65.

Campbell, J. A., Gunn, A. A. and McLaren, I. F. (1966) Acute obstruction of the colon. *J. R. Coll. Surg. Edin.*, **1**, 231–239.

Frisell, J., Ihre, T., Lundh, G. *et al.* (1981) Colonic stricture as a complication of the colon. *Acta Chir. Scand.*, **147**, 609–612.

Kang, J. Y. and Doe, W. F. (1979) Unprocessed bran causing intestinal obstruction. *BMJ*, **i**, 1249–1250.

Koruth, N. M., Hunter, D. G., Krukowski, Z. H. *et al.* (1985) Immediate resection in emergency large bowel surgery: a 7 year audit. *Br. J. Surg.*, **72**, 703.

Mair, W. S. J., McMahon, M. J. and Goligher, J. C. (1976) Stenosis of the colon in acute pancreatitis. *Gut*, **17**, 692–695.

Russell, J. C., Welch, J. P. and Clark, D. G. (1983) Colonic complications of acute pancreatitis and pancreatic abscess. *Am. J. Surg.*, **146**, 558–564.

7.2.4 ACUTE FUNCTIONAL COLONIC OBSTRUCTION, OR ILEUS OF THE COLON, OR ACUTE PSEUDOMECHANICAL OBSTRUCTION OF THE COLON

The clinical picture of 'paralytic' ileus is well known. It is often a complication of peritonitis or retroperitoneal trauma and produces a functional obstruction of both small and large intestine (p. 258). A similar 'ileus of the colon' (Dorudi *et al.*, 1992) can occur in which the patient presents the typical picture of large-bowel obstruction, but no mechanical cause can be found. Some call this 'Ogilvie's syndrome' because he gave an early description of a chronic form of the condition due to retroperitoneal malignant infiltration (Ogilvie, 1948). Surgeons have generally adopted the term 'pseudo-obstruction' or 'pseudomechanical obstruction' (Dudley *et al.*, 1958), although it is open to the serious objection that an obstruction of the colon is certainly present and can sometimes lead, like a mechanical obstruction, to caecal rupture and faecal peritonitis. However, it is probably a term that has come to stay.

In the majority of patients, the colonic dilatation appears to be a complication of one of many diseases or injuries, such as a cerebrovascular accident, or following a spinal injury or caesarean section (Table 7.4).

Recognition of these different conditions is important because the occurrence of major colonic distension associated with one of them should always lead to suspicion of a

Table 7.4 Conditions associated with functional obstruction of the colon

Inflammatory	Intra-abdominal especially acute gall bladder disease
	Systemic infection with bacteraemia
	Pneumonia
Vascular	Cerebrovascular accident
	Myocardial infarction
	Heart failure
	Subarachnoid haemorrhage
Trauma	Pelvic and spinal fractures
	Retroperitoneal haematoma
	Pregnancy
	Postpartum, especially after caesarean section
Postoperative	Hip replacement and bone grafting operations
	Abdominal surgery, especially retroperitoneal
Malignant disease	Affecting retroperitoneum
	Disseminated disease
Metabolic derangement	Renal failure
	Electrolyte disturbances
	Diabetes mellitus
	Parkinsonism
	Myxoedema
Idiopathic	Some drugs, e.g. antidepressants and phenothiazines

functional colonic obstruction. However, in 15–20% of patients no predisposing condition can be found.

If all large-bowel obstructions presenting to a surgical unit are recorded (Koruth *et al.*, 1985), between 5% and 8% prove to have a functional basis. However, since many cases of pseudo-obstruction are treated in orthopaedic or obstetric units, while others do not produce sufficiently severe complaints to warrant a surgical consultation, it is difficult to estimate the true incidence.

Some hours, or a day or two, after the onset of these predisposing conditions (Table 7.4), the patient notices a rapidly increasing degree of abdominal distension. Some complain of colicky abdominal pain and others will vomit. Almost all are constipated and do not pass flatus. Most are generally unwell and in a few the abdomen is so tense that breathing is difficult, quick and shallow. On percussion the abdomen is hyper-resonant but is not particularly tender. However, when the caecum becomes so distended that splitting of the wall occurs, tenderness and guarding are usually found. Obstructive bowel sounds are quite often heard. The rectum is generally empty on digital examination.

Plain abdominal X-rays show a very marked degree of gaseous distension of the right and transverse colon, and in a typical case there is a 'cut-off' in the gas column at the splenic flexure or in the sigmoid colon. Small-bowel distension is not usually very noticeable, in marked contrast to 'paralytic' ileus. In a minority, the whole colon is distended down to the rectum. Generally, there are noticeably fewer fluid levels than would be seen in a mechanical obstruction, and haustral markings are often retained. However, the degree of distension is impressive and particular attention should be given to the caecum, where there is a real danger of rupture. Lowman and Davis (1956) studied caecal diameters in obstructed and normal patients and concluded that anyone in whom the diameter was more than 9 cm was in danger of perforation. Much greater diameters, up to 20 and even 23 cm (Keenan *et al.*, 1985), may be seen without any signs of rupture. Occasionally, the erect film will show free gas under the diaphragm when the caecum has already ruptured. It is probably wise to regard 12 cm as an upper limit beyond which decompression is needed.

As long ago as 1960, Morton *et al.* emphasized how helpful a gentle emergency barium enema could be to demonstrate absence of mechanical obstruction. Quite a limited examination is sufficient to show the contrast flowing freely past an apparent point of obstruction. If gastrografin is used this is sometimes followed by the passage of flatus and faeces.

A contrast enema examination is valuable in three possible ways.

1. It can confirm the diagnosis of function obstruction when that is already suspected.
2. The examination may show that there is in fact a mechanical obstruction.
3. Most importantly, it will show in a number of patients who are thought to be mechanically obstructed that no such blockage exists (for details, see p. 268).

This information can save a number of fruitless laparotomies and is of special relevance in the idiopathic cases, which can bear a particularly close resemblance to neoplastic colon obstruction. However, when a contrast enema is carried out, Corder (1986) warns that persistent sigmoid spasm can, on rare occasions, mimic neoplastic obstruction.

Treatment

As soon as the diagnosis is suspected, it is important to stop all intake and to initiate continuous nasogastric suction through a sump-type nasogastric tube, so that swallowed air is aspirated. Fluid is given intravenously and any anaemia or electrolyte imbalance is corrected. In addition to these measures it is necessary to treat the precipitating acute illness. In a few patients chronic conditions, e.g. myxoedema, may be associated with colonic dilatation.

Sometimes a gentle sigmoidoscopy, with passage of a flatus tube into the dilated sigmoid, can provide useful decompression. In a minority of patients who already have signs of actual or threatened caecal perforation (based on signs of peritoneal irritation and caecal diameter), laparotomy must be undertaken forthwith. But in most patients, time must be given to await the results of the earlier mentioned treatments. This is achieved by the patient being assessed by the same team twice daily, when fresh X-rays showing caecal diameter can be viewed.

If there is no improvement, and if the caecal diameter remains greater than 9–10 cm, colonoscopic deflation should be considered (Strodel and Brothers, 1989; Dorudi *et al.*, 1992). The use of this method depends on the availability of a skilled colonoscopist, because this procedure may be difficult and is potentially dangerous. It is difficult because of the lack of bowel preparation and potentially dangerous because excess use of air insufflation to help the advance of the instrument may further increase the pressure within the caecum (Munro and Youngson, 1983; Bode *et al.*, 1984). It is helpful to give one or two cleansing saline enemas before the colonoscopy, and thereafter lavage is used (to wash away the faeces and secure a view) as the instrument is advanced. Once dilated colon is entered, large volumes of gas and several litres of liquid faeces may be aspirated (Munro and Youngson, 1983) with obvious improvement in the condition of the patient.

The abdominal signs and X-rays require continued observation because improvement is not always maintained after decompression. The knowledge from an opaque enema or colonoscopy that there is no distal obstruction may be helpful in assisting deflation by sympathetic blockade with guanethidine, followed by prostigmine or bethanechol, as in the treatment of ileus (see p. 259). The success of this method (Munro and Youngson, 1983; Bullock and Thomas, 1984) raises interesting parallels between those patients in whom distension is largely confined to the colon and patients with ileus, in whom both large and small bowel are dilated and obstructed.

If the caecum reaches about 12 cm in diameter, despite the decompression efforts of colonoscopy, then serious consideration must be given to exposing the caecum through the right iliac fossa muscle-splitting or muscle-dividing incision, and performing a caecostomy. If at any time the signs suggest caecal perforation then a vertical laparotomy incision will be needed because peritoneal cleansing and thorough antibiotic lavage will be required, as well as deflation of the caecum. Preliminary decompression can then generally be obtained by guiding a wide tube or sigmoidoscope up the rectum into the dilated colon. If the caecum has reached the stage of perforation, it must be assumed that there is a substantial interference with blood supply (p. 297). Whenever caecal viability is in question, resection by right hemicolectomy will be required. If there is heavy faecal contamination it will be wise to fashion an ileostomy, with the transverse colon brought out separately as a mucous fistula. This is the safer approach and restoration of continuity can be undertaken some weeks later, if and when the patient becomes fit.

Reports on the results of caecostomy are unanimous about its value as a means of decompressing functional obstruction of the caecum, and many also comment on the unsatisfactory results after transverse colostomy. This is an interesting reversal of the situation in neoplastic obstruction, for which tube caecostomy gives such poor results.

In carrying out a caecostomy *via* a right iliac fossa incision (approximately 4 cm in length depending on the patient's subcutaneous fat thickness), a number of technical details are important. The incision should be made at the classical site of McBurney's point (one-third along the line joining the anterior superior iliac spine with the umbilicus). The incision should be oblique and either a muscle-dividing or muscle-splitting approach can be taken to the peritoneal surface. Great care must be used in opening the peritoneal cavity to prevent injury to the greatly distended caecum. Once the bowel wall is viewed, it is wise to suck off as much gas as possible by needle aspiration. This will permit the deflated caecum to prolapse through the incision in the abdominal wall. We have found it safer to then sew the caecal wall to the skin in a circumferential fashion so that the use of tubes and purse-string sutures can be avoided. The caecal contents are then aspirated and irrigated, and a stoma appliance is applied snugly around the orifice. An alternative method is that the prolapsed deflated caecal wall is brought out through the incision, a double purse-string suture is placed and a 26–30 FG De Pezzer catheter (with the distal half of the bulb removed) is introduced to drain and irrigate the caecum. However, although this is often recommended, its record is a poor one, because of failure of drainage, and an open 'blow-hole' caecostomy is safer because it is more reliable (Grierson *et al.*, 1975).

The amount of gas and faecal fluid that drains through the caecostomy varies greatly, but the major objective, to preserve the viability of the caecum, will have been attained. The flow chart devised by Keenan *et al.* (1986) provides a useful summary for clinical management (Figure 7.17).

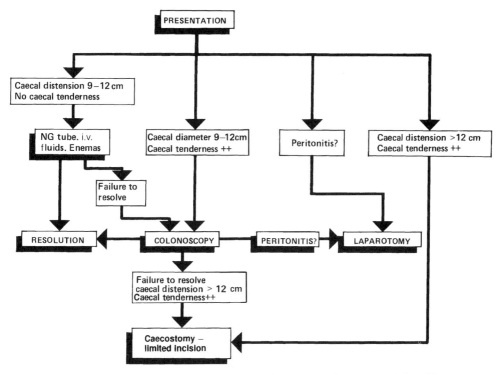

Figure 7.17 Methods of management of acute functional obstruction (after Keenan et al 1986).

Once the cause of the pseudomechanical obstruction has resolved, the caecostomy site usually closes. If a fistula persists the 'stoma' can be mobilized, excised and sutured, and the bowel returned to the abdomen, once the patient is fit and well. However, quite frequently the stoma site becomes reactivated as the 'process' of pseudomechanical obstruction waxes and wanes, particularly in the idiopathic variety.

The aetiology of these functional obstructions of the colon remains uncertain. It is possible to list the conditions associated with their occurrence (Table 7.4) but difficult to see the relationships between them. However, they all appear to affect the autonomic control of colonic movement and this notion receives some support from the successful use of pharmacological sympathetic blockade (Neely, 1970). Otherwise, no explanation can be offered for the idiopathic cases in which the obstructions arise without any detectable previous injury or illness. It is in these patients that the consistent use of an emergency contrast enema examination is particularly useful because these conditions can so closely resemble neoplastic colonic obstruction.

REFERENCES

Bode, W. E., Beart, R. W., Spencer, R. J. *et al.* (1984) Colonoscopic decompression for acute pseudo-obstruction of the colon (Ogilvie's syndrome). *Am. J. Surg.*, **147**, 243–245.

Bullock, P. R. and Thomas, W. E. G. (1984) Acute pseudo-obstruction of the colon. *Ann. R. Coll. Surg. Engl.*, **66**, 327–330.

Corder, A. P. (1986) Pseudo-obstruction. *BMJ*, **292**, 1463.

Dorudi, S., Berry, A. R. and Kettlewell, M. G. (1992) Acute colonic pseudo-obstruction. *Br. J. Surg.*, **79**, 99–103.

Dudley, H. A. F., Sinclair, I. S. R., McLaren, I. F. *et al.* (1958) Intestinal pseudo-obstruction. *J. R. Coll. Surg. Edin.*, **3**, 206–217.

Grierson, E. D., Storm, F. K., Shaw, W. *et al.* (1975) Caecal rupture due to colonic ileus. *Br. J. Surg.*, **62**, 383–386.

Keenan, R. A., Logie, J. R. C. and Munro, A. (1986) Acute pseudo-obstruction of the colon in late pregnancy and the puerperium. Paper read to meeting of Royal College of Surgeons of Edinburgh, Inverness.

Koruth, N. M., Hunter, D. C., Krukowski, Z. H. *et al.* (1985) Immediate resection in emergency large bowel surgery: a 7 year audit. *Br. J. Surg.*, **72**, 703–707.

Lowman, R. M. and Davis, L. (1956) An evaluation of cecal size in impending perforation of the cecum. *Surg. Gynecol. Obstet.*, **103**, 711–718.

Morton, J. H., Schwartz, S. I. and Gramiak, R. (1960) Ileus of the colon. *Arch. Surg.*, **81**, 425–434.

Munro, A. and Youngson, G. G. (1983) Colonoscopy in the diagnosis and treatment of colonic pseudo-obstruction. *J. R. Coll. Surg. Edin.*, **28**, 391–393.

Neely, J. (1970) Pseudo obstruction of the large bowel. *BMJ*, **ii**, 793–794.

Ogilvie, H. (1948) Large intestine colic due to sympathetic deprivation. *BMJ*, **ii**, 671–673.

Strodel, W. E. and Brothers, T. (1989) Colonoscopic decompression of pseudo-obstruction and volvulus. *Surg. Clin. North Am.*, **69**, 1327–1335.

7.3   ACUTE SIGMOID DIVERTICULAR DISEASE

The presence of diverticula in the colon (diverticulosis) is common in the older citizens of Northern Europe, Australasia and North America. Among those over 60 years of age, one in three will be affected (Manousos *et al.*, 1967), but it is very unusual to find diverticula in the colons of individuals under 40 years of age. In the great majority the diverticula are confined to the left colon, mainly in the sigmoid. Only 6% of over 500 patients with symptomatic diverticular disease had generalized colonic diverticulosis (Parks, 1969): their average age, at 55 years, was 10 years below that of the majority with localized disease and this distribution may have a congenital basis.

In the vast majority, diverticulosis is clearly an acquired condition, characterized by a remarkable thickening of the muscular layers of the distal colon (Morson, 1963), with herniations of the mucosa occurring mainly at points of weakness, where the arteries pierce the muscular wall (see Figure 8.11). Recent work shows increased elastic tissue in the longitudinal taenia coli. The work of Painter (1964) is now generally accepted, which points to the generation of exceptionally high pressures within segments of colon, which in turn produce pulsion diverticula. Painter and Burkitt (1975) have assembled an impressive array of data suggesting that the low-fibre diet of Western peoples is associated with these high pressures. It is an observed fact that inhabitants of Third World countries who eat a diet rich in natural fibre very rarely show signs of diverticular disease.

In spite of the fact that so many older people have colonic diverticula, the frequency of complications requiring admission to hospital is low. In Goteborg, Sweden, Haglund *et al.* (1979) found that the overall admission rate for diverticulitis was only 33 patients each year to a hospital serving 500 000 people. In the Grampian region of Scotland, with a population of 450 000, the annual number of admissions for perforated diverticulitis was seven (Kyle and Davidson, 1975), and in Goteborg it was between five and six.

Consequently, even in a large hospital serving a population of nearly half a million, individual surgeons will only gradually build up experience of complicated diverticular disease (Table 7.1).

Presentation

There have been many more recent attempts to describe, classify and categorize diverticulitis but the full account of Telling and Gruner in 1917 of the complications of colonic diverticulosis remains relevant today. Broadly these are of four kinds.

- About two-thirds of the patients have acute diverticulitis (see below).
- About one in ten have intestinal obstruction, which may be due to adhesions and kinking of small bowel, or occlusion of the sigmoid (p. 301).
- Another 10% present with significant rectal haemorrhage (p. 376).
- The remaining 10–15% present less acutely, but still with serious disease. This is due to low-grade sepsis in diverticula causing chronic pericolic inflammation which, at its most severe, culminates in the development of a fistula into the bladder or the vagina, or occasionally other viscera. These patients have a serious complaint but rarely present as an emergency.

7.3.1   ACUTE PYOGENIC DIVERTICULITIS

Pathology

The basic pathology of this condition is an acute infection arising in one or more diverticula obstructed by a faecolith that has become impacted in the neck of the diverticulum. Infection of mucus trapped within the diverticulum sets up an acute inflammatory reaction, which goes on to the formation of an acute pyogenic pericolic abscess. The next stage depends on the situation of the diverticulum and the virulence of the infection.

Acute phlegmonous diverticulitis is the result of a spreading low-grade cellulitis, mainly in the mesocolon, which originated in a pericolic abscess within the mesentery of sigmoid or descending colon. This leads to oedematous thickening of the colon and appendices epiploicae, and the formation of a tough indurated colonic and pericolic mass. The mesentery is very thick and the mass is usually stuck to the surrounding parietes and other tissues. The left ureter is very likely to be adherent to the back of the mass. A fibrinous reaction on the serosal surface of the mass is likely but there is little or no pus formation.

On abdominal examination the pelvic colon is easily palpable and tender but, in contrast to the patient with non-suppurative diverticular disease, the patient is usually unwell and febrile.

This is an important form of acute diverticulitis to recognize because the acute inflammation is likely to subside with antibiotics, bed rest and a fluid diet, or intravenous fluids.

However, this form of acute diverticulitis can be the forerunner of a true **pericolic abscess**. Here the inflammatory reaction has progressed locally to form a collection of pus, usually originating within the mesocolon but extending to become adherent to, and enclosed by, the adjacent abdominal and pelvic wall, omentum and loops of small bowel. This forms a localized acutely tender mass, usually in the left lower quadrant. Although most patients with pericolic sepsis resolve with antibiotics, some patients progress to form sizeable collections of pus which no amount of antibiotic treatment will resolve; the patient becomes febrile and toxic, and drainage is necessary. Although these abscesses contain pus rather than faeces, a faecal fistula often develops after drainage.

The most serious form of pericolic abscess is the one that forms relatively quickly, in the presence of more virulent bacteria, so that there is no time for firm adhesions to form before, as in perforated acute appendicitis, the abscess leaks into the peritoneal cavity, causing either a local or a generalized peritonitis. This may take several forms.

- **A localized peritonitis** with a small, sometimes unidentifiable, perforation in the wall of the acutely inflamed sigmoid. There is usually no communication with the lumen of the colon because the narrow neck of the diverticular abscess that has burst is occluded by oedema. This is one of the types of acute pyogenic diverticulitis that can be expected to settle with antibiotics and intravenous fluids.

  However, it is important to remember always that an exactly similar situation can arise from perforation of a carcinoma, so, although it is clearly beneficial for an unfit elderly patient to be spared a laparotomy for a self-limiting condition, it is essential that the colon be investigated thoroughly as soon as is reasonable.

- If the abscess was larger, and the pus that leaked out provided a virulent inoculation of the peritoneum with faecal bacteria, then a **diffuse purulent peritonitis** can develop and spread throughout the peritoneal cavity. This will be reflected in the appearance of an ill, toxic patient with the signs of generalized peritonitis.

- The most dangerous situation arises when the pressure within a pericolic abscess rises so quickly that ischaemic necrosis of the wall of the colon results in a sizeable perforation, 1–2 cm in diameter, with irregular edges, which opens directly into the lumen of the colon and allows heavy faecal contamination of the peritoneum. Among patients with generalized peritonitis, some 20–25% will have a **faecal peritonitis** (Pheils *et al.*, 1982) and only quick and effective treatment can help them. They are likely to show the signs of a very severe generalized peritonitis and of bacteraemia, so energetic resuscitation and intravenous antibiotic treatment is vital, followed as soon as practicable by laparotomy.

Very occasionally the mesocolic cellulitis leads to interruption, presumably by thrombosis, of the colic vessels and actual **gangrene of a segment** of the colon results. This must be managed in the same way, and a similar picture may be seen in **stercoral perforation** (p. 317), and occasionally in perforation of **radiation-damaged bowel** (p. 234).

Clinical picture

Critical assessment of the symptoms and signs of these patients is of the greatest importance in planning treatment because only a minority require laparotomy: Haglund *et al.* (1979) performed laparotomy on only 97 (25%) of 392 patients who presented with their first attack of acute pyogenic diverticulitis, but for most of these 97 patients operative treatment was literally life-saving. However, the average age of patients coming to operation is in the late 60s; 40% have cardiovascular disease and 30% are overweight (Kyle, 1968) so it is important to avoid operation where it is not essential for recovery.

It is common for patients with diverticular disease to complain of pain in the left iliac fossa and to have a recurrent palpable, thickened, tender pelvic colon, although they are generally in normal health. However, in acute pyogenic diverticulitis there is usually little previous history (Haglund *et al.*, 1979; Nagorney *et al.*, 1985) and the symptoms start acutely. In about 75% a typical history is of a patient in the late 60s or 70s who, over the space of 2–3 days, feels increasing pain in the left iliac fossa, and is constipated, anorexic, feverish and generally unwell. On examination the patient looks unwell, a little dehydrated, with a dirty tongue and a fever, and there is tenderness with, occasionally, a mass in the left iliac fossa. There may be guarding in the overlying abdominal wall but the rest of the abdomen is relaxed and not tender. There is likely to be a leucocytosis and rectal examination is generally negative, but a tender mass may be felt in the pouch of Douglas.

These findings suggest acute diverticulitis, possibly with a pericolic abscess or cellulitis which should settle with treatment.

Very rarely the patient is admitted when it is evident that there is a large pericolic abscess, which is usually sited out towards the flank, is acutely tender and may be associated with reddening of the overlying skin. Large abscesses, if neglected, may track up under the diaphragm or into the scrotum.

The 20–25% of patients with perforated diverticulitis have a more acute onset. After only hours or a day or so of left lower quadrant pain, there is a sudden exacerbation of pain, which may become generalized, although in some patients it is maximal in the right lower quadrant (Dawson *et al.*, 1965). When the perforation is large, with faecal contamination, the signs rapidly spread to involve the whole abdomen and these patients soon show signs of bacteraemic shock. Among the 121 patients with perforated diverticulitis and generalized peritonitis operated on by Nagorney *et al.* (1985), 80% presented with acute left-sided pain and developed signs of generalized peritonitis, and 20% came in with signs of bacteraemia, rigors, hypotension and severe generalized peritonitis. In 44% plain films showed gas under the diaphragm. Other important clinical features of this group were that two-thirds had other major disabilities such as cardiorespiratory disease or diabetes, and 24 patients were on long-term corticosteroid therapy. The laparotomy showed that 44% had a spreading peritonitis from a ruptured pericolic abscess; 42% had gross faecal contamination of the peritoneal cavity.

When clinical features alone are used to determine the need for operation in patients with presumed perforated diverticulitis the diagnosis is correct in only one-third (Dawson *et al.*, 1965). Contemporary practice requires a more conservative approach with early investigation to confirm a provisional diagnosis of acute diverticulitis.

Treatment

There was a striking change in the approach to the treatment of acute diverticulitis during the 1980s with a deliberate move towards a more conservative non-operative approach for the majority of patients, allied to a more aggressive surgical policy for those patients requiring laparotomy (Ryan, 1983; Krukowski *et al.*, 1985).

This was based on the observations that:

- many patients with initially severe acute diverticulitis settle on medical treatment, provided they are not complicated by generalized peritonitis;
- when operation is indicated for acute perforated diverticulitis the results are better if the perforated colon is resected rather than defunctioned by proximal colostomy.

One paper (Krukowski *et al.*, 1985) spells out an important corollary of these trends, in these words: 'The infrequency of acute diverticulitis, the variable nature of its complications, and the several treatment options, make management decisions difficult. We therefore do not think that the emergency care of such patients should be delegated, as it often is, to junior surgical trainees'.

The principles of management include the importance of assessing the patient generally and treating, so far as possible, important coincidental conditions such as heart failure, arrhythmias and anaemia. Those patients with established sepsis are appreciably dehydrated and rehydration needs careful control: it is helpful to measure hourly urine output and, in some, central venous pressure.

Whenever diffuse peritonitis is present, especially when faecal peritonitis is suspected because of signs of bacteraemic shock, these patients should if at all possible be admitted to an HDU or ITU area where controlled expansion of blood volume by electrolyte and colloid solutions will go hand in hand with immediate intravenous administration of effective doses of antibiotics (p. 143).

Obstruction

A small number of patients with diverticulitis develop a dense fibrotic stricture following an episode of sepsis and the progressive obstruction of the colon presents in a manner indistinguishable from an obstructing carcinoma. Management is essentially the same. When the diagnosis of left-sided colonic obstruction is made on the clinical findings and plain abdominal radiographs the site of obstruction must be confirmed by an urgent contrast study. Although the benign nature of the stricture may be suspected because of the absence of mucosal destruction and the tapering nature of the stricture it is normally confirmed only after resection, opening the specimen and examining the mucosa.

Small-bowel obstruction may result from adhesion of small bowel to an inflammatory mass in the lower abdomen and the clinical presentation of small-bowel obstruction can be more striking than the underlying colonic pathology.

7.3.2   INVESTIGATION

Rectal examination is important but sigmoidoscopy may be omitted unless the patient has to undergo laparotomy, in which case it must be done before opening the abdomen: discomfort is minimized if this is carried out after inducing general anaesthesia. This avoids the embarrassment of overlooking significant but coincidental anorectal problems, particularly a rectal neoplasm. Plain abdominal and chest radiographs may give indirect evidence of diverticulitis, with abnormal soft tissue shadows, pneumoperitoneum and bowel distension.

In patients with an uncomplicated clinical picture of mild diverticulitis the clinical features alone may permit effective management with minimal investigation (Rege and Nahrwold, 1989; Thompson and Bailey, 1990). For the majority of patients, however, in whom urgent laparotomy for generalized peritonitis is not indicated, the appropriate course after resuscitation and institution of antibiotic therapy is to confirm the clinical diagnosis of acute diverticulitis with either a water-soluble contrast enema or CT scan as soon as convenient: normally within 48 hours of admission. Barium should be avoided despite its superior radiological definition because of the possibility of extravasation and difficulty in clearing the bowel if surgery becomes necessary.

Imaging in acute diverticulitis was reviewed by McKee *et al.* (1993). The water-soluble contrast enema shows pathology from the luminal aspect and may show bowel wall thickening, mucosal oedema, irregularity and occasional leakage of contrast. Extravasation, if present, is usually localized to an abscess cavity but free perforation into the peritoneal cavity is sometimes seen. The urgent enema can be limited to the left side of the colon when this confirms the diagnosis but formal colonoscopy or barium enema when the acute episode has resolved is mandatory. The urgent enema is only an aid to management and coexistent carcinoma within an inflammatory mass or elsewhere in the colon must be excluded subsequently. It should be remembered that colon cancer is found in 20–25% of resected specimens when the left colon is resected as an emergency for presumed diverticular disease (Krukowski and Matheson, 1984).

Routine CT scanning is more widely used in North America for the assessment of the acute abdomen but its role, in a more selective manner, in the assessment of more complicated cases is being increasingly appreciated elsewhere (Ambrosetti, 1997). In acute diverticulitis CT demonstrates bowel wall thickening, (non-communicating) abscesses and extraluminal disease better than a contrast enema. Systematic review of the literature, however, shows that it is no more accurate than a water-soluble contrast study in terms of diagnosis (McKee *et al.*, 1993) and subjects patients to a higher dose of radiation. The value of CT is in assessing severity which is, in turn, of prognostic value both in the short and long term (Ambrosetti, 1997; Table 7.5). We reserve contrast-enhanced CT for difficult cases in whom diagnosis or management decisions have not been clear on the basis of a single contrast enema and usually after 2–3 days when a decision for or against surgery is proving difficult.

Although extravasation of contrast, whether seen on enema or CT, increases the likelihood of operation during the acute admission it is not an absolute indication for operation (Kourtesis *et al.*, 1988; Ambrosetti *et al.*, 1994), which should always be based on clinical rather than radiological criteria.

Ultrasound scanning may be useful in acute diverticulitis but operator variability reduces its utility as the first investigation in acute diverticulitis. Furthermore, the requirement for subsequent definitive assessment of the bowel with barium enema or colonoscopy remains. Ultrasound, however, can be useful in following the progression of inflammatory masses and abscesses. It is interesting to speculate on the reasons for the apparently higher rate of

Table 7.5 Radiological assessment of severity of diverticulitis and prognosis (after Ambrosetti, 1997)

	Mild	Severe
CT	Bowel wall thickness > 5 mm	+ *either* Abscess *or* Extraluminal air *or* Extravasation of contrast
Contrast enema	Segmental luminal narrowing Tethered mucosa Extrinsic mass effect	+ *either* Extraluminal air *or* Extravasation of contrast
Failure of conservative therapy	4%	30%

ultrasound-guided percutaneous drainage of diverticular abscesses reported in North America, which is an extreme rarity in our practice.

7.3.3 TREATMENT

Great care is required in the interpretation of papers reporting management of patients with diverticulitis because the variability of the septic process and the relative rarity of the most severe forms of generalized and faecal peritonitis (Krukowski and Matheson, 1984) means that authors may include both patients with mild disease and those with the potentially lethal variants. The brisk correspondence following the paper of Wedell *et al.* (1997), which advocates single-stage surgery for all patients with complicated diverticulitis, is characteristic.

The treatment of acute diverticulitis, however, can be logically considered by addressing three questions: when to operate, when to resect and when to anastomose (Krukowski, 1998). The management of acute diverticulitis is directed towards the control of peritoneal sepsis and when this can be accomplished medically the risks of emergency colonic surgery are eliminated. However, the timely identification of the minority of patients who either require urgent operation or fail to settle on conservative management requires fine clinical judgement. It can be surprising for the surgical novice to observe the rapid clinical improvement in patients with apparently extensive peritoneal signs due to diverticular sepsis in response to fluid resuscitation, antibiotics and analgesia.

The choice of antibiotics is based on a broad-spectrum agent or combination directed at the Gram-negative aerobes and Gram-positive anaerobes responsible for gut-derived sepsis. The specific agents chosen vary with the severity of the infection, local protocols and bacterial sensitivities. Oral agents suffice for mild attacks and the combination of trimethoprim (200 mg b.d.) and metronidazole (400 mg b.d.) or co-amoxiclav (625 mg q.i.d.) are suitable. For more severe sepsis requiring parenteral antibiotics the choice again lies between a combination of antibiotics and a single agent. Although some authorities consider the combination of gentamicin and metronidazole to be obsolete this is not our experience. The once-daily dosage regime for gentamicin (7 mg/kg body weight) has greatly simplified therapy and when gentamicin resistance in coliform organisms is not an issue there appears to be no more rapidly bactericidal agent. The long half-life of metronidazole means that this can be given as a 500 mg infusion twice or three times daily. Alternatively the gentamicin may be replaced with a third-generation cephalosporin (cefotaxime 1g or 2g i.v. t.i.d.).

When to operate?

When there are signs of generalized peritonitis and free gas, urgent laparotomy, after resuscitation and institution of antibiotic therapy, for a diagnosis of generalized peritonitis of unknown origin is both appropriate and indeed life-saving. Equally clearly, an obviously minor attack clearly does not require urgent surgery but for the remainder with moderately severe peritonitis a trial of conservative therapy is appropriate and resolution of even extensive signs of peritonitis can be expected in the majority. The threshold for surgery is imprecise and based on the degree of confidence relating to the diagnosis and response to treatment. If operation is performed too frequently a large proportion of patients with an inherently good prognosis will be included in the operative group and a spuriously low mortality may result. This is well illustrated by Haglund and colleagues (1979) who found that, in 392 patients admitted with acute diverticulitis, 97 (25%) underwent emergency operation. Within this group 31 patients had phlegmonous inflammation without suppuration or perforation and the mortality was 3%. In the 66 patients with evidence of perforation the mortality was 33%. When the threshold for operation is set too low more patients with mild disease and a good prognosis are subjected to surgery and, provided the postoperative complication rate is low, an erroneous perception of the role of surgery may be engendered.

Regular assessment of the response to treatment is essential and the clinical diagnosis must be confirmed by appropriate imaging. We persevere with conservative treatment for 3 days before deciding that sufficient resolution has not occurred. This approach requires consistency in the observer and a continuity in care that contemporary work patterns may make difficult. Accurate documentation and liaison then become increasingly important.

Extravasation on contrast enema or CT scan increases the likelihood of surgery during the emergency admission but a surprising number of patients will settle without acute intervention, permitting subsequent single-stage elective surgery (Ambrosetti *et al.*, 1994; Ambrosetti, 1997).

When to resect

When urgent surgery is reserved for failure of conservative management or generalized or faecal peritonitis then the need for resection of the sigmoid colon is clear. Control of sepsis under these circumstances demands eradication of the source, both from the circulation and the peritoneal cavity, by resection of the affected colon and mesocolon. The review by Krukowski and Matheson (1984) of patients with the most severe sepsis demonstrated a lower mortality (11%) with radical surgery in which the affected colon is resected compared with conservative procedures (27%) in which the colon is not excised and surgical therapy depends on drainage and proximal colostomy. Although it should be apparent that not all patients treated conservatively died or that all patients treated conservatively lived the balance is so strongly in favour of radical surgical therapy that the clear recommendation was eradication of the source of sepsis by resection of the sigmoid colon for severe sepsis.

The question of resection is more problematic when operation has been premature or when the diagnosis of acute diverticulitis is unexpected, which can follow a preoperative misdiagnosis of gynaecological or appendicular sepsis. An acutely inflamed colon may also be found on laparoscopy performed for assessment of the acute abdomen, particularly in women and under these circumstances resection is not indicated. Inappropriate resection confers the risk of anastomotic leakage or unnecessary stoma formation. The correct action is antibiotic peritoneal lavage, closure of the abdomen and postoperative antibiotics but this requires confidence and experience in the assessment of the situation. The inexperienced tend to err on the side of intervention with inappropriate drains, stomas or resection. Although such actions may be thought life-saving, the mortality, morbidity, inconvenience and potential for a second major laparotomy outweigh the risks of non-resection of the inflamed but unperforated colon.

When to anastomose

If the indications for operation were correct the decision on timing of anastomosis can also be difficult and contentious. There is a trend to single stage treatment, i.e. resection with immediate anastomosis, for complicated diverticulitis but it is important to distinguish between surgery performed in the convalescent period as an elective or semi-elective procedure after successful conservative therapy for an acute episode and the true emergency. It is possible to combine these groups into a report with an overall very low mortality and morbidity while containing a high mortality in the small group of patients requiring emergency surgery (Weddel *et al.*, 1997). Hartmann's procedure has been regarded as the safest option for left-sided colonic emergencies over the last 25 years by eradicating the source of sepsis and avoiding anastomotic leakage, albeit at the cost of a left iliac fossa colostomy. The resulting single-barrelled left lower quadrant stoma has the additional merit that, should it prove permanent, it is relatively easily managed compared to the increased bulk and double lumen of a transverse colostomy.

Nevertheless increasing confidence in immediate anastomosis after left colonic resection, usually with on-table irrigation in emergency surgery, is increasing the use of single-stage definitive surgery in patients at low risk of anastomotic failure after resection for perforated diverticulitis. Low-risk means that the patient is fully resuscitated and stable and that a senior anaesthetist and competent surgeon are present. The postoperative care and supervision must be of a high standard to identify and treat the cardiovascular instability and hypoxaemia that lead to anastomotic failure. When these requirements are not fulfilled considerations of safety should override surgical enthusiasm and anastomosis should be avoided in favour of Hartmann's procedure.

Operative strategy

Optimal preoperative preparation of the patient undergoing laparotomy for advanced intraperitoneal sepsis, with clinical assessment supplemented by appropriate monitoring, must continue through to the postoperative period.

Incision

As for all major emergency abdominal surgery a midline incision has the advantages of simplicity, reliable closure and low wound infection rate if appropriate precautions are used (Krukowski and Matheson, 1988). When there is a possibility of a stoma in the left lower quadrant it is sensible to make the skin incision to the right of the umbilicus. Simple mechanical precautions to minimize contamination of the wound by infected intraperitoneal material contribute to a low wound infection rate. For example: before the peritoneum is opened widely the abdominal wall is elevated to allow aspiration of pus and contaminated peritoneal fluid before it percolates over and inoculates the wound. In the presence of suppuration and potential for faecal contamination of the operative field there is much to be said for the use of wound towels, plastic ring wound protector and institution of a 'red danger towel' technique.

This is a situation in which a long incision is important. Struggling through a small incision restricts access and creates tissue trauma by excessive retraction. Poor exposure leads to inadequate surgery with incomplete assessment of peritoneal sepsis, and incomplete peritoneal toilet and lavage and makes the necessary colonic mobilization more difficult. Access to all quadrants of the abdomen permits accurate assessment of the extent of the inflammatory process.

Although the operation is for presumed benign disease, a limited wedge excision of a few centimetres of sigmoid colon is unwise because it risks leaving disease and results in any stoma or anastomosis being made in inflamed tissue. If resection of the colon is dictated by the extent of inflammation, adequacy of arterial pulsation at the point of division and awareness of the possibility of cancer means that mobilization of the left colon should be equivalent to a radical cancer operation. Mobilization of the splenic flexure permits tension-free formation of a stoma or anastomosis. The possibility that the inflammatory mass or perforated segment contains a carcinoma makes radical excision of the inflamed mesocolon with high ligation of the inferior mesenteric artery a sensible manoeuvre. There need be no concern that opening intact tissue planes will disseminate infection with routine tetracycline lavage.

If there is gross faecal loading of the colon and rectum, this must be evacuated, even when Hartmann's procedure is performed, to avoid stercoral obstruction or even perforation proximal to a stoma. Access to the rectum is required in emergency left-sided colonic procedures and the operating surgeon must take responsibility for placement of the patient in the Lloyd-Davies position.

Hartmann's procedure

When conditions preclude safe anastomosis the divided left colon is brought out through a trephined wound in the left lower quadrant through the rectus abdominis muscle, which reduces the rate of parastomal herniation. Closure of the lateral space is not necessary and simplifies subsequent restoration of bowel continuity. The rectal stump can be closed by cross-stapling or suturing, although our experience (including closure of the rectal stump after total colectomy for inflammatory bowel disease) suggests fewer leaks in sutured cases. An open sutured technique also permits evacuation of faeces which stapling can incorporate in the closure. A single layer of continuous 2/0 or 3/0 serosubmucosal monofilament absorbable suture is supplemented with two long non-absorbable sutures at the lateral ends to aid future identification of the rectal stump.

Immediate anastomosis

The need for mechanical preparation of the bowel by on-table colonic irrigation is unproven in that there are no, and are unlikely to be any, randomized trials of sufficient power to demonstrate unequivocally a difference in leak rate with and without lavage. What it does achieve is near-perfect cleansing and has aesthetic if unproven clinical appeal. The appendix or, if absent, the terminal ileum is intubated with a Foley catheter through which 3 litres of warmed saline is infused. The effluent is collected by a collecting system inserted proximal to the segment of colon to be resected. When available, a custom system collects the effluent, failing which corrugated anaesthetic tubing is inserted into the colon proximal to the diseased area and tied in place with nylon tape. If the rigid corrugated tube is used this usually results in siphoning with suction of the bowel wall into the tube as irrigation proceeds. This is abolished by inserting a 16 FG needle into the tubing to allow air in and abolish the low pressure inducing the siphon (p. 280).

The rectum should be irrigated through a proctoscope before division of the rectum between the sacral promontory and peritoneal reflection. After division of the proximal colon to include the site of insertion of the irrigation tube an open single-layer serosubmucosal end-to-end colorectal anastomosis is made with interrupted 3/0 sutures.

Antibiotic lavage

We remain convinced of the importance of peroperative irrigation of the peritoneal cavity and abdominal parietes with tetracycline solution in reducing wound and intraperitoneal infection rates (Krukowski and Matheson, 1988). Tetracycline at this concentration (1000 mg/l 0.9% saline) is active against all bacterial pathogens. Several litres may be required to achieve thorough peritoneal toilet and lavage is repeated at the end of the procedure. The midline incision is closed with a continuous mass suture with 1/0 polydioxanone, with further lavage of the subcutaneous space before primary skin closure. This strategy, even in such 'dirty' surgery, is associated with a low wound infection rate and delayed primary closure is not required at a first laparotomy. Postoperative antibiotics are continued for only 3 days provided peritoneal contamination has been eliminated.

REFERENCES

Ambrosetti, P. (1997) Diverticulitis of the left colon, in *Recent Advances in Surgery 20*, (ed. I. Taylor and C. D. Johnson), Churchill Livingstone, Edinburgh, pp. 165–160.

Ambrosetti, P., Robert, J., Witzig, J. A. *et al.* (1994) Acute left colonic diverticulitis: a prospective analysis of 226 consecutive cases. *Surgery*, **115**, 546–550.

Dawson, J. L., Hanon, I. and Roxburgh, R. A. (1965) Diverticulitis coli complicated by diffuse peritonitis. *Dis. Colon Rectum.*, **28**, 71.

Haglund, U., Hellberg, R., Johnsen, C. and Hulten, L. (1979) Complicated diverticular disease of the sigmoid colon: an analysis of short and long term outcome in 392 patients. *Ann. Chir. Gynaecol.*, **68**, 41–46.

Krukowski, Z. H. (1998) Diverticular disease, in *Colorectal Surgery*, (ed. R. K. S. Phillips), W. B. Saunders, London, pp. 123–140.

Krukowski, Z. H. and Matheson, N. A. (1984) Emergency surgery for diverticular disease complicated by generalized and faecal peritonitis: a review. *Br. J. Surg.*, **71**, 921–927.

Krukowski, Z. H. and Matheson, N. A. (1988) Ten-year computerized audit of infection after abdominal surgery. *Br. J. Surg.*, **75**, 857–861.

Krukowski, Z. H., Koruth, N. M. and Matheson, N. A. (1985) Evolving practice in acute diverticulitis. *Br. J. Surg.*, **72**, 684–686.

Kyle, J. (1968) Prognosis in diverticulitis. *J. R. Coll. Surg. Edin.*, **13**, 136.

Kyle, J. and Davidson, A. I. (1975) The changing pattern of hospital admission for diverticular disease of the colon. *Br. J. Surg.*, **62**, 537–541.

McKee, R. F., Deignan, R. W. and Krukowski, Z. H. (1993) Radiological investigation in acute diverticulitis. *Br. J. Surg.*, **80**, 560–565.

Manousos, O. N., Truelove, S. C and Lumsden, K. (1967) Prevalence of colonic diverticulosis in general population of Oxford Region. *BMJ*, **iii**, 762.

Morson, B. C. (1963) The muscle abnormality in diverticular disease of the sigmoid colon. *Br. J. Radiol.*, **36**, 385.

Munson, K. D., Hensien, M. A., Jacob, L. N. *et al.* (1996) Diverticulitis: a comprehensive follow-up. *Dis. Colon Rectum*, **39**, 318–322.

Nagorney, D. M., Adson, M. A. and Pemberton, J. H. (1985) Sigmoid diverticulitis with perforation and generalised peritonitis. *Dis. Colon Rectum*, **28**, 71.

Painter, N. S. (1964) The aetiology of diverticulosis of the colon. *Ann. R. Coll. Surg. Engl.*, **34**, 98.

Painter, N. S. and Burkitt, D. P. (1975) Diverticular disease of the colon, a 20th century problem. *Clin. Gastroenterol.*, **4**, 3–22.

Pheils, M. T., Chapuis, P. H., Bokey, E. L. *et al.* (1982) Diverticular disease: a retrospective study of surgical management 1970–1980. *Austr. N.Z. J. Surg.*, **52**, 53.

Rege, R. V. and Nahrwold, D. L. (1989) Diverticular disease. *Curr. Probl. Surg.*, **26**, 128–132.

Ryan, P. (1983) Changing concepts in diverticular disease. *Dis. Colon Rectum*, **26**, 12.

Telling, W. H. M. and Gruner, O. C. (1917) Acquired diverticula, diverticulitis and peri-diverticulitis of the large intestine. *Br. J. Surg.*, **4**, 468.

Thompson, D. A. and Bailey, H. R. (1990) Management of acute diverticulitis with abscess. *Semin. Colon. Rectal Surg.*, **1**, 74–80.

Wedell, J., Banzhaf, G., Chaoui, R. *et al.* (1997) Surgical management of complicated colonic diverticulitis. *Br. J. Surg.*, **84**, 380–383

7.4 ACUTE INFLAMMATORY BOWEL DISEASE

Although inflammatory bowel disease is a common condition, attacks of severe generalized colitis are fairly unusual, but when it occurs there is a real threat to life. Expert assessment and treatment is needed but experience of this emergency is necessarily limited: Ritchie *et al.* (1984) found that a district general hospital may admit only two or three such patients in a year.

7.4.1 ACUTE ULCERATIVE AND CROHN'S COLITIS

Acute severe colitis occurs in both ulcerative colitis (UC) and Crohn's disease (CD). In a study of UC in North-east Scotland Sinclair *et al.* (1983) traced 537 patients but only 59 had panproctocolitis with a severe acute attack in 39. In the same region, 41% of patients with CD have colorectal involvement (Kyle, 1992) but only 6% require operation for fulminant colitis, although many more present with a severe illness.

From the clinical point of view acute UC and Crohn's colitis present in a very similar way, although operative decisions and prognosis are clearly affected.

For the family doctor, who sees many cases of gastroenteritis, recognition of a severe attack requires judgement. Failure of acute diarrhoea to settle, continued fever, abdominal pain and distension, and blood in the stools are signals for urgent admission to hospital. Similar severe attacks can occur in *Salmonella* and *Campylobacter* infections but stool and blood cultures will soon identify these.

Once in hospital, it is important for hospital staff to quickly assess the situation and to diagnose the problem promptly. Many 'scoring' indices have been produced, but none has surpassed that of Truelove and Witts in 1955:

- severe diarrhoea (more than six stools per day);
- macroscopic blood in stools;
- fever (mean evening temperature over 37.5°C or a temperature of 37.8°C on two days out of four);
- tachycardia (mean pulse rate over 90/min);
- anaemia (Hb < 11 g/dl);
- ESR more than 30 mm in the first hour.

To this we would add a low serum albumin of less than 30 g/l and rapid weight loss. These are sure signs that the illness is severe and having a profound metabolic effect on the patient.

Every one of these criteria does not have to be entirely satisfied, but they identify a group who are at risk of developing serious complications. Most will settle with intensive medical treatment but some 20–35% are likely to need emergency – or more urgent – surgery.

Joint approach

The need for joint care between gastroenterologist and surgeon at an early stage cannot be overemphasized. Even with such shared care it can be difficult to distinguish those who need immediate surgery and to recognize those who merit a trial of medical treatment. It is even more difficult to make a decision, at the correct time, that intensive medical treatment has failed and surgery is indicated.

Perhaps the best combination in this situation is a physician fully aware of the merits of early surgery and a surgeon who is mindful of the difficulties and dangers of operation but convinced of the need to avoid delay when surgery is needed.

We have had a team approach for many years. The team has been expanded to include a stomatherapist, a dietician and also a few former patients. This has allowed us to counsel both patient and worried relatives regarding the implications and dangers of major surgery and the need for a stoma which may be permanent.

Pathology

An understanding of the pathophysiology of the condition of fulminant colitis is important if one is to appreciate why these patients are so ill.

Hulten *et al.* (1977) in Gothenburg showed that in severe pancolitis there is a two- to sixfold increase in colonic blood flow, which can be as high as 1500 ml/min. There is widespread and deep ulceration, so the effects can be compared with extensive burns or scalds, depending on the extent and depth of ulceration. From these areas of ulceration and granulation there is a loss of serosanguinous exudate and desquamated epithelium, which results in rapid loss of protein and blood. The absorptive function of intact mucosa is lost, resulting in copious stools containing blood, pus and mucus. Hypoalbuminaemia occurs rapidly because appetite is lost and the consequence is a malnourished patient who will rapidly become dehydrated and anaemic. Crile and Thomas in 1951 gave a vivid description of the process by likening it to 'an extensive third-degree burn covered with a faecal poultice'. The risk of bacteraemia is ever-present. as shown by Jalan *et al.* (1969), who cultured Gram-negative bacteria from the blood of nine of 38 severely ill colitic patients.

Apart from producing a patient who is weakened, ill and toxic, the constant worry is that the colitis progresses to a 'disintegrative colitis', the useful term coined by Brooke and Sampson (1964) to indicate that ulceration has penetrated so deeply that perforation is likely. When such inflammation spreads through the muscular wall (Sampson and Walker, 1960), so weakening it, the process may progress to dilatation (megacolon). Much of the skill in managing these patients correctly lies in recognizing those showing the early signs of progression to the irreversible disintegrative stage requiring colectomy.

Clinical assessment

- A severe attack may occur in the first presentation of IBD, or during a relapse. It is often thought that the first attack is more serious, but this may be because a relapse is more speedily recognized and treated. Patients may give a history of progressive illness over some weeks, but some patients with a pancolitis can deteriorate rapidly and within a short period can become desperately ill. A few patients will present with severe haemorrhage.

- Certain factors have been recognized as being **promoters** of dilatation of the bowel in cases of toxic colitis. Anticholinergic agents, antidiarrhoeal medication, hypokalaemia and contrast radiology (Fazio, 1980) have been incriminated. To this can be added colonoscopy which requires air insufflation to distend the bowel; it is our practice to refrain from this.
- The **general appearance** of the patient is an important clinical sign in itself. The impression gained each morning and each evening as one greets the patient is as important an index of progress as the information gained from the temperature, pulse and blood pressure charts, important signs as these are. Fluid input and output are measured and a chart aimed at recording frequency, weight and character of the stool passed is kept. Inspection of the stools is important. A fall in their number and weight is not necessarily a good sign if accompanied by increasing distension.
- The **full blood count, electrolyte and albumin concentrations** are recorded daily, and a low albumin is a clear indication of the severity of the disease. Stool is cultured, as infections such as *Campylobacter* and *Clostridium difficile* may complicate the picture.
- **Abdominal examination** is vital if early signs of perforation or impending perforation are to be detected. It has to be emphasized that this task may be very difficult. Patients are usually receiving narcotics, steroids and other immunosuppressants, which may mask the true situation (Re Mine and McIlraith, 1980). Corticosteroids are effective antipyretics and modify the normal response of the parietal peritoneum. Fewer than one in three patients will show guarding. When pain is a prominent feature, it is a worrying complaint because it is not a feature typically present in toxic colitis. Distension is usually due to gas in distended bowel, but may be present if perforation has occurred into the peritoneal cavity. Then areas of tenderness and guarding will be found, and rebound tenderness, which is best sought by percussion. Auscultation is of limited value, but normal peristaltic sounds are unlikely to be heard in peritonitis.
- **Rectal examination** is useful. It may show signs of perianal Crohn's and the velvety feel of the mucosa in proctitis may be revealed. A gentle limited sigmoidoscopy is almost certain to show inflamed mucosa, but this will not necessarily be diagnostic as infective causes may look identical.
- **Plain abdominal radiology** is very important in diagnosing and following the progress of these patients. The value of such a simple investigation should not be underestimated. Fresh films should be taken each morning and evening while the initial effects of intensive medical treatment are being observed. The films should be seen immediately after each clinical examination. The following appearances may be seen: in severe colitis, the colon is generally empty of faeces and contains a fair amount of gas so air-contrast pictures are readily obtained (McConnell *et al.*, 1958). As alluded to earlier, barium enemas are unnecessary and dangerous.
  - Mucosal and mural oedema may be recognized in the thickened wall of the colon. Small, 1 cm nodular, rounded mucosal folds outlined against the gas are often seen, giving a scalloped thumbprint appearance.
  - 'Mucosal islands' as described by Brooke and Sampson in 1964 may be seen when there is deep widespread ulceration. The few islands of surviving oedematous mucosa may be identified as multiple pale circles, contrasted against the darker gas shadows. Brooke emphasized the value of this sign, which is only seen when ulceration is widespread and deep, and perforation is imminent: he described an example of this sign being neglected for as little as 12 hours, allowing perforation to occur.

– Dilatation of the colon is likely to occur, which, although appreciated on clinical examination, is best assessed by plain radiology. There is no agreement on the diameter that defines the presence of 'megacolon' (a term first used by Marshak *et al.* in 1950) but it is generally accepted that a transverse colon diameter measuring 6 cm in the presence of severe colitis is worrying, and the diagnosis is established if the diameter reaches 8 or 9 cm. Megacolon is probably due to the severity of the inflammation weakening the muscularis, although oedema and kinking may produce an element of obstruction. Modest degrees of dilatation without mucosal islands may resolve with intensive medical treatment, but perforation becomes an immediate threat once dilatation reaches 10 cm or more. Megacolon appears in severe Crohn's colitis, although rather less often than in UC.

– Pneumoperitoneum is a clear sign of perforation, but two-thirds of perforations are sealed (Goligher *et al.*, 1970). Absence of free gas does not, therefore, exclude perforation.

Management

The first task of physician and surgeon is to identify the small number of patients who require immediate colectomy. Indications are:

- perforation of the colon;
- massive rectal haemorrhage (p. 374) that requires continuing blood transfusion;
- disintegrative colitis, as evidenced by the 'mucosal island' sign;
- gross megacolon, defined as a diameter of 10 cm or greater, has such a high risk of perforation that it is safer to proceed to emergency colectomy. In lesser degrees of megacolon Binder *et al.* (1974) found it safe to treat the patient aggressively for 24–48 hours.

For these patients a few hours must be spent over correction of dehydration, hypovolaemia, anaemia and electrolyte depletion. Parenteral antibiotics are commenced. There is no indication for giving corticosteroids but in the patient already receiving them they must be continued. A urinary catheter and a central venous line will be needed in these critically ill patients. Technique is considered on p. 324.

Intensive medical treatment

Nine out of ten patients do not require immediate surgery, and are started on intensive medical treatment. The details were worked out by Dr S C Truelove in Oxford (Truelove and Jewell, 1974; Truelove *et al.*, 1978) and have been widely adopted.

The patient is placed at complete rest in bed, with restricted fluids by mouth. Intravenous fluids are adapted to correct fluid and electrolyte deficiencies: stool volumes can measure 1.5–3.0 litres per day. Blood transfusions are usually needed, and parenteral antibiotics are given in full dosage. Prednisolone is given intravenously. Some suggest that intravenous hyperalimentation is needed, but McIntyre *et al.* (1986) showed that a light, nourishing diet could safely be given by mouth with equally good results.

A careful clinical and radiological reassessment is made of the patient at least twice a day, so far as possible by the same physician and surgeon. Some are clearly better within 24 hours and among the 80–90% of patients who start on this treatment some 60–70% respond and go into remission. Among the other 20% there is a poor response or they deteriorate

(Truelove *et al.*, 1978). Lennard-Jones *et al.* (1975) found that when, after 24 hours of treatment, a patient was still passing eight stools per day, had a temperature over 38°C and a pulse rate of over 100/min, there was an 80% chance of emergency surgery being required in the next few days. A serum albumin of less than 30 g/l makes this more likely.

Consequently, the criteria that indicate failure of medical treatment are a combination of:

- the 'end of the bed' impression that the patient is not so well;
- a sustained or rising tachycardia;
- abdominal pain;
- local tenderness and a suggestion of guarding; corticosteroids modify abdominal signs so in peritonitis guarding is not the reliable sign that it usually is;
- radiological signs of increasing distension and mucosal islands.

It is important to constantly remember that the signs of failure of medical management may be muted. It is again emphasized that nothing takes the place of examining the patient two or three times per day.

What should be done for the patient who after a few days of intensive treatment is neither better nor worse? Goligher *et al.* (1970) reported on 258 cases of severe colitis who proceeded to surgery who had not improved after 5–7 days on active aggressive medical treatment. They had a mortality rate of 7%. When treatment ran on for 12–15 days before deciding on surgery, the mortality was 20%. Truelove *et al.* (1978) came to the same conclusion and after treating 100 severe attacks in 87 patients they laid down the principle that 'absence of decisive improvement after 5 days of intensive treatment is an indication for emergency colectomy'. Some 25 patients came into this category and had an urgent colectomy, without a death.

Truelove and Marks (1981) felt that by adhering closely to their 5-day rule they prevented some patients from developing megacolon. We have adopted the rule that if there has been no improvement within 5–7 days then surgery should be performed; in an older patient, and when in serious doubt over progress, it is probably wiser to shorten this to 3–4 days.

Emergency and urgent surgery

These patients are extremely ill and the aim of emergency surgery is to keep it as simple as possible to give the patient the optimal chance of making a good recovery. General consensus among surgeons is to perform subtotal or total colectomy with retention of the lower sigmoid or rectal stump.

These techniques have several benefits.

- The great bulk of the disease is removed.
- There is no anastomosis which may leak.
- The histology at the time of operation is often unknown. Retaining the rectum allows a free choice of a later restorative procedure in either UC or CD and it also avoids a major addition to the operation.
- There are now few indications for emergency proctocolectomy, unless serious bleeding is seen to be coming from the rectum itself.

Emergency colectomy and ileostomy

It has been our practice to fit patients with anti-embolism stockings at the time of admission. Also, they will receive subcutaneous heparin in an attempt to prevent deep venous thrombosis and fatal pulmonary embolism, the risks of which are increased in inflammatory bowel disease. A urinary catheter is inserted when the patient is anaesthetized and the anaesthetist inserts a central venous line.

There are great advantages in placing the patient in lithotomy–Trendelenburg position. It gives access to all parts of the abdomen, makes retraction easier and allows access to the rectum.

A long midline incision is preferred and has the advantage of leaving both iliac fossae free for stoma formation at the time of operation or later, should revision be needed.

When the abdomen is opened there may be an established peritonitis and there is often considerable colonic distension, which may be dangerously tense. It is then necessary to deflate the colon as the first step of the operation. This has two important advantages. Once deflated, the bowel is easier to handle and the risk of tearing the bowel is much reduced. The other advantage is that one of the hazards of emergency colectomy – the opening-up of sealed perforations, which cannot be avoided – does not result in serious peritoneal contamination.

The method of decompression used in our unit was specifically devised for this event. A 28 or 30 FG Foley catheter is inserted *via* the ileum or appendix stump and, with the help of the Y-piece, it can be threaded up the proximal colon and its contents sucked out (Figure 7.9). An operating sigmoidoscope is placed in the rectum *via* the anus, and a wide tube is passed up it to evacuate distal colon. If necessary warm saline is allowed to flow *via* a Y-connection attached to the Foley catheter. The fluid flows gently along the colon and the bloodstained faecal fluid is collected *via* the wide sigmoidoscope into a suitable container.

If the distension is purely gaseous it may be overcome by wedging a large hypodermic needle into a suction tube. It is then inserted into the transverse colon *via* a taenia coli and suction applied.

Once the danger of major perforation is over and the bowel is decompressed the small bowel should be examined for other sites of Crohn's disease, although this finding is fortunately unusual in cases needing emergency colectomy.

Colectomy can then proceed, commencing with mobilization of the proximal colon. Throughout great care is needed because the inflamed colon is easily torn. The ileocolic artery is preserved in case a pouch is needed in the future. During mobilization of the transverse colon it is often wise to remove the greater omentum along with the colon as it may be sealing perforations: it is divided a short distance below the gastroepiploic arcade, each omental branch being ligated. This opens the lesser sac and allows access to the transverse mesocolon, which can be dealt with step by step by dividing each branch to the middle colic artery. The splenic flexure can then be approached. Gentleness and patience are needed. As suggested on page p. 280, it helps for the surgeon to stand between the legs if the Lloyd-Davies position is being used, and both the transverse and the descending colon should be mobilized, to allow gentle traction on both limbs of the splenic flexure (Figures 7.6 and 7.7).

It then remains to divide the mesentery of the splenic flexure and descending colon, ligating and dividing the branches of the inferior mesenteric artery, until the sigmoid colon is mobilized down to the rectosigmoid junction. Transillumination of the mesentery can add to the accuracy of this operation.

It remains to decide at which level the distal division should be made. There are two main options.

1. The sigmoid colon is divided, ensuring that the blood supply is intact, and closed with a de Martel clamp. It can then be brought out to produce a mucous fistula through the lower part of the wound without tension, the clamp being allowed to slough off several days later. Most patients do well using the technique, but a longer segment of diseased bowel is left behind and it may lead to a wound infection.

2. The technique we prefer is to close the rectum as one would perform a modified Hartmann's procedure. Again, the blood supply to the upper rectum is preserved and the area is closed with a right angled clamp. The rectum is then irrigated. A rectal tube that is connected to a bag of 0.2% chlorhexidine solution is placed in the rectum *via* a proctoscope, and guided to the apex of the rectum, and the rectum is washed out. Once satisfied that the rectum is 'clean' the surgeon closes the rectum. It is our preference to do this by using absorbable sutures instead of staples. It is our belief that stapling can 'crack' the diseased tissue and cause dehiscence. Suturing allows the surgeon to have a tactile appreciation of the closure as the sutures are drawn tight.

    We reported the results of closure of the rectum in 62 patients with colitis. Three out of 16 patients who had stapled closure had suture line dehiscences, but there was only one dehiscence in the remaining 46 patients who had a hand-sewn closure (McKee *et al.*, 1995).

The abdomen is finally thoroughly irrigated with 0.1% tetracycline solution. It is **most** important to check on every ligature and raw area for bleeding points. The spleen is carefully examined for an unnoticed tear in its capsule, especially if the bowel has been adherent. Postoperative haemorrhage is a real risk in this operation.

It remains to construct a good ileostomy. The major requirements are as follows.

*   **A good site in the right abdominal wall**. If appropriate, the patient is asked to wear an ileostomy appliance half full of water to allow it to hang. A belt is attached and the patient is asked to stand. Once the site is chosen, the site is marked. This is easy to do in the elective situation, but may well be difficult in the emergency situation, and the best possible estimate has to be made. The belt will need to lie at or below the waist line and this can be gauged by eye. The site for the stoma is then placed in this line and as far as possible from both the right anterior superior iliac spine and the umbilicus. It should lie in the centre of a flat area of skin to which an ileostomy appliance can readily be fixed. The main concern of the patient is for the appliance to be secure, and if it is to stay in place it must not impinge on bony points, scars and depressions. If a patient has an ugly puckered scar from a previous appendicectomy wound then the ileostomy may be brought out on the left side.

    When the appropriate site has been chosen the skin is tented up using tissue forceps and a disc of skin 2 cm in diameter is removed by cutting across the base of the tent. This results in the excision of a neat circle of skin. The fat is separated and a cruciate incision is made through the sheath of the rectus muscle, which is then gently split with scissors. With suitable retraction the peritoneum is identified and opened. This should allow the terminal ileum to be brought out without undue compression and yet leave no room for herniation of bowel alongside it. It is important to be careful not to tear the inferior epigastric artery.

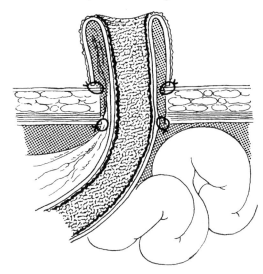

Figure 7.18 Construction of terminal spout ileostomy, illustrating the 4/0 sutures that anchor the seromuscular layer of the ileum to the rectus sheath.

The majority of the patients are thin, but in a small minority the patient may be obese, especially if on steroids. It may be difficult to bring the ileostomy through the abdominal wall and form a nice spout. In these circumstances we staple the end of the ileum so that there is no need to bring the de Martel clamp through the abdominal wall.

- In the circumstances of emergency colectomy it is possible that the ileostomy may need to be taken down to allow reconstructive surgery such as ileorectal anastomosis or a pouch operation. The ileum is therefore brought directly out, across the peritoneal cavity. The wide space thus left between the ileostomy and the lateral wall of the iliac fossa is so wide that we have not seen a hernia through it.

The ileum is drawn out gently and a good pulse is seen in the mesentery, and the orientation is checked so as not to produce a twist. Approximately 4–6 cm of ileum is left to project outside the abdomen. Six 4/0 braided nylon sutures attach the seromuscular coat of ileum to anterior rectus sheath. Great care must be taken not to pick up mucosa lest a fistula result (Figure 7.18).

- **A final check is made of the abdominal cavity**. It is thoroughly lavaged and closed using a mass closure technique with 1 PDS. In over 100 laparotomies for colitis there has not been a case of wound dehiscence. The skin is closed with a subcuticular absorbable suture before forming the spout. The wound is cleaned and covered with a fresh pack.

It remains to construct a good ileal spout. The de Martel clamp is removed, two Babcock intestinal forceps are passed down the lumen for 3–4 cm and the mucosa is grasped. The cut end of ileum is then everted to produce a spout measuring 3–4 cm. This is done by placing a 2/0 chromic catgut suture on a curved trocar-pointed needle in such a way as to triangulate the stoma. The suture runs from the mucosal edge into the seromuscular wall of the ileum and then subcuticularly. Three such sutures are placed, one directly opposite the mesentery and the other two at right angles to this. These are tied and the ileum is everted to produce a neat spout. The gaps between these sutures are closed by several mucocutaneous sutures. The appliance is applied, ensuring a good fit over the stoma. The modern plastic bag allows the surgeon to inspect the finished stoma and detect any hint of ischaemia.

Outcome

In Aberdeen 206 emergency and urgent (within 5 days) operations have been performed for IBD. Among 160 patients with UC, four required a panproctocolectomy for severe bleeding with advanced rectal disease. In 156 subtotal or total colectomy and ileostomy was performed, with closure of the rectosigmoid area in 136, and with 20 having lower sigmoid brought out as a mucous fistula. The indications for operation were toxic megacolon in 35 and fulminant colitis in 121. In 30 (19%) patients the operation was done within 24 hours of admission (three deaths) and in 130 during the first 5 days (two deaths); three deaths were due to cardiorespiratory disease and two followed multiorgan failure secondary to peritonitis. The overall mortality rate was 2.4%, and for wound infections 6%. In the 46 patients with Crohn's colitis, all had a colectomy with rectal preservation; there were four deaths in patients who arrived with advanced peritonitis.

Leizonmarck *et al.* (1989) in Stockholm reported 185 acute operations for severe UC performed during 1955–1984. At first many panproctocolectomies were done but by 1980–1984 most patients had a subtotal colectomy, with a view to a later pouch operation. Mortality had fallen from 38% in 1960–1964 to 1.6% in 63 patients in 1980–1984.

Nearly all deaths now occur in patients who only reach hospital at a late stage. Early admission by family doctors, and close consultation between physicians and surgeons, are the chief keys to success in treating complicated IBD.

REFERENCES

Binder, S. C., Patterson, J. F. and Glotzer, D. J. (1974) Toxic megacolon in UC. *Gastroenterology*, **66**, 909–915.

Brooke, B. N. and Sampson, P. A. (1964) An indication for surgery in acute ulcerative colitis. *Lancet*, **ii**, 1272–1273.

Crile, G. and Thomas, C. Y. (1951) Treatment of acute toxic ulcerative colitis by ileostomy and simultaneous colectomy. *Gastroenterology*, **19**, 58–68.

Fazio, V. W. (1980) Toxic megacolon in ulcerative colitis and Crohn's disease. *Clin. Gastroenterol.*, **9**, 389–407.

Goligher, J. C., Hoffman, D. C. and de Dombal, F. T. (1970) Surgical treatment of severe attacks of ulcerative colitis with special references to the advantages of early operation. *BMJ*, **iv**, 703–706.

Hulten, L., Lindhafen, J. and Lundgren, O. (1977) Regional intestinal blood flow in ulcerative colitis and Crohn's disease. *Gastroenterology*, **72**, 388–396.

Jalan, K. N., Sircus, W., Card, W. I. *et al.* (1969) An experience of ulcerative colitis: I. Toxic dilatation in 55 cases. *Gastroenterology*, **57**, 68–82.

Kyle, J. (1992) Crohn's in north and northern isles of Scotland: an epidemiological review. *Gastroenterology*, **103**, 392–399.

Leizonmarck, C. E., Brostrom, O., Monsen, V. *et al.* (1989) Surgical treatment of ulcerative colitis in Stockholm county 1955–84. *Dis. Colon Rectum*, **32**, 918–926.

Lennard-Jones, J. E., Ritchie, J. K., Hilder, W. *et al.* (1975) Assessment of severity in colitis. *Gut*, **16**, 579–584.

McConnell, F., Hanelin, J. and Robbins, L. L. (1958) Plain film diagnosis of fulminating ulcerative colitis. *Radiology*, **71**, 674–682.

McIntyre, P. B., Powell-Tuck, J., Wood, S. R. *et al.* (1986) Controlled trial of bowel rest in the treatment of severe acute colitis. *Gut*, **27**, 481–485.

McKee, R., Keenan, R. A. and Munro, A. (1995) Colectomy for acute colitis: Is it safe to close the rectal stump. *Int. J. Colorectal Dis.*, **10**, 222–224.

Marshak, R. H., Lester, L. J. and Friedman, A. I. (1950) Megacolon: a complication of ulcerative colitis. *Gastroenterology*, **16**, 768–772.

Re Mine, S. G. and McIlraith, D. C. (1980) Bowel perforation in steroid-treated patients. *Ann. Surg.*, **192**, 581–586.

Ritchie, J. K., Ritchie, S. M., McIntyre, P. B. *et al.* (1984) Management of severe acute colitis in district hospitals. *J. R. Soc. Med.*, **77**, 465–471.

Sampson, P. A. and Walker, P. C. (1961) Dilatation of the colon in ulcerative colitis. *BMJ*, **ii**, 1119–1123.

Sinclair, T. S., Brunt, P. W. and Mowat, N. A. G. (1983) Non-specific proctocolitis in North Eastern Scotland: a community study. *Gastroenterology*, **85**, 1–11.

Truelove, S. C. and Jewell, D. P. (1974) Intensive intravenous regime for severe attacks of acute colitis. *Lancet*, **ii**, 1067–1070.

Truelove, S. C. and Marks, C. G. (1981) Toxic megacolon: pathogenesis, diagnosis and treatment. *Clin. Gastroenterol.*, **10**, 107–117.

Truelove, S. C. and Witts, L. J. (1955) Cortisone in ulcerative colitis: final report on therapeutic trial. *BMJ*, **ii**, 1041–1048.

Truelove, S. C., Lee, E. G., Willoughby, C. P. *et al.* (1978) Further experience in the treatment of severe attacks of ulcerative colitis. *Lancet*, **ii**, 1086–1108.

7.4.2 ACUTE INFECTIVE ENTERITIS AND COLITIS

Both the common bacterial causes of adult gastroenteritis, *Salmonella* and *Campylobacter* spp., usually cause an enteritis, but have a lesser effect on the colon.

***Campylobacter* enteritis** is particularly likely to be seen by surgeons because after prodromal fever, headache and malaise, patients complain of profuse diarrhoea and considerable abdominal pain (Skirrow, 1977). This is generally central and colicky but it may shift to the right iliac fossa and then these patients are admitted as surgical emergencies. The pain is clearly quite distressing, but the signs are usually not sufficient to call for laparotomy (p. 53).

However, a small proportion of patients with ***Salmonella* and *Campylobacter* enteritis** develop a colitis, pass blood, pus and mucus, and on sigmoidoscopy show an oedematous granular bleeding rectal mucosa (Lambert *et al.*, 1979; Mandal and Schofield, 1992).

Occasionally these changes progress to a degree that strongly resembles acute ulcerative colitis, and Schofield (1982) recorded 20 patients seen over 8 years with toxic dilatation of the colon, of whom eight had UC, six had CD, and six had acute *Salmonella* colitis: all were severely ill with a transverse colon greater than 8 cm in diameter. The patients with infective colitis had a short history of less than 3 weeks, and only two of the six had blood in the stools. Sigmoidoscopy showed a proctitis in all, but it was more severe in patients with IBD than infective colitis. Schofield particularly remarks on the quick improvement shown on intravenous fluids only among the six infective patients. However one of the six showed increasing signs of peritoneal irritation and had a laparotomy: the colon was greatly dilated but did not look like IBD, although an area of transverse colon was not viable and had to be exteriorized as a colostomy.

We have had one such case in which the signs compelled us to undertake laparotomy, and a Hartmann-type resection was performed.

It is important to bear this possibility in mind, to take stool cultures in all patients with acute colitis and in patients with a history only of days to observe the effect of intravenous fluid for a few hours before embarking on corticosteroid treatment.

***Yersinia enterocolitica* infection** can also involve the colon and, rarely, toxic megacolon (Stuart *et al.*, 1986). They suggest that when a patient presents with toxic dilatation, without a history of IBD, it is important to culture the stools and estimate antibody titres for these common bacterial causes of enterocolitis.

Amoebic colitis is generally treated on an outpatient basis, but in its severe form can carry a very high mortality. Luvuno *et al.* (1982, 1985) in Durban, South Africa, have made a particular study of fulminant amoebic colitis. Many of their patients are seriously malnourished and some have tuberculosis, so mortality can be very high. Both perforation and megacolon can complicate severe colitis and by a combination of angiography and histology Luvuno has shown that the basic pathology is amoebic invasion of the vasa recta, with thrombotic occlusion of the vessel. This produces transmural necrosis, which may be completely sealed off by an adhesive wrap of omentum, or it may produce a free perforation. Lesser degrees of ischaemia may produce megacolon. In these very sick patients Luvuno *et al.* (1985) prefer to do an ileostomy and washout and decompress the colon, rather than perform a colectomy, provided free perforation has not occurred.

REFERENCES

Lambert, M. E., Schofield, P. F., Ironside, A. G. *et al.* (1979) *Campylobacter* colitis. *BMJ*, **i**, 857–859.

Luvuno, F. M., Mtshali, Z. and Baker, L. W. (1982) Treatment options in fulminating amoebic colitis: an autopsy study. *S. Afr. J. Surg.*, **20**, 269–274.

Luvuno, F. M., Mtshali, Z. and Baker, L. W. (1985) Vascular occlusion in the pathogenesis of complicated amoebic colitis: evidence for an hypothesis. *Br. J. Surg.*, **72**, 123–127.

Mandal, B. K. and Schofield, P. F. (1992) Tropical colonic diseases. *BMJ*, **305**, 638–641.

Schofield, P. F. (1982) Toxic dilation and perforation in inflammatory bowel disease. *Ann. R. Coll. Surg. Engl.*, **64**, 318–320.

Skirrow, M. B. (1977) *Campylobacter* enteritis: a 'new' disease. *BMJ*, **ii**, 9–11.

Stuart, R. C., Leahy, A. L., Cafferkey, M. T. *et al.* (1986) *Yersinia* enterocolitis infection and toxic megacolon. *Br. J. Surg.*, **73**, 590.

7.5 PSEUDOMEMBRANOUS OR ANTIBIOTIC-ASSOCIATED COLITIS

A few years after the introduction of antibiotics some patients developed severe diarrhoea after an abdominal operation that had required antibiotic cover. This was often ascribed to overgrowth of a virulent strain of *Staphylococcus aureus*. If sigmoidoscopy was performed some membrane was seen on the rectal mucosa.

It is now known that such attacks can occur not only in postoperative patients but in those taking an antibiotic for a medical illness. For some years it has been recognized that *Clostridium difficile* can be isolated from the stools of patients with severe diarrhoea who have received an antibiotic, broad-spectrum penicillins, cephalosporins or clindamycin being those commonly identified. These agents alter the normal bacterial flora of the colon and allow *C. difficile* to colonize the bowel and produce an enterotoxin (Bradbury and Barrett, 1997).

In a typical case profuse watery diarrhoea occurs, with the passage of much mucus. There may be abdominal pain and tenderness and the patient is clearly unwell and febrile. In a severe attack there is marked small- and large-bowel distension with mucosal oedema and thumb-printing.

Sigmoidoscopy reveals the characteristic whitish-yellow plaques, 3–10 mm in diameter, scattered over glistening, oedematous rectal mucous membrane. The organism can be cultured from faeces, and there are now assays (ELISAs) that detect the toxin in stools and are completed in 3 hours.

Once confirmed, any antibiotic being administered is stopped. Metronidazole is the treatment of choice, given by mouth 250 mg 6-hourly, or intravenously in a dose of 500 mg 8-hourly. Vancomycin is equally effective but more expensive and best kept in reserve: it has to be given orally or *via* a nasogastric tube, 200 mg 6-hourly.

This treatment is usually effective but a close watch must be kept because a few patients develop toxic megacolon, and some perforate. Subtotal colectomy and ileostomy is the operation that has given the best results (Bradbury and Barrett, 1997).

We have had two such patients. In one elderly patient a Hartmann-type of distal colon resection was performed. The other patient was a young woman who had taken co-trimoxazole for cystitis and who developed acute severe diarrhoea 5 days later. She rapidly deteriorated and developed a distended tender abdomen and we strongly suspected a perforation. At operation we fortunately carried out a further sigmoidoscopy, which showed typical scattered plaques on an inflamed rectal mucosa. Anxiety about perforation made us open the abdomen and the whole colon was acutely inflamed and oedematous, with a considerable amount of free fluid. Feeling that the colitis would probably settle, a split ileostomy was established. Convalescence was slow and complicated by a gastric stress ulcer with massive haemorrhage, which required a very urgent gastrectomy. The ileostomy was later closed when the colon had returned to normal.

REFERENCE

Bradbury, A. W. and Barrett, S. (1997) Surgical aspects of *Clostridium difficile* colitis (review). *Br. J. Surg.*, **84**, 150–159.

7.6   ISCHAEMIA OF THE COLON

This is fortunately not a common event, because ischaemia of the large bowel is particularly serious, its intrinsic mural damage being potentiated by the rich bacterial population in the lumen. The whole subject is extensively reviewed by Marston (1986). The causes can be broadly classified into (1) specific causes and (2) spontaneous ischaemia.

7.6.1   SPECIFIC CAUSES

Extrinsic pressure on the blood supply occurs in some cases of volvulus (p. 289), and on the occasions when the colon is involved in a strangulated hernia. This may occur in large scrotal inguinal hernias and in paraumbilical hernias. The effects of strangulation of colon are not so acutely noticeable as they generally are in small bowel; pain is not so marked and vomiting tends to occur late, but the dangers are just as great. These are considered further on p. 223.

Surgical ligation of the inferior mesenteric artery occurs whenever an aortic aneurysm is resected and usually the sigmoid survives by perfusion through the marginal artery, but colonic ischaemia is a well-recognized complication, and close attention is paid to colonic perfusion at the end of the reconstruction. In 2137 aortoiliac reconstructions, Brewster *et al.* (1991) saw 19 cases of colonic ischaemia characterized by onset of severe pain and bloody diarrhoea, and requiring urgent re-operation, for resection of ischaemic colon and colostomy. In marginal cases, without abdominal signs, colonoscopy will show mucosal oedema and discoloration in the sigmoid colon.

Trauma to the abdomen may damage the mesocolon, either directly by a penetrating wound, or by crushing in a blunt injury (p. 418).

Reference has already been made to the effect of rising intraluminal pressure in large-bowel obstruction (p. 267).

7.6.2 SPONTANEOUS ISCHAEMIA

'A possible cause of acute structural change in the colon is deprivation of arterial blood. Episodes of ischaemia involving the heart or brain are common enough, and it would be surprising if similar events did not occasionally take place in the intestine, particularly the large intestine whose blood supply is comparatively precarious' (Marston *et al.*, 1966).

There is increasing evidence that this statement was fully justified. Acute obstruction of the inferior mesenteric artery itself, comparable to the much more familiar superior mesenteric obstruction, is a rare event, but it has become clear over the last 20 years that the small vessels of the colon are open to a number of influences. Blood flow is slower in the large bowel than in the small intestine, it is diminished by colonic activity and it is influenced by the emotions (Boley *et al.*, 1978).

The reason for diminished flow may be small-vessel disease or the effects of low flow in, for example, hypovolaemic shock, cardiac failure, digitalis intoxication or, it may be, venous thrombosis (possibly associated with the use of oral contraceptives).

The most important aspect of this type of colonic ischaemia is that observation shows that the damage may be either recoverable or irreversible (Robert *et al.*, 1993).

If the interruption of flow is recoverable the colon may suffer some damage but the integrity of the colon wall will not be affected and the patient can be treated conservatively: this has come to be known as 'ischaemic colitis' (Marston *et al.*, 1966). The interruption of flow that is sufficiently extensive and prolonged to produce full-thickness damage to the colon wall has been named 'gangrene of the colon'.

7.6.2.1 Acute gangrene

This is a rare but distinct condition that presents as a very acute illness, requires speedy action and carries a high mortality. It can be distinguished from acute obstruction of the superior mesenteric artery, and of the inferior artery, in which damage is limited to the left colon.

A typical patient is middle-aged or elderly, and is often under treatment for hypertension or ischaemic heart disease. However, these patients are usually in their normal state of health when they are suddenly taken with severe lower abdominal pain and vomiting. The pain spreads and grows worse and the patient is obviously acutely ill, so they reach hospital within hours. Within 4–6 hours of onset they are pale, cyanosed, cold and hypotensive, with signs usually of generalized, but sometimes of localized, peritonitis. It is evident that they require urgent resuscitation and laparotomy.

When the abdomen is opened, all show a considerable volume of foul-smelling turbid free fluid, and the colon shows areas of obvious full-thickness ischaemia. Tate *et al.* (1965), who describe a classical case, particularly noted a sharp line of demarcation between healthy and ischaemic bowel at the ileocaecal valve, and in the midsigmoid area, thus clearly showing that the ischaemia was not due to superior or inferior mesenteric artery obstruction. Extensive areas of green gangrenous change were seen, with the consistency of blotting-paper, and some intervening areas of viable colon. These are well illustrated by Killingback and Williams (1961): in six patients only one patient had complete involvement of the colon, while patches of gangrene were scattered through the colon in the others. There is general agreement that pulsation in the mesocolic vessels is normal. If the interior of the colon is examined immediately after resection it is evident that mucosal destruction is much more severe and continuous than are the changes on the serosal surface.

Microscopy shows necrosis of the mucosa and intense polymorph infiltration and inflammation in the submucosa. Gram staining shows invasion of mucosa and submucosa by enormous numbers of Gram-positive bacilli that are morphologically like clostridia. Tate *et al.* (1965) obtained a pure growth of *C. welchii* from their specimen. Whitehead (1971) remarks on the frequency of intravascular thrombi in the small vessels within the wall of the colon.

Killingback and Williams (1961) name this condition 'necrotizing colitis', Tate *et al.* (1965) call it '*Clostridium welchii* colitis', Whitehead (1971) calls it 'ischaemic enterocolitis' and Hunt (1977) refers to 'gangrenous ischaemic colitis' to distinguish this syndrome from the form of ischaemic colitis generally recognized (see below).

Most workers on the subject believe that for some reason colonic perfusion is reduced and this allows invasion of the colonic wall by virulent faecal clostridia to take place. The only example we have seen was probably secondary to a low-flow state occurring in a patient with Gram-negative bacteraemia from a urinary tract infection, and in this patient gas was visible within the wall of the colon in the preoperative X-ray.

When seen these patients will generally be thought to have perforated diverticular disease, or mesenteric arterial obstruction. It is clear that rapid resuscitation is required, with intravenous fluids and colloid, parenteral antibiotics and nasal oxygen. Central venous pressure readings will be helpful, and dopamine may be required.

Laparotomy will be undertaken as soon as possible and it will at once be evident that a length of colon is gangrenous. This should be quickly resected and a thorough tetracycline lavage performed. Close attention must be given to the point of division of the bowel. It is not enough to see mesenteric pulsation because larger vessels are usually patent. Resection must be taken back to a point in both proximal and distal bowel where the mucosa is a good colour and there is active bleeding from the cut edge of the submucosa. The only safe way of terminating this operation is to exteriorize the two ends through separate incisions.

These patients will clearly need to be nursed in an intensive therapy unit, and will often require respiratory assistance for several days.

Killingback and Williams (1961) resected all their six patients, and Hunt (1977) all his five patients, and six of the 11 survived. It is clear that speedy resection and formation of stomata is essential, and it is unwise to consider these patients too ill to withstand resection.

7.6.2.2 'Ischaemic colitis'

This term is not entirely accurate but it is widely used and is generally understood as a definition of a clinical entity. Boley *et al.* (1963), who were the first to describe it, called it 'reversible vascular occlusion of the colon' and this emphasizes the fact that in some patients the signs produced by ischaemia gradually resolve, with the bowel returning to normal. However, in others there is permanent damage, with the ischaemic bowel wall surviving to heal by fibrosis and formation of a stricture.

Almost all patients are over 60 years, and many have arterial disease in the cardiac or peripheral vessels. In a typical case there is sudden onset of cramping pain in the lower abdomen, mainly in the left side. There is often tenesmus and soon some bright or dark red blood and clots are passed *per rectum*. There may be tenderness over the left colon but the patient does not appear ill, and recordings are generally normal. Rectal examination and sigmoidoscopy show altered blood in the rectum, but rarely any mucosal abnormality: occasionally some submucosal haemorrhage is seen at the rectosigmoid junction. This is a notably different picture from the brisk rectal haemorrhage that occurs in angiodysplasia and diverticular disease, which is more profuse and not accompanied by abdominal pain (p. 374).

If colonoscopy is performed, the affected segment of colon shows bluish, oedematous bulging mucosa in the affected segment. The chief diagnostic test is an urgent contrast enema, which shows a narrowed colon with characteristic 'thumb printing' of its outline, produced by the oedematous mucosa bulging into the lumen; this is usually centred on the splenic flexure and involves varying lengths of transverse or descending colon. This change appears 3–4 days after the onset, and may remain for days or weeks.

Once seen, this is a very recognizable clinical picture and because it is generally a self-limiting event ischaemic colitis can be treated conservatively, with the expectation that pain and bleeding will settle in a day or two.

On a few occasions there have been signs of peritonism and resection has provided pathological material (Brown, 1972): this shows scattered mucosal ulcers, with a striking thickening of the submucosa due to oedema and later granulation tissue and fibrosis. It is this fibrosis which, in about half the patients, goes on to the formation of a localized stricture. A barium enema should be performed after 6–8 weeks: in some the colon will have returned to normal, in others the lumen shows a funnel-shaped, smooth narrowing, without any shouldering suggestive of carcinoma, or rose-thorn ulcers suggestive of Crohn's disease. Most strictures are asymptomatic.

The nature of the vascular lesion remains obscure. Ischaemic colitis is an acute illness that generally affects healthy individuals, and its most striking feature is its evanescent character, with improvement in the striking changes seen in barium enema over the space of a few days.

There is considerable animal experimental evidence that these changes occur after interruption of the mesocolic vessels. A few cases have been described in women on oestrogen-containing contraceptive pills (Marcuson and Farman, 1971), and other cases are associated with sudden diminution in mesenteric perfusion due to haemorrhagic hypovolaemia, or to atrial fibrillation. These factors may precipitate a thrombosis that has an acute effect on the mucosa and submucosa, which are more susceptible to ischaemia than the muscularis, which is able to survive as the collateral circulation improves. The reason for the frequent localization of these changes at the splenic flexure is not certain; it may be related to the variable anatomy of the marginal artery at the splenic flexure (arc of Riolan).

The treatment of the great majority of patients with ischaemic colitis is expectant. A provisional diagnosis is made on the basis of the characteristic history, and the patient is kept under close observation in hospital. It is most unusual (Marston, 1986) for such a patient to progress to gangrene and require urgent laparotomy. However, one of Hunt's (1977) 17 patients came to operation when clear signs of peritonitis developed 2½ days after the onset of pain. The course of the healing process in the colon is followed by barium enema. Colonoscopy may prove to have a part of play in this.

If a stricture develops and produces significant obstruction this is dealt with on its merits. In the 142 patients reported by Boley *et al.* (1978) 67% settled, 13% developed a stricture and 20% developed gangrene.

Ischaemic proctitis is rare (Boley *et al.*, 1978), probably because there is an excellent triple blood supply through the superior, middle and inferior rectal arteries. We saw an example (Orr and Jones, 1982) in a 66-year-old man with a history of myocardial infarction and hypertension. He complained of acute lower abdominal pain and fresh rectal bleeding. He had lower abdominal tenderness and on sigmoidoscopy necrotic blue-black rectal mucosa was seen, with a coarse, lumpy surface up to the rectosigmoid junction, above which normal mucosa was seen. He was a very poor subject for laparotomy and fortunately settled on intravenous fluids, with gentamicin and metronidazole. After a month there was a tight stricture 1 cm in diameter 5 cm from the anus, which required dilatation on several occasions over 6 months before finally resolving.

REFERENCES

Boley, S. J., Schwartz, S., Lish J. *et al.* (1963) Reversible vascular occlusion of the colon. *Surg. Gynecol. Obstet.*, **116**, 53–60.

Boley, S. J., Brandt, L. J. and Veeth, F. J. (1978) Ischemic disorders of the intestines. *Curr. Probl. Surg.*, **15**(4), 6–85.

Brewster, D. C., Franklin, D. P., Cambria, R. P. *et al.* (1991) Intestinal ischemia complicating abdominal aortic aneurysm surgery. *Surgery*, **109**, 447–454.

Brown, A. R. (1972) Non-gangrenous ischaemic colitis: a review of 17 cases. *Br. J. Surg.*, **59**, 463–473.

Hunt, D. R. (1977) Surgical management of gangrenous ischaemic colitis: report of 5 cases. *Dis. Colon Rectum*, **20**, 36–39.

Killingback, M. and Williams, K. L. (1961) Necrotizing colitis. *Br. J. Surg.*, **49**, 175–185.

Marcuson, R. W. and Farman, J. A. (1971) Ischaemic disease of the colon. *Proc. R. Soc. Med.*, **64**, 1080–1083.

Marston, A. (1986) *Vascular Disease of the Gut*, Edward Arnold, London.

Marston, A., Pheils, M. T., Thomas, M. L. *et al.* (1966) Ischaemic colitis. *Gut*, **7**, 1–15.

Orr, G. and Jones, P. F. (1982) Ischaemic proctitis followed by stricture. *Br. J. Surg.*, **69**, 433–434.

Robert, J. H, Mentha, G. and Rohner, A. (1993) Ischaemic colitis: two distinct patterns of severity, *Gut*, **34**, 4–6.

Tate, G. T., Thompson, H. and Willis, A. T. (1965) *Clostridium welchii* colitis. *Br. J. Surg.*, **52**, 194–197.

Whitehead, R. (1971) Ischaemic enterocolitis: an expression of the intravascular coagulation syndrome. *Gut*, **12**, 912–917.

7.7 ANORECTAL EMERGENCIES

7.7.1 ACUTE PERIANAL HAEMATOMA

The name in common currency for this condition is imprecise and it has been more accurately described as a 'clotted perianal venous saccule'. This acutely painful condition is very common. The mechanism for inducing the clot in the dilated subcutaneous anal vein is obscure but is often associated with a strain. A tense, blue, shiny, circumscribed swelling arises at the anal verge, usually on the left or right side, although occasionally in the midline. There is often a little ecchymosis of the surrounding skin. This lump is very tender and is usually continuously uncomfortable for the patient, becoming acutely painful if sat upon and during defecation.

The diagnosis is usually easy because the signs are quite characteristic. If a hasty inspection is made, it is possible to think that there is a prolapsed strangulated internal haemorrhoid, but in these circumstances the oedematous anal skin is usually more widely involved, and if this skin is gently drawn back the dark lower pole of the prolapsed haemorrhoid will be seen.

An immediate diagnosis can be made and prompt surgical treatment can give complete relief. The patient is placed in the left lateral position, and it is helpful if an assistant can lift the overhanging right buttock upwards, to open the natal cleft. The skin is shaved and cleaned. After local infiltration with 1% lignocaine, the 'haematoma' can be painlessly incised in a radial direction, releasing the tense clot. The cavity is simply left open with a light dressing laid on top. The patient is asked to bathe regularly for a few days, and the wound quickly granulates and heals.

If treatment is not given in the first 2–3 days the haematoma will begin to resolve and pain will lessen. It is then no longer an urgent matter to operate because the main reason for operation is to relieve the severe and continuing discomfort. Resolution is usually complete, given time. A few individuals appear to be predisposed to the formation of these clots. Any internal haemorrhoids should be treated by injection of phenol in almond oil, but this does not always prevent recurrence.

7.7.2 ACUTELY PROLAPSED AND STRANGULATED HAEMORRHOIDS

This is a painful condition that can be speedily relieved by the right treatment.

The initial event is prolapse of a pre-existing internal haemorrhoid, the lower pole of which comes to lie well outside the anal sphincter. This condition is painful, so the sphincter involuntarily tightens around the prolapsed haemorrhoid and venous return is interrupted. The haemorrhoid becomes increasingly congested, cyanotic and swollen and, with the obstruction of venous drainage through the branches of the inferior haemorrhoidal veins, oedema of the perianal skin also occurs. A deep trench divides the strangulated haemorrhoids from the oedematous perianal skin, and this appearance is characteristic.

If diagnosed at an early stage, i.e. within a matter of a few hours, prolapsed haemorrhoids should be treated by manual reduction. The patient lies in the left lateral position, a gauze pad is placed over the haemorrhoids and pressure is applied with the extended index, middle and ring fingers. The patient is asked to concentrate on breathing deeply and steadily while pressure, gentle at first, is gradually increased. There should be no hurry to achieve reduction, because the initial pressure helps to reduce oedema: then, if the piles are not too rigid, they will reduce within the anal canal. There is a tendency for prolapse to recur and the patient should be advised to take a laxative and stay in bed for 48 hours. Defecation may cause the piles to prolapse again but the patient should take a hot bath and, lying on the side, replace the piles: this is usually much easier once the initial prolapse has been reduced and oedema has subsided. The thrombosed vessels in the pile undergo fibrosis and this may lead to a natural resolution of the haemorrhoids. The patient should be reviewed over the following weeks and any residual haemorrhoids should be injected.

When the haemorrhoid has been prolapsed for some time the oedema in the tissues makes the whole area so rigid, and the anal sphincter is so tightly contracted, that reduction is virtually impossible. By this time the lower pole of the haemorrhoid is usually gangrenous. The classical treatment for this situation was bed rest, which often extended over a week or two. However, a gentle rectal examination shows that in the great majority of patients the pedicle of the haemorrhoid is quite soft and, as Smith (1967) pointed out, ligation is quite practical. Immediate haemorrhoidectomy is now standard treatment and is associated with much more rapid recovery.

Technique for emergency haemorrhoidectomy

The injection of bupivacaine with adrenaline reduces both peroperative bleeding and postoperative pain but does distort the anatomy even further, with an increased risk of excising too much tissue. The anus is gently dilated and most surgeons now prefer the cutting diathermy needle to scissors for the dissection. A conscious effort must be made to remove the minimum of skin, and it is particularly important to preserve good skin bridges. The external and internal sphincters must be clearly identified and excessive traction, which risks pulling internal sphincter muscle fibres into the excised tissue, guarded against. If the dissection proceeds into the lower rectum the size of the resulting pedicle requiring transfixion and division becomes progressively smaller and the apex lies above and not in the anal canal. The size of the haemorrhoidal masses excised reduces progressively, commencing, usually, with the left lateral and largest mass. There is a particular risk of the prolapsed haemorrhoids forming a circumferential deformity and it is preferable to err on the side of too conservative an excision of skin and mucosa rather than risk later anal stenosis. This may result in the immediate postoperative appearance of very oedematous bridges after a classical open haemorrhoidectomy but this will resolve fairly quickly although residual skin tags may require later trimming. Alternatively a 'closed' haemorrhoidectomy may be performed, which requires less excision of perianal skin with immediate suture of the anal mucosa and skin. While this can appear much more attractive immediately postoperatively we lack conviction that the final result differs substantially from healing by secondary intention.

In either case there is immediate relief of pain, although analgesics and laxatives must be prescribed postoperatively. A combination of senna and lactulose or Fybogel is suitable after an emergency procedure. Patients can go home within 1–2 days but it is often necessary to stay until after the first bowel movement on the third or fourth day, which can be painful and require opiate analgesia.

This emergency has a reputation for being complicated by portal pyaemia, but this does not appear to have any basis in contemporary experience. However, it is important to examine the perineum carefully before operating. Rarely, the whole pile becomes infected, with involvement of the pedicle, and then any attempt at dissection must be performed under antibiotic cover and only by a surgeon familiar with this type of procedure.

7.7.3 ANORECTAL ABSCESSES

This is a common and painful emergency that results in about 7000 hospital admissions annually in England and Wales, with many more patients being treated as outpatients. These abscesses often cause patients considerable trouble over several days before they arrive at hospital. Buchan and Grace (1973) found that, among the 183 patients they studied (of whom 80% were men), almost 50% had had pain for more than 5 days.

There is a tendency for there to be some delay between onset and eventual surgical drainage. It is a common experience for these patients to have had antibiotic therapy for some days. This is not effective treatment for a collection of pus and surgical incision is an urgent matter because: the patient suffers a great deal of pain; the risk of internal discharge, predisposing to fistula formation, is real; and finally, in the debilitated long-stay patient, such inappropriate management can be a preliminary to spreading perineal gangrene. The skin overlying anorectal abscesses is tough, so waiting for spontaneous drainage tends to be a slow and uncomfortable, as well as a hazardous, form of treatment.

There is general agreement that the majority of anorectal abscesses commence with infection of an anal gland (Figure 7.19).

Many of these glands lie in the loose tissues of the intersphincteric plane, in which it is easy for infection to spread. Commonly this occurs downwards, to form a **perianal abscess**. Less frequently, the infection penetrates the internal sphincter to produce an **ischiorectal abscess** (Figure 7.20). Rarely, infection spreads upwards, above the levator ani, to form a **pelvirectal abscess**.

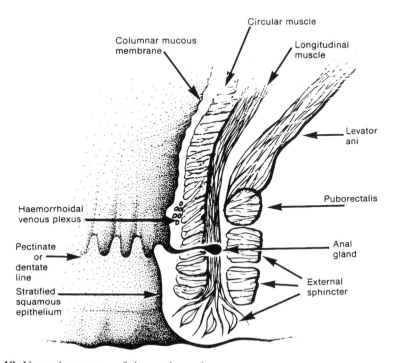

Figure 7.19 Normal anatomy of the anal canal.

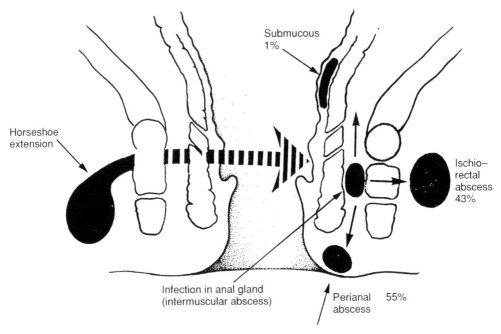

Figure 7.20 Sites and incidence of the principal anorectal abscesses (after Jones and Siwek, 1986).

Perianal abscess

This is the commonest abscess, accounting for 56% of those seen in Cardiff hospitals (Buchan and Grace, 1973). They are readily diagnosed, presenting as an obvious tense, shiny, red swelling immediately beside the anus. Tenderness is acute and defecation painful. However, if the finger is gently passed into the rectum along the opposite wall of the anal canal there is no deep mass or tenderness. Sometimes a perianal abscess extends forward towards the labia or scrotum in the subcutaneous plane.

Incision and drainage
These abscesses can usually be effectively dealt with by a simple radial incision and it is unnecessary to carry out 'deroofing' except for excision of frankly necrotic skin. Any loculi in the cavity are broken down by gentle curettage, debridement with a swab on an artery forceps and irrigation. The cavity should not be 'packed' and application of a light absorbent dressing to capture serosanguinous discharge with twice-daily bathing is followed by rapid healing. Most patients can be treated in a department equipped for day-stay surgery.

Incision, drainage and primary closure
Although such abscess cavities usually heal quickly by granulation, recovery can be expedited and consumption of resources reduced if the well-established practice of incision, drainage and primary suture is followed. The value of this policy has been documented for many years (Ellis, 1960) but it is a curious phenomenon that few centres adopt it until they have themselves carried out a study to confirm its validity (Stewart *et al.*, 1985; Abraham *et*

al., 1997). Following incision and drainage as described the incision is closed with interrupted vertical mattress sutures, which should obliterate the cavity. For large cavities and those extending anteriorly the skin is closed and a suction drain inserted. The original requirement for systemic antibiotics has been modified and there is good evidence that 24 hours of antibiotics is as effective as 4 days (Lundhus and Gottrup, 1993). Indeed, we have shown that it is not necessary to provide routine antibiotic cover for primary closure in the abscess of spreading cellulitis (Stewart *et al.*, 1985). We, like all others, found healing time to be reduced from 25 days to 7, and time off work from 2 weeks to less than a week, with primary closure.

Incision, drainage and fistulotomy

Sometimes careful inspection of the anal canal reveals that there is a coexistent fistula, and Buchan and Grace (1973) found one in 39 of 115 patients, although they correctly remark that it is not difficult to make a false track. Unless an obvious very low subcutaneous intrasphincteric track is found it is probably better to leave any possible track alone. Although some authors have recommended aggressive treatment of fistulas at the emergency operation this is unnecessarily hazardous. Tang and colleagues (1996) have studied this question: they have shown that there is very little difference in the recurrence rate between those patients with no obvious fistula and those with an opening demonstrated at the time of incision and drainage. Furthermore in a randomized trial of patients with a definite fistula comparing simple incision and drainage with immediate fistulotomy, only three of 21 patients treated by drainage alone developed recurrent sepsis compared with none in the 24 treated by immediate fistulotomy. Clearly a conservative policy with treatment as indicated at postoperative review is appropriate for most patients.

Ischiorectal abscess

Although this is a familiar term that is used to describe all anal abscesses, only some 40% are truly ischiorectal in position (Figure 7.20). These abscesses are more deeply placed than perianal abscesses and are consequently not easy to see, causing only a slight fullness and reddening of the skin over the fossa. Diagnosis depends on a gentle rectal examination showing that one ischiorectal fossa is soft and painless whereas the other is tense and tender. These patients are often febrile and unwell by the time the diagnosis is made. Ischiorectal abscesses have a particular tendency to extend posteriorly around the anal canal to involve the opposite ischiorectal fossa, thus forming a 'horseshoe' extension.

These abscesses can generally be treated in a manner similar to a perianal abscess although the depth of the cavity may require gentle intermittent irrigation twice daily for 24–48 hours postoperatively. This avoids the need for wide excision of the overlying skin to permit 'healing from below', which might otherwise be necessary. It is striking how quickly even a large cavity will contract if the traditional desire to 'pack' an abscess cavity can be resisted. It is equally possible to close the skin and use a suction drain in a large cavity. The traditional wider excision of overlying skin when the abscess is extensive and deep, and especially with a horseshoe extension may still be required. While healing may be more protracted, the outcome is usually secure.

In complicated abscesses it may be necessary to take the patient back to theatre for examination under anaesthesia after 4–5 days. This may reveal an undrained loculus. A fistulous track that has become evident as oedema has subsided may be suitable for laying open at this stage, provided it lies below the dentate line. If there are doubts about the track it is wiser to allow inflammation to settle and review the patient in the outpatient clinic.

Pelvirectal or supralevator abscess

A pelvirectal or supralevator abscess is a rarity, and no example was seen among Buchan and Grace's (1973) 183 patients. The patient is likely to be unwell and febrile, with rectal pain, The only sign is an area of tenderness on high rectal examination, and it may be possible to define a mass on bimanual examination. An ultrasound scan may be helpful in defining the area. The abscess may arise from upward spread of infection from either an intersphincteric abscess or an ischiorectal abscess. In the latter case the ischiorectal abscess is drained in the usual way, and then an exploring needle on a syringe is passed up through the levator ani: it is useful to use the other index finger as a guide within the rectal ampulla. If the abscess is entered and pus withdrawn, then a sinus forceps can be passed alongside the needle into the abscess and opened out to allow drainage.

Submucous abscess

A submucous abscess (or a high intermuscular abscess) is occasionally seen (about 1% incidence). The patient complains of pain in the rectum, and may well present after the abscess has burst, with discharge of pus *per rectum*. Rectal examination reveals a tender lump in the rectal wall, above the anorectal ring, or an indurated area with a central ulcer.

With the patient in lithotomy position the area is carefully palpated, paying particular attention to the possibility of any other collection above or below levator ani. A Parks speculum is passed and the area is visualized. An undrained abscess is best opened with the diathermy needle because this area is very vascular.

Recurrence

Recurrence of anorectal suppuration is not unusual. Some 25% of Buchan and Grace's (1973) 147 patients who were followed up required re-admission, 15 for recurrent abscesses, 10 for fistula and 12 for both an abscess and a fistula.

Perianal abscesses generally do well with simple incision, but it is important for an experienced surgeon to treat the other abscesses. The advantages of reviewing a difficult situation at examination under anaesthesia after 4–5 days should be remembered.

7.7.4   ACUTE ANAL FISSURE

This emergency can usually be diagnosed from the history. A few days previously the patient felt sharp anal pain following defecation. Pain and throbbing continued for some time after completion of defecation. The next attempt at defecation was viewed with apprehension and proved to be acutely painful, the pain again persisting for some hours.

Examination shows an apprehensive patient who holds the anus in tight spasm. Digital examination is acutely painful and may be impossible in the acute phase. If the buttocks are separated, the fissure can usually be seen, in the midline posteriorly, extending from the anal verge to the dentate line.

When this situation obtains it is best to desist from further attempts to examine the anus in the outpatient clinic. If pain is intolerable the patient should be admitted, examined under anaesthesia and sigmoidoscopy performed (we have seen just such a case in which examination under the anaesthetic revealed a low rectal carcinoma, which had not been felt in outpatients). The acute fissure is a soft, bruised-looking crack on the posterior surface of the anal canal with a typical sentinel skin tag and hypertrophied anal papilla. In this situation it is reasonable to proceed to lateral subcutaneous internal anal sphincterotomy. If symptoms are less acute conservative measures are usually effective: a regime of hot baths, extra bran morning and evening, and passage of an anal dilator lubricated with local anaesthetic jelly immediately before bathing (so that the lignocaine jelly is washed away). Jensen (1986) has shown that regular use of sitz baths and bran relieves the pain of 75% of patients with acute fissures within a week and 87% are healed in 3 weeks. More recently there has been interest in the use of topical glyceryl trinitrate (0.2–0.4%) ointment (Lund *et al.*, 1996), which is successful in abolishing the internal anal sphincter spasm, promotes healing in the majority of patients and avoids the permanent division of internal sphincter fibres necessary for surgical sphincterotomy. For the few in whom healing has not occurred after 6 weeks, a lateral sphincterotomy will promptly terminate the symptoms provided anal spasm persists. It is important to differentiate between the low pressure chronic fissure and the acute anal fissure that benefits from either chemical or surgical sphincterotomy.

REFERENCES

Abraham, N., Doudle, M. and Carson, P. (1997) Open versus closed surgical treatment of abscesses: a controlled clinical trial. *Austr. N.Z. J. Surg.*, **67**, 173–176.

Buchan, R. and Grace, R. H. (1973) Anorectal suppuration: the results of treatment and factors influencing the recurrence rate. *Br. J. Surg.*, **60**, 537–540.

Ellis, M. (1960) Incision and primary suture of abscesses in the anal region. *Proc. R. Soc. Med.*, **53**, 652–654.

Jensen, S. L. (1986) Treatment of first episodes of acute anal fissure. *BMJ*, **292**, 1167–1169.

Lund, J. N., Armitage, N. C. and Scholefield, J. H. (1996) Use of glyceryl trinitrate ointment in the treatment of anal fissure. *Br. J. Surg.*, **83**, 776–777.

Lundhus, E. and Gottrup, F. (1993) Outcome at three to five years of primary closure of perianal and pilonidal abscess. A randomised, double-blind clinical trial with a complete three-year followup of one compared with four days' treatment with ampicillin and metronidazole. *Eur. J. Surg.*, **159**, 555–558.

Smith, M. (1967) Early operation for acute haemorrhoids. *Br. J. Surg.*, **54**, 141–144.

Stewart, M. P. M., Laing, M. R. and Krukowski, Z. H. (1985) Treatment of acute abscesses by incision, curettage and primary suture without antibiotics: a controlled clinical trial. *Br. J. Surg.*, **72**, 66–67.

Tang, C. L., Chew, S. P. and Seow-Choen, F. (1996) Prospective randomized trial of drainage alone vs. drainage and fistulotomy for acute perianal abscesses with proven internal opening. *Dis. Colon Rectum*, **39**, 1415–1417.

8

Acute gastrointestinal haemorrhage

8.1 INTRODUCTION

During the early 1930s the mortality of acute haemorrhage from the stomach or duodenum treated in hospital was 20–25%. Apart from bed rest and a meagre diet little was done, and many died from dehydration, anaemia and malnutrition. Then, in 1935 Marriott and Kerwick devised a technique for drip blood transfusion, and Meulengracht (1934) in Denmark showed that it was much better to treat patients with bleeding from a peptic ulcer with ample fluids and a soft, nourishing diet. These two advances were given a trial in London by Avery Jones (1939) and during 1941–1946 he pursued, in a special unit, a consistent policy of using liberal blood transfusion and a good diet in 563 patients with peptic ulcer haemorrhage, with a mortality of 7% (Jones, 1947). For their time, these results were remarkable.

At the same time a major surgical advance was under way. In those days surgeons visited the autopsy room regularly, and Finsterer (1939) in Vienna, Gordon-Taylor (1937) in London and Yudin (1937) in Moscow were all impressed by the repeated sight of an open, eroded artery, lying in the base of a peptic ulcer, from which the patient had bled to death. Clearly, nothing would avail in these cases except an attempt at surgical haemostasis. A number of these patients were young, otherwise fit and in active employment, so there was good reason to test the effect of emergency partial gastrectomy, and in 1939 Finsterer could report 71 such operations with only three deaths.

This work led in the 1940s and 1950s to an extended trial of surgical treatment, and more attention was being paid to the other main cause of haematemesis – oesophageal varices – and to the wide variety of conditions that cause major haemorrhage from the rectum. More recently, developments in all aspects of alimentary tract endoscopy have produced great advances in diagnosis and treatment throughout this field of emergency work.

Over the past 50 years, three studies of acute gastrointestinal haemorrhage among the defined population of the North-east of Scotland have been made, and they provide a useful illustration of the effect of these developments. All gastrointestinal emergencies arising in a population of some 450 000 people are treated in one group of hospitals in Aberdeen, so collection of information can be comprehensive and accurate. Two studies surveyed all patients admitted with haematemesis and melaena – one was made in 1949 on admissions during 1941–1948 (Needham and McConachie, 1950) and a prospective study was done

Emergency Abdominal Surgery. Edited by Peter F. Jones, Zygmunt H. Krukowski and George G. Youngson. Published in 1998 by Chapman & Hall, London. ISBN 0 412 81950 3.

Table 8.1 Origins of upper gastrointestinal haemorrhage in 1098 patients investigated 1991–1993 (Masson *et al.*, 1996)

	No.	%
Duodenal ulcer	275	25.0
Oesophagitis/ulcer	180	16.4
Gastric ulcer	151	13.8
Mallory–Weiss	113	10.3
Gastric erosions	90	8.2
Varices	59	5.4
Gastric and oesophageal cancer	27	2.5
Duodenitis	21	1.9
Others	59	5.4
No cause found	67	6.1
No endoscopy	56	5.1

during 1967 and 1968 (Johnston *et al.*, 1973). These patients were admitted to the receiving ward on duty, but in the third study, during 1991–1993, all patients with suspected bleeding from the upper and the lower alimentary tract were admitted to a six-bedded bleeding unit, with a 24-hour endoscopy service and trained nursing and medical staff (Masson *et al.*, 1996).

During 1941–1948 blood transfusion was liberally used in the treatment of 476 patients with bleeding from a peptic ulcer, but only 11 operations were performed and overall mortality was 14%. During 1968/69 817 consecutive patients with haematemesis and melaena were studied: among the 511 patients with a peptic ulcer (of whom 75 had an emergency operation) the mortality was 8.6%, but overall the death rate remained high, at 13.7%. During the 2 years 1991–1993, 1098 patients had upper, and 252 lower, alimentary bleeding confirmed: 95% were endoscoped within 24 hours, and a management protocol was followed that included endoscopic and surgical haemostasis. Tables 8.1 and 8.2 show the diagnoses made, and with this directed approach overall mortality had fallen to 4.1%, a result in line with reports from other bleeding units (Hunt *et al.*, 1983; Holman *et al.*, 1990; Sanderson *et al.*, 1990); however, in many hospitals rates remain at 10–14% (Rockall *et al.*, 1995). The need for these units is underlined by the existence of several major risk factors.

1. There has been a steady rise in the age of these patients. In Aberdeen in 1941–1948 only 29% of patients were over 60, in 1968/69 this figure was 49% and during 1991–1993 55% were over 60, 37% were over 70 and 19% were over 80 years of age. More patients over 60 have a 'significant' bleed (66%) than a 'trivial' one. Many have chronic respiratory and cardiovascular disease, which makes them less able to withstand haemorrhage and the demands of an operation. It is now very unusual for a death to occur in a patient under the age of 60, except in variceal haemorrhage (p. 366).

However, the growth in the proportion of older patients is only partly accounted for by an ageing population. Aspirin and non-steroidal anti-inflammatory drugs (NSAIDs) are particularly likely to be taken by older patients, and they have a definite association with alimentary tract bleeding (p. 346): in 1968/69 they had been used by 28% of patients but by 1991–1993 they had been used by 46%.

Table 8.2 Diagnosis and severity of bleed in 251 patients with confirmed lower gastrointestinal haemorrhage (Bramley *et al.*, 1996)

Disease	Significant haemorrhage	Trivial haemorrhage	Total	%
Origin not found	29	35	64	25
Diverticulosis	40	20	60	24
Infective	2	24	26	10
Haemorrhoids	1	21	22	9
Angiodysplasia	15	2	17	7
Cancer	8	5	13	5
Polyp	3	9	12	5
Colitis				
Ischaemic	5	5	10	4
Crohn's	7	2	9	4
UC	2	5	7	3
Other	7	4	11	4.5
	119 (47%)	132 (53%)		

None of these factors can be significantly altered, and they underline the need for expert and coordinated care for these patients.

2. About two-thirds of patients admitted with haematemesis and melaena stop bleeding spontaneously; a few will have had a severe bleed but almost all this group will recover. Prognosis is very different among those who show signs of **further haemorrhage** (FH), which can take two forms.

- In spite of adequate resuscitation the patient shows signs of continuing blood loss.
- The patient settles after admission and treatment but then, after an interval, has a fresh haematemesis or develops signs of internal bleeding. Recurrence usually occurs within 48 hours, but may be delayed for several days.

The dangers of FH were highlighted in Aberdeen in 1941–1948 when the mortality among 124 patients with FH was 41%, but was only 4.3% in those who settled. Among the 51 deaths in the FH group, 41 died from uncontrollable haemorrhage, and in 32 who came to post-mortem an eroded artery was seen in the base of the peptic ulcer in 24. In 1968/69, when more emergency surgery was performed, comparable mortality figures were 28.8% and 7.8%.

In those days FH was detected by close clinical observation and measurement of losses through haematemesis and melaena. Blood transfusion rates and indications for surgery were judged accordingly. Nowadays early endoscopy gives objective evidence of continued loss, or warning signs of probable recurrence (p. 352).

The basic pathology seen by Finsterer and his friends remains the same. Swain *et al.* (1986) examined the histology of 27 gastric ulcers that had been removed by gastrectomy for FH. After injection of the specimens with barium and gelatin, radiography showed that all the arteries traversed the floor of the ulcers and, in both acute and chronic ulcers, erosion had always involved the side of the vessel, so intimal retraction as a natural mode of haemostasis was ruled out. Luminal diameter at the bleeding point averaged 0.6 mm, and calculation showed that such a vessel could transmit over 1 litre of blood in an hour.

In the 1991–1993 series in Aberdeen, 95% were endoscoped within 24 hours – many much sooner – and, among the 435 patients with peptic ulceration, 244 (58%) showed signs of recent haemorrhage (SRH). These patients were closely watched and were seen by a surgeon. Endoscopic injection therapy (p. 355) was not used, but in 75 (30%) early surgery was needed to secure arrest of FH: surgical mortality was 8% and overall mortality in the 244 patients was 7%. Comparable mortality in 1968/69 was 28%, and in that report particular attention was drawn to the dangers of procrastination in seeking surgical advice. This was eliminated by the protocol in the bleeding unit, and much of this improvement was due to this.

3. At all ages some causes of haemorrhage carry a particularly serious prognosis. This is especially true for variceal bleeding (p. 366), because most of these patients have advanced liver disease. Gastro-oesophageal cancer that presents with bleeding also carries a high mortality.

4. An important group of patients are those who begin to bleed after they have been admitted to hospital for a different reason, and who are apt to be overlooked unless prospective recording covers all wards. In 1991–1993 16% of all patients treated in the bleeding unit were transferred to it having been already admitted to another ward: their mortality rate was 18%, compared to an overall rate of 2.4% among the 73% of patients who were directly referred as emergencies by their general practitioner (the remaining 11% were admitted by the Accident and Emergency Department).

In the majority of **patients who remain haemodynamically stable**, a full history and a thorough physical examination, including rectal examination, are needed, blood samples are withdrawn, an intravenous crystalloid transfusion is set up, and they are placed under observation. Upper gastrointestinal endoscopy is undertaken within 24 hours.

Among patients who remain stable, it is necessary to maintain close observation over several days among those in whom endoscopy reveals SRH (p. 353). They can receive fluids and an attractive diet, but there is little evidence that specific medical intervention has any effect on peptic ulcer bleeding, including the use of H_2-receptor antagonists. Inhibition of fibrinolysis, using tranexamic acid, has been studied but did not affect rebleeding and operation rates, and has not been widely adopted (Henry and O'Connell, 1989).

Somatostatin has also been tested because it can reduce both acid secretion and splanchnic blood flow, but apart from some evidence that it may be useful in torrential bleeding from gastric erosions (Jenkins *et al.*, 1992), the trials have been disappointing. The prostaglandin misoprostol appears to have some promise, and there is one small trial which indicates that it may reduce the need for emergency surgery to arrest bleeding (Birnie *et al.*, 1991).

Thus the available evidence indicates that pharmacological treatment makes little difference to the outcome in acute non-variceal upper alimentary haemorrhage (NVH).

8.2 AETIOLOGY

8.2.1 PEPTIC ULCER

By far the commonest cause of significant NVH is peptic ulceration, and there have been important recent developments in our understanding of the aetiology of this condition, particularly with regard to the role of *Helicobacter pylori*. For many years, it was thought that ulceration arose purely from an imbalance between the protective mechanisms of the gastric mucosa and the effect of acid and pepsin, and because this theory still has relevance it is worth reiterating.

The mucosa lining the fundus and much of the body of the stomach secretes acid and pepsin, but in normal circumstances the mucosa remains intact, and this is due to several defensive mechanisms, which largely prevent the diffusion of hydrogen ions back from the lumen into the mucosa. Gastric mucus is a relatively viscous layer that adheres to the mucosa and confines the bicarbonate, which is secreted by the surface epithelial cells: this is only the equivalent of 5% of acid production, but because the bicarbonate is held beneath the mucus layer it provides a pH gradient from about 2.0 in the lumen up to about 6.0 at the cell surface. The membrane of the mucosal cells, and the junctions between the cells, are relatively impermeable to acid; also, the acid that does diffuse into the cell is neutralized by an effective buffer mechanism (O'Brien, 1985). These three mechanisms, which defend the luminal aspect of the mucosal cells, all depend in turn on an intact microcirculation to supply the interstitial aspect of the cells with oxygen and with the nutritional elements of extracellular fluid.

Thus, the mucosa of the stomach can be damaged in two ways, by swallowed harmful substances or by circumstances that impair the gastric blood supply. Non-steroidal anti-inflammatory drugs (NSAIDs) such as aspirin and indomethacin are the classical harmful drugs, and their effects have been extensively studied. In 1938 Douthwaite and Lintott performed gastroscopy on 16 subjects who had each swallowed 900 mg aspirin: 13 showed hyperaemia of, and haemorrhage into, the mucosa of the fundus. It appears that NSAIDs directly damage the mucosa and, by inhibition of prostaglandin synthesis, repair mechanisms are impaired, with consequent development of erosions (Lanza, 1991). The underlying submucosal vessels may be damaged, so there may be overt haemorrhage (Davenport, 1967). Measurements show that when an adult takes 600 mg aspirin four times a day, about 5 ml of blood can be recovered from the stools (Wood *et al.*, 1962).

The actual role of these drugs in inducing gastric haemorrhage has proved difficult to establish. In a study from Aberdeen, three times as many men and twice as many women had taken aspirin before admission for bleeding as had been taken by 300 controls, who were interviewed in beds adjacent to the patients who bled (Needham *et al.*, 1971). This difference was highly significant among patients with duodenal and gastric ulcers, and those with erosive gastritis, but not among patients with oesophageal varices. There was little difference in alcohol consumption between those who had bled and the controls but among the small group who had consumed both aspirin and alcohol there was a notable excess of bleeding, and the two drugs together clearly had a synergistic effect.

It is now clear, however, that the main aetiological factor in peptic ulceration is the organism *Helicobacter pylori*. This organism is a pathogen that inhabits the mucus layer that overlies the gastric epithelial cells, and it was first identified and cultured in 1983 by Warren and Marshall. Since then, it has been shown that there is a strong association between the risk of developing peptic ulcers and infection of the gastric and duodenal mucosa with *H. pylori*, and for both duodenal and gastric ulcers there is evidence from randomized controlled trials that eradication of infection greatly reduces the rates of relapse after healing induced by antisecretory drugs (Marshall, 1994).

In bleeding peptic ulcer, therefore, the most important aetiological factors are drugs of the non-steroidal anti-inflammatory type or infection with *H. pylori*. It is important to establish whether or not *H. pylori* is implicated in an individual case, as this will determine long-term treatment. The simplest way to achieve this is to take an antral biopsy at the time of endoscopy and to carry out a urease test, which involves placing the biopsy in a preprepared gel containing urea and a pH indicator. It is also advisable to send a further biopsy for histology, as the organisms can easily be seen by the histopathologist.

8.2.2 OTHER CAUSES OF NON-VARICEAL HAEMORRHAGE

Stomal ulcer. Bleeding from a stomal ulcer is unusual, and accounts for only 1–2% of all acute UGIH. The diagnosis will be suspected because of the history of gastric surgery. Only about one-quarter are chronic symptomatic ulcers, the remainder being acute superficial haemorrhagic erosions along the suture line (Hunt *et al.*, 1979).

Carcinoma of the stomach is also the source of 1–2% of acute gastric haemorrhage. Although eight of the 15 patients reported by Hunt *et al.* (1982) required urgent surgery, only three lesions had been identified as a carcinoma at endoscopy. Carcinoma has to be considered as a possibility in any bleeding gastric ulcer and these eight neoplasms were among a total of 61 gastric ulcers requiring an emergency operation for haemorrhage.

A **leiomyoma** in the stomach has a typical appearance of a smooth mass projecting into the lumen, surmounted by an ulcer with signs of recent bleeding. A leiomyoma may arise in the duodenal loop and be more difficult to identify, especially at the duodenojejunal flexure. Local excision in the stomach is usually a simple procedure but can be difficult in the duodenum, where it may encroach on the pancreatic and bile ducts.

Haemobilia is considered on p. 466. Unusual causes of NVH are well illustrated by a patient who bled intermittently from a pseudoaneurysm in the head of the pancreas resulting from chronic pancreatitis. This presented with repeated episodes of haematemesis and he had several normal endoscopies. The diagnosis was finally made by coeliac axis angiography and, after failed attempts at embolism, the patient was cured by a Whipple's operation. Very occasionally a carcinoma of the head of pancreas or of the bile duct can invade the duodenal wall and lead to acute haemorrhage.

Meckel's diverticulum and diverticula of the small bowel may also cause bleeding but these conditions are covered in Chapters 3 and 6.

Blood diseases may be associated with acute UGIH. There may be a history of previous bleeding episodes, or of a bleeding diathesis such as haemophilia, when clotting time will be prolonged. Prolongation of the bleeding time will occur in thrombocytopenic purpura. Occasionally bleeding occurs in patients on anticoagulant treatment.

Pseudoxanthoma elasticum is a hereditary connective tissue disorder characterized by loss of elasticity in the tissues. As a consequence the skin of the neck and abdominal wall tends to lie in folds and is yellowish and coarse in texture. Rarely, the loss of the elastic lamina in the arteries leads to rupture of a vessel in the stomach or in the intestines.

Aortointestinal fistulae are rare and dangerous sources of severe bleeding and are considered in Chapter 14 (p. 523).

Mallory–Weiss syndrome. In 1929 Mallory and Weiss reported five patients whom they had seen at the Boston City Hospital, who, 'after a long and intense alcoholic debauch, developed massive gastric haemorrhage with haematemesis'. All had experienced persistent nausea, retching and vomiting before the onset of haematemesis. Four came to post-mortem, which showed two to four definite fissure-like lesions of the mucosa, characteristically arranged around the circumference of the cardiac opening into the stomach.

With the introduction of endoscopy more of these tears are seen and incidence has risen from 1% to 6–8% and in some reports it has been as high as 14% (Graham and Schwartz, 1977). There is a wide age range, from the teens up to the 70s. About two-thirds of patients are men. Between 50% and 60% give a typical history of retching and vomiting before bleeding commences. About one-half have recently imbibed a large volume of alcohol and about one-quarter have taken analgesics (Stern *et al.*, 1979).

The natural tendency of gastro-oesophageal tears is to heal, and after 2–3 days there is a linear ulcer covered in slough and healing is complete in 8–10 days. However, in some the tear has opened a sizeable submucosal vessel and arteriolar haemorrhage continues. A blood transfusion is required by about 40% of patients, and most need 3–6 units. In a small minority that averages around 10% of all tears, bleeding is severe and continuous enough to require surgical arrest. It is unusual for patients to die from Mallory–Weiss tears and the few who do so are generally elderly patients with serious concomitant disease.

Stress ulceration, first described as such by Selye in 1935, covers a range of conditions in which the gastric mucosa is damaged by a deficiency in blood supply. Two names are particularly associated with stress ulceration: those of Curling and Cushing. In 1842 Curling described 10 cases of duodenal ulcer in burn patients, and in 1932 Harvey Cushing reported on a number of patients who suffered gastroduodenal haemorrhage after operations on the pituitary or cerebellum. Thus the term 'Curling's ulcer' has come to mean ulceration associated with burns and 'Cushing's ulcer' ulceration associated with head injury. It must be appreciated, however, that most stress ulceration does not follow the pattern, described by Curling and Cushing, of deep, penetrating ulcers. Rather, multiple erosions, similar to those seen in drug-induced disease, are the rule. This pattern of ulceration is commonly seen after multiple injuries and in patients in intensive care units. It has become common practice to treat such patients with prophylactic H_2-receptor antagonists (Nash *et al.*, 1994), although more recent evidence suggests that sucralfate is superior because of the lower incidence of respiratory infection (Wyncoll *et al.*, 1997).

However, in a recent study of 2252 patients admitted to intensive care units in Canada, the two important risk factors for bleeding were respiratory failure and coagulopathy (Cook *et al.*, 1994). Of patients with one or both of these factors 4% developed significant UGIH, whereas of the others only 0.1% bled. The authors concluded that prophylactic measures could safely be restricted to patients who require mechanical ventilation or who have a coagulopathy.

Dieulafoy's ulcer, or exulceratio simplex, is a small, solitary gastric mucosal ulceration with an eroded artery in its base. Its aetiology is unclear but it is thought to represent a vascular dysplasia rather than a peptic ulcer (Juler *et al.*, 1984). It is relatively uncommon but, in a Swiss series of 480 patients endoscoped for UGIH, 28 (5.8%) were found to have a Dieulafoy lesion (Baettig *et al.*, 1993). It can be dangerous in that bleeding is often profuse, and the lesion can be difficult to find both at endoscopy and at operation. It is usually situated in the fundus or high on the lesser curve and is detected by palpation, rather than inspection (p. 361).

Reflux oesophagitis is a common condition and can cause a slow loss of blood from the raw surface. Sometimes the eroded surface of the lower oesophageal mucosal folds can be seen on endoscopy to be the site of acute haemorrhage, but this almost always settles with medical measures. If a considerable degree of bleeding continues it is important to look for another cause. Very occasionally a peptic ulcer develops in **Barrett's columnar-lined oesophagus.** This can cause a difficult situation, with a deep ulcer fixed by extensive fibrosis in the lower oesophagus. Resection in the face of continued haemorrhage will involve a combined abdominal and right thoracic approach, as for an Ivor Lewis oesophagectomy.

8.3   CLINICAL FEATURES

When a patient presents with the complaint of vomiting blood or passing blood *per rectum*, it is necessary to establish that it is actually blood that has been voided. Sometimes this is all too evident, because the patient is shocked, or blood is vomited or a melaena stool is passed at the time of admission. A history solely of 'coffee-grounds' vomiting cannot be accepted as evidence of bleeding without confirmation because not all vomit which is so described actually contains blood: rectal examination showing a melaena stool, or passage of a nasogastric tube and examination of the aspirate may be needed before the fact of upper tract bleeding can be established. A period of observation may be required in a stable patient with only a history of vomiting blood, before a diagnosis of UGIH can be confirmed or discarded.

Some patients will already be known to have oesophageal varices, because they are particularly liable to recurrent bleeding. A past history of dyspepsia or ulceration at some time is obtained in 80–90% of patients who bleed from a peptic ulcer; however, more than half these patients experience no digestive symptoms immediately before their haemorrhage, and these patients show a considerably higher mortality rate. This absence of a dyspeptic history must not be allowed to influence management. Very few patients bleed from an aortointestinal fistula, but it is essential to think of this possibility in any patient with a history of insertion of an abdominal aortic prosthesis.

A report of a previous barium meal or endoscopy may be available in about 50% of patients with haemorrhage from a peptic ulcer (Needham *et al.*, 1971), but in only a little over half the patients do the radiological site of ulceration and the actual site of bleeding correspond.

The important effects of NSAIDs and other drugs need to be considered and a carefully taken history of drug and alcohol intake is of great importance. It is interesting to consider to what extent the increasing number of elderly patients treated for UGIH is due to the widespread use of NSAIDs in this age group.

Physical examination is of the greatest importance in finding signs of hypovolaemia and shock and in assessing the general health of the patient (especially cardiac and respiratory disease which can affect the operative risk). Abdominal signs are usually few. A palpable spleen or cutaneous signs of liver failure are important in suggesting that the patient may have portal hypertension. Tenderness and guarding in the epigastrium will suggest that there may be the grave complication of simultaneous haemorrhage and perforation in a peptic ulcer. A scar may raise the possibility of previous gastric or aortic surgery. Auscultation is always helpful – continued bleeding is accompanied by characteristic active liquid bowel sounds. The presence of an aortic aneurysm may be revealed or confirmed by palpation, and by hearing an arterial bruit. It is essential to carry out a rectal examination, and to look at a sample of the stool. It is important for nursing staff to retain stool specimens in the sluice room, so that they can be inspected.

A full blood count, clotting screen and biochemical profile should always be requested. The serum urea and creatinine are of interest. Although the serum urea rises within the first 24 hours, it usually drops back to normal in the second 24 hours. Protein (and therefore blood) is absorbed in small bowel, so a colonic haemorrhage does not affect the serum urea (Snook *et al.*, 1986).

8.4 INITIAL MANAGEMENT

Patients bleeding from the oesophagus, stomach or duodenum give a history of haematemesis, melaena or rectal bleeding. It is important to bear the last of these in mind, because the patient with profuse fresh rectal haemorrhage, especially when accompanied by haemodynamic instability, may well be bleeding from the upper gastrointestinal tract. In assessing such a patient there are three important questions to answer in the first few minutes:

1. **Is the airway clear?** It may be necessary to evacuate vomit or clot from the upper airway.
2. **Is there evidence of active bleeding?** This may be difficult to ascertain, but in the patient who is voiding fresh blood it must be likely.
3. **Is there evidence of hypovolaemia?** Pulse rate and blood pressure must be measured at the first opportunity and even when these signs are normal the signs of peripheral vasoconstriction should be sought.

   Management should then continue as follows.

1. **Vascular access** should be established with a wide-bore (14 FG) cannula, and blood cross-matched.
2. **If the patient is haemodynamically stable**, obtain a full history, carry out a thorough examination and arrange for an upper gastrointestinal endoscopy on the next available list, preferably within 24 hours.
3. **If the patient is haemodynamically unstable**, resuscitation must take priority. A reasonable approach is to institute and continue with rapid fluid replacement therapy as long as the systolic blood pressure is less than 100 mmHg and the pulse rate greater than 100/min. In elderly patients or in those with cardiac disease, the central venous pressure (CVP) should be monitored. It must be stressed that a CVP catheter should be inserted or supervised by an experienced surgeon or anaesthetist and monitoring carried out in an adequate environment such as a high-dependency unit. A urinary catheter should also be inserted, and the urine volume should be maintained at not less than 30 ml/h.

   Fluid replacement can start with 500 ml of physiological saline over the first 15 minutes, followed by 500 ml of colloid (e.g. gelatin) over the next 15 minutes. Resuscitation should then continue with blood at 1 unit every 15 minutes. If the blood pressure fails to rise or falls, this infusion rate must be increased accordingly, but when the patient becomes stable (BP > 100 mmHg and pulse < 100/min) rapid infusion must be stopped and maintenance fluids only given. If the CVP is being measured, then rapid infusion should proceed until it reaches more than 5 cmH$_2$O.

   If the CVP remains greater than 12 cmH$_2$O and the BP greater than 100 mmHg, then overload has occurred and a diuretic (40 mg of frusemide) should be given intravenously. Frusemide should not be given solely to increase urine output, as this will have the effect of exacerbating hypovolaemia. If the CVP remains greater than 12 cmH$_2$O, and BP is less than 100 mmHg, then there is a degree of cardiac failure, and intensive care is necessary. It is advisable to start an infusion of an inotrope (dopamine at 5 mg/kg/min) while this is being arranged.

   If it proves difficult to stabilize the patient using these measures, urgent investigation to locate the bleeding point and decide on further management is then necessary.

8.5 INVESTIGATION

The mainstay of the investigation of acute upper gastrointestinal bleeding is flexible endoscopy. Therefore this section concentrates largely on endoscopy and is divided into the following sections: (1) endoscopy equipment; (2) technique in acute bleeding; (3) endoscopic appearances in acute bleeding; and (4) other diagnostic techniques.

8.5.1 ENDOSCOPY EQUIPMENT

Most modern endoscopy units have video-endoscopy equipment, and for routine gastro-intestinal endoscopy this has major advantages. It affords an excellent view to all the members of the team, which is of great importance for endoscopic intervention where the assistant has to coordinate with the endoscopist, and it greatly facilitates teaching. In addition, the working channels of the endoscope are held away from the endoscopist's face, which reduces the risk of blood or secretions splashing into the eyes.

Unfortunately, however, video-endoscopy equipment is not ideal for examining the bleeding patient. In the presence of large amounts of blood the image can become very dark owing to saturation of the 'red channel' of the chip camera, and this can seriously hamper both diagnosis and therapy. Thus, while video-endoscopy may be suitable for upper gastrointestinal haemorrhage, it is useful to have a fibreoptic instrument for demanding situations.

The endoscope itself must be chosen with a view to the particular circumstances. The slim 'paediatric' instrument is very manoeuvrable, but its 2.8 mm working or biopsy channel limits the use of therapeutic accessories, and does not allow good suction. The bigger double-channel endoscope allows good suction and washing through the unoccupied channel when an accessory is in use, but it is uncomfortable for the patient and cumbersome when trying to reach relatively inaccessible lesions. A useful compromise is an endoscope with a single wide (3.7 mm) working channel and a separate forward washing channel: this allows good suction and the passage of a wide range of therapeutic instruments.

Other important pieces of equipment include a lavage tube, a pharyngeal overtube, washing devices and therapeutic accessories. The lavage tube is occasionally required when the stomach is full of clot, and the most useful device is a wide-bore (40 FG if possible), soft tube with an open end. The pharyngeal overtube is a 30 cm tube with a flange at one end to prevent it from slipping into the mouth. This can be passed over the endoscope when lavage is needed; it both facilitates repeated changes between the endoscope and the lavage tube and protects the airway. The simplest washing method is to insert the nozzle of a 20 ml syringe filled with water directly into the working or washing channel of the endoscope and to empty its contents in one rapid action. Another technique is to use a water toothbrush modified by a foot switch. The outlet can then be attached to the working or washing channel. Finally, it is important to have all the therapeutic accessories that might be required immediately to hand.

8.5.2 ENDOSCOPY TECHNIQUE IN ACUTE BLEEDING

Even when not urgent, endoscopy should take place within 24 hours of admission, as the chances of making a diagnosis diminish rapidly after this time. Usually, endoscopy takes place with benzodiazepine sedation, but in the patient who is vomiting large quantities of blood, general anaesthesia with cuffed endotracheal intubation should be considered. When sedation is adequate, careful monitoring is still required, and the patient's pulse and blood

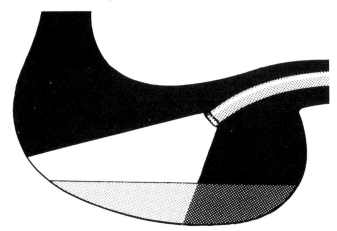

Figure 8.1 In the left lateral position blood pools in the fundus away from areas in which most ulcers are seen.

pressure should be measured regularly. Pulse oximetry should be regarded as mandatory, as arterial desaturation is a particular risk during a prolonged procedure with a large-diameter endoscope. For this reason it is also wise to administer oxygen throughout the procedure, either nasally or by means of a specially designed mouth-guard.

The endoscopy should take place on a bed or trolley that can tip into either the head-up or head-down position. The examination should start with the patient in the left lateral position, as this encourages blood to pool in the fundus of the stomach, where ulcers are uncommon (Figure 8.1). If it becomes necessary to view the fundus, this can be done by turning the patient on to the right side and tipping the trolley head-up so that the blood falls into the antrum.

When the endoscope has been passed beyond the gastro-oesophageal junction, it is not uncommon to encounter a daunting mass of blood and clot. However, as long as the stomach is allowed to distend in response to insufflation and the above guidelines are followed, a moderate amount of blood in the stomach rarely prevents an adequate view of the responsible lesion. Often clot will be seen overlying an ulcer, and it is important to wash this to ascertain whether or not it is adherent; this has implications for prognosis and treatment, and gentle washing will rarely precipitate haemorrhage.

Occasionally, however, there will be too much blood in the stomach to allow and adequate examination, and lavage will be necessary. With a pharyngeal overtube in place, the 40 FG. lavage tube is passed into the stomach and direct suction is applied. This may clear enough blood and clot to allow the examination to proceed, but if not, a formal lavage is carried out by rapidly pouring in a litre of water *via* a funnel. This will break up clot, which can then be siphoned out by placing the tube in a dependent position.

8.5.3   ENDOSCOPIC APPEARANCES OF THE BLEEDING ULCER

The endoscopic appearance of a peptic ulcer that has bled or is still bleeding provides valuable prognostic information, which can be used to predict outcome and risk of rebleeding. Various classification systems have been used, and the most popular has been that

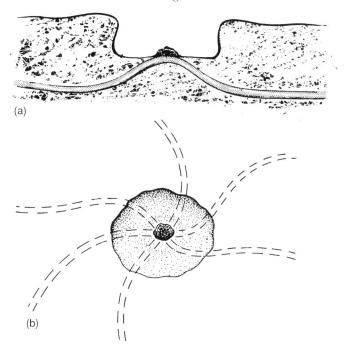

Figure 8.2 **(a)** The vessel in the base of an ulcer loops up to the surface and is plugged by thrombus, forming a so-called 'visible vessel'. **(b)** From its appearance on endoscopy the course of a vessel is not predictable – it could follow any of the indicated routes.

proposed by Forrest and others which distinguishes between active bleeding, a non-bleeding visible vessel and adherent clot (Forrest *et al.*, 1974). Unfortunately, however, there is considerable interobserver variation in the interpretation of these appearances (Laine *et al.*, 1994), indicating that the descriptive terms lack precision. It is nevertheless important to be able to describe the 'stigmata of recent haemorrhage', and the categories given below are widely recognized.

Active arterial bleeding indicates erosion of an artery or arteriole, and although studies have indicated that this type of bleeding may stop in up to 40% of cases (Steele, 1989), it is regarded as a clear indication for endoscopic or surgical intervention.

Active non-pulsatile bleeding or oozing from the base of an ulcer implies ongoing bleeding from a partially occluded vessel and is associated with a 20–30% chance of continued bleeding. It must be distinguished from contact bleeding from the edge of an ulcer which is of no significance.

A visible vessel is best defined as a raised lesion in the base of an ulcer. This may represent either an exposed vessel or an organized thrombus plugging a hole in the underlying vessel (Figure 8.2), and is important as it carries a significant risk of rebleeding if untreated. The precise risk is difficult to ascertain because of the disagreement among endoscopists as to what constitutes a visible vessel, but it is probably in the region of 30–50%.

Adherent blood clot may be difficult to distinguish from a visible vessel but, as the underlying pathology is the same, making the distinction is not absolutely necessary.

Flat red or black spots indicate dried blood in the slough of the ulcer base and are of little significance, with a rebleeding rate of less than 5%.

These stigmata change fairly rapidly, and a recent study from China by Yang *et al.* (1994) has indicated that visible vessels disappear in a mean of four days. Given the implications of a visible vessel, it is unwise to discharge a patient from hospital until endoscopic evidence of regression is seen, regardless of whether or not endoscopic therapy has been used.

8.5.4 OTHER DIAGNOSTIC TECHNIQUES

When endoscopy by an experienced endoscopist fails to provide the diagnosis, other approaches are required. If blood is not seen in the stomach, and the patient is haemodynamically unstable with continuing signs of bleeding, a decision has to be made on how to identify a more distal site of bleeding. This is discussed in the section on severe rectal haemorrhage (p. 374).

8.6 ENDOSCOPIC TREATMENT

Endoscopic haemostasis for peptic ulcer bleeding is now well established, and randomized trials have demonstrated the ability of several treatment modalities to reduce rebleeding and the need for emergency surgery.

8.6.1 TECHNIQUES OF ENDOSCOPIC HAEMOSTASIS

At the present time, the main endoscopic techniques available for controlling peptic ulcer bleeding are laser photocoagulation, bipolar diathermy, heater probe, injection sclerotherapy and adrenaline injection. Each of these will now be considered in turn.

Laser photocoagulation

Laser photocoagulation is simply a method of delivering heat energy to tissue. The laser that has been used almost exclusively for peptic ulcer bleeding is the neodymium–yttrium–aluminium–garnet (Nd–YAG), as this appears to achieve sufficient tissue penetration to coagulate vessels of appropriate size. The main reported dangers of laser therapy are perforation and exacerbation of the bleeding, but these can be minimized by good technique. The laser is also hazardous for staff: everyone involved has to wear special filter goggles to prevent retinal damage; and the room used has to be specially modified. These problems, together with the cost of the laser unit, its relative immobility and the rather indifferent results reported in randomized trials, have resulted in laser therapy being replaced by simpler methods.

Bipolar diathermy

Diathermy also relies on heat generated by electric current flowing through tissue near the electrode. Only bipolar diathermy has been used – to avoid deep thermal injury – but results have often shown little benefit, and diathermy has been superseded by the heat probe.

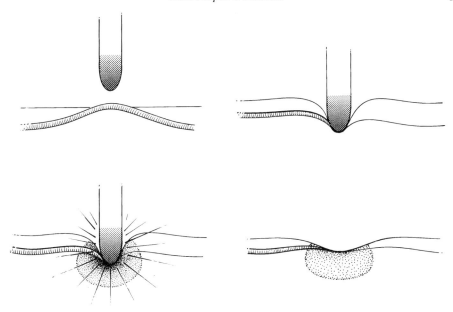

Figure 8.3 Coaptive coagulation. The heat probe compresses and occludes the vessel; when heat is applied the vessel is thrombosed along with surrounding tissue.

Heat probe

The heat probe has a coated metal tip which contains a coil that can rapidly generate a temperature of 150°C. In use it relies, like bipolar diathermy, on coaptive coagulation, in which the walls of the vessel are brought together by external pressure while heat is applied. If the pressure stops the bleeding the probe must be in the correct position, and loss of heat through blood flow is minimized (Figure 8.3). The largest probe (3.2 mm) is preferable.

The probe incorporates a channel for washing and when a good view of the bleeding point is obtained, pressure is applied and three or four pulses of 30 joules are delivered.

Adrenaline injection

Adrenaline injection probably achieves immediate haemostasis by virtue of the tamponade effect of the injected fluid, but the permanent effect depends on vasospasm and platelet activation encouraging the formation of platelet and fibrin thrombus within the vessel lumen (Pinkas *et al.*, 1995). A solution of 1 in 10 000 is most often used, delivered by means of a needle of the type used for sclerotherapy for oesophageal varices.

When an active bleeding point is identified, the ulcer is washed and the needle, already flushed through with the adrenaline solution, is passed through the working channel of the endoscope with the point withdrawn into the sheath. As soon as the needle is seen emerging from the endoscope, the assistant pushes out the needle point. The needle is then inserted into the base of the bleeding point, and the assistant injects 0.5 ml of the adrenaline solution. Some force is required and if the injection is very easy the needle is probably not in the tissue. If the bleeding does not stop immediately, a second 0.5 ml should be injected at the same site and the needle should be moved to a slightly different site to repeat the process. When the bleeding has stopped more adrenaline should be injected around the bleeding point in four to six 0.5 ml aliquots. A non-bleeding visible vessel can be treated in the same manner. Injection therapy is particularly useful where adherent clot obscures the bleeding point, as it is quite easy to pass a needle through the clot to allow injection of the ulcer base. Exacerbation of the bleeding is not a significant problem, presumably because of the combined tamponade and vasoconstriction.

Adrenaline injection appears to be very safe, with no recorded instances of perforation. Tachycardia and hypertension can occur, however, and, although fatal arrhythmias have not been reported, it is a sensible precaution to use ECG monitoring in addition to pulse and blood pressure recording during the procedure.

Injection sclerotherapy

The sclerosants that have been used in non-variceal haemorrhage include absolute alcohol, 1% polidocanol, 5% ethanolamine and 3% sodium tetradecyl sulphate (STD). Alcohol acts by dehydration and fixation of tissue whereas the others are detergents which cause endothelial damage; the intended end result is obliteration or thrombosis of the feeding vessel in the ulcer.

If there is active bleeding it is usual to control this with adrenaline injection as above and then to surround the bleeding point with aliquots of sclerosant – 0.1 ml for alcohol or 0.5 ml for the other sclerosants. Like adrenaline, sclerotherapy appears to be safe, although there have been a few case of extensive necrosis of the stomach wall after injection of the left gastric artery (Levy *et al.*, 1991).

Combined therapy

Chung *et al.* (1997) have reported a trial of combined adrenaline injection and heat probe treatment, randomly compared with adrenaline injection alone.

8.6.2 RESULTS OF ENDOSCOPIC TREATMENT

In about 80% of patients UGIH stops without intervention, so it is important for techniques of endoscopic therapy to have been subjected to randomized trials. Before drawing conclusions from these trials, however, it is important to understand which end-points are being studied.

Mortality is the most important but, as this is likely to be around 5% in interested centres, it would take a very large trial to demonstrate a convincing improvement in death rate. The next most important is probably need for emergency surgery; this can be associated with a mortality of up to 20% (Welch *et al.*, 1986), and any intervention that can reduce urgent operation rates is likely to result in reduction in morbidity and mortality. Rebleeding is less reliable as an end-point as it does not necessarily represent a clinically significant outcome if it does not result in surgery or death. Unfortunately, however, rebleeding is the only end-point that is reported in many of the published trials; these can be divided into those that have compared endoscopic haemostasis with no endoscopic therapy, and those that have compared different techniques.

Heat probe

In heat probe treatment, there have been four randomized controlled trials with 'no endoscopic treatment' arms. Two of these showed no benefit (Steele, 1989), and one demonstrated a reduction in rebleeding but no effect on surgery rates (Fullarton, 1989). However, Jensen (1990) demonstrated significant reductions in rebleeding and the need for emergency surgery in high-risk patients with arterial bleeding or visible vessels. In this report, Jensen emphasized the need for the large (3.2 mm) probe, firm tamponade of the vessel and the use of four 30 J pulses.

Adrenaline injection

Adrenaline injection of actively bleeding ulcers has been widely used and it is clear that adrenaline injection alone can be effective. There has been one randomized trial of 1:10 000 adrenaline *versus* no endoscopic treatment in actively bleeding ulcers carried out by Chung *et al.* in Hong Kong (1988), which showed reductions in the need for emergency surgery, blood transfusion and hospital stay. Chung *et al.* (1997) conducted a randomized trial in 276 patients with actively bleeding ulcers: 136 received adrenaline injection only and 140 had adrenaline injection and heat probe treatment. Overall results were similar, with initial haemostasis in 98% and 99% in the two groups. Emergency surgery was required in 14 of the adrenaline group and eight of the combined group. When 58 patients with spurting haemorrhage were analysed two of 31 in the combined group required emergency surgery compared with eight of 27 who received adrenaline only.

Injection sclerotherapy

The use of absolute alcohol is very popular, especially in Japan. There has been one comparative study which has suggested that it can reduce emergency surgery rates (Pascu *et al.*, 1989).

   The sclerosant polidocanol has also been widely used, and a trial showed a reduction in the need for emergency surgery (Panes *et al.*, 1987). Trials of adrenaline followed by 5% ethanolamine showed reductions in rebleeding and non-significant trends towards less emergency surgery (Oxner *et al.*, 1992).

Comparison between different methods

There is now no doubt that endoscopic haemostasis should be employed. It is effective in producing initial control of active bleeding, reducing clinical rebleeding and reducing the need for emergency or urgent surgical intervention. Furthermore, a recent meta-analysis by Cook *et al.* (1992) has indicated that endoscopic therapy can significantly reduce mortality.

   Making a decision as to which type of endoscopic therapy to use is more difficult, however, and when examining the different trials it is very important to take account of the type of lesion that has been treated. When trials are studied in which the control patients were treated non-surgically until they fulfilled criteria that were independent of endoscopic appearances, it is found that patients with active arterial bleeding came to surgery in about 60% of cases. Those with active oozing or non-bleeding visible vessels required surgery in about 25% and 40% of cases respectively. When the results of adequately documented trials are put together, it becomes clear that diathermy, heat probe and injection techniques can reduce the requirement for surgery to around 15% (Steele, 1989). The indications are that adrenaline injection and heat probe treatments will be those preferred, and a combination of these techniques may be optimal.

8.7 SURGICAL TREATMENT

Despite the important advances in endoscopic intervention outlined above, there remains a small group of patients who require surgical intervention as a life-saving procedure. This is becoming a major problem, as few surgeons in this country now have extensive experience of operating for peptic ulcer disease, and the emergency that does not respond to endoscopic treatment usually represents a significant surgical challenge. It is therefore vital that an experienced surgeon, who is used to operating on the stomach and duodenum, is involved in all surgery for upper gastrointestinal bleeding and that the operation is not delegated to an unassisted junior member of staff.

Indications for surgery

Prior to the introduction of endoscopic haemostasis the decision as to whether or not to operate for bleeding peptic ulcer could be difficult. When active bleeding was seen at the time of endoscopy this was usually taken as an absolute indication for surgery. However, it was more common to find that the patient had stopped bleeding at the time of endoscopy, and the surgeon had to decide between waiting for clinical evidence of rebleeding or performing 'prophylactic' surgery as advocated by Finsterer and Tanner.

The most important factors in predicting rebleeding appeared to be the presence of significant endoscopic stigmata of recent haemorrhage, an ulcer on the posterior wall of the duodenum or high on the lesser curve of the stomach, age over 60 years and shock or anaemia on admission (Hunt, 1987). In 1984, Morris *et al.* published the results of a randomized study comparing a policy of delayed surgery with early surgery. The criteria for early surgery were one rebleed in hospital, four units of plasma expander or blood in 24 hours, endoscopic stigmata or a previous history of peptic ulcer with bleeding. In the delayed group the criteria consisted of two rebleeds in hospital or eight units of blood or plasma expander in 24 hours. For patients over the age of 60 years, early surgery was associated with a lower mortality, and despite doubts as to the appropriateness of the endoscopic stigmata chosen and the very high operation rate, this study does emphasize the need for prompt surgical intervention in high-risk elderly patients.

Since the widespread adoption of endoscopic haemostasis, the decision as to when to operate has become easier to make. If initial control of active bleeding is impossible endoscopically, surgery is mandatory. If rebleeding occurs after successful delivery of endoscopic treatment then immediate surgery should be undertaken unless the patient is clearly unfit. Some consider that re-treatment after clinical rebleeding is safe, but good evidence for this is lacking. In this author's experience such a policy can be very dangerous, frequently leading to a patient being presented for surgery in suboptimal condition. Some endoscopists advocate routine re-endoscopy within 24 hours of endoscopic haemostasis, with retreatment if indicated. This has been tested in a small randomized trial, which showed a non-significant benefit (Villaneuva *et al.*, 1994), and it is possible that this approach might improve the results of endoscopic treatment. This must not, however, be confused with the re-treatment of overt clinical rebleeding.

If clinical rebleeding is to be used as an indication for surgery, it is important to have clear criteria to define rebleeding, especially as melaena can continue for several days following a major bleed. If a patient remains haemodynamically stable without rapid fluid replacement and does not have a fresh haematemesis or a drop in haemoglobin after initial resuscitation, then rebleeding can be discounted. If there is any doubt as to whether a patient has re-bled, repeat diagnostic endoscopy should be carried out before committing the patient to surgery.

8.7.1 TECHNIQUES

The bleeding duodenal ulcer

The majority of bleeding duodenal ulcers that require surgery are chronic posterior wall ulcers involving the gastroduodenal artery. A longitudinal duodenotomy is made immediately **distal** to the pyloric ring, and active arterial bleeding is controlled with finger pressure. If necessary the duodenotomy can be extended proximally through the pyloric ring to obtain adequate access but, unless a vagotomy is to be carried out (see below), the pylorus should be preserved.

When the stomach is distended with blood and clot this must be emptied by suction, expression or extraction with sponge-holding forceps. Failure to do so will impair access, limit visualization of bleeding points and risk aspiration of regurgitated blood on reversal of anaesthesia. If access if still difficult, mobilization of the duodenum laterally (Kocher's manoeuvre) may help.

Whether there is active bleeding or a non-bleeding exposed artery it is important to obtain secure control of the vessel. This is best achieved using a small (23 mm diameter), heavy, round-bodied or taper-cut semicircular needle with No. 0 or No. 1 size suture material. This type of needle is ideal for the restricted space and the tough fibrous tissue encountered at the base of a chronic ulcer. The material should be a synthetic absorbable, of reasonable strength duration (e.g. polydioxanone). The vessel must be under-run using two deeply placed sutures – one above the bleeding point and one below (Figure 8.4).

Using the small needle suggested minimizes the risk of damaging underlying structures, particularly the bile duct. The duodenotomy may be closed in the same direction as it was made (a single layer of 3/0 PDS is suitable) but, if a truncal vagotomy has been performed, a pyloroplasty should be constructed. This involves dividing the pyloric ring, if not already done, and closing the defect as a modified Finney pyloroplasty (p. 29). The modified Finney technique is particularly useful if a long pyloroduodenotomy has been necessary because it results in less tension on the suture line than with a Heinecke–Mickulicz pyloroplasty. If it is impossible to achieve safe closure the duodenotomy can be closed longitudinally and a gastrojejunostomy performed.

Occasionally, the first part of the duodenum is virtually replaced by a giant ulcer, and once opened it is impossible to repair. It is then necessary to proceed to a partial gastrectomy once the vessel has been secured. The right gastric and gastroepiploic vessels are ligated and divided, and the stomach is separated from the ulcer with a combination of sharp and blunt

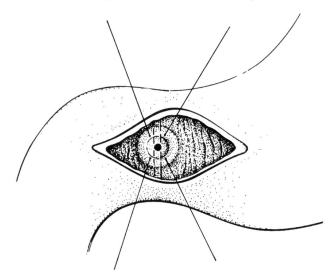

Figure 8.4 Securing a bleeding gastroduodenal artery (dotted lines) in the base of a deep duodenal ulcer. Two transversely running sutures under-run the vessel above and below the bleeding point.

dissection. If gastric resection is limited to antrectomy this should be supplemented with a vagotomy, and continuity restored by a gastrojejunostomy (p. 27). The difficulty then lies in closing the duodenal stump.

Mobilizing the duodenum posteriorly in an attempt to achieved conventional closure is hazardous and should not be attempted. It is preferable to employ Bentley's method (Bentley, 1952) where the anterior wall of the duodenum is plicated on to the edge of the fibrotic ulcer base with interrupted sutures (Figure 8.5).

If necessary, a second layer of sutures can be inserted in the same way, rolling the anterior wall of the duodenum on to the ulcer base. Drainage is rarely indicated but can be achieved by a T-tube brought out through the healthy side wall of the second part of the duodenum. Occasionally, the duodenum cannot be sutured safely and a tube duodenostomy may salvage this situation: the open end of the duodenum is loosely closed around a large-bore drain or Foley catheter to create a controlled duodenal fistula. This can be removed after 3 weeks, when the resulting fistula will close rapidly provided there is no distal obstruction of the duodenum.

The bleeding gastric ulcer

Haemostasis in a bleeding gastric ulcer can be achieved by gastrotomy and under-running of the vessel, excision of the ulcer or, conventionally, by partial gastrectomy, particularly for a large antral ulcer. However, with effective endoscopic haemostasis, by far the commonest situation requiring surgery is the chronic high lesser curve ulcer involving the left gastric artery. The procedure is then partial gastrectomy with excision of the lesser curve (Pauchet's manoeuvre; Figure 8.6), but for secure haemostasis, a formal gastrectomy may be unnecessary and excision of the lesser curve and ulcer may suffice.

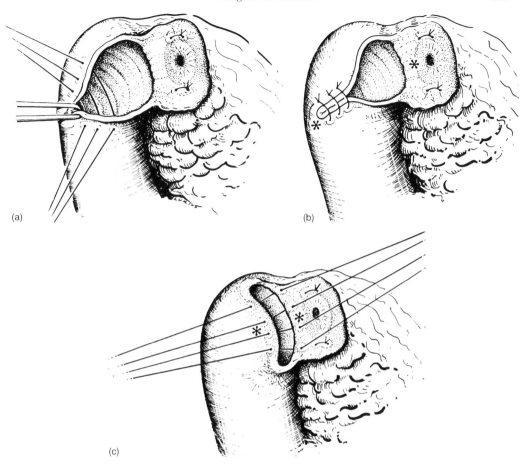

Figure 8.5 Bentley's (1952) method of duodenal closure. **(a)**, **(b)** The anterior wall of the duodenum is cut as long as possible. It is closed with sutures until its length equals that of the posterior wall, which is densely adherent to the distal edge of the ulcer. **(c)** Two sutures are inserted on either side of the two stars; when tightened these will bring the two stars together by rolling the anterior wall into the duodenal lumen. The closure is completed with further sutures, which take deep bites of the distal edge of the ulcer and of the anterior duodenal wall. All sutures are inserted, and then tied.

There is a distinct risk that the ulcer is a carcinoma, so histological examination of the specimen is essential. Of 61 bleeding gastric ulcers treated by urgent operation eight were carcinomas (Hunt *et al.*, 1982).

In a patient with a large gastric ulcer with a visible vessel, it is tempting to merely under-run the vessel. Unless the patient will be put at risk by ulcer excision, this should be resisted as it is associated with a high risk of rebleeding. On the other hand, the tiny ulcer with an exposed vessel – the 'Dieulafoy lesion' – can be treated appropriately in this way. In this condition, the ulcer can be difficult to identify at operation, even if it has been seen at endoscopy. Rather than trying to see the lesion, it is better to palpate the suspicious area with the finger tip, when the protruding vessel can be felt as a distinct 'bristle'.

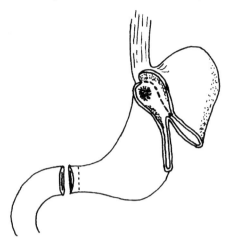

Figure 8.6 Pauchet's manoeuvre. The figure shows the line of the whole incision. It is often wise to make the upper half of the incision and then suture the new lesser curve before making the lower half of the incision.

Simple ulcer excision may be the treatment of choice (Figure 8.7) but is not a minor procedure, and has to be carried out with great care.

The lesser curve must be mobilized completely, often pinching the ulcer off the posterior abdominal wall and dividing the left gastric vessels, which may be incorporated in an inflammatory mass. The stomach wall is then divided around the ulcer, making the incision in healthy tissue. When an anterior gastrotomy is required to find the ulcer or to obtain initial haemostasis, it should be made so that it can be incorporated in the excision. The defect in the lesser curve is closed with an initial mucosal suture to obtain secure haemostasis followed by a separate serosubmucosal, suture both of continuous 3/0 polydioxanone.

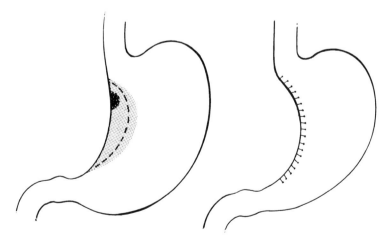

Figure 8.7 Formal excision of a high lesser curve ulcer.

Occasionally, with massively bleeding multiple erosions throughout the stomach, it is necessary to carry out a total gastrectomy and it is important to reduce gastric blood flow as quickly as possible. The first steps should be to ligate and divide the right gastric and gastroepiploic vessels, divide the duodenum, lift up the stomach and ligate and divide the left gastric vessels. The rest of the operation can then be done at relative leisure.

The bleeding oesophageal ulcer

Arterial bleeding from the oesophagus is usually due to reflux oesophagitis or a Mallory–Weiss tear. It is very unusual for either of these to come to surgery, as both tend to settle spontaneously and, if they do not, adrenaline injection almost always achieves permanent haemostasis (Park *et al.*, 1994).

However, if a Mallory–Weiss tear does require surgery, it is usually accessible through the abdomen, certainly in a thin subject. The oesophagus is mobilized, and the gastro-oesophageal junction exposed through a high anterior longitudinal gastrotomy. It is then possible to see and under-run the tear in the mucosa. In the fat patient, access to the lower oesophagus is easier through a left thoracotomy, and this approach should be used for true lower oesophageal bleeding from oesophagitis that does not respond to injection therapy. In this case it may be possible to gain control *via* an oesophagotomy, but oesophagectomy is occasionally necessary.

8.7.2   CHOICE OF PROCEDURE

Vagotomy

For many years the standard treatment for a bleeding duodenal ulcer was under-running of the bleeding point, truncal vagotomy and drainage, and, when a gastrectomy was necessary, a vagotomy was often added. The rationale behind this approach was to provide definitive therapy and thereby minimize the risk of life-threatening recurrence. Over the past 10 years or so, however, changes in the management of peptic ulcer disease have brought about a major change in attitude to this problem.

Firstly, the side effects of truncal vagotomy led to the development of the highly selective vagotomy (HSV; Johnston, 1975), and it has been suggested that, after local control of bleeding, HSV should be the definitive procedure. However, the results of HSV are highly operator-dependent, and few surgeons now have extensive experience of the operation. This, along with the time-consuming nature of the operation, makes it impractical in most emergency situations.

More importantly, the medical treatment of peptic ulcer has improved greatly over the years. Although ineffective in stopping bleeding, antisecretory therapy in the form of the H_2-receptor antagonists or the proton-pump inhibitors is effective in securing ulcer healing. In addition, the pathogenic role of *H. pylori* is now firmly established, in duodenal ulcer at least, and successful eradication therapy reduces the risk of recurrent ulcer to very acceptable levels.

For these reasons, the need for truncal vagotomy in acute bleeding may be questioned and securing haemostasis is sufficient treatment in the majority of patients. It is then mandatory to ensure that the patient is properly treated and investigated postoperatively; in practical terms this usually comprises a 1-week eradication course for *H. pylori* coinciding with discharge from hospital. If it is important to establish the *H. pylori* status this must be done off all medication, because antisecretory agents can lead to false-negative results. The urea breath test is convenient and obviates the need for another endoscopy.

Occasionally, the surgeon will come across the patient who has had multiple courses of treatment and attempts at *H. pylori* eradication who bleeds from an ulcer. In this case a vagotomy is definitely indicated, but should only be carried out by a surgeon experienced in the technique.

Control of ulcer bleeding

In the duodenum, this inevitably involves under-running of the bleeding vessel, and, vagotomy aside, the only choice then is between closure of the duodenotomy and gastrectomy. The ideal course of action is usually obvious and determined by the size of the ulcer. In gastric ulcer the decision can be more difficult. Two groups have found that simple under-running for bleeding gastric ulcer produced satisfactory results (Teenan and Murray, 1990; Schein and Gecelter, 1989). However, in a randomized trial comparing minimal surgery with conventional ulcer surgery, Poxon *et al.* (1991) found that patients treated by under-running alone were more likely to suffer fatal rebleeding. In this trial 62 patients had the bleeding point under-run with parenteral ranitidine; 67 patients had either vagotomy and pyloroplasty or a partial gastrectomy. Some 16 (26%) of the 62 patients died and 13 (19%) of the 67, and the cause of the excess deaths on conservative management was rebleeding.

The optimal operation for bleeding peptic ulcer depends on the individual circumstances, and varies with the clinical situation and the experience of the surgeon. The priority is to save life by securing haemostasis by whatever means are most appropriate. In the event of recurrence of major bleeding postoperatively the involvement of a surgeon experienced in major gastric resection is mandatory.

REFERENCES

Baettig, B., Haecki, W., Lammer, F. *et al.* (1993) Dieulafoy's disease: endoscopic treatment and follow up. *Gut*, **34**, 1418–1421.

Bentley, F. H. (1952) Surgical management of the penetrating posterior wall duodenal ulcer. *Br. J. Surg.*, **40**, 107–110.

Birnie, G. C., Fenn, G. C., Shield, M. J. *et al.* (1991) Double blind comparative study of Misoprostol with placebo in acute upper gastrointestinal bleeding. *Gut*, **32**, A1246.

Chung, S. C. S., Leung, J. W. C., Steele, R. J. C. *et al.* (1988) Endoscopic adrenaline injection for actively bleeding ulcers: a randomised trial. *BMJ*, **296**, 1631–1633.

Chung, S. C. S., Lau, J. Y. W., Sung, J. J. Y. *et al.* (1997) Randomised comparison between adrenaline injection alone and adrenaline injection plus heat probe treatment for actively bleeding ulcers. *BMJ*, **314**, 1307–1311.

Cook, D. J., Guyatt, G. H., Salena, B. J. *et al.* (1992) Endoscopic therapy for acute non-variceal upper gastrointestinal haemorrhage: a meta-analysis. *Gastroenterology*, **102**, 139–148.

Cook, D. J., Fuller, H. D., Guyatt, G. H. *et al.* (1994) Risk factors for gastrointestinal bleeding in critically ill patients. *N. Engl. J. Med.*, **330**, 377–381.

Curling, T. B. (1842) On acute ulceration of the duodenum in cases of burns. *Med. Chir. Trans. Lond.*, **25**, 260.

Cushing, H. (1932) Peptic ulcers and the interbrain. *Surg. Gynecol. Obstet.*, **55**, 1–34.

Davenport, H. W. (1967) Salicylate damage to the gastric mucosal barrier. *N. Engl. J. Med.*, **276**, 1307–1312.

Douthwaite, A. H. and Lintott, G. A. M. (1938) Gastroscopic observation of the effect of aspirin and certain other substances on the stomach. *Lancet*, **ii**, 1122–1125.

Finsterer, H. (1939) Surgical treatment of acute profuse gastric haemorrhage. *Surg. Gynecol. Obstet.*, **69**, 291–298.

Forrest, J. A. H., Finlayson, N. D. C. and Shearman, D. J. V. (1974) Endoscopy in gastrointestinal bleeding. *Lancet*. **ii**, 394–397.

Fullarton, G. M., Birnie, G. C., MacDonald, A. *et al.* (1989) Controlled trial of heater probe treatment in bleeding peptic ulcers. *Br. J. Surg.*, **76**, 541–544.

Gordon-Taylor, G. (1937) The problem of bleeding peptic ulcer. *Br. J. Surg.*, **25**, 403–425.

Graham, D. Y. and Schwartz, J. T. (1977) Spectrum of the Mallory–Weiss tear. *Medicine*, **57**, 307–318.

Henry, D. A. and O'Connell, D. L. (1989) Effects of fibrinolytic inhibitors on mortality from upper gastrointestinal haemorrhage. *BMJ*, **298**, 1142–1146.

Holman, R. A. E., Davis, M., Gough, K. R. *et al.* (1990) Value of a centralised approach in the management of haematemesis and melaena. *Gut*, **31**, 504–508.

Hunt, P. S. (1987) Bleeding gastroduodenal ulcers: selection of patients for surgery. *World J. Surg.*, **11**, 289–294.

Hunt, P. S., Dowling, J., Korman, M. *et al.* (1979) Bleeding stomal ulceration. *Austr. N.Z. J. Surg.*, **49**, 15–18.

Hunt, P. S., Hansky, J. and Korman, M. (1982) Bleeding carcinomatous ulcer of the stomach. *Med. J. Austr.*, **1**, 494.

Hunt, P. S., Francis, J. K., Hansky, J. *et al.* (1983) Reduction in mortality from upper gastrointestinal haemorrhage. *Med. J. Austr.*, **2**, 552–555.

Jenkins, S. A., Taylor, B. A., Nott, D. M. *et al.* (1992) Management of massive upper gastrointestinal haemorrhage from multiple sites of peptic ulceration with somatostatin and octreotide – a report of five cases. *Gut*, **33**, 404–407.

Jensen, D. M. (1990) Heat probe for haemostasis of bleeding peptic ulcers: techniques and results of randomised controlled trials. *Gastrointest. Endosc.*, **36**, S42–S49.

Johnston, D. (1975) Operative mortality and post-operative morbidity of highly selective vagotomy. *BMJ*, **iv**, 545–547.

Johnston, S. J., Jones, P. F., Kyle, J. *et al.* (1973) The epidemiology and course of gastrointestinal haemorrhage in North-East Scotland. *BMJ*, **iii**, 655–660.

Jones, F. A. (1939) Haematemesis and melaena: observation on the use of continuous drip transfusions. *BMJ*, **i**, 915.

Jones, F. A. (1947) Haematemesis and melaena with special reference to bleeding peptic ulcer. *BMJ*, **ii**, 441–446.

Juler, G. L., Labitzke, H. G., Lamb, R. *et al.* (1984) The pathogenesis of Dieulafoy's gastric erosion. *Am. J. Gastroenterol.*, **79**, 195–200.

Laine, L., Freeman, M. and Cohen, H. (1994) Lack of uniformity in evaluation of endoscopic prognostic features of bleeding ulcers. *Gastrointest. Endosc.*, **40**, 411–417.

Lanza, F. L. (1991) NSAID induced gastroduodenal injury. *Gastroenterology*, **101**, 555–557.

Levy, J., Khakoo, S., Barton, R. *et al.* (1991) Fatal injection sclerotherapy of a bleeding peptic ulcer. *Lancet*, **37**, 504.

Mallory G. K. and Weiss, S. (1929) Haemorrhages from lacerations of the cardiac orifice of the stomach due to vomiting. *Am. J. Med. Sci.*, **178**, 506.

Marshall, B. J. (1994) *Helicobacter pylori*. *Am. J. Gastroenterol.*, **89**, S116–S128.

Marriott, H. L. and Kerwick, A. (1935) Continuous drip blood transfusion. *Lancet*, **i**, 977–981.

Masson, J., Bramley, P. N., Herd, K. *et al.* (1996) Upper gastrointestinal bleeding in an open access dedicated unit. *J. R. Coll. Phys. Lond.*, **30**, 436–442.

Meulengracht, E. (1934) Treatment of haematemesis and melena with food. *Acta Med. Scand. Suppl.*, **59**, 375.

Morris, D. L., Hawker, P. C., Brearley, S. *et al.* (1984) Optimal timing of operation for bleeding peptic ulcer: prospective randomised trial. *BMJ*, **288**, 1277–1280.

Nash, J., Lambert, L. and Deakin, M. (1994) Histamine H_2-receptor antagonists in peptic ulcer disease. Evidence for a prophylactic use. *Drugs*, **47**, 862–871.

Needham, C. D. and McConachie, J. A. (1950) Haematemesis and melaena. *BMJ*, **ii**, 133–138.

Needham, C. D., Kyle, J., Jones, P. F. *et al.* (1971) Aspirin and alcohol in gastrointestinal haemorrhage. *Gut*, **12**, 819–821.

O'Brien, P. (1985) The pathogenesis, prevention and treatment of stress ulceration, in *Gastrointestinal Haemorrhage*, (ed. P. S. Hunt), Churchill Livingstone, Edinburgh, p. 60.

Oxner, R. N. G., Simmonds, N. J., Gertner, D. J. *et al.* (1992) Controlled trial of endoscopic injection treatment for bleeding from peptic ulcers visible vessels. *Lancet,* **339**, 966–968.

Panes, J., Vivier, J. Forne, M *et al.* (1987) Controlled trial of endoscopic sclerosis in bleeding peptic ulcers. *Lancet,* **ii**, 1292–1294.

Park, K. G. M., Steele, R. J. C. and Masson, J. (1994) Endoscopic adrenaline injection for benign oesophageal ulcer haemorrhage. *Br. J. Surg.,* **81**, 1317–1318.

Pascu, O., Draghici, A. and Acalovachi, I. (1989) The effect of endoscopic haemostasis with alcohol on the mortality rate of nonvariceal upper gastrointestinal haemorrhage: a randomised prospective study. *Endoscopy,* **36**, S53–S55.

Pinkas, H., McAllister, E., Norman, J. *et al.* (1995) Prolonged evaluation of epinephrine and normal saline solution injections in an acute ulcer model with a single bleeding artery. *Gastrointest. Endosc.,* **41**, 51–55.

Poxon, V. A., Keighley, M. R. B., Dykes, P. W. *et al.* (1991) Comparison of minimal and conventional surgery in patients with bleeding peptic ulcer: a multicentre trial. *Br. J. Surg.,* **78**, 1344–1345.

Rockall, T. A., Logan, R. F. A., Devlin, H. B. *et al.,* (1995) Incidence of and mortality from acute upper gastrointestinal haemorrhage in the United Kingdom. *BMJ,* **311**, 222–226.

Sanderson, J. D., Taylor, R. F. H., Pugh, S. *et al.* (1990) Specialised gastrointestinal units for the management of upper gastrointestinal haemorrhage. *Postgrad. Med. J.,* **66**, 654–656.

Schein, M. and Gecelter, G. (1989) Apache II score in massive upper gastrointestinal haemorrhage from peptic ulcer: prognostic value and potential clinical applications. *Br. J. Surg.,* **76**, 733–736.

Selye, H. (1935) Stress ulcer. *Nature,* **138**, 32.

Snook, J. A., Holdstock, G. E. and Bamforth, J. (1986) Value of a simple biochemical ratio in distinguishing upper and lower sites of gastrointestinal haemorrhage. *Lancet,* **i**, 1064–1065.

Steele, R. J. C. (1989) Endoscopic haemostasis for non-variceal upper gastrointestinal haemorrhage. *Br. J. Surg.,* **76**, 219–225.

Stern, A. I., Korman, M. G., Hunt, P. S. *et al.* (1979) Mallory–Weiss lesion as a cause of upper gastrointestinal bleeding. *Austr. N.Z. J. Surg.,* **49**, 13–18.

Swain, C. P., Storey, D. W., Bown, S. G. *et al.* (1986) Nature of the bleeding vessel in recurrently bleeding gastric ulcers. *Gastroenterology,* **90**, 595–608.

Teenan, R. P. and Murray, W. R. (1990) Late outcome of undersewing alone for gastric ulcer haemorrhage. *Br. J. Surg.,* **77**, 811–812.

Villanueva, C., Balanzo, J., Torras, X. *et al.* (1994) Value of second-look endoscopy after injection therapy for bleeding peptic ulcer: a prospective and randomised trial. *Gastrointest. Endosc.,* **40**, 34–39.

Warren, J. R. and Marshall, B. (1983) Unidentified curved bacilli on gastric epithelium in active chronic gastritis. *Lancet,* **i**, 1273–1275.

Welch, C. E., Radkey, G. V. and von Ryll-Gryska, P. (1986) A thousand operations for ulcer disease. *Ann. Surg.,* **204**, 454–467.

Wood, P. H. N., Harvey-Smith, E. A. and Dixon, A. S. (1962) Salicylates and gastrointestinal bleeding. *BMJ,* **i**, 669–675.

Wyncoll, D. L. A., Roerts, P. C., Beale, R. J. *et al.* (1997) H_2 blockers in the intensive care unit: ignoring the evidence? *BMJ,* **314**, 1013.

Yang, C. C., Shin, J. S., Lin, X. Z. *et al.* (1994) The natural history (fading time) of stigmata of recent haemorrhage in peptic ulcer disease. *Gastrointest. Endosc.,* **40**, 562–566.

Yudin, S. S. (1937) Transfusion of stored cadaver blood. *Lancet,* **ii**, 361–366.

8.8   ACUTE VARICEAL HAEMORRHAGE

8.8.1   AETIOLOGY

Haematemesis due to rupture of oesophageal varices, although accounting for only 3–5% of acute UGIH in the UK, is one of its most worrying forms. It is difficult to treat, and the cirrhotics, who make up most of this population, are generally unfit before the bleed further impairs hepatic function. As many as 30–40% die after the first bleeding episode. The incidence is probably on the increase, although not yet at the level of about 10% found in Australia and of 15–20% of all upper tract haemorrhages seen in the USA. Alcoholic cirrhosis, the principal cause of varices, is certainly on the increase; in Birmingham, England, incidence trebled over the years 1959–1976 (Saunders *et al.,* 1981). It is therefore necessary to be well prepared for these patients, who can bleed very fiercely and deteriorate very rapidly.

Portal hypertension is due to impaired flow in the portal venous circulation. As a consequence, venous channels open up and dilate as they develop a communication with the systemic veins in the abdominal wall and principally, through the peri-oesophageal veins, with the azygous venous channels. Pressure within the portal venous system is high either because the vein itself is blocked outside the liver or because there is obstruction within it; the cause of the obstruction has a great bearing on prognosis.

The non-cirrhotic causes are generally associated with reasonable or normal hepatic function.

- **Portal or splenic vein thrombosis** is the commonest of the non-cirrhotic extrahepatic obstructions seen in Western countries, and occurs mainly in young people.

Within the liver capsule there are three main causes of presinusoidal obstruction.

- **Schistosomiasis** is widespread throughout Africa and in parts of Asia and South America.
- **Congenital hepatic fibrosis** (p. 118) and **primary biliary cirrhosis** are two fairly unusual causes of portal hypertension.
- **Cirrhosis of the liver** still accounts for 80–90% of cases of portal hypertension in most countries. About two-thirds of cases are alcoholic in origin, about one-quarter are cryptogenic, and a few are the sequelae of hepatitis or examples of chronic active hepatitis. In all these patients there is impairment of hepatic function, and in many this is severe even before it is aggravated by the effects of haemorrhage and hypovolaemia. Consequently, a number of patients with variceal haemorrhage present with ascites or jaundice and may suffer from episodes of encephalopathy, making them exceptionally poor risks for any form of treatment.

The reason for the abrupt onset of bleeding from oesophageal varices that have been present for months or years is not known. There is a zone that extends for 2–5 cm above the oesophagogastric junction in which the oesophageal veins are exceptionally exposed, where they lie largely in the lamina propria. Normally these veins are about 1 mm in diameter, but in portal hypertension they distend to 3–4 mm and are separated from the lumen by epithelium only 0.2 mm thick. In gastric mucosa, and in the oesophagus above this zone, the veins lie at a deeper level, in the submucosa, so these histological findings help to explain why rupture of the veins is localized in the lowest few centimetres of the oesophagus (Beswick and Butler, 1951). Considering the remarkably exposed position of the varices in the lowermost part of the oesophagus and the extreme thinness of the covering epithelium, it seems remarkable that they do not bleed more often. When they do, Spence *et al.* (1984) have calculated that if there is only a pinhole opening in a subepithelial vein, 1.0–1.5 litres of blood can be lost each hour.

8.8.2 CLINICAL FEATURES

Quite often the patient is already known to have varices, and may have bled on previous occasions. The most useful warning physical sign is splenomegaly, which Bull *et al.* (1979)

showed to be highly significant. Signs such as ascites, gynaecomastia, spider naevi, palmar erythema and prominent abdominal wall veins suggest liver disease. The liver itself may or may not be palpable. The protein 'meal' from the blood in the bowel may precipitate hepatic encephalopathy.

8.8.3 MANAGEMENT OF VARICEAL HAEMORRHAGE

Medical therapy

The patient with variceal haemorrhage (VH) should be assessed and resuscitated as for NVH, but there are some special considerations that have to be taken into account. The bleeding is often torrential, and clotting abnormalities are common, so it is important to send blood for a clotting screen and for fresh frozen plasma and platelet concentrate to be ordered immediately. Large volumes of crystalloid must be avoided because this exacerbates the ascites and peripheral oedema associated with portal hypertension and liver failure. The patient is at risk of hepatic coma, and appropriate preventative measures should be taken: opiates should not be used, blood glucose levels must be monitored and a 10% glucose infusion should be used to correct hypoglycaemia. To reduce the amount of protein in the gut, oral lactulose (10 ml q.i.d.) and neomycin (1 g q.i.d.) are given to reduce the production of toxic metabolites by bacterial flora.

The main pharmacological agents that have been used to control acute VH are vasopressin and somatostatin or its analogues. Vasopressin is a splanchnic vasoconstrictor, and infusion at 0.5–0.6 units/min will reduce portal pressure sufficiently to control acute variceal bleeding in 50–70% of cases. The side effects of vasoconstriction, notably angina and cardiac arrhythmias, can be a problem, and its use has been abandoned in many centres. Somatostatin and its longer-acting analogue octreotide are much more selective in terms of their action on mesenteric smooth muscle, and there is good evidence from a randomized trial from Hong Kong that a 50 μg bolus of octreotide followed by an infusion at 50 μg/h may be as effective at controlling acute haemorrhage as sclerotherapy (Sung *et al.*, 1993).

The risk of rebleeding from varices may be reduced by the long-term administration of beta-blockers such as propranolol, but this has no place in the treatment of the acute bleed. Their negative inotropic and chronotropic effects may indeed compromise the hypovolaemic patient.

Endoscopic therapy

Background
Injection sclerotherapy is long established as an effective endoscopic means of controlling VH, and was first performed by Crafoord and Frenckner in 1936. However, it is only since enthusiasm for open portosystemic shunting waned in the 1970s that it has really come into its own.

Endoscopic sclerotherapy certainly controls acute VH; although only 25% of patients admitted with VH will actually be seen to have active bleeding at the time of endoscopy, about 60% of the remainder will have further bleeding while in hospital (Mitchell *et al.*, 1982). Several studies demonstrate the ability of sclerotherapy to greatly improve on these figures (Johnston and Rodgers, 1973; Terblanche *et al.*, 1979a), and sclerotherapy has been shown to be more effective than balloon tamponade in a randomized, controlled trial (Paquet and Feussner, 1985).

Opinion as to the timing of injection for the acute bleed is divided between (1) immediate injection and a period of resuscitation combined with vasoactive therapy or (2) tamponade followed by semi-elective injection. Published evidence supports the former approach; Prindiville and Trudeau (1986) found that immediate emergency injection gave significantly better control of the bleeding than delayed endoscopic therapy.

A single session of sclerotherapy, however, carries a high risk of recurrent bleeding (Terblanche *et al.*, 1979b) and several sessions are necessary to achieve obliteration of the varices and acceptably low recurrence rates (Larson *et al.*, 1986). Even so, recurrent bleeding after endoscopic treatment remains a problem, and there has been a return to elective portosystemic shunting when long-term control is difficult (Shields, 1991).

All patients who have suffered VH should be treated endoscopically at least initially; but the frequency of repeat injections is uncertain. Westby *et al.* (1984) found that injections at weekly rather than 3-week intervals resulted in more rapid obliteration of the varices.

Which sclerosant to use is also debatable. In several trials, 5% ethanolamine has been compared with 3% sodium tetradecyl sulphate (STD), and, although both are effective in controlling VH, STD obliterated the varices in fewer sessions (Chan *et al.*, 1993).

An alternative endoscopic treatment of VH is banding. In this technique, described below, elastic 'O' rings similar to those used to band haemorrhoids are applied to the varices using special equipment which is attached to the endoscope. This is extremely promising, and studies suggest that it may be at least as effective as sclerotherapy but with fewer complications (Stiegmann *et al.*, 1989; 1990). It is of particular value in the management of fundal varices for which injection therapy is less effective.

Sclerotherapy

It is important to choose the correct endoscope if varices are suspected. For sclerotherapy, a twin-channelled endoscope is ideal for three reasons. Firstly, suction and irrigation are still available with the injector needle in place. Second, the size of the instrument is useful in obtaining a degree of tamponade, and thirdly, the two channels provide flexibility in obtaining the correct position for the needle.

The most commonly used sclerosants are 3% STD, 5% ethanolamine, 1% polidocanol and absolute alcohol. Injection needles are available in many different designs and sizes, but it is agreed that the disposable type should be used in all cases to eliminate the risk of disease transmission. When an oil-based sclerosant such as ethanolamine is used, it is necessary to employ a needle of at least 23 gauge.

In most circumstances it is possible to inject varices under sedation, and the flexible endoscope has supplanted the need for rigid oesophagoscopy. There has been some debate as to whether injection should be performed directly into the varices or around them, but it is now generally agreed that the intravariceal technique leads to more rapid obliteration of the varices (Sarin *et al.*, 1987).

When varices are seen at endoscopy, it is still important to carry out a full examination of the stomach and duodenum if possible, as a significant proportion of patients with varices bleed from some other lesion. Active bleeding from a varix is usually seen as a jet of blood, but if no active bleeding is seen, varices can be assumed to have been the site if no other lesions are found in the upper gastrointestinal tract. If one of the varices is bleeding actively, this should be treated first by puncturing it just proximal to the bleeding point and injecting 1–2 ml of sclerosant. Further injections should then proceed upward from the oesophagogastric junction at 2 cm intervals in all the variceal columns until a maximum of 15 ml of sclerosant have been used.

When massive bleeding obscures the view, the endoscope should be inserted into the stomach, and as much blood as possible should be aspirated. The shaft of the instrument will compress the varices, and is left in position for at least 5 minutes. The endoscope is then withdrawn slowly, with the patient in a head-up position if possible, and it is then usually feasible to obtain a view that is clear enough to place the injection precisely. Occasionally, the bleeding is too profuse, and under these circumstances the insertion of a Sengstaken–Blakemore tube becomes necessary (see below). The endoscopy can be repeated at 24–48 hours.

If the sclerotherapy is successful in controlling the haemorrhage, repeat sclerotherapy should be carried out at weekly intervals until the varices have been obliterated, and check endoscopy with repeat injections as necessary at 6-monthly intervals thereafter. Serious complications are relatively rare, but ulceration does occur in about 50% of cases. Stricture formation occurs after multiple injections in about 5% of cases, but can usually be managed by endoscopic dilatation. Perforation of the oesophagus is rare, but may occur if large amounts of sclerosant are used over a short period of time.

Banding

The technique of endoscopic banding is being used increasingly in acute variceal haemorrhage. The special equipment and the technique are fully described by Stiegman. The equipment required (the Stiegmann–Goff ligator) is made up of an outer cylindrical adapter, which fits on to the tip of the endoscope, an inner cylinder preloaded with an elastic 'O' ring and a trip wire for pulling the inner cylinder into the outer adapter to release the ring. When the use of banding is anticipated, it is necessary to use an overtube to allow easy passage of the device and facilitate multiple loadings and re-insertions.

Balloon tamponade

Balloon tamponade of varices is necessary when endoscopic therapy and octreotide infusion prove ineffective in controlling acute haemorrhage. The most commonly used device is the Sengstaken–Blakemore tube or one of its variations. This comprises a gastric balloon of about 400 ml capacity, an oesophageal balloon and aspiration channels both distal and proximal to the balloons.

The first step is to check the balloons for leaks. After thorough lubrication, the tube can then be inserted through the mouth or the nose; the latter may seem unduly painful, but is in fact much more comfortable for the patient once in place. The large gastric balloon must be in the stomach before inflating; this is confirmed by insufflating air down the gastric aspiration channel balloon and auscultating over the stomach. The gastric balloon is inflated to about 350 ml using either water or air. If water is used, contrast medium is added so that the position of the balloon can be checked on X-ray; if air is used, the balloon will be seen on a penetrated chest X-ray. If air is being used, this should be insufflated in series with a sphygmomanometer to ensure that the pressures that are being developed are not too high.

Once the gastric balloon is inflated, traction is applied to interrupt the blood flow into the varices at the gastro-oesophageal junction (Figure 8.8).

The traction can then be maintained by taping the tube to the bridge of the nose if the nasal route has been used. If the oral route has been used traction is provided by using pulley and

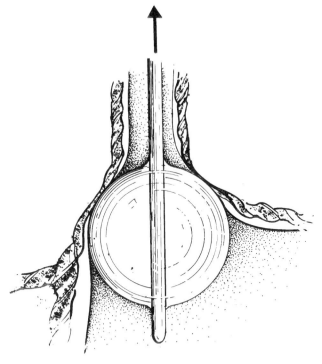

Figure 8.8 The gastric balloon of the Sengstaken–Blakemore tube compressing varices at the gastro-oesophageal junction.

weight, which makes the procedure more complex. It is not usually necessary to use the oesophageal balloon but, if active bleeding continues, this should be connected to a sphygmomanometer and inflated to a pressure of 20–40 mmHg.

Balloon tamponade is very much a temporary measure, and traction should be released after a maximum period of 24 hours to avoid necrosis of the gastro-oesophageal junction. This should be done in the endoscopy room, and if the bleeding has stopped, the tube can be removed and immediate endoscopic therapy delivered.

Oesophageal surgery for variceal bleeding

Very occasionally all the above measures fail, and direct oesophageal surgery is necessary. Direct under-running of oesophageal varices has been supplanted by the use of the circular end-to-end anastomosis stapling gun, and the best approach is through an upper midline abdominal incision. Mobilization of the oesophagus is more difficult than normal because of the surrounding high-pressure venous collaterals. These must be individually isolated, ligated and divided. The phreno-oesophageal ligament is divided just above the 'white line' to gain access to the posterior mediastinum and the oesophagus is mobilized circumferentially, preferably under vision, by careful blunt dissection using a pledget on a Roberts forceps, taking care to keep anterior to the posterior vagal trunk. The objective is to clear the lower 4–5 cm of oesophagus and ligate all vascular channels entering it. The anterior vagal trunks

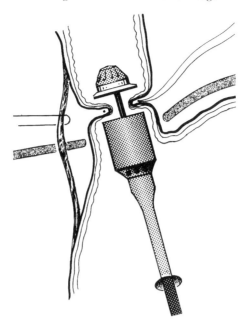

Figure 8.9 Insertion of the circular end-to-end stapler prior to oesophageal transection for varices. The posterior vagus is held aside. The invaginating ligature has been tied.

are mobilized and held aside, and a strong silk ligature is passed around the oesophagus above the oesophagogastric junction. A small gastrotomy is made in the upper aspect of the anterior gastric wall and a 31 mm circular stapler in the 'open' position is inserted through the gastrotomy into the lower oesophagus. The silk ligature is tied firmly around the shaft of the stapling head (Figure 8.9), and the device is closed and fired, simultaneously transecting and rejoining the oesophagus so that the portosystemic flow through the lower oesophageal veins is interrupted.

It is usual to withhold oral intake until anastomotic integrity has been confirmed by contrast study after 7 days. Spence and Johnston (1985) reported 100 consecutive stapling operations, 25 of which were done as an emergency; there were no anastomotic leaks.

When it is gastric varices that are bleeding, this is more difficult to control surgically. When this becomes necessary, the stomach has to be opened *via* a high gastrotomy and the variceal columns under-run with a continuous suture. For any direct surgery to varices, the patient should come to the theatre with a Sengstaken tube in place, and the balloon should only be let down at the last moment so that the stomach is not full of blood.

Portosystemic shunting

The purpose of portosystemic shunting is to lower portal pressure by diverting portal blood into the systemic circulation. The most common surgical procedures that have been employed to achieve this have been the direct portocaval shunt or the selective 'Warren' shunt in which the splenic vein is anastomosed to the left renal vein so that the short gastric veins are decompressed into the systemic system. Although good results have been reported from specialist centres for these operations, they are widely associated with a high operative mortality, and with increasingly good results from endoscopic therapy they have tended to lose favour.

The advent of a new technique has brought shunting back into the arena as a viable option for variceal bleeding. The transjugular intrahepatic portosystemic stent-shunt (TIPSS) is inserted by interventional radiological techniques that involve passing a sheath over a guidewire *via* the internal jugular vein into the right or middle hepatic veins. A stylet is then passed through the sheath to puncture a branch of the portal vein within the liver, the tract between the hepatic vein and portal vein is dilated with an angioplasty balloon, and an expanding metal stent (Wallstent) is inserted to keep the tract open.

The results of this procedure indicate that it may be useful in the control of refractory variceal bleeding, but in common with the other methods of portosystemic shunting it is associated with the development of encephalopathy in patients with severe liver disease. In addition, shunt dysfunction may occur over a 6–12-month period in a proportion of patients (Jalan *et al.*, 1995).

REFERENCES

Beswick, T. S. L. and Butler, H. (1951) Fatal haematemesis, from oesophageal varices in presence of large portacaval anastomosis. *BMJ*, **ii**, 5212.

Bull, J., Keeling, P. W. N. and Thompson, R. P. H. (1979) Palpable spleen and bleeding oesophageal varices. *BMJ*, **ii**, 1328–1329.

Chan, A. C., Chung, S. C., Sung, S. Y. *et al.* (1993) A double-blind randomised controlled trial comparing sodium tetradecyl sulphate and ethanolamine in the sclerotherapy of bleeding oesophageal varices. *Endoscopy*, **29**, 513–517.

Crafoord, C. and Frenckner, P. (1939) New surgical treatment of varicose veins of the oesophagus. *Acta Oto-laryngol.*, **27**, 422–429.

Jalan, R., Redhead, D. N. and Hayes, P. C. (1995) Transjugular intrahepatic portosystemic stent-shunt in the treatment of variceal haemorrhage. *Br. J. Surg.*, **82**, 1158–1164.

Johnston, G. W. and Rodgers, H. W. (1973) A review of 15 years experience in the use of sclerotherapy in the control of acute haemorrhage from oesophageal varices *Br. J. Surg.*, **60**, 797–800.

Larson, A. W., Cohen, H., Zweiban, B. *et al.* (1986) Acute oesophageal variceal sclerotherapy: results of a prospective randomised controlled trial. *J.A.M.A.*, **255**, 497–500.

Mitchell, K. A., MacDougall, B. R. D., Silk, D. B. A. *et al.* (1982) A prospective reappraisal of emergency endoscopy in patients with portal hypertension. *Scand. J. Gastroenterol.*, **17**, 965–968.

Paquet, K. J. and Feussner, H. (1985) Endoscopic sclerosis and oesophageal balloon tamponade in acute haemorrhage from oesophageal varices: a prospective controlled randomised trial. *Hepatology*, **5**, 580–583.

Prindiville, T. and Trudeau, W. (1986) A comparison of immediate versus delayed endoscopic injection sclerosis of bleeding oesophageal varices. *Gastrointest. Endosc.*, **32**, 385–388.

Sarin, S. K., Nanda, R., Sachdev, G. *et al.* (1987) Intravariceal versus paravariceal sclerotherapy: a prospective, controlled, randomised trial. *Gut*, **28**, 657–662.

Saunders, J. B., Walters, J. R. F., Davies, P. *et al.* (1981) A 20-year prospective study of cirrhosis. *BMJ*, **282**, 263–266.

Shields, R. (1991) Bleeding oesophageal varices and the surgeon. *Br. J. Surg.*, **78**, 513–515.

Spence, R. A. J. and Johnston, G. W. (1985) Results in 100 consecutive patients with stapled oesophageal transection for varices. *Surg. Gynecol. Obstet.*, **160**, 323–325.

Spence, R. A. J., Sloan, J. M. and Johnston, G. W. (1984) Histologic factors of the oesophageal transection ring as clues to the pathogenesis of bleeding varices. *Surg. Gynecol. Obstet.*, **159**, 253–259.

Stiegmann, G. V., Goff, J., Sum, J. H. *et al.* (1989) Endoscopic variceal ligation: an alternative to sclerotherapy. *Gastrointest. Endosc.*, **35**, 431–434.

Stiegmann, G., Goff, J., Korula, J. *et al.* (1990) Endoscopic variceal ligation vs sclerotherapy for bleeding oesophageal varices: early results of a prospective randomised trial. *Gastrointest. Endosc.*, **36**, 118.

Sung, J. J., Chung, S. C., Lai, C. W. *et al.* (1993) Octreotide infusion or emergency sclerotherapy for variceal haemorrhage. *Lancet*, **342**, 637–641.

Terblanche, J., Northover, J. M. A., Bornman, P. *et al.* (1979a) A prospective evaluation of injection sclerotherapy in the treatment of acute bleeding from oesophageal varices. *Surgery*, **85**, 239–245.

Terblanche, J., Northover, J. M. A., Bornman, P. *et al.* (1979b) A prospective controlled trial of injection sclerotherapy in the long-term management of patients after oesophageal variceal bleeding. *Surg. Gynecol. Obstet.*, **148**, 323–333.

Westby, D., Melia, W. M., MacDougall, B. R. D. *et al.* (1984) Injection sclerotherapy for oesophageal varices: a prospective randomised trial of different treatment schedules. *Gut*, **25**, 129–132

8.9   SEVERE RECTAL HAEMORRHAGE

This can be one of the most demanding abdominal emergencies, for several different reasons.

- It mostly affects elderly patients, who have a reduced tolerance for sudden blood loss. Among 252 such patients in Aberdeen, two-thirds were over the age of 60, and 85% of the major bleeds occurred in this age group, of whom 20% were admitted in a state of cardiovascular collapse (Bramley *et al.*, 1996).
- Rectal haemorrhage can arise from a considerable variety of causes, and there are often real difficulties in identifying the bleeding point in a patient with continuing loss.
- Only 20% of patients with acute alimentary tract haemorrhage present with copious loss of fresh blood *per rectum*. This means that the individual surgeon does not build up much experience with which to meet a demanding situation, so it is important to have a well-considered plan with which to meet these situations.

Figure 8.10 and Table 8.2 show some of the commoner conditions which present in this way. That there are difficulties in reaching a diagnosis is shown by the fact that in 25% of cases the origin of the bleeding was not found.

8.9.1   AETIOLOGY

The causes of rectal haemorrhage in childhood have been considered on page p. 119. When this occurs in the teens or early 20s it is, as in childhood, most likely to be due to peptic ulceration in a Meckel's diverticulum, with intestinal haemangiomata, duplications and, occasionally, inflammatory bowel disease as other possibilities. Beyond 30 years, bleeding from a Meckel's diverticulum becomes very unlikely, and other causes become more frequent (Figure 8.10).

It is always necessary to remember that free bleeding from a source in the **upper alimentary tract** can present solely with rectal haemorrhage, e.g. from a penetrating duodenal ulcer. It is unusual for this to occur without haematemesis, but this possibility makes such a difference to the direction of treatment that it must be confirmed or eliminated in the patient who is hypovolaemic. Gastroscopy must be performed, although if this is not immediately available aspiration of clear bile *via* an nasogastric tube is a reasonable alternative.

Before considering colonic diverticulosis and angiodysplasia, there are a number of more unusual sources of bleeding to be remembered.

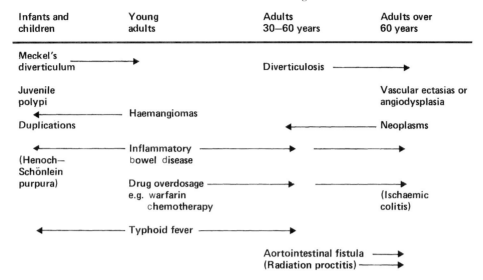

Figure 8.10 Some causes of severe rectal haemorrhage. The condition is listed in the age range in which it is most often seen. Arrows indicate possible occurrence at other ages.

Internal haemorrhoids must not be overlooked because they can on occasion give rise to severe, even life-threatening bleeding. Careful proctoscopy is needed because blood collects at the rectosigmoid, and this may suggest a more proximal site for the bleeding.

Rectal varices, secondary to portal hypertension, must be distinguished from haemorrhoids. They form from the development of communications between the superior, middle and inferior rectal veins. They therefore extend up the rectum in the submucosal plane, and outward from the anus toward the buttocks. Occasionally a vein bursts, causing severe bleeding, and this can be arrested by transanal suture with an over-and-over absorbable suture (McCormack *et al.*, 1984).

Inflammatory bowel disease occurs over a wide age range, but it is unusual for ulcerative colitis or Crohn's disease to produce rapid rectal bleeding.

Ischaemic colitis has a characteristic picture of acute left-sided abdominal pain followed by brisk rectal bleeding (p. 333).

Neoplasms of the small and large bowel, both benign and malignant, do not often bleed freely. However, careful digital examination of the rectum must never be omitted, because a low neoplasm in a blood-filled rectum can easily be missed at sigmoidoscopy.

Pelvic radiotherapy can cause long-term damage to the rectum and the intestines. Radiation proctitis is a recognized cause of rectal bleeding. The small intestine in the pelvis usually shows progressive fibrosis (p. 234), but there can be ulceration and serious bleeding (Taverner *et al.*, 1982).

Benign solitary ulcer of the rectum can cause sufficiently severe bleeding to require urgent local suture and a temporary colostomy (Haycock *et al.*, 1983).

Infective enteritis and colitis, including amoebic dysentery and pseudo-membranous colitis, often produce bloody diarrhoea, but rarely free bleeding, although deep ileal ulceration in typhoid fever can erode a major vessel.

Jejunal diverticulosis is an occasional cause, and Taylor (1969) saw a man of 79 who required 15 units of blood over 48 hours: laparotomy revealed bleeding from a diverticulum 6 cm in diameter (p. 257).

Aortointestinal fistula (p. 523) must be considered in any patient who has undergone aortic surgery: in about half these patients loss is only through the rectum even though most fistulae involve the duodenojejunal area.

Occasionally patients whose **anticoagulant therapy** is out of control present with rectal haemorrhage, and a clotting screen should always be performed. The majority of patients who bleed on anticoagulants are found to have a surgical source.

Diverticulosis of the colon can be demonstrated in about half the population of Western Europe and North America who are over 65, but fewer than 5% are afflicted with rectal haemorrhage. Unlike acquired diverticulitis, which largely affects the sigmoid colon, diverticulosis occurs throughout the colon, and 50–60% of diverticula lie in the right half (Boley *et al.*, 1981). Meyers *et al.* (1976) made a histological study of 10 patients with massive diverticular bleeding. Figure 8.11 shows that a diverticulum forms by the mucosa pushing through the gap in the circular muscle through which a branch of the marginal artery passes from beneath the serosa to the submucosal plane; in this process the vessel is pushed in front of the bulging mucosa and consequently comes to be stretched over the fundus of the diverticulum.

Some injury causes erosion of the mucosa and penetration of the side of the vessel, commonly at the fundus, sometimes at the neck of the diverticulum: as in gastroduodenal ulceration (p. 344), erosion of the side of a vessel prevents haemostasis by intimal retraction. Diverticulosis is usually asymptomatic until the patient feels an urgent need to defaecate, passes a large amount of red blood mixed with faeces, and feels weak and sweaty. About half these patients are in a stable condition when they reach hospital, and they pass little more blood. Management of the other half, who suffer further bleeding, is considered below.

The vascular ectasias or angiodysplasia of the colon occur almost entirely in patients over the age of 60, and some 80% lie in the caecum and ascending colon. They are flat or slightly raised, red, rounded or stellate patches in the mucosa, which are difficult to see because they are only 2–10 mm in diameter. The lesion is defined as 'an ectasia of normal

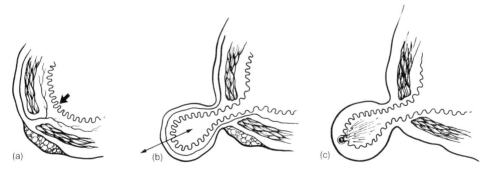

Figure 8.11 Bleeding diverticular disease. (**a**) Site of development of a diverticulum in relation to vasa recta. (**b**) The artery is pushed outwards, over the fundus of the diverticulum, as it develops. (**c**) A section through the plane shown by the arrow in (b), demonstrating the close relationship of the vasa recta to the mucosa, allowing erosion of the side of the vessel by injury from the lumen.

pre-existing intestinal submucosal veins and overlying mucosal capillaries' (Foutch, 1993). The suggestion is that muscle spasm repeatedly obstructs venous drainage, leading to the ectasia, and this occurs where luminal tension is highest – in the wide caecum and ascending colon (LaPlace's law). There is an association with aortic stenosis and chronic respiratory disease. Bleeding occurs into the lumen of the colon and can be very persistent. A few of these ectasias are found in terminal ileum and more distally in the colon.

8.9.2 MANAGEMENT

As in all forms of acute gastrointestinal haemorrhage, these patients need full assessment and many need immediate treatment for hypovolaemia (p. 350). All need careful supervision because in an unpredictable number bleeding will recommence at a later time. There are rarely any abdominal signs. Rectal examination, proctoscopy and sigmoidoscopy by an experienced clinician are the first steps, and often gastroduodenoscopy is indicated (p. 374). In those who remain stable, colonoscopy is performed as soon as feasible, and planned mesenteric angiography, and scanning of red cells labelled with technetium, may be helpful.

In the group that experiences further haemorrhage, many eventually settle, and they are well managed by close observation and measured transfusion. The emergency surgeon is concerned with the small but worrying group who have received 4 or 5 units of blood and are still unstable and continuing to bleed. Of the 252 patients in Aberdeen, 21 required an urgent operation to secure haemostasis. It is for this group, in whom it can be difficult to find the bleeding point, that the surgeon needs to have a considered plan ready.

It is usually unhelpful to attempt colonoscopy because the colon is so full of blood that there is no useful or safe way of proceeding. Much has been reported about the value of inferior and superior mesenteric arteriography, and this has proved a valuable way of demonstrating a bleeding point, particularly in referral centres that see a number of patients with recurrent bleeding from an undetected source (Thomson *et al.*, 1987). However, thought must be given to the practicalities of this investigation in an elderly patient with serious bleeding. It is essential that it is performed by a radiologist with considerable experience of emergency angiography, and allowance must be made for the fact that it usually takes $1\frac{1}{2}$ hours to perform.

This means that a responsible surgeon must accompany the patient and devote full attention to the transfusion and the general welfare of the patient. When blood is shed at more than 0.5–1.0 ml/min a bleeding point may be seen, and if it lies in the colon it may be localized. The problem is that too often a useful result is not obtained. Colacchio *et al.* (1982) in New York carried out 89 emergency angiographies but only 39 yielded a helpful result, and Cussons and Berry (1989) found that in nine urgent angiograms only one was useful, and an average of 6 units of blood was given during the examination. In Aberdeen, 47% of the angiograms performed were unhelpful. (Sometimes a coeliac axis angiogram is required when haemobilia or pancreatic bleeding is suspected.)

With this record, with an elderly patient who has received 4 units of blood and is still bleeding, it may be wiser to proceed at once to laparotomy. This is a situation that requires an experienced anaesthetist and surgeon. The patient is placed in the Lloyd-Davies position. If a thorough examination of the upper alimentary tract proves negative, and there is no obvious abnormality in the blood-filled colon, colonoscopy after colonic wash-out is indicated. A 14 FG Foley catheter is inserted into the side of the appendix, or terminal ileum, the balloon is inflated and it is attached to a drip apparatus. Some 2–4 litres of warm saline are used to wash out the clots and blood through a wide proctoscope. The colonoscope is inserted and guided round to the caecum with the help of the abdominal assistant. An area of fresh bleeding is sought, the lesion identified, the site marked with a stitch, and an appropriate resection can then be performed. The colon will be clean and an anastomosis will usually be possible (Batch *et al.*, 1988).

If the small bowel is full of blood, and no lesion can be seen or felt, enteroscopy can be performed by passing a 160 cm colonoscope: the oral route can be used, with manual guidance round the duodenum, or it is introduced through an enterotomy (Desa *et al.*, 1991).

Suggestions have been made for endoscopic treatment of the bleeding point, but this has little to offer in acute colonic bleeding. It is unlikely to be applicable to bleeding from within a diverticulum, and local treatment of an ectasia in the thin-walled caecum would be hazardous.

Reliance on simple and tested methods is wise in these elderly patients, and can yield reasonable results. The overall mortality rate in Aberdeen was 5.1%: one patient was under 60 years of age. There were five operative deaths, and the median age of these patients was 82 (Bramley *et al.*, 1996).

REFERENCES

Batch, A. J. G., Pickard, R. G. and de Lacey, G. (1981) Preoperative colonoscopy in massive rectal bleeding. *Br. J. Surg.*, **68**, 64.

Boley, S. J., Brandt, L. J. and Frank, M. S. (1981) Severe lower intestinal bleeding. *Clin. Gastroenterol.*, **10**, 65–91.

Bramley, P. N., Masson, J. W., McKnight, G. *et al.* (1996) The role of an open access bleeding unit in the management of colonic haemorrhage. *Scand. J. Gastroenterol.*, **31**, 764–769.

Colacchio, T. A., Forde, K. A., Patsos, J. *et al.* (1982) Impact of modern diagnostic methods on the management of active rectal bleeding. *Am. J. Surg.*, **143**, 607–610.

Cussons, P. D. and Berry, A. R. (1989) Comparison of the value of emergency mesenteric angiography and intraoperative colonoscopy with antegrade colonic irrigation in massive rectal haemorrhage. *J. R. Coll. Surg. Edin.*, **34**, 91–93.

Desa, L. A., Ohri, S. K., Hutton, K. A. R *et al.* (1991) Role of intraoperative enteroscopy in obscure gastrointestinal bleeding of small bowel origin. *Br. J. Surg.*, **78**, 192–195.

Foutch, P. G. (1993) Angiodysplasia of the gastrointestinal tract. *Am. J. Gastroenterol.*, **88**, 807–818.

Haycock, C. E., Suryanavayan, G., Spiller, C. R. *et al.* (1983) Massive haemorrhage from benign solitary ulcer of rectum. *Am. J. Gastroenterol.*, **78**, 83–85.

McCormack, T. T., Bailey, H. R., Simms, J. M. *et al.* (1984) Rectal varices are not piles. *Br. J. Surg.*, **71**, 163.

Meyers, M. A., Alonso, D. R., Gray, G. F. *et al.* (1976) Pathogenesis of bleeding colonic diverticulosis. *Gastroenterology*, **71**, 577–583.

Taverner, D., Talbot, I. C., Carr-Locke, D. L. *et al.* (1982) Massive bleeding from the ileum: a late complication of pelvic radiotherapy. *Am. J. Gastroenterol.*, **77**, 29–31.

Taylor, M. T. (1969) Massive haemorrhage from jejunal diverticulosis. *Am. J. Surg.*, **118**, 117–120.

Thompson, J. M., Salem, R. R., Hemingway, A. P. *et al.* (1987) Specialist investigation of obscure gastrointestinal bleeding. *Gut*, **28**, 47–51.

9

Emergency surgery of the pancreatobiliary system

9.1 ACUTE PANCREATITIS

The clinical entity of acute pancreatitis (AP) was well recognized over a century ago (Senn, 1886). Over the decades, a wide variety of conditions with varying presentations have been grouped under AP. Its incidence appears to have increased and it is now generally recognized, and diagnosis confirmed, shortly after admission. However, because there is no specific treatment to terminate the acute attack, only supportive measures can be offered and prognosis remains uncertain. The clinical course may range from a mild, self-limiting condition to a fulminating illness with serious complications. Despite recent advances in diagnosis and management, AP continues to be a serious illness with an overall mortality of 5–10%. In emergency abdominal surgery, these patients can present some of the most challenging problems in diagnosis and treatment.

9.1.1 INCIDENCE

Acute pancreatitis is rare in childhood and adolescence but thereafter the incidence rises steadily and is maximal at 60–80 years of age. Alcohol-related cases are predominantly seen in men below 60 years, while incidence of AP due to gallstones increases steadily with age, with a female-to-male ratio of 5:3. A number of studies have shown that the incidence may be increasing, but it is likely that much of this apparent increase may be due to increasing awareness and improvements in diagnosis (O'Sullivan et al., 1972; Trapnell and Duncan, 1975). When the years 1961 and 1985 are compared, the Scottish Hospitals statistics show an 11-fold rise in AP in males (from 69 to 750 patients/year) and fourfold in females (from 112 to 484 patients/year; Wilson and Imrie, 1990). In the Bristol area, AP increased from 55 per million per annum during 1968–1973 to 90 per million during 1974–1979 (Corfield et al., 1985a). In the Grampian region of Scotland there was an annual incidence in 1983–1985 of 242 cases per million (Thomson et al., 1987). The seriousness of this condition was emphasized by two regional surveys which showed that the overall mortality for the first

Emergency Abdominal Surgery. Edited by Peter F. Jones, Zygmunt H. Krukowski and George G. Youngson. Published in 1998 by Chapman & Hall, London. ISBN 0 412 81950 3.

attack of AP was 20% in Bristol (Corfield *et al.*, 1985a) and 15% in the Grampian region (Thomson *et al.*, 1987).

The two main causes of AP are gallstones and chronic alcoholism. The proportion of cases due to these two causes varies markedly between countries, and between regions within countries. In North America 60–70% of cases are alcohol-related (Ranson, 1979). The proportion of alcohol-induced AP in Sweden rose in the 1970s to 66% (Svensson *et al.*, 1979). In Australia some 30% of patients with AP have consumed excess alcohol (Emslie, 1967). Within the UK there are marked differences in incidence, and alcohol is reported to be a less common cause for AP. In the Grampian region a study of 359 patients during 1983–1985 showed that 15% of attacks were alcohol-related, and 46% were due to gallstones. Alcohol was a factor in 3% of women and 26% of men (Thomson *et al.*, 1987).

9.1.2 AETIOLOGY

Gallstone disease and overindulgence in alcohol are the most important causes of AP and together account for 90% of cases. **Biliary calculi** are responsible for 20–50% of AP. The pathology of AP was described by Fitz in 1889, and Opie in 1901 established a clear association between calculi in the biliary tract and AP. It is an accepted fact that recurrent pancreatitis frequently occurs if gallstones are not removed after the first attack of AP, whereas recurrence is very unusual if the biliary tree has been cleared of stones. Acute pancreatitis affects 6–8% of patients with symptomatic gallstones (Neoptolomos, 1993). The frequency rate of AP is inversely proportional to the size of stones. Houssin *et al.* (1983) found that 20% of patients with microlithiasis (< 3 mm), 5% of patients with small stones (3–10 mm), 3% of patients with medium-sized stones (10–20 mm) and 1% of patients with larger stones (> 20 mm) suffered from AP. It seems likely that migrating small stones may produce transient obstruction at the ampulla and induce pancreatitis. Gallstones were recovered from the stools of 90% of patients after an attack of pancreatitis (Acosta and Ledesma, 1974; Kelly, 1976).

Armstrong *et al.* (1985) studied 769 consecutive patients undergoing cholecystectomy for cholelithiasis. Some 59 (7.7%) had AP and were compared with the other 710 patients. The AP patients had smaller stones, a wider cystic duct and nearly twice as many stones in the bile duct as the controls: pancreatic duct reflux during cholangiography occurred in 62% compared with 15% of controls. The earlier an operation is performed after an attack of AP, the greater the number of stones that are found in the bile duct. There is also evidence that, if operation is carried out within 48 hours of an attack of AP, a stone will be found lodged in the ampulla of Vater in 70% of patients (Acosta *et al.*, 1978; Kelly, 1980). Acosta *et al.* (1978) found that, if cholecystectomy was delayed for 5–7 days for clinical recovery from AP, then only 5% of patients had a stone impacted in the ampulla. It seems reasonable to suppose that in the 75% of patients who make a quick recovery from gallstone-related AP, there is an early spontaneous passage of stone(s) from the biliary/pancreatic confluence, allowing resolution of the pancreatitis.

The relationship between **chronic heavy ingestion of alcohol** and AP is well established. The incidence varies in different populations and seems to correlate with the amount of alcohol consumed. It is more common in men and a history of daily heavy drinking or 'binge' drinking is common (Durbec and Sarles, 1978) and makes recurrence particularly likely. The exact mechanism of alcohol-induced pancreatitis is unclear but there are several theories (Malagelada, 1986). The toxic–metabolic hypothesis suggests that alcohol has a direct cytotoxic effect on pancreatic acinar cells. The ductal plug theory postulates hypersecretion of protein in alcoholics resulting in formation of protein plugs in small ductules. Finally, the theory based on flow/reflux disturbances affecting the main pancreatic duct, the sphincter of Oddi and the duodenum suggests that hindrance to the flow of pancreatic juice, and/or reflux of duodenobiliary contents into the pancreatic duct may result from alcohol-induced dysfunction of the sphincter of Oddi. Abstinence is rewarded in these patients by cessation of attacks.

Abnormalities in lipid metabolism and hyperlipidaemia are commonly seen in patients with alcohol-induced AP.

Secondary acute pancreatitis is uncommon but carries a relatively high mortality. Imrie *et al.* (1978b) reported an incidence of 8% and this type occurred after an operation, injury or diagnostic investigation. Combined with a retrospective survey, a total of 50 cases were studied. Out of 30 postoperative cases, 26 had operations on the biliary tract, but in 15 patients reported by Bragg *et al.* (1985) only four operations were on the biliary tree and the others were: small-bowel resection, 4; colectomy, 3; partial gastrectomy, 2; splenectomy involving trauma to the spleen, 1; and resection of an aortic aneurysm, 1.

The operation does not have to be in the abdomen. Patients who require cardiorespiratory bypass are recognized as occasional sufferers from AP. Haas *et al.* (1985) saw 12 examples in 5400 cardiac operations, nine having severe attacks with pancreatic necrosis, and these required extensive debridement and drainage. Inadequate perfusion may be a factor in these patients. Among the other 20 patients studied by Imrie *et al.* (1978b), 12 cases of AP followed abdominal trauma and eight were sequelae to investigations. Blunt injury to epigastrium was responsible in 11 out of 12 post-traumatic cases and five required laparotomy, though none had removal of pancreas. The investigations causing secondary AP were endoscopic retrograde cholangiopancreatography (ERCP) – five examples in 115 examinations – and translumbar aortography – three cases in 700.

The diagnosis of secondary acute pancreatitis can be difficult. Pain and vomiting in a postoperative patient and a quiet and distended abdomen, or high nasogastric aspirates, are not at first considered remarkable. Some patients have few complaints, but are just not as well as they should be. If there is any doubt, serum amylase should be estimated. If elevated it is important to adopt the appropriate measures. The difficulty of diagnosis tends to lead to delay and is partly responsible for the relatively high mortality: 30% of postoperative cases (Imrie *et al.*, 1978b). Another factor is the relatively high incidence of complications such as abscess and pseudocyst formation.

Some **drugs** are associated with attacks of AP: corticosteroids, azathioprine, thiazide diuretics, oestrogens and sulphonamides are particularly implicated. An accurate drug history is important and suspected drugs should be withdrawn.

Virus infections with mumps or Coxsackie B may play a small part. Imrie *et al.* (1977a) found a rising titre for one or other virus in five out of 116 patients with AP.

The association with **pregnancy** is rather dubious (Trapnell and Duncan, 1975). Most of these patients have gallstones and it may be no more than chance that the attack of AP occurs during pregnancy or the puerperium.

Other rare causes of AP are **hyperparathyroidism** and **occult pancreatic carcinoma**. **Ascariasis** can cause mechanical obstruction of the ampulla and is an important condition in developing countries (Louw, 1966; Laung *et al.*, 1986).

Hereditary pancreatitis is an extremely rare form of the disease and is thought to be responsible for about 1% of cases in children and young patients. A mutation in chromosome 7q35 is believed to be responsible for failure of the normal inactivation of trypsin within the pancreas (Whitcomb *et al.*, 1996).

9.1.3 CLINICAL PICTURE

Almost all patients with AP present with the sudden onset of acute upper abdominal pain, mainly in the epigastrium. It often begins after a big rich meal or a bout of drinking. Pain usually spreads across the upper abdomen, may radiate into the flanks and tends to bore through to the back. It may be felt substernally. The pain is usually constant and may be of great severity. Repeated vomiting is characteristic, but it is not copious and is colourless, unlike obstructive vomiting. Less commonly, AP may present with minimal pain and rarely it may even be painless – a situation liable to cause delay in recognition and increased fatality (Lankisch *et al.*, 1991).

The appearance of patients varies widely, ranging from relatively well-looking to extremely ill with features of shock and toxicity. Some are in great pain and tend to sit or lie curled up. Tachypnoea is common and cyanosis may be present. The presence of mild jaundice may suggest cholelithiasis and an associated swinging pyrexia indicates acute cholangitis. In severe cases there is significant loss of blood and inflammatory exudate into the retroperitoneal space and signs of hypovolaemia (pale, cold skin, tachycardia and hypotension) are obvious. This loss can be of the order of 5–6 litres.

Some patients are much less distressed and it is a mistake to assess the potential severity of AP on first impressions.

Acute pancreatitis, like early mesenteric infarction, is one of the emergencies in which severe pain is not accompanied by the marked abdominal signs which the distress of the patient would lead the examiner to expect. In most patients there is some tenderness in the epigastrium but guarding is slight. This is because the pancreas is retroperitoneal and a generalized peritoneal exudate will take time to cause signs of peritoneal irritation. However, some patients may present severe generalized tenderness and rigidity and when this occurs it is not surprising that 25% of such patients would be suspected of having a perforated peptic ulcer. In severe AP the signs of paralytic ileus are often present.

The appearance of bruising by extravasated blood in the flank (Turner, 1920) and at the umbilicus (Cullen, 1918) is a rare and serious sign, denoting considerable retroperitoneal haematoma. Dickson and Imrie (1984) surveyed 770 patients with AP and found Grey Turner's sign in nine, Cullen's sign in another nine and five patients showed both signs. In most, the sign(s) appeared around the fourth day; 20 of the 23 had a severe form of AP, eight died and over 90% suffered serious complications.

Respiratory complications are frequently associated with AP. Pleural effusion is present in 10–20% of patients. Progressive pulmonary changes from diminished air entry to pulmonary oedema and pneumonitis may lead on to full adult respiratory distress syndrome (ARDS). Clinical signs tend to underestimate the degree of hypoxia and it is essential to measure arterial blood gases. Imrie *et al.* (1977b), in a consecutive series of 84 patients with AP, showed that during the first week of illness 45% had a severe degree of hypoxia ($P_aO_2 < 8.0$ kPa or 60 mmHg) and this degree of hypoxia did not produce obvious distress. However mortality among the severely hypoxic group was more than twice that of a group whose P_aO_2 remained over 9.0 kPa (70 mmHg). All patients with AP need their arterial oxygen levels measured during the first five days of illness, and everyone over 60 years or with the P_aO_2 below 9 kPa requires supplementary humidified oxygen.

9.1.4 DIAGNOSIS

Acute pancreatitis is now commonly recognized and there are few patients with acute upper abdominal pain in whom it is not considered as a differential diagnosis. If the index of suspicion is low, the diagnosis may be missed. Wilson and Imrie (1988) found that the diagnosis had been missed in 42% of fatal attacks of AP.

Serum amylase

The serum amylase is significantly raised in 95% of patients with AP and this test should confirm the suspected diagnosis in most cases. In the Phadebas test which is generally used in the UK the normal range in serum is 70–300 IU/l. (In USA the Somogyi unit has a normal range of 200–1000 u/dl). In the presence of a typical clinical presentation, and with serum amylase concentration greater than four times the normal (> 1200 IU/l), the diagnosis of AP is reasonably certain. The serum amylase concentration remains elevated for 2–3 days after the onset of symptoms. If there is a delay in presentation, the serum amylase concentration may be normal at the time of admission. This problem may be overcome by estimation of urinary amylase concentration. In AP the urinary amylase is usually above 3000 IU/l (normal < 1000 IU/l) and it is particularly useful in 4% of patients with alcohol-induced AP who have hyperlipidaemia; the serum amylase is then difficult to estimate. Two difficult situations must be considered.

- In some cases of AP the **serum amylase may be below 1200 IU/l**. This can happen because the amylase level rises and falls quickly, so, during the first 3–4 hours and after 24 hours from onset, the serum amylase may be quite low. In very early cases it is worth repeating the test after a few hours and in later cases estimation of urinary amylase is helpful.
- **Raised serum amylase in conditions other than AP.** Minor elevation of serum amylase (300 IU/l–1000 IU/l) can occur in a number of other illnesses, such as acute biliary colic, cholecystitis, ischaemia of small intestine, upper abdominal injury and perforated peptic ulcer (Thomson, 1984). Hyperamylasaemia is seen in 30% of peptic perforations but the amylase level is usually below 1040 IU/l (Imrie *et al.*, 1974).

Occasionally the clinical picture of a patient with high serum amylase (> 1200 IU/l) is atypical for AP and may give rise to confusion in management. Among 401 consecutive patients with a high serum amylase Hendry *et al.* (1987) found 30 who did not have AP and whose mean serum amylase was 2200 IU/l. Of these, 11 had gastroduodenal perforations and five had ischaemic small bowel. Others had acute hepatitis (2), myocardial infarction (2), an appendix abscess and diabetic ketoacidosis. In three the rise occurred after ERCP, without evidence of pancreatitis. In 113 patients with a serum amylase in excess of 1200 IU/l, 90 had AP but 10 required an urgent operation for perforation or ischaemic bowel (McGowan and Wills, 1964). In another important group 12 had previously had a partial gastrectomy: 10 had afferent loop obstruction requiring operative release. If a patient who has had a gastrectomy presents with the picture of AP, the diagnosis of obstruction of the afferent loop must be considered (p. 213). It is vital to be watchful when the clinical picture is not typical of AP. Other investigations like plain abdominal radiography, peritoneal aspiration, liver function tests, blood and urine sugar and ketone levels, and electrocardiogram may help in differentiation.

Serum calcium

Low serum calcium is a common feature of severe pancreatitis and is caused by hypoalbuminaemia producing a fall in circulating protein-bound calcium. However clinical tetany is very rare (Allam and Imrie, 1977). It is the hypoalbuminaemia that needs correction.

Hyperglycaemia

A transient rise in blood glucose is sometimes seen in severe cases and it is important to check the blood sugar and use insulin therapy as required. Some patients become permanently diabetic after severe AP, and a recent report showed that the incidence may be as high as 50%; the risk is worse in the alcohol group (Doepel *et al.*, 1993).

Radiology

Plain abdominal X-ray has very little to offer in the diagnosis of AP but it may be of value in excluding other causes of acute abdomen. Chest X-ray can show a range of changes. Left-sided pleural effusion is common and severe cases may show features of diffuse alveolar oedema – a sign of adult respiratory distress syndrome.

Ultrasonography

Ultrasound imaging is useful as it is non-invasive, inexpensive and portable but its value in AP is limited because of the associated gaseous distension of the gastrointestinal tract. It is however useful in the detection of gallstones and complications of pancreatitis such as pseudocysts and abscess formation.

Computed tomography

Computed tomography is the most accurate method of imaging for evaluation of patients with AP (Block *et al.*, 1986). It is now used more widely for assessment of severe pancreatitis. Acute oedematous pancreatitis is characterized by focal or diffuse enlargement of pancreas, blurring of margins and intra- or peripancreatic fluid collections.

Diagnostic peritoneal lavage

In spite of routine estimation of serum amylase in patients with an acute abdomen, there are some patients with diffuse abdominal tenderness and guarding where the surgeon is in serious doubt as to the wisdom of relying on a high serum amylase reading and the diagnosis of AP is uncertain. In such a situation, diagnostic peritoneal lavage should be considered as an alternative to laparotomy. A peritoneal dialysis catheter is introduced through a small subumbilical incision using local anaesthesia. The tip of the catheter is advanced into the pelvis and peritoneal fluid is aspirated. Peritoneal lavage is performed using a litre of warm saline. Peritoneal fluid and lavage return fluid should be examined for colour, odour, amylase content, microscopy and bacteriological culture. High concentrations of amylase in peritoneal fluid have been seen in a variety of acute abdominal conditions and hence it is unsuitable for diagnostic purposes. The peritoneal fluid in patients with AP ranges from pale yellow to dark chocolate brown (prune juice) in colour, is odourless and contains no bacteria or fibres of animal or vegetable origin (see next section). The presence of uncharacteristic colour, faecal or purulent odour or organisms or fibres means that the diagnosis of AP is incorrect. Mayer and McMahon (1985) reported 2% of patients to have had a false diagnosis of AP which was corrected by the use of peritoneal lavage: the true diagnoses were perforated peptic ulcer, perforated common bile duct and necrosis of small and large bowel due to ischaemia and the serum amylase ranged from 1240–9510 IU/l.

9.1.5 ASSESSMENT OF SEVERITY OF ACUTE PANCREATITIS

Acute pancreatitis is a disease of remarkable variability, ranging from mild cases with a benign course to severe illness leading to multiorgan failure, sepsis and death. The accurate assessment of severity in the early stages is difficult; however, early recognition is essential for appropriate monitoring and relevant treatment. Clinical evaluation alone can be misleading. Prospective studies have shown that early clinical evaluation is successful in identifying only 34–39% of severe AP (McMahon *et al.*, 1980; Corfield *et al.*, 1985b).

During the 1970s Ranson (1979) described the first multiple factor grading system. He analysed many observations on patients with AP, looking for results that would quickly distinguish those who were destined to develop a serious attack. He selected 11 measurements, mostly biochemical tests, that provided good discrimination. Imrie *et al.* (1978a) simplified the system to eight measurements listed in Table 9.1.

Table 9.1 Prognostic measurements in acute pancreatitis (Glasgow scoring system; Osborne *et al.*, 1981); the presence of three or more factors indicates a severe attack

1. White cell count $> 15 \times 10^9/l$

2. $P_aO_2 < 8.0 \, kPa$

3. Plasma constituents:
Glucose	$> 10 \, mmol/l$
Urea	$> 16 \, mmol/l$ maintained over 6 hours of rehydration
Lactic dehydrogenase	$> 600 \, IU/l$
Aspartate aminotransferase	$> 200 \, IU/l$
Uncorrected calcium	$< 2 \, mmol/l$
Albumin	$< 32 \, g/l$

Imrie believed that early hypoxaemia of P_aO_2 <8 kPa was the most valuable single predictor. Using this system, Blamey *et al.* (1984) reported the outcome on 405 patients with AP due to various causes. The overall outcome was predicted accurately in 72% of cases; 31% of severe episodes (three or more factors present) were associated with death or serious complications, in contrast to 8% of episodes judged to be mild. The disadvantage of this system is that some delay must occur, at least 24 hours, before all the test results are available.

Peritoneal lavage

Peritoneal lavage offers a valuable alternative and has some advantage because assessment is carried out at the time of admission (McMahon *et al.*, 1980). Pancreatitis is graded as severe if there is more than 10 ml of free fluid and its colour is dark, or if the lavage return is darker than pale straw colour (matched with a colour chart provided). Corfield *et al.* (1985b) reported a prospective comparison of the prognostic indices in 436 attacks of AP in 418 patients. At the time of admission, prognostic factors were assessed as described in Table 9.1 and were repeated 2 days later. In 155 patients the attack was considered to be too mild to merit insertion of a peritoneal catheter but this was performed in 252 attacks. There was one accidental puncture of caecum, which was repaired at laparotomy with good recovery. Peritoneal lavage predicted 69 attacks to be severe and 52 of these proved to be severe, with 21 deaths. In 183, the lavage was negative and four developed a serious complication but there were no deaths. However it is important to note that, in the 155 attacks that were thought at the time of admission to be too mild to merit insertion of a catheter, 25 developed major complications and eight died. After 48 hours the laboratory criteria accurately identified two-thirds of the patients who would prove to have a severe attack.

The special value of the peritoneal lavage is in the patient with fairly marked abdominal signs: it allows speedy identification of two very important groups of patients:

- the few who appear to have AP, with a serum amylase over 1200 IU/l, but who in fact have a perforation or ischaemic bowel and need urgent laparotomy;
- the fulminant case, who almost always produces typical prune juice aspiration and who needs immediate transfer to the intensive therapy unit.

C-reactive protein (CRP)

The acute-phase proteins are a group of proteins synthesized by the liver in response to a variety of stimuli, such as tissue trauma, inflammation, infection, ischaemia and malignancy. They have wide-ranging but mostly protective functions that modulate the host response at the site of inflammation and counteract adverse effects of proteolytic enzymes. CRP is a non-specific acute-phase protein that is seen in a number of conditions including AP. The serum level rises within a few hours of pancreatitis and peak levels are observed in 24–48 hours (Wilson *et al.*, 1989). A persistently raised CRP is suggestive of continuing inflammation with the associated risk of complications. A peak level of more than 210 mg/l on days 2–4 after admission offered simple and accurate discrimination between mild and complicated episodes.

Modified APACHE II score

The disease-specific multifunctional scoring systems for grading the severity of an attack of pancreatitis (Ranson and Glasgow systems) have limitations of delay for 48 hours, pre-existing disease states are not accounted for, and they cannot be used to monitor the disease course or response to treatment. The acute physiology and chronic health evaluation (APACHE) scoring system takes account of pre-existing illness and allows repeated assessment during the course of illness. The APACHE II system uses 12 routinely available physiological and laboratory measurements that are weighted for age and pre-admission health status (Knaus *et al.*, 1985). An APACHE II score of more than 9 has been used to distinguish between mild and severe attacks of AP with a sensitivity of 82% and specificity of 76% (figures comparable to the Ranson and Glasgow scoring systems; Wilson *et al.*, 1990). No deaths occurred in patients with a score of less than 10 and only 6% of these developed complications. After 48 hours, APACHE II scoring was more accurate than Ranson and Glasgow scoring.

9.1.6   MANAGEMENT OF THE ACUTE ATTACK

Because no system of prediction of outcome is wholly reliable, it is an essential part of the care of all patients with AP that active observation is continued, on at least a twice-daily basis, until the attack has settled.

About 80% of all patients will make an uneventful recovery with relatively little treatment. Oral intake is withheld and all patients require intravenous fluids for a day or two. Vomiting is relieved by insertion of a nasogastric tube and gastric aspiration. Pethidine or physeptone may be combined with diazepam or nitrazepam for analgesia; morphine can cause spasm of the sphincter of Oddi and is not usually recommended, but it is effective and may be used along with an antispasmodic like hyoscine butylbromide. It is important to know the urine output and if there is any difficulty in passing urine, a urethral catheter should be inserted and hourly urine output charted. Baseline laboratory measurements are performed and a prognostic risk score (Table 9.1) is calculated, which will help in identifying a severe attack of pancreatitis. Assessment of severity of the illness at presentation is critical to appropriate clinical management. In a recent audit of deaths from AP, 42% of patients who died were insufficiently assessed by objective criteria and the true severity of an attack was underestimated (Mann *et al.*, 1994).

9.1.6.1   Mild attacks

These patients are managed in a general ward and the majority of patients with mild AP will improve on simple supportive measures and invasive monitoring is not necessary. Basic measurements of cardiopulmonary function, fluid balance and temperature are carried out. Recording of central venous pressure is not routine but it may be indicated in patients with cardiac problems. Blood gas analysis should be performed in all patients and repeated daily for 2–3 days, and indices of haematology and biochemistry should be repeated daily for 48 hours to determine any worsening in the severity score of the attack (Table 9.1). The onset of organ failure such as pulmonary or renal insufficiency puts the patient into the severe category. After 24–48 hours, it will be clear in many patients that they are steadily improving and acute measures may be discontinued, as seems appropriate.

9.1.6.2 Severe attacks

Patients classified as having a severe attack of acute pancreatitis are best managed in an intensive therapy unit or high-dependency ward where full cardiorespiratory monitoring is available. Central venous pressure recording is routine; if there are features of shock or pulmonary insufficiency, an arterial line is valuable for frequent blood gas analysis and blood pressure monitoring. Continuous ECG monitoring is usual and patients are closely watched for features of multisystem failure. Laboratory tests and chest X-rays are carried out daily or more frequently. Bedside review by the same surgical staff – so far as possible – is made at least twice daily.

Intravenous fluids

Anyone suspected of hypovolaemia will require a carefully chosen sequence of intravenous fluids, which will include plasma and plasma expanders and may need to include blood if there are features of blood loss or retroperitoneal haemorrhage. In a severe attack of AP, there is loss of protein-rich fluid into the peripancreatic space. There is also widespread capillary leak of serous fluid into the extravascular space in tissues remote from the pancreas, including the lungs and subcutaneous tissue. This can result in a profound fall in serum albumin concentration and plasma has to be used freely to replace this. This is also usually the correct way to manage hypocalcaemia.

Effective management of fluid loss is critical and appropriate measures of evaluation like central venous pressure monitoring and hourly urine output measurement (0.5 ml/kg/h) help in determining the adequacy of fluid replacement. Suboptimal fluid administration can lead either to renal failure or fluid overload and cardiorespiratory embarrassment, especially in the elderly. Persisting oliguria in spite of correction of hypovolaemia is an early sign of renal impairment and judicious use of low-dose dopamine ($2-4\,\mu g$/kg/h) and diuretics such as mannitol (200 ml of 10% mannitol) or frusemide may help to avoid renal shut down. By adopting these methods Imrie *et al.* (1978a) were able to reduce the incidence of renal failure from 14.5% to 3%. If these measures fail, peritoneal or haemodialysis should be considered (Gordon and Calne, 1972).

Respiratory insufficiency

The importance and frequency of respiratory insufficiency in AP is well recognized (Imrie and Whyte, 1975). Pulmonary complications were the most important feature leading to death in a Mayo Clinic study of patients who died within 7 days of an onset of AP (Renner *et al.*, 1985). One of the difficulties is that patients, who are by no means all elderly, may show little effect beyond some tachypnoea, and chest radiographs can look normal. It is therefore vital to perform arterial blood gas analysis in all patients daily during the first 2–3 days of an attack and more frequently in those who are classified as severe. Imrie *et al.* (1977b) did this during the first week of illness for 84 patients with AP and 68 patients with other abdominal emergencies such as appendicitis, perforated peptic ulceration and intestinal obstruction. In the AP group, 45% had marked hypoxaemia ($P_aO_2 < 8.0\,kPa$ or 60 mmHg) and in another 35% P_aO_2 levels were below 9.0 kPa. Mortality among the severely hypoxic group (13%) was more than double the figure among those whose P_aO_2 remained over 9.0 kPa (6%). When humidified oxygen was given through a mask, the arterial oxygenation generally improved considerably, but it was important to continue estimating the arterial blood gases and keep a close watch on physical signs and chest radiographs: ten patients developed a pleural effusion and five had atelectasis.

If humidified oxygen does not lead to an improvement of P_aO_2 above 8.0 kPa (60 mm) the advice of an anaesthetist will be required and mechanical ventilation may be needed.

The heart is under considerable strain in older patients and cardiac assessment is an important part of initial and recurring examinations. Digoxin seems to exert a useful effect and sometimes dopamine is of value.

Antibiotics

There is no evidence that prophylactic antibiotics have any value in a mild attack of AP. However antibiotic therapy may be logical when there is evidence of gallstones and infection within the biliary tree. The issue is more contentious in the severe form of AP. Previous reports suggested that prophylactic antibiotics made no difference to the overall outcome (Finch *et al.*, 1976). However these studies were performed in patients with milder forms of the attack and the antibiotics used were subsequently shown to be unable to cross the blood–pancreas barrier (Buchler *et al.*, 1992). Pharmacokinetic studies of systemic broad-spectrum antibiotics in human pancreatic tissue have shown that acylureidopenicillins, third-generation cephalosporins, quinolones and imipenem are able to penetrate human pancreatic tissue in bactericidal concentrations but aminoglycosides do not (Buchler *et al.*, 1992). Recent clinical studies have shown that antibiotics like imipenem, cefotaxime and cefuroxime are able to improve the prognosis significantly (Pederzoli *et al.*, 1993; Luiten *et al.*, 1995; Sainio *et al.*, 1995). There is now increasing evidence that early effective antibiotic prophylaxis is beneficial, and this should form part of the standard treatment for severe acute pancreatitis.

Peritoneal lavage

Peritoneal lavage has been considered as a useful method to remove products of tissue breakdown that were thought to have an adverse effect on patients with AP. There have been many reports of trials of peritoneal lavage, some of which suggested that it had a useful effect during the early stages of a severe attack (Ranson, 1979; Stone and Fabian, 1980). These were conducted in small numbers and, although immediate improvement was a feature of both trials, mortality was not materially affected.

A carefully controlled trial of therapeutic lavage in 413 patients has shown no detectable advantage (Mayer *et al.*, 1985); 91 attacks were graded as severe and received intensive treatment, 46 of these patients acted as controls (34 had 1 litre of diagnostic lavage to assess severity) and the remaining 45 patients were randomly allocated to therapeutic lavage, which meant that they received 2 litre cycles of dialysing fluid hourly over 72 hours; to each litre 4 mmol of potassium chloride and 250 IU of sodium heparin was added. There were 12 deaths in the lavage group and 13 in the controls. Infected pancreatic collections developed in 11 patients in each group. Patients having lavage lost 44 g of protein daily and required 3 litres of plasma intravenously over the first 3 days, compared to 400 ml in the control group. A disadvantage of this trial may be that most patients were only admitted to hospital 24–28 hours after the onset of pancreatitis, and it was 30–40 hours after onset when lavage was commenced. Even so, therapeutic lavage does not appear to have much effect. The two American trials, which produced a more striking immediate improvement, were nearly all conducted in alcohol-related cases but only 20% of patients in the British trial were in this category, and this could be significant.

Specific treatment

Currently there is no useful specific treatment for acute pancreatitis. The extensive trials of aprotinin and glucagon, for which claims had been made, did not show any benefit (Welbourn *et al.*, 1977; Imrie *et al.*, 1978a). Somatostatin is known to inhibit pancreatic exocrine secretion and has been recommended for the treatment of AP but a controlled study failed to show any clear benefit (Usadell *et al.*, 1980). A recent comparison where somatostatin was given at a dose of 3.5 μg/kg/h by continuous intravenous infusion for periods of 72–100 hours showed more rapid pain relief and lower morbidity but the difference did not achieve statistical significance (D'Amico *et al.*, 1990).

Proinflammatory cytokines such as platelet activating factor (PAF) have been implicated in the pathogenesis of systemic complications of acute pancreatitis. A recent randomized trial of lexipafant, a potent inhibitor of PAF, in patients with severe acute pancreatitis showed significant reduction in organ failure score in the treated group, along with trends towards a reduction in mortality and reduced incidence of systemic complications (McKay *et al.*, 1997). The size of the study was insufficient to draw firm conclusions but the results are encouraging and lexipafant may have a role in the treatment of severe acute pancreatitis.

Nutrition. Patients with the mild form of pancreatitis normally settle within 2–3 days, when oral fluids may be started. It is usually possible to go quite quickly on to a light diet. In the severe attacks, oral feeding is not possible for a prolonged period and support is provided by intravenous nutrition. If laparotomy is necessary as part of management, a fine tube jejunostomy feeding can be established as an alternative to parenteral nutrition.

The place of surgery

There are three reasons for operating on patients with acute pancreatitis during the period of the first emergency admission.

1. Diagnostic uncertainty

It is unusual to undertake an urgent laparotomy in order to confirm or exclude the diagnosis of AP. Occasionally, in the absence of typical X-ray features, it may be impossible to clinically differentiate AP from peptic ulcer perforation or intestinal obstruction. Rather than deciding on immediate laparotomy, a diagnostic peritoneal tap/lavage (p. 384) with examination of the aspirate will usually show whether operation is indicated. In some patients laparotomy may be the only safe policy to establish the diagnosis. If the findings at laparotomy indicate gallstone-related pancreatitis, it may be safe and appropriate to excise the gallbladder. If the pancreatitis is of the severe type it is safer to limit the operation to opening and draining the lesser sac and performing a cholecystostomy (Ranson, 1979). The presence of cholangitis or bile duct calculi may be best managed by T-tube drainage of the bile duct.

2. Operation for complications

Pancreatic necrosis Pancreatic necrosis and associated complications are leading causes of mortality in AP. Several natural history studies show that approximately 15% of patients admitted with AP develop pancreatic necrosis and the risk of mortality is 9–40% (Fenton-Lee and Imrie, 1993). When severe pancreatitis leads to pancreatic necrosis the process is initially ischaemic, because of impairment of lobular microcirculation, and aseptic. The inflammatory exudate which then forms around the necrotic tissue is very likely to become infected with alimentary tract organisms and the presence of necrotic pancreas further encourages the septic process. The autodigestive mechanism of fat necrosis in and around the pancreas and retroperitoneum aids the spread of sepsis into the mesocolon, perinephric fat and retroperitoneal tissues in both flanks and iliac fossae.

The clinical features of pancreatic necrosis are essentially those of severe AP with worsening abdominal signs and general systemic deterioration. The prognostic scoring systems do not correlate well, but the C-reactive protein is generally more than 210 mg/l. The use of contrast-enhanced computed tomography (CECT) has been a major advance in the evaluation of patients with severe AP; thin tomographic sections of the pancreas are obtained during infusion of intravenous contrast medium, which allows identification of pancreatic perfusion defects. These contrast-deficient areas correlate well with the anatomical extent of pancreatic necrosis and the clinical outcome. The positive predictive value for CECT for the presence of pancreatic necrosis is nearly 90% (Kemppainen *et al.*, 1996; Kivisaari *et al.*, 1984).

Secondary infection of the necrosed pancreas is a serious complication. Widdison and Karanjia (1993) estimated that 30% of pancreatic necrosis may become infected. The mortality associated with infection may rise fourfold (Beger *et al.*, 1986). The bacteria commonly responsible for secondary infection of pancreatic necrosis are Gram-negatives of enteric origin. By relying solely upon clinical features, it is impossible to distinguish between sterile pancreatic necrosis and infected necrosis. The diagnosis is best achieved by CT-guided fine needle aspiration of the necrotic site. The aspirate is immediately examined by Gram staining and culture (Gerzof *et al.*, 1987). Management of a patient suspected of pancreatic necrosis and/or infection may require serial CT examinations, fine needle aspiration and microbiology of areas of necrosis.

The role of surgery in the management of patients with pancreatic necrosis and infection is an evolving subject. During the last decade, there were proponents for early pancreatic resection, in the first week (Alexandre and Guerrieri, 1981; Aldridge *et al.*, 1985; Nordback *et al.*, 1986), but mortality rate was 30–60% and viable pancreatic tissue was often found in the resected specimen. There is increasing evidence that sterile pancreatic necrosis can be safely managed by non-operative treatment (Bradley and Allen 1991; Karimgani *et al.*, 1992). Bradley and Allan (1991) found that, in a prospective 2-year study of 194 patients with acute pancreatitis, 38 had confirmed features of pancreatic necrosis on CECT. Of the 38 patients, 27 developed infected necrosis during the period of observation and underwent necrosectomy and drainage; 11 patients had persistently sterile pancreatic necrosis (including six with pulmonary or renal failure) and were successfully managed without surgery. These observations suggest that sterile pancreatic necrosis, even in the presence of organ failure, is not an absolute indication for surgical intervention.

All patients with pancreatic necrosis must be managed in an intensive care unit with full support and special attention given to pulmonary, renal and cardiocirculatory dysfunction. It is important to be vigilant in the recognition and treatment of metabolic and haematological disorders and all patients should receive appropriate antibiotics (p. 389).

Under close observation it becomes clear that laparotomy is needed in those patients with pancreatic necrosis who develop signs of an 'acute abdomen', who deteriorate very rapidly or develop signs of sepsis (Beger *et al.*, 1988). Mortality rate increases sixfold when sterile pancreatic necrosis becomes infected; hence early diagnosis of infection is vital. The most appropriate method of diagnosis of infected necrosis is by CT-guided fine needle aspiration of the suspected area. As infection can develop at an early stage, aspiration should be performed in patients with persisting or deteriorating systemic complications.

Once the diagnosis of infected pancreatic necrosis is made the treatment is debridement (necrosectomy) and drainage. Attempts at percutaneous radiological drainage of infected pancreatic necrosis have been tried without much success (Adams *et al.*, 1990). There is general agreement that surgical debridement is essential. However, controversy continues to exist regarding timing of the operation and the optimal form of surgical drainage. Several studies have shown that early surgical intervention (within the first week) may be associated with increased risk of infection, haemorrhagic complications and mortality (de Beaux *et al.*, 1995; Mier *et al.*, 1997). A study from Edinburgh (de Beaux *et al.*, 1995) showed that all five patients who underwent necrosectomy within 2 weeks of diagnosis died and perioperative haemorrhage was a major factor in mortality. In contrast, there were five (21%) deaths in 24 patients when necrosectomy was performed after 2 weeks. Postoperative haemorrhage was seen in only one of these patients and was successfully controlled by a second laparotomy.

The best exposure for necrosectomy is obtained through a bilateral subcostal incision. The gastrocolic ligament is divided and the whole length of pancreas and adjoining retroperitoneum are explored using blunt techniques. Finger dissection of the necrotic pancreas and removal of non-viable tissue is helped by flushing the cavity with 0.1% tetracycline in saline solution. The necrotic cavity may be quite extensive: it may reach beyond the duodenal loop into the right flank and extend behind the ascending colon. On the left the process may track down behind the descending colon to the left iliac fossa, and posteriorly into the perinephric fat (Figure 9.1).

Close attention must be given to the circulation in large and small intestine as involvement of mesocolon and mesentery by transmural infarction is common, necessitating intestinal resection, proximal diversion and a distal mucous fistula.

Once thorough debridement has been achieved, a decision regarding drainage has to be made. Controversy continues to exist regarding the optimal form of surgical drainage. The traditional method of treatment is necrosectomy followed by closed abdominal drainage and re-exploration when required. Postoperative mortality of 30–40% is common and re-exploration for persistent intra-abdominal infection is required in one-third of these patients (D'Egidio and Schein, 1991). An alternative approach to closed abdominal drainage after debridement is to place large-bore drainage tubes into the lesser sac for continuous high-volume postoperative lavage to continue the debridement of the ongoing necrotic process (Beger *et al.*, 1988; Figure 9.1). The overall mortality of this form of management is around 20% (D'Egidio and Schein, 1991). Farkas *et al.* (1996) from Hungary have reported excellent results using this method of treatment. During a 7-year period, 123 patients with infected pancreatic necrosis underwent necrosectomy and postoperative lavage at a mean of 18.5 days after the onset of pancreatitis. The lavage was continued for a mean of 39.5 days with a median of 6.5 litres of saline per day. The overall hospital mortality was 7% and reoperation was required in 17% for a mixture of septic and haemorrhagic complications.

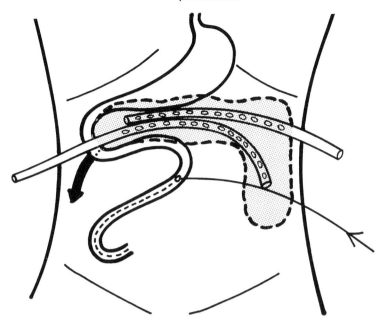

Figure 9.1 Diagram showing the extent of a peripancreatic abscess, with drains *in situ*. The arrow indicates the direction in which the abscess may extend over the right kidney and behind the ascending colon. A feeding jejunostomy has been inserted at the time of drainage.

A third form of management after necrosectomy is open packing, where the pancreatic cavity is packed with gauze swabs and the abdomen is left open or partially closed, and planned re-exploration is performed frequently for continued debridement. Prior to packing, it is useful to spread non-adhesive paraffin gauze in the base of the cavity, over any exposed vessels and transverse colon to minimize injury to surrounding structures (Bradley, 1987). Others have avoided packing and opted for a synthetic mesh or a zip in the abdominal fascia for easy re-entry for repeated lavage (Walsh *et al.*, 1988). The overall mortality of this method of management is 21% and complications such as intestinal fistulation, haemorrhage and wound problems are frequent. Bradley (1993a), an enthusiast for this management, reported a mortality of 14% in 71 patients but serious morbidity was present in 40%.

There is a place for each of these three forms of management and surgical approach should be tailored to the findings at operation and the clinical course. Traditional closed drainage is best suited for localized septic collections without significant necrosis; lesser sac lavage is ideal for limited infected necrosis (less than half of pancreas); and open packing may be the optimal treatment when there is extensive and spreading necrosis.

Pancreatic abscess Pancreatic abscess occurs in 1–4% of patients with acute pancreatitis. According to the modern classification, a pancreatic abscess is a walled-off collection of pus around the pancreas without much evidence of pancreatic necrosis (Bradley 1993b). It may develop as an infected pseudocyst or may present as a result of bacterial colonization of minor devitalized tissue, 3–5 weeks after the onset of pancreatitis. Abdominal pain, tenderness and a palpable mass are commonly noted and the diagnosis is confirmed by CT scanning. Treatment consists of antibiotic therapy and image-guided percutaneous placement of a drain.

Colonic complications These are unusual but can cause considerable problems in management: peripancreatic necrosis and sepsis may precipitate thrombosis in the middle colic vessels. Abcarian *et al.* (1979) reported 10 examples seen during the management of 1000 patients with acute pancreatitis; three patients showed features of pseudo-obstruction of the colon and one suffered a typical attack of ischaemic colitis which resolved. Two patients with large pancreatic abscess developed signs of peritonitis, which were due to necrosis of the transverse colon; one survived after transverse colectomy and proximal colostomy. In two patients a pseudocyst ruptured into the colon with severe concomitant rectal haemorrhage. Following drainage of a pancreatic abscess, two patients developed intestinal fistulae. The diagnosis of intestinal necrosis may not be easy but should be suspected when the triad of abdominal mass, sepsis and gastrointestinal haemorrhage is seen in a patient with acute pancreatitis. Management is by resection of the involved segment and proximal enterostomy. In spite of early and aggressive treatment, mortality is often greater than 50% (Bouillot *et al.*, 1989).

Pseudocysts Pseudocyst formation is a well-known complication of acute pancreatitis. It occurs in about 15% of alcohol-related attacks but only in about 5% of attacks associated with gallstones. D'Egidio and Schein (1992) proposed a classification which is useful in understanding the pathology and helps in management decisions. Type I or acute 'postnecrotic' pseudocysts occur after an episode of acute pancreatitis, and rarely communicate with the pancreatic duct, which retains its normal anatomy. They usually develop within 2 weeks of the onset of an attack. These cysts should be monitored by serial scans and intervention should be reserved for those that increase in size or persist beyond 4 weeks, or develop complications such as infection, obstruction, rupture or haemorrhage. Spontaneous resolution occurs in half the number of cases. Type II, also postnecrotic pseudocysts, occur after an episode of acute-on-chronic pancreatitis. The pancreatic duct is diseased but not strictured and duct–pseudocyst communication is seen frequently. Internal drainage is usually required. Type III, defined as 'retention' pseudocysts, occur with chronic pancreatitis and are often associated with duct strictures and pseudocyst–duct communication.

The formation of an acute pseudocyst is suspected when inflammatory features of acute pancreatitis continue beyond the first week and a mass (often painful) may be palpable in the epigastrium; CT or ultrasonic scan will confirm the diagnosis. On routine ultrasonography Bradley *et al.* (1976) found acute fluid collections in the lesser sac in 57% of patients with acute pancreatitis. The late pseudocyst, a localized fluid collection with clearly defined wall, is seen in only 2–7% of patients with acute pancreatitis.

The management of pseudocysts should vary according to the clinical situation. Acute peripancreatic collections will often resolve spontaneously. If the patient is asymptomatic, an initial 6-week period of observation is justified; thereafter small cysts (<6 cm) can be observed safely but larger cysts should be treated by internal drainage. Acute cysts that become symptomatic, enlarge or get infected during the period of observation are best treated by ultrasound-guided external drainage by the radiologist. Mature pseudocysts are traditionally treated by surgical internal drainage either into the stomach or into a Roux loop of jejunum. Retrogastric pseudocysts are ideally treated by anastomosis to the posterior wall of stomach (cystogastrostomy) but very large or distally placed cysts are better drained by Roux loop cystojejunostomy (Newell *et al.*, 1990). Non-operative endoscopic and radiological methods of internal drainage have been described but at present there is little evidence that the methods are superior to operative internal drainage (Szentes *et al.*, 1991). The expansion of laparoscopic techniques in recent years has widened the surgical options for treatment of pancreatic pseudocysts. Laparoscopic cystogastroscopy and laparoscopically assisted cystojejunostomy have been described, but a more promising concept is the innovative technique of intraluminal laparoscopic pseudocyst drainage. Specially designed trocars are inserted into the dilated gastric lumen and the remainder of the operation is performed inside the stomach. Gagner (1994) reported 14 patients with good results: mean hospital stay was 4 days, mean operating time 85 minutes and there was one conversion.

Pancreatic haemorrhage   This is an uncommon but potentially lethal complication of acute pancreatitis. Haemorrhage into the gastrointestinal tract, retroperitoneum or peritoneal cavity occurs in 1–3% of acute pancreatitis. The bleeding is due to vascular necrosis or rupture of a pseudoaneurysm (more common), and the clinical presentation varies depending on the site and rate of bleeding. Any of the peripancreatic arteries can be involved. The bleeding may be episodic and slow or massive with circulatory collapse. The diagnosis should be suspected in patients with spontaneous retroperitoneal, intrasplenic or intrahepatic haematomas in the presence of pancreatitis. While contrast-enhanced CT scan may provide useful diagnostic information, selective angiography will confirm the site of bleeding. Angiographic embolization of the offending vascular site provides control in a difficult clinical situation and may even be definitive treatment in selected patients. However, if haemorrhage is associated with pancreatic necrosis or pseudocyst, these patients will in addition require laparotomy and appropriate management.

3. Operation in gallstone pancreatitis

Advances in the techniques of laparoscopic surgery, endoscopic retrograde cholangiography (ERC) and endoscopic sphincterotomy (ES) have led to major changes in the management of biliary pancreatitis. The traditional approach was to treat an acute attack, discharge the patient when appropriate and re-admit 6–8 weeks later for cholecystectomy. The major disadvantage in this arrangement is that recurrence of pancreatitis can occur during this waiting period. Osborne *et al.* (1981) reported 147 patients with AP and gallstones, of whom 100 were discharged without an operation: 20 suffered a further attack of AP while awaiting the elective operation. Mayer at al (1984) put 37 patients on the waiting list for interval biliary surgery and four returned with recurrent AP, of whom one died. Recognizing the potential dangers of interval biliary surgery, some surgeons adopted a policy of urgent operation. Acosta *et al.* (1978) explored 46 patients at 6–48 hours after onset and found a stone impacted at the ampulla of Vater in 33: there were four deaths. Kelly (1980) similarly operated on 24 patients and an impacted ampullary stone was found in 15; seven were removed by supraduodenal choledochotomy and eight by duodenotomy and sphincterotomy. Three patients died of haemorrhagic pancreatitis. There are several reports that showed very early surgery to be dangerous and inadvisable.

Many patients, however, are candidates for early biliary surgery, performed at about the end of the first week, when the attack of AP has settled. Before operation can be considered it is necessary to establish the presence of gallstones, and this can be achieved by a combination of ultrasonography and ERCP. Laparoscopic cholecystectomy is the procedure of choice for the treatment of symptomatic gallstones. Some reports suggest that this procedure can be performed safely as soon as the symptoms of AP resolve. Tate *et al.* (1994) found that laparoscopic cholecystectomy performed at a median of 7 days after admission was successful in 88% of patients but the operation was more difficult when compared with controls. The major difficulty was in the dissection of Calot's triangle. A wide cystic duct is to be expected in such patients and metal clips are unsafe. They recommend externally tied ligature in continuity to secure the cystic duct.

4. Endoscopic management

The early reports on the use of ERC and ES in the management of gallstone pancreatitis were isolated retrospective analyses. There were justifiable fears and concerns not only regarding the usual complications of bleeding and perforation but also over the possibility of provoking the ongoing pancreatitis. Further studies have allayed these concerns and there is a growing confidence that when used carefully the endoscopic technique is safe in the acute situation and is beneficial to a defined group of patients with gallstone pancreatitis. Two prospective randomized studies have addressed this issue. Neoptolemos *et al.* (1988) randomly allocated 121 patients to either conservative treatment or urgent endoscopic intervention; 59 had ERCP within 72 hours and sphincterotomy performed if duct stones were found. The other 62 patients were followed conservatively. Overall, a significant reduction in morbidity rate (12%) was seen in the endoscopically treated group when compared to the control group (24%). The patients were also stratified according to the modified Glasgow criteria. In patients with a mild attack, regardless of the form of treatment, there was very little morbidity and no mortality. However, the patients with severe disease showed marked response to ERC/ES, with a morbidity rate of 24% versus 61% and a mortality rate of 4% versus 18%. Patients with severe pancreatitis were more likely to have common bile duct stones on ERC than those with mild pancreatitis (63% versus 25%). Patients undergoing early ERC also had a shorter hospital stay (9.5 days to 17.0 days). Patients with mild pancreatitis did not appear to benefit from early intervention. Fan *et al.* (1993) reported a similar study where 195 patients with AP were randomized to either ERC and possible ES or conservative treatment and selective ERC if they deteriorated clinically. The endoscopic treatment was performed within 24 hours of admission. Of these, 127 were shown to have common duct stones. Patients with severe pancreatitis had superior results after endoscopic management (morbidity 23%, mortality 12%) in comparison to conservative treatment (morbidity 58%, mortality 23%).

These two studies show that in expert hands urgent endoscopic intervention is a safe and efficacious treatment for patients with severe gallstone pancreatitis. It is important to stress the timing of ERC, especially in severe pancreatitis. Undue delay may make cannulation of the ampulla very difficult or even impossible because of severe duodenal oedema. Patients with mild gallstone pancreatitis who fail to improve or show signs of clinical deterioration can benefit from ES. In the elderly or unfit patients with biliary pancreatitis, endoscopic treatment is of particular value in reducing the risk of recurrent pancreatitis and the gallbladder may be left alone.

Patients with mild gallstone pancreatitis generally respond well to conservative treatment and they should be investigated for bile duct stones. In the absence of ductal stones, the definitive treatment is laparoscopic cholecystectomy. If stones are found, the options are preoperative ES followed by laparoscopic cholecystectomy, open operation and stone clearance or laparoscopic cholecystectomy and duct exploration.

REFERENCES

Abcarian, H., Eftaiha, M., Kraft, A. R. and Nyhus, L. M. (1979) Colonic complications of acute pancreatitis. *Arch. Surg.*, **114**, 995–1001.

Acosta, J. M. and Ledesma, C. L. (1974) Gall stone migration as a cause of acute pancreatitis. *N. Engl. J. Med.*, **290**, 484–487.

Acosta, J. M., Rossi, R., Galli, O. M. R. *et al.* (1978) Early surgery for acute gallstone pancreatitis: evaluation of a systematic approach. *Surgery*, **83**, 367–370.

Adams, D. B., Harvey, T. S. and Anderson, M. C. (1990) Percutaneous catheter drainage of infected pancreatic and peripancreatic fluid collections. *Arch. Surg.*, **125**, 1554–1557.

Aldridge, M. C., Ornstern, M., Glazer, G. and Dudley, H. A. F. (1985) Pancreatic resection for severe acute pancreatitis. *Br. J. Surg.*, **72**, 796–800.

Alexandre, J. H. and Guerrieri, M. T. (1981) Role of total pancreatectomy in the treatment of necrotizing pancreatitis. *World J. Surg.*, **5**, 369–377.

Allam, B. F. and Imrie, C. W. (1977) Serum ionised calcium in acute pancreatitis. *Br. J. Surg.*, **64**, 665–668.

Armstrong, C. P., Taylor, T. V., Jeacock, J. *et al.* (1985) The biliary tract in patients with acute gall stone pancreatitis. *Br. J. Surg.*, **72**, 551–555.

Beger, H. G., Bittner, R., Block, S. *et al.* (1986) Bacterial contamination of pancreatic necrosis. *Gastroenterology*, **91**, 433–438.

Beger, H. G., Buchler, M., Bittner, R. *et al.* (1988) Necrosectomy and postoperative local lavage in necrotizing pancreatitis. *Br. J. Surg.*, **75**, 207–221.

Blamey, S. L., Imrie, C. W., O'Neill, J. *et al.* (1984) Prognostic factors in acute pancreatitis. *Gut*, **25**, 1340–1346.

Block, S., Maier, W., Bittner, R. *et al.* (1986) Identification of pancreatic necrosis in severe acute pancreatitis: imaging procedures versus clinical staging. *Gut*, **27**, 1035–1042.

Bouillot, J. L., Alexander, J. H., Vuong, N. P. (1989) Colonic involvement in acute necrotizing pancreatitis: Results of surgical treatment. *World J. Surg.*, **13**, 84–87.

Bradley, E. L. III (1987) Management of infected pancreatic necrosis by open drainage. *Ann. Surg.*, **206**, 542–550.

Bradley, E. L. III (1993a) A fifteen year experience with open drainage for infected pancreatic necrosis. *Surg. Gynecol. Obstet.*, **177**, 215–222.

Bradley, E. L. III (1993b) A clinically based classification system for acute pancreatitis: summary of the International Symposium on Acute Pancreatitis, Atlanta, Georgia, September 11th–13th, 1992. *Arch. Surg.*, **128**, 586–590.

Bradley, E. L. III and Allen, K. (1991) A prospective longitudinal study of observation versus surgical intervention in the management of necrotizing pancreatitis. *Am. J. Surg.*, **161**, 19–25.

Bradley, E. L. III, Gonzalez, A. C. and Clements, L. J. (1976) Acute pancreatic pseudocysts: Incidence and implications. *Ann. Surg.*, **184**, 734–737.

Bragg, L. E., Thompson, J. S., Burnett, D. A. *et al.* (1985) Increased incidence of pancreas-related complications in patients with postoperative pancreatitis. *Am. J. Surg.*, **150**, 694–697.

Buchler, M., Malfertheiner, P., Friess, H. *et al.* (1992) Human pancreatic tissue concentration of bactericidal antibiotics. *Gastroenterology*, **103**, 1902–1908.

Corfield, A. P., Cooper, M. J. and Williamson, R. C. N. (1985a) Acute pancreatitis: a lethal disease of increasing incidence. *Gut*, **26**, 724–729.

Corfield, A. P., Cooper, M. J., Williamson, R. C. N. *et al.* (1985b) Prediction of severity in acute pancreatitis: prospective comparison of 3 prognostic indices. *Lancet*, **ii**, 403–407.

Cullen, T. S. (1918) A new sign in ruptured extrauterine pregnancy. *Am. J. Obstet. Dis. Women*, **78**, 457.

D'Amico, D., Favia, G., Biasiato, R. *et al.* (1990) The use of somatostatin in acute pancreatitis: results of a multicentre trial. *Hepato-gastroenterology*, **37**, 92–98.

De Beaux, A. C., Palmer, K. C. and Carter, D. C. (1995) Factors influencing morbidity and mortality in acute pancreatitis: an analysis of 279 cases. *Gut*, **37**, 121–126.

D'Egidio, A. and Schein, M. (1991) Surgical strategies in the treatment of pancreatic necrosis and infection. *Br. J. Surg.*, **78**, 133–137.

D'Egidio, A. and Schein, M. (1992) Pancreatic pseudocysts: a proposed classification and its management implication. *Br. J. Surg.*, **78**, 981–984.

Dickson, A. P. and Imrie, C. W. (1984) The incidence and prognosis of body wall ecchymosis in acute pancreatitis. *Surg. Gynecol. Obstet.*, **159**, 343–347.

Doepel, J., Eriksson, J., Halme, L. *et al.* (1993) Good long-term results in patients surviving severe acute pancreatitis. *Br. J. Surg.*, **80**, 1583–1586.

Durbec, J. and Sarles, H. (1978) Multicenter survey of the aetiology of pancreatic diseases: relationship between the relative risk of developing chronic pancreatitis and alcohol, protein and lipid consumption. *Digestion*, **18**, 337–341.

Emslie, R. G. (1967) A pattern of acute pancreatitis. *Austr. N.Z. J. Surg.*, **37**, 36–39.

Fan, S. T., Lai Mok, F. P. T., Lo, C. M. *et al.* (1993) Early treatment of acute biliary pancreatitis by endoscopic papillotomy. *N. Engl. J. Med.*, **328**, 228–232.

Farkas, G., Marton, J., Mandi, Y. *et al.* (1996) Surgical strategy and management of infected pancreatic necrosis. *Br. J. Surg.*, **83**, 930–933.

Fenton-Lee, D. and Imrie, C. W. (1993) Pancreatic necrosis: assessment of outcome related to quality of life and cost of management. *Br. J. Surg.*, **80**, 1579–1582.

Finch, W. T., Sawyers, J. L. and Schenker, S. (1976) A prospective study to determine the efficacy of antibiotics in acute pancreatitis. *Ann. Surg.*, **183**, 667–670.

Fitz, R. H. (1889) Acute pancreatitis. *Med. Record NY*, **35**, 197–204.

Gagner, M. (1994) Laparoscopic transgastric cystogastrostomy for pancreatic pseudocyst. *Surg. Endosc.*, **8**, 239–242.

Gerzof, S. G., Banks, P. A., Robbins, A. H. *et al.* (1987) Early diagnosis of pancreatic infection by computed tomography guided aspiration. *Gastroenterology*, **93**, 1315–1320.

Gordon, D. and Calne, R. Y. (1972) Renal failure in acute pancreatitis. *BMJ.*, **iii**, 801–802.

Haas, G. S., Warshaw, A. L., Daggett, W. M. *et al.* (1985) Acute pancreatitis after cardiopulmonary bypass. *Am. J. Surg.*, **149**, 508–515.

Hendry, W. S., Thomson, S. R., Scott, S. T. *et al.* (1987) Significant hyperamylasaemia in conditions other than acute pancreatitis. *J. R. Coll. Surg. Edin.*, **32**, 213–216.

Houssin, D., Castaing, D., Lemoine, J. and Bismuth, H. (1983) Microlithiasis of gall bladder. *Surg. Gynecol. Obstet.*, **157**, 20–24.

Imrie, C. W. and Whyte, A. S. (1975) A prospective study of acute pancreatitis. *Br. J. Surg.*, **62**, 490–494.

Imrie, C. W., Whyte, A. S. and Frew, E. M. S. (1974) A pattern of serum amylase concentration in the initial 24 hours after perforation of duodenal ulcers. *J. R. Coll. Surg. Edin.*, **19**, 370–403.

Imrie, C. W., Ferguson, J. C., Somerville, R. G. (1977a) Coxsackie and mumps virus infection in a prospective study of acute pancreatitis. *Gut*, **18**, 53–56.

Imrie, C. W., Ferguson, J. C., Murphy, D. *et al.* (1977b) Arterial hypoxia in acute pancreatitis. *Br. J. Surg.*, **64**, 185–188.

Imrie, C. W., Benjamin, I. S., Ferguson, J. C. (1978a) A single centre double blind trial of Trasylol therapy in primary acute pancreatitis. *Br. J. Surg.*, **66**, 337–341.

Imrie, C. W., McKay, A. J., Benjamin, I. S. *et al.* (1978b) Secondary acute pancreatitis: aetiology, prevention, diagnosis and management. *Br. J. Surg.*, **65**, 399–402.

Karimgani, I., Porter, K. A., Langevin, R. E. *et al.* (1992) Prognostic factors in sterile pancreatic necrosis. *Gastroenterology*, **103**, 1636–1640.

Kelly, T. R. (1976) Gallstone pancreatitis: pathophysiology. *Surgery*, **80**, 488–492.

Kelly, T. R. (1980) Gallstone pancreatitis: the timing of surgery. *Surgery*, **88**, 345–350.

Kemppainen, V., Sainio, R., Haapiainen, L. *et al.* (1996) Early localisation of necrosis by contrast-enhanced computed tomography can predict outcome in severe acute pancreatitis. *Br. J. Surg.*, **83**, 924–929.

Kivisaari, L., Somer, K., Standertskjold-Nordenstam, C. G. *et al.* (1984) A new method for diagnosis of acute haemorrhagic-necrotising pancreatitis using contrast-enhanced CT. *Gastrointest. Radiol.*, **9**, 27–30.

Knaus, W. A., Draper, E. A., Wagner, D. P. *et al.* (1985) APACHE II: a severity of disease classification system. *Crit. Care Med.*, **13**, 818–829.

Lankisch, P. G., Schirren, C. A. and Kunze, E. (1991) Undetected fatal acute pancreatitis: why is the disease so frequently overlooked? *Am. J. Gastroenterol.*, **86**, 322–326.

Laung, J. W. C., Chung, S. C. S. and King, W. W. K. (1986) Round worm pancreatitis: endoscopic worm removal without papillotomy. *Br. J. Surg.*, **73**, 925.

Louw, J. R. (1966) Abdominal complications of *Ascaris lumbricoides* infestation in childhood. *Br. J. Surg.*, **53**, 510–521.

Luiten, E. J. T., Hop, W. C. J., Lange, J. F. *et al.* (1995) Controlled clinical trial of selective decontamination for the treatment of severe acute pancreatitis. *Ann. Surg.*, **222**, 57–65.

McGowan, G. K. and Wills, M. B. (1964) Diagnostic value of plasma amylase, especially after gastrectomy. *BMJ.*, **i**, 160–162.

McKay, C. J., Curran, F., Sharples, J. N. *et al.* (1997) Prospective placebo-controlled randomized trial of lexipafant in predicted severe acute pancreatitis. *Br. J. Surg.*, **84**, 1239–1243.

McMahon, M. J., Playforth, M. J. and Pickfor, J. R. (1980) A comparative study of methods for the prediction of severity of attacks of acute pancreatitis. *Br. J. Surg.*, **67**, 22–25.

Malagelada, J. R. (1986) The pathophysiology of alcoholic pancreatitis. *Pancreas*, **1**, 270–278.

Mann, D. V., Hershman, M. J., Hittinger, R. *et al.* (1994) Multicentre audit of death from acute pancreatitis. *Br. J. Surg.*, **81**, 890–893.

Mayer, A. D. and McMahon, M. J. (1985) The diagnostic and prognostic value of peritoneal lavage in patients with acute pancreatitis. *Surg. Gynecol. Obstet.*, **160**, 507–512.

Mayer, A. D., McMahon, M. J., Benson, E. A. *et al.* (1984) Operations upon biliary tract in patients with acute pancreatitis: aims, indications and timing. *Ann. R. Coll. Surg. Engl.*, **66**, 179–183.

Mayer, A. D., McMahon, M. J., Corfield, A. P. *et al.* (1985) Controlled clinical trial of peritoneal lavage for the treatment of severe acute pancreatitis. *N. Engl. J. Med.*, **312**, 399–404.

Mier, J., Leon, E. L., Castillo, A. *et al.* (1997) Early versus late necrosectomy in severe necrotizing pancreatitis. *Am. J. Surg.*, **173**, 71–75.

Neoptolemos, J. P. (1993) Endoscopic sphincterotomy in acute gall stone pancreatitis. *Br. J. Surg.*, **80**, 547–549.

Neoptolemos, J. P., Carr-Locke, D. L. and London, N. J. M. (1988) Controlled trial of urgent ERCP and endoscopic sphincterotomy versus conservative treatment for acute pancreatitis due to gallstones. *Lancet*, **ii**, 979–983.

Newell, K. A., Liu, T., Aranha, G. V. *et al.* (1990) Are cystogastostomy and cystojejunostomy equivalent operations for pancreatic pseudocysts? *Surgery*, **108**, 635–640.

Nordback, I., Auvinen, O., Pess, T. *et al.* (1986) Complications after pancreatic resection for acute necrotizing pancreatitis. *Acta Chir. Scand.*, **152**, 49–54.

Opie, E. L. (1901) Etiology of acute haemorrhagic pancreatitis. *Bull. Johns Hopkins Hosp.*, **12**, 182.

Osborne, D. H., Imrie, C. W. and Carter, D. C. (1981) Biliary surgery in the same admission for gallstone associated acute pancreatitis. *Br. J. Surg.*, **68**, 758–761.

O'Sullivan, J. N., Nobrega, F. T., Morlock, C. G. *et al.* (1972) Acute and chronic pancreatitis in Rochester, Minnesota 1940–1969. *Gastroenterology*, **62**, 373–379.

Pederzoli, P., Bassi, C., Vesentini, S. *et al.* (1993) A randomized multicentre trial of antibiotic prophylaxis of septic complications in acute necrotising pancreatitis with imipenem. *Surg. Gynecol. Obstet.*, **176**, 480–483.

Ranson, J. H. C. (1979) Acute pancreatitis, in *Current Problems in Surgery XVI, No. 11*, (ed. M. M. Ravitch), Year Book Medical Publishers, Chicago, IL, pp. 5–83.

Renner, I. G., Savage, W. T., Pantoja, J. L. *et al.* (1985) Death due to pancreatitis. A retrospective analysis of 405 autopsy cases. *Dig. Dis. Sci*, **30**, 1005–1018.

Sainio, V., Kemppainen, E., Puolakkainen, P. *et al.* (1995) Early antibiotic treatment in acute necrotising pancreatitis. *Lancet*, **346**, 663–667.

Senn, N. (1886) *The Surgery of the Pancreas*, W. J. Dorman, Philadelphia, PA, p. 71.

Stone, H. H. and Fabian, T. C. (1980) Peritoneal dialysis in the treatment of acute alcoholic pancreatitis. *Surg. Gynecol. Obstet.*, **150**, 878–882.

Svensson, J. O., Norback, B., Bokey, E. L. *et al.* (1979) Changing patterns in aetiology of pancreatitis in an urban Swedish area. *Br. J. Surg.*, **66**, 159–161.

Szentes, M. J., Traverso, L. W., Kozarek, R. H. *et al.* (1991) Invasive treatment of pancreatic fluid collections with surgical and non-surgical methods. *Am. J. Surg.*, **161**, 600–605.

Tate, J. J. T., Lau, W. Y. and Li, A. K. C. (1994) Laparoscopic cholecystectomy for biliary pancreatitis. *Br. J. Surg.*, **81**, 720–723.

Thomson, H. J. (1984) Clinical significance of moderate elevation of serum amylase. *J. R. Coll. Surg. Edin.*, **29**, 303–306.

Thomson, S. R., Hendry, W. S., McFarlane, G. A. *et al.* (1987) Epidemiology and outcome of acute pancreatitis in North East of Scotland. *Br. J. Surg.*, **74**, 398–401.

Trapnell, J. E. and Duncan, E. H. L. (1975) Patterns of incidence in acute pancreatitis. *BMJ.*, **ii**, 179–183.

Turner, G. G. (1920) Local discoloration of the abdominal wall as a sign of acute pancreatitis. *Br. J. Surg.*, **7**, 394.

Usadell, K.-H., Leuschner, U., Ubrela, K. K. *et al.* (1980) Treatment of acute pancreatitis with somatostatin; a multicentre double-blind trial. *N. Engl. J. Med.*, **303**, 999–1002.

Walsh, G. L., Chiasson, P., Hedderich, G. *et al.* (1988) The open abdomen. The Marlex mesh and zipper technique method of managing intraperitoneal infection. *Surg. Clin. North Am.*, **68**, 25–40.

Welbourn, R. B., Armitage, P., Gilmore, O. J. A. *et al.* (1977) Death from acute pancreatitis. MRC multicentre trial of glucagon and aprotinin. *Lancet,* **ii**, 631–635.

Whitcomb, D. C., Gororry, M. C., Preston *et al.* (1996) Hereditary pancreatitis is caused by a mutation in the cationic trypsinogen gene. *Nature Genet.*, **14**, 141–145.

Widdison, A. L. and Karanjia, N. D. (1993) Pancreatic infection complicating acute pancreatitis. *Br. J. Surg.*, **80**, 148–154.

Wilson, C. and Imrie, C. W. (1988) Deaths from acute pancreatitis: why do we miss the diagnosis so frequently? *Int. J. Pancreatol.*, **3**, 273–282.

Wilson, C. and Imrie, C. W. (1990) Changing patterns of incidence and mortality from acute pancreatitis in Scotland, 1961–1985. *Br. J. Surg.*, **77**, 731–734.

Wilson, C., Heads, A., Shenkin, A. *et al.* (1989) C-reactive protein, antiproteases and complement factors as objective markers of severity in acute pancreatitis. *Br. J. Surg.*, **76**, 177–181.

Wilson, C., Heath, D. I. and Imrie, C. W. (1990) Prediction of outcome in acute pancreatitis: a comparative study of APACHE II, clinical assessment and multiple factor scoring systems. *Br. J. Surg.*, **77**, 1260–1264.

9.2   EMERGENCY SURGERY OF THE BILIARY TRACT

It is useful to distinguish between biliary colic, which does not require urgent surgical treatment, and acute cholecystitis, which quite often does.

9.2.1   BILIARY COLIC

This is a term that has come to stay although, if colic is taken to mean a cramping pain that comes and goes, it is not an accurate description. It does, however, correctly imply a severe pain of fairly sudden onset.

In a typical attack there is acute severe pain sited just below the xiphoid process. This increases over the space of 30 minutes to 1 hour until it is excruciatingly severe and the patient constantly seeks a fresh position in an attempt to ease the pain. It is often felt across the upper abdomen, especially under the right costal margin, and may be felt in the back around the tip of the right scapula. There may or may not be vomiting. The patient looks pale and sweaty and the pulse rate may rise, but there is no evidence of shock. There is little change in the severity of the pain, but after a few hours it eases, although in some there is no relief until an analgesic is given. French and Robb (1963) made a prospective study of 50 patients who were later proved to have gallstones and found that in 45 the attack followed this general pattern. Only one experienced pain that came and went; in 10 pain was maximal under the right costal margin. Gunn and Keddie (1972) found that an attack lasted on average about 16 hours, and 25% of their patients had severe pain under the left as well as the right ribs.

It is interesting to ask what causes this pain. The presence of an impacted stone in the cystic duct is a familiar finding during planned cholecystectomy, but there has been no pain for days or weeks, so mere presence of a stone in the cystic duct is not painful. Presumably impaction of a stone in Hartmann's pouch or cystic duct, at a time when the gallbladder is full of bile, causes painful contractions of the biliary smooth muscle, and produces this typical clinical picture. The commonest site of pain is, as might be expected, in the midline and this is useful in differential diagnosis from acute cholecystitis.

There may or may not be tenderness in the region of the gallbladder, which may occasionally be palpable. If one of the stones has escaped into the common bile duct there may be jaundice.

The lack of abdominal physical signs usually allows exclusion of other acute abdominal diseases, acute pancreatitis being the emergency most closely imitated. The distribution of pain and normal blood pressure make a coronary thrombosis unlikely. However, cardiac irregularities and acute biliary tract disease can go together. Dyspnoea is common and the lungs need careful examination.

Management

Biliary colic is usually an aseptic phenomenon which is self-limiting and unassociated with cholecystitis. This outcome cannot, however, be anticipated during an attack and it is necessary to maintain active observation.

It is often necessary to relieve the severe pain. Morphine is known to produce spasm of the sphincter of Oddi and is not usually recommended but it may be used along with an antispasmodic agent like hyoscine butylbromide; pethidine or pentazocine are more commonly used. The pain usually subsides quickly. If tenderness disappears and the patient remains comfortable a diagnosis of biliary colic is made. Ultrasonography, if performed within 24 hours of onset of symptoms, will show a distended gallbladder and the presence of stone in the cystic duct area.

Most patients are apprehensive about suffering another attack of biliary colic and welcome interval cholecystectomy, but this must be decided separately for each individual. In a few patients the pain of biliary colic will settle and a palpable but not tender gallbladder will continue to be felt. This is likely to be a mucocele and it will generally require early planned cholecystectomy.

9.2.2   ACUTE CHOLECYSTITIS

Acute cholecystitis presents, like biliary colic, with acute epigastric and right upper quadrant pain, but is generally less sudden and severe in onset. In the elderly it can commence in a slow and unimpressive manner and this is unfortunate because acute cholecystitis can quickly progress to a dangerous condition.

It almost always occurs in a gallbladder that is already the site of stone formation. Glenn and Thorbjarnarson (1963) found that only 5.5% of 1130 patients did not have stones, and 1% harboured a carcinoma of the gallbladder. Most often the precipitating factor is the impaction of a stone in Hartmann's pouch or, less frequently, the cystic duct. Gradually the mildly infected bile in the gallbladder becomes purulent, tension rises, and the threat of perforation is real.

Incidence in women is only a little higher than in men. Mitchell and Morris (1982a) found a female:male ratio of 1.7:1 during the 1970s, with a rising incidence in the number of women under 40 and men over 50 years of age. They suggested that the rise among young women was associated with the use of an oral contraceptive, and found that takers of the pill had a much higher incidence of stones in the common bile duct. Acute cholecystitis is now the third commonest cause of acute abdominal pain requiring admission to surgical wards (de Dombal, 1980).

Clinical picture

Cope (1970) gives an interesting description of his own attack of acute cholecystitis. He experienced sudden severe deep pain in the epigastrium and complete anorexia. He retired to bed and found that he could feel his gallbladder, which was the size of a small golf ball but not tender. His pain eased and some 3–4 hours later the gallbladder was no longer palpable. However, 9 hours after onset, pain and tenderness in the right hypochondrium was felt and this was still present, with slight fever, 24 hours later. Operation was then advised and an acutely inflamed gallbladder, containing 15 pigmented stones and already partially necrotic, was removed.

In some patients the central pain caused by the impaction of the stone is forgotten and then the history is a rather vague one of onset of pain in the right upper quadrant associated with anorexia and nausea. The degree of virulence of the infection in the gallbladder makes a considerable difference to the outcome. A severe virulent infection can lead to rapid rise of tension within the gallbladder, which forces the stone further into Hartmann's pouch: infective and pressure ischaemia of the gallbladder wall develops, and perforation can occur in 24–48 hours. If there is insufficient time for adhesions of omentum and intestine to form round the gallbladder, a spreading peritonitis can result. This sequence is fortunately unusual, and in most cases the virulence of the infection is less, tension rises gradually, and with the movement of the patient the stone falls back into the gallbladder and the purulent contents of the gallbladder can drain down the cystic duct. In 80–85% of patients an episode of acute cholecystitis resolves spontaneously in this way.

The length of history can therefore vary considerably from a matter of hours to several days. Most patients feel nauseated and unwell, but only a minority are obviously acutely ill with a high fever and tachycardia. The pain of breathing makes a number of patients appear breathless. The main finding is an area of tenderness under the right costal margin, usually accompanied by muscle guarding. The degree of tenderness and guarding varies. In a few there are signs of local or more generalized peritonitis. The guarding can make palpation difficult but in about one-third of patients the distended gallbladder can be felt with gentle palpation. Some patients are, or become, jaundiced. This may be due to stones in the common bile duct but often appears to be due to pressure on the duct from the distended gallbladder.

Although this appears to be a fairly specific clinical condition, many other conditions may simulate these clinical features. Schofield *et al.* (1986) found that 36 of 100 patients who appeared at admission to have acute cholecystitis did not, after investigation, have gallbladder disease: five had acute renal disease (pyelonephritis or hydronephrosis), four had pancreatitis, three acute hepatitis, three a duodenal ulcer, six had neoplasms of liver, pancreas, stomach and gallbladder, and others had emergencies such as appendicitis, diverticular disease, congestive cardiac failure and pleurisy. In 11 no specific diagnosis could be made. The Curtis–Fitz-Hugh syndrome (p. 536) must also be remembered because its incidence appears to be increasing.

Conversely, in some patients with acute cholecystitis the provisional diagnosis is appendicitis, and this is especially likely to occur in obese patients in whom it is difficult to localize signs, so appendicitis, which is four times more common than cholecystitis, is favoured. In a few patients the provisional diagnosis may be perforation of a peptic ulcer because they show signs of peritonitis. Lennon and Green (1983) found that 29 of 177 patients with acute cholecystitis had a perforated gallbladder, with signs of generalized peritonitis in 15 and six showing signs of septic shock. In these circumstances appendicitis, peptic ulcer perforation or perforated diverticular disease are all possible diagnoses and not easy to differentiate; this is not of great importance because they all require urgent laparotomy.

In a small number of patients the serious condition of **acute obstructive cholangitis** occurs. The patient presents with acute epigastric pain, jaundice and a high fever, associated with rigors. These patients are obviously ill and are liable to progress quickly to septic shock due to developing bacteraemia. Almost all of the patients have stones in the common bile duct causing some obstruction, which allows the intestinal bacteria in the duct to multiply rapidly. This dangerous condition requires speedy recognition, resuscitation with intravenous fluids, a full dose of third-generation cephalosporin and metronidazole, and emergency operation or endoscopy to remove the stones and drain the common bile duct. In expert hands the results of endoscopic treatment are superior to open surgery (Lai, 1990).

In the majority of patients the signs are localized and the general tendency is for resolution to occur over the next few days. This cannot, however, be anticipated and it is essential for active observation to continue. Most patients require intravenous fluids for a day or two, antibiotics and an appropriate analgesic. Clear fluids in restricted amounts are allowed by mouth.

During this time plain abdominal X-rays, examination of urine, serum amylase and liver function tests will be performed, and will contribute to the differential diagnosis.

Between 10% and 15% of patients who are under observation will show persistent or worsening signs around the gallbladder and over the space of 24–48 hours they will join the group who present with signs of peritonitis and require urgent laparotomy. Among the large majority who settle under observation it is now the custom to consider early cholecystectomy. It is important to confirm the diagnosis before laparotomy.

Ultrasonography is the most widely used method of investigating the gallbladder. In a patient who is not excessively fat or distended with intestinal gas, an experienced radiologist can detect the presence or absence of gallstones, increased thickness of the wall of gallbladder, 4 mm or more, an anechoic layer in the wall due to oedema, distension or perforation of the gallbladder, and widening of the common bile duct; faint echoes may be picked up within the gallbladder due to fibrinous particles. In 56 cases of proven acute cholecystitis, Sovia *et al.* (1986) found characteristic sonographic signs in 52: gallstones were present in another three, and oedema and distension of the gallbladder in another, so all 56 showed conclusive or suggestive signs that could be interpreted in the light of clinical findings.

Cholescintiscan is another method used for diagnosis of acute cholecystitis. The principle is that 99^m-technetium-labelled hydroxyiminodiacetic acid (HIDA), when given intravenously, is excreted by the liver into the biliary ductal system even in the presence of jaundice. Normally, the scan outlines the liver and extrahepatic biliary tree, including the gallbladder. In acute cholecystitis, the gallbladder is not seen on the scan but bile duct and/or duodenum are visualized. The implication is that the cystic duct is obstructed. When this finding is combined with signs typical of acute cholecystitis it is very significant. Gill *et al.* (1985) have shown that scintigraphy is more accurate than ultrasonography. However, the test is not helpful if there is any obstruction to the common bile duct by a stone, and false positives can occur in alcoholics, in patients on parenteral nutrition and in acute pancreatitis.

Infusion cholecystography has been used to demonstrate cystic duct obstruction (Dykes *et al.*, 1984); however it is less accurate than biliary scintigraphy for diagnosis of acute cholecystitis and cannot be used when serum bilirubin is more than 50 μmol/l.

Treatment

W. S. Halsted was among the first to advocate early surgery for acute cholecystitis and his diary for 1881 (quoted by MacCallum, 1930) records his most memorable patient: 'I was summoned to Albany Hospital by telegram to see my mother··· . I found her very ill, slightly jaundiced, with tumefaction and great tenderness in the region of the gallbladder. So at 2 am I operated, incised the gallbladder which was distended with pus, and extracted seven stones.' This vivid passage summarizes many features of acute cholecystitis, and shows that early surgery can be successfully practised. Halsted's mother lived for another 2 years. When Halsted's pupil, G. J. Heuer, started work at the New York Hospital he adopted a policy of operating on patients with acute cholecystitis within a day or two of admission (Glenn and Heuer, 1946). Between 1932 and 1947, 586 patients underwent early surgery, 87% having a cholecystectomy. In 13% who were seriously ill because of delay or perforation, a cholecystostomy was performed, often under local infiltration anaesthesia (Glenn, 1948). In spite of a remarkably low mortality rate of 2.9%, the policy was much criticized, and the debate about the merits of early over delayed surgery has continued ever since.

The course followed by an attack of acute cholecystitis determines treatment. In 80–90% of patients the signs are well localized, and with rest in bed and a day or two on intravenous fluids most show steady improvement: this is usually due to disimpaction of a stone lodged in Hartmann's pouch. Antibiotics are not necessarily indicated. When investigation confirms the presence of gallstones, and these patients have become asymptomatic and fit for operation, there is a strong case for proceeding to cholecystectomy on the next available operating list.

- In a number of these patients the operation reveals advanced disease with an area of gangrene.
- Experience shows that operative difficulties are generally less in the week after an attack than if operation is delayed.
- If there is a delay, between 15% and 25% of patients have to be readmitted as an emergency with recurrence of acute cholecystitis (Fowkes and Gunn, 1980).

Early operation has been on trial for some years and there is convincing evidence that it is safe and generally advantageous for the patient (Mitchell and Morris 1982b).

Some 10% of patients have only local signs at the time of admission but, under observation, their condition and signs worsen. These patients prove to have obstructive cholecystitis with an area of gangrene in the wall, or an empyema has formed. Another 10–15% will show these signs on admission, and will require an urgent operation as soon as intravenous fluids, parenteral antibiotics and other resuscitative measures have rendered them fit for operation. A few patients will never become fit for operation, but for most three options are available. Open operation or laparoscopic cholecystectomy will be chosen for most patients, and that choice will depend, as discussed below, on local opinion and facilities. The third method, percutaneous cholecystostomy, has recently been introduced by the interventional radiologists, and offers a relatively low-risk method of draining the gallbladder in gravely ill patients who are unlikely to withstand a laparotomy.

Open operation

Preoperative preparation   When an emergency operation is needed for perforation of the gallbladder, biliary peritonitis or acute obstructive cholangitis, only a few hours are available for intensive resuscitation.

If early operation is adopted as a policy, there are 2 or 3 days in which to make sure that dehydration is corrected and renal function is satisfactory. With the increasing number of elderly men it is particularly important to provide physiotherapy to improve respiratory function, and to correct any cardiac abnormalities.

If it is necessary to operate on the jaundiced patient it is vital to ensure that renal function is optimal. An intravenous infusion should run during the night before operation so that the necessary restriction of oral intake does not result in dehydration, urine output *via* a catheter is checked during operation, and it is generally wise to give 200–300 ml of 10% mannitol during the operation.

Operation   Nowadays the diagnosis has usually been confirmed by ultrasonography or other methods so it is reasonable to use a subcostal incision, which gives the best access to the gallbladder: Kocher in fact devised this incision in 1878 for the approach to the acutely inflamed gallbladder. The exception to this proposal occurs when the diagnosis is in doubt or when there are signs of generalized peritonitis. Then a vertical incision is indicated.

Procedure   When the peritoneum is opened there are usually many fibrinous adhesions around the tense, discoloured gallbladder, which are easily separated. When there is a localized leak from a perforated gallbladder 500–700 ml of turbid bile may be aspirated. If the gallbladder is still intact, it is common to see areas of ischaemia in the wall. It is wise to introduce a wide-bore needle gently into the gallbladder and aspirate as much of the contents as possible, sending a sample for culture. This allows tissue forceps to be placed on the fundus to draw out the gallbladder and approach Hartmann's pouch. In most cases a large stone can be felt there and it is often possible to dislodge this stone up into the gallbladder so that a Babcock's forceps can be placed on Hartmann's pouch. This enables the dissection of the cystic duct to proceed in the usual manner. In the majority of patients the cystic duct can be clearly defined and intraoperative cholangiography performed just as in elective cholecystectomy, and the remainder of this operation does not require description. We have now had an extensive experience of early cholecystectomy and the difficulties are neither more nor less severe than those encountered in elective operations. Stones in the common duct are also removed by standard methods, although T-tube drainage of the duct may be used a little more freely.

However, in a few patients it is clear that it is impossible to make a satisfactory dissection beyond Hartmann's pouch, which may be firmly fused by fibrous adhesions to the front of the bile duct.

Cholecystostomy is a valuable and safe alternative in these circumstances, and is also useful if an inexperienced surgeon is faced with operating without assistance, or the patient is very sick and speed is important. The fundus is opened, the fluid contents are sucked out and then all the stones are evacuated. If there are many small stones it is wise to irrigate the cavity with syringe and catheter to make sure that all have been removed. An 18 or 20 FG Silastic Foley catheter is then inserted (after passing it through a suitably sited stab incision in the abdominal wall), the balloon is inflated and the incision closed around the catheter.

Sometimes this procedure has to be modified because the fundus of the gallbladder is necrotic. The preferable way of dealing with a necrotic gallbladder is clearly to perform cholecystectomy, but if the cystic duct cannot be safely dissected it is still possible to perform partial excision of the necrotic parts, and leave about half the gallbladder *in situ*, with a catheter sewn into it. There are occasions when only the Hartmann's pouch can be left, which is then oversewn and a drain is placed close to the area. These devices are preferable to hazardous attempts to complete cholecystectomy.

In the course of performing 87 emergency operations, Jarvinen and Hastbacka (1980) used a cholecystostomy on 15 occasions. The catheter is placed on open drainage and may or may not yield bile. A cholangiogram can be attempted in 10–14 days and may give valuable information about the bile duct. The catheter can generally be removed after 2–3 weeks and it is unusual for any continuing leakage to occur. Subsequently, most patients remain free of symptoms and it is rather unusual to have to perform a later cholecystectomy.

Laparoscopic cholecystectomy for acute cholecystitis

Laparoscopic cholecystectomy is the treatment of choice for most patients with symptomatic gallstones. The advantages over open cholecystectomy have been well accepted. During the initial experience with laparoscopic cholecystectomy, acute cholecystitis was considered to be a contraindication (Cuschieri *et al.*, 1991). The reasons for the disquiet were: friability of the inflamed and oedematous tissue; difficulty in displaying the anatomy; and the potential risk of damage to surrounding vital structures. With greater experience in laparoscopic surgery, better equipment and enhanced techniques, there are increasing reports of a growing interest in laparoscopic treatment of acute cholecystitis (Flowers *et al.*, 1991; Wilson *et al.*, 1992).

The role of laparoscopic surgery in the acute situation remains controversial. Almost all the reports have stressed the fact that inherent dangers are high. It is not a technique suitable for the inexperienced. The incidence of major bile duct injuries is increased in the early phase of a surgeon's training in laparoscopic cholecystectomy. Scott *et al.* (1992), in a review of over 12 000 patients, showed that more than two-thirds of the major duct injuries occurred during the surgeon's first 25 laparoscopic cholecystectomies. Even in the hands of the experienced, when compared to the planned operation, laparoscopic surgery for acute cholecystitis is often difficult, more lengthy and conversion to open biliary surgery high. Conversion rates of over 30% are frequent (Cox *et al.*, 1993; Rattner *et al.*, 1993). Several aspects of the laparoscopic management of acute cholecystitis merit special consideration. Zucker *et al.* (1993) discussed these aspects while describing their experience in 83 patients. In patients with abdominal distension the open method of port insertion is safer and more appropriate than the closed method. Additional ports are required for adequate retraction. The wide-angle (30–50°) telescope provides better visualization and is more versatile in the acute situation. Partial decompression of the gallbladder by aspiration improves the operative exposure and allows better grasping and handling of the gallbladder. It also minimizes the incidence of inadvertent perforation and bile/stone spillage. Complete emptying is not helpful as it is more difficult to dissect a flaccid gallbladder away from the liver. Larger and better grasping forceps are at times required for effective handling of a very thick-walled gallbladder. The anatomy of the porta hepatis is often distorted by inflammatory reaction and oedema, and the cystic duct and bile duct may appear much larger than normal. Complete dissection and visualization are essential prior to ligation or division of any presumed ductal or vascular structure. The routine use of intraoperative cholangiography will confirm the anatomy of the bile duct and exclude choledocholithiasis. The most common cause for intraperitoneal bleeding is failure to ligate and divide the posterior branch of the cystic artery and it is good practice to control both branches of the cystic artery prior to the dissection of the gallbladder. The titanium clips that are generally used are not always safe in the acute situation and laparoscopic sutures or pre-tied ligatures are safer. The specimen retrieval bags are often used to collect spilled gallstones or to remove infected tissues, and postoperative drainage is frequently necessary.

Zucker *et al.* (1993) reported a 27% (22 patients) conversion to open operation in their series and the reasons for conversion were: difficulty in safe dissection of the junction between cystic duct and common bile duct due to adhesions and/or inflammation in 12 patients; gangrene of gallbladder or associated abscess in five patients; tense, distended gallbladder and poor exposure in two patients; the finding of choledocholithiasis in two patients and a pancreatic pseudocyst in one patient. The rate of conversion was five times greater when compared with elective surgery (27.7% versus 5.2%). They believe that a low threshold for conversion to open laparotomy is important to reduce the risk of major complications. The mean postoperative hospital stay for the laparoscopic group was 3.3 days and 6.8 days for patients undergoing conversion to laparotomy. There was no mortality or major bile duct injury.

It is important to emphasize that the above results were obtained from the work carried out by a very experienced and interested group. A higher incidence of complications, including a bile duct injury rate of 1.5%, has been reported (Kum *et al.*, 1994).

A recent report from Hong Kong (Chung *et al.*, 1996) compared early laparoscopic cholecystectomy in acute cholecystitis with delayed treatment. There were 27 patients in the early and 25 in the delayed groups. Their conversion rate was 7.4% but there were no major complications.

Laparoscopic cholecystectomy has a place in the management of patients with acute cholecystitis. Technically it is more demanding and potential risks are high. Modifications in the technique are essential and the operator should have sufficient skill and experience to deal with the complex situation. Safety has to be the paramount concern, which may mean an increased willingness for conversion to open surgery.

Percutaneous treatment of acute cholecystitis
The treatment of critically ill patients with worsening acute cholecystitis is a challenging situation. Emergency cholecystectomy in gravely compromised patients with severe concurrent diseases is fraught with danger. Although cholecystostomy under local anaesthesia is an option, the morbidity of a laparotomy and the technical difficulties of the operation itself are inescapable. Less invasive, percutaneous, transhepatic or transperitoneal radiological techniques of gallbladder puncture and drainage provide a distinct advantage in this situation (Eggermont *et al.*, 1985; Dunham *et al.*, 1985). Under ultrasound guidance, using local anaesthesia, and often by the bedside, a catheter can be placed inside the gallbladder that enables diagnosis as well as therapy.

The success rate of percutaneous gallbladder intubation is high and procedure-related immediate complications are rare. The transhepatic route is preferable to the transperitoneal as it minimizes the risk of intraperitoneal bile leak and accidental bowel injury. Catheter dislodgement is a problem in 5–10% of patients, mostly as a result of confusion and agitation of the patient, and difficulty in catheter fixation. In the majority of patients, septic features are rapidly under control, permitting a planned approach to further treatment.

Melin *et al.* (1995) described their experience of percutaneous cholecystostomy (transhepatic 17, transperitoneal five) in 22 consecutive patients. All were considered to be extremely high-risk patients (mean Apache II score 16), 14 were in the intensive care unit and 21 of 22 were ultimately shown to have severe acute cholecystitis (acalculous 11, calculous 10). Following insertion of the catheter under local anaesthesia, the features of acute cholecystitis resolved within 24–48 hours in 18 (82%) patients but nine died within 60 days, six from co-morbid complications. Of the remaining 13 patients, three had planned cholecystectomy, three had successful non-operative treatment for removal of stones and in seven the gallbladder drain was removed (five acalculous) without a problem for a mean follow-up of 19 months.

Verbanck *et al.* (1993) reported the results of ultrasound-guided transhepatic gallbladder puncture and aspiration, without insertion of a catheter, in a similar group of 18 high-risk patients with acute cholecystitis. Under local anaesthesia aspiration of the gallbladder was performed at the bedside using a 14 FG needle; if the aspirate was purulent or cloudy, the gallbladder was rinsed with saline until clear. Following aspiration there were no complications. In 17 of the 18 patients symptoms improved; 13 remained free from biliary infections during a mean follow up period of 14 months and four had uncomplicated cholecystectomy 6–10 weeks later for recurrent cholecystitis.

It would therefore seem that, when faced with the difficult problem of worsening acute cholecystitis in a critically ill patient, the interventional radiologist may have a definite role in the management of the emergent situation. In such high-risk patients ultrasound-guided percutaneous, transhepatic aspiration or drainage of the gallbladder is a safe and efficient method of temporary management.

9.2.3   ACUTE EMPHYSEMATOUS CHOLECYSTITIS

This is an unusual but well-defined form of acute cholecystitis which was first accurately described by Lobinger in 1908. He found a gallbladder distended by gas, with palpable gas-crepitation in its wall. The condition is well reviewed by May and Strong (1971).

These patients present in the same manner as other patients with acute cholecystitis, although almost all patients are men and often they appear unusually toxic. The diagnosis is made when plain radiography of the abdomen reveals a gas-distended gallbladder around which there is often a thin halo of gas; in the erect film there is a fluid level. Sometimes these changes are seen on the films taken on admission but in a number of patients they only develop after patients have been managed conservatively for some days.

It is not clear why gas collects under pressure. Stones were present in only one of the three cases described by May and Strong (1971). Wilson (1958) reviewed the literature and found that stones were present in about half the cases. There was usually a positive anaerobic culture of *Clostridium*, either *C. welchii* or *C. perfringens*, or of *E. coli*. There is a suggestion from May and Strong (1971) that occlusion of the cystic artery may be a factor.

If the typical radiological appearance is seen it would seem wise to proceed with cholecystectomy. The three cases described by May and Strong were all treated conservatively but when explored later gangrene of the gallbladder was found in each case.

9.2.4 ACUTE ACALCULOUS CHOLECYSTITIS

Acute cholecystitis generally occurs in a gallbladder occupied by one or more stones, but in 5–6% of cases a specific form of cholecystitis occurs in the absence of stones. It can occur at any age and these patients are, for one reason or another, already severely ill. Children are dehydrated from gastroenteritis or have suffered severe burns or trauma (p. 111), adults are generally recovering from a major operation or injury, or have had a serious cardiovascular or respiratory illness.

In all these patients normal eating and drinking has more or less ceased and some are receiving parenteral nutrition, so there is likely to be relative stasis of bile: they are often dehydrated so the bile may be more viscous than normal. Some have been hypovolaemic and/ or hypoxic, so the perfusion of the gallbladder may have been impaired.

Herlin *et al.* (1982) examined 11 cholecystectomy specimens and could find no evidence of obstruction in any, although the wall was gangrenous in 10 and the bile unusually dark and viscous. Infection does not play a large part because only three of seven gallbladders yielded a positive culture.

The result is that, in a small number of patients who are already seriously ill, the changes of acute cholecystitis develop and cause similar symptoms and signs to those of calculous cholecystitis.

Diagnosis is made difficult by the fact that the patient is often recovering from a major operation, or an injury, and has considerable discomfort. However, both Howard (1981) and Fox *et al.* (1984) found that 50% of their patients had a gangrenous gallbladder so the signs can be severe enough to focus attention on the gallbladder. The time of occurrence varies but Flancbaum *et al.* (1985) found that in their 18 post-traumatic cases the onset was delayed on average for 25 days. The 11 patients of Herlin *et al.* (1982) developed cholecystitis between 9 and 40 days after operation or injury.

The problem is that this is such an unusual condition that it does have to be actively considered as a possibility. Then cholescintigraphy or ultrasonography can be undertaken; Fox *et al.* (1984) found that the radionuclide scan was positive in 14 of 15 cases but ultrasound only detected nine out of 14.

Because there tends to be some delay in diagnosis, and there is such a high incidence of gangrene, this is a serious complication in patients who are already ill: 14 of the 18 patients by Flancbaum *et al.* (1985) were hypotensive and 16 had required long periods of mechanical ventilation. Although cholecystectomy is urgently required, the care of these sick patients calls for a high degree of skill in both anaesthetist and surgeon. In some reports the mortality rate is 18–20%, but Fox *et al.* (1984) recorded only six deaths among their 68 patients.

9.2.5 TORSION OF THE GALLBLADDER

This is a rare event seen mostly in elderly women and so it may be on the increase as more people live longer.

Torsion of the gallbladder can only occur if it hangs free. Two anatomical anomalies permit torsion. In the more common type, the gallbladder is suspended from the liver on a narrow mesentery that is sufficiently long to allow torsion. In the rarer type, the gallbladder is not attached to the liver and lies free in the peritoneal cavity, suspended only by the cystic duct and artery, both of which may have a short mesentery.

The majority of cases have a rather acute onset of pain with rapid development of a tense, tender mass under the right costal margin. Accurate diagnosis is rarely made preoperatively, as the clinical features are frequently mistaken for acute cholecystitis, appendicitis or perforated peptic ulcer (Levene, 1958).

The acute local signs are likely to lead to urgent laparotomy and this is necessary because these gallbladders are gangrenous by the time they are removed. The cholecystectomies have proved to be easy and, in spite of their advanced age, these patients generally make a quick recovery.

9.2.6   BILE PERITONITIS

The escape of bile into the peritoneal cavity is a fairly unusual cause of peritonitis, but bile produces a severe form of chemical injury to the peritoneum which will be accentuated when the bile is infected. It has in the past carried a high mortality (Ellis and Cronin, 1960). There are three main causes: perforated acute cholecystitis, perforation of the gallbladder after injury and spontaneous rupture of the biliary tree.

Perforation of, or leakage from, the gallbladder or biliary tree after operation or injury

It is not unusual to see bile drain along the tube left in the gallbladder bed after cholecystectomy and this is generally due to **damage to a subvesical bile duct**. This accident is generally avoidable and is only harmful if drainage of the gallbladder is not routinely provided. At first as much as 300 ml of bile can drain in 24 hours, but this soon diminishes and ceases in a few days. It is possible for the ligature on the cystic duct to slip, but this is rare. Much more serious is accidental damage to the common hepatic or bile duct. These sources of bile peritonitis are almost entirely avoidable by careful operative technique.

Leakage of bile after **withdrawal of a T-tube** is a rare but very worrying complication of biliary tract surgery. It is now universal practice to obtain a normal T-tube cholangiogram before withdrawing the tube on the 12th postoperative day. In about one in every 120 removals (Corbett *et al.*, 1986) the patient complains within minutes of severe pain in the right upper quadrant, which fairly quickly spreads over the abdomen. The patient looks pale and unwell, is obviously in severe pain and shows the signs of local or general peritonitis. There is no doubt about the diagnosis in these patients and they require prompt laparotomy, peritoneal lavage and closure of the bile duct.

The occurrence of this mishap appears to be quite capricious. Use of latex rubber T-tubes is now universal, and they appear to be of standard quality, so it is obscure why, in less than 1% of patients, adhesions fail to develop and bile can leak from the defect in the common bile duct into the general peritoneal cavity. Corbett *et al.* (1986) conducted an extensive investigation but could not explain the unpredictable occurrence of this complication. They collected 68 examples: 51 required laparotomy and there were four deaths. Very occasionally a choledochoduodenostomy may develop a leak.

Occasionally, bile peritonitis follows **percutaneous liver puncture**, performed for biopsy or for transhepatic cholangiography. This is more or less confined to patients who have obstructive jaundice with dilated intrahepatic bile ducts. Morris *et al.* (1975) encountered one case of bile peritonitis requiring laparotomy in 127 liver biopsies with a Menghini needle. These patients make a good recovery following laparotomy, peritoneal lavage and placement of a drain beside the liver wound. If the leakage of bile is from a percutaneous transhepatic cholangiogram performed for investigation of jaundice, it may be appropriate to deal with the cause of obstructive jaundice at the same time; for example, stones are removed from the bile duct, cholecystectomy is performed and drainage is provided to the area of leak as well as to the biliary tree. If malignant obstruction of the bile duct is present it may be useful in an emergency to establish a tube cholecystostomy only, to decompress the biliary tree and to plan to return after a week or two for a definitive operation.

Blunt or penetrating injury to the gallbladder or bile ducts is a rare cause of bile peritonitis (p. 467).

Spontaneous rupture of the biliary tree

This is a rare but well-documented cause of bile peritonitis, which is reviewed by Billington and Hargreaves (1984). There are several theories about the cause, all of which mainly concentrate on a congenital weakness of the bile ducts. The rupture tends to occur at the junction of the cystic and common hepatic ducts and it is important to visualize the posterior as well as the anterior aspect of the bile duct during the search for the source of bile leakage. Gough *et al.* (1976) describe a patient with multiple small stones in the gallbladder and perforation of the unobstructed common hepatic duct: although a 4 mm stone was protruding from the rupture, it could not have exerted pressure on the duct, which apparently ruptured at a point of weakness.

The **clinical presentation** of bile peritonitis is usually acute because of the highly irritant effect of bile on the peritoneum: the signs of a spreading local or general peritonitis cannot be overlooked. Kune and Sali (1980) draw attention to some cases that present in an insidious manner. There may be a sudden pain under the right costal margin, but this eases and the patient only presents after several days of discomfort. There is likely to be some abdominal distension and tenderness in the region of the gallbladder. Pulse rate is particularly likely to be raised to 100–140/min, which is out of proportion to the general clinical picture. Diagnostic paracentesis and ultrasonography are then likely to be particularly helpful in clarifying the diagnosis.

The important feature of **treatment** is to evacuate the bile and provide external drainage. Some patients will require a short period of resuscitation before laparotomy. The cause of the biliary leak is dealt with appropriately, thorough peritoneal lavage performed and T-tube and other drainage provided as required.

9.2.7 IATROGENIC COMPLICATIONS OF ENDOSCOPIC SPHINCTEROTOMY

Endoscopic biliary sphincterotomy (ES) was first described in 1974 (Classen and Denling, 1974). The technique has been widely accepted for removal of bile duct stones. In the era of laparoscopic cholecystectomy, ES is often preferred to surgical exploration of the common bile duct. Sphincterotomy is also performed to help the placement of stents in the treatment of malignant or benign strictures. Significant complications occur in about 10% of patients with an overall mortality of 1.5–3.0% (Lesse *et al.*, 1985; Lambert *et al.*, 1991; Cotton *et al.*, 1991; Freeman *et al.*, 1996). Most complications are apparent within 24 hours and some will require emergency operation. An awareness of the potential complications is vital for prompt and effective treatment.

Contrary to the conventional opinion, various reports have shown that the presence of periampullary diverticula do not increase the risk of sphincterotomy (Vaira *et al.*, 1989; Shemesh *et al.*, 1990). However, a small or normal-sized bile duct increases the risk. The technique of precut, where the papilla is dissected off the surrounding mucosa prior to sphincterotomy, is more prone to complications. The skill of the endoscopist is also important: complication rates are substantially higher among endoscopists doing their first 20 procedures (Bilbao *et al.*, 1977). A multicentre audit showed that clinicians performing an average of more than one sphincterotomy per week had fewer complications than lower-volume centres (Freeman *et al.*, 1996). Complications cannot always be avoided, with haemorrhage, pancreatitis, perforation of duodenum and cholangitis being the most frequent.

Haemorrhage

Post-sphincterotomy bleeding is a relatively frequent complication. In a multicentre audit, Cotton *et al.* (1991) reported an overall incidence of 2.5–5%; operative intervention was required in 22% with a mortality rate of 13%. Bleeding is usually obvious immediately after sphincterotomy but can be delayed for hours or even days. The risk of bleeding can be higher when the sphincterotomy is enlarged at a second procedure within a few days or weeks (Goodall, 1985).

Most patients with bleeding can be managed by conservative measures. The indication for surgical intervention is not different from other causes of upper gastrointestinal bleeding. If bleeding is seen at the time of sphincterotomy the endoscopist will usually attempt control of the bleeding site by diathermy coagulation or by submucosal injection of adrenaline. Some have suggested repeated endoscopic management (Freeman *et al.*, 1996) or balloon tamponade (Cotton *et al.*, 1991). Saeed *et al.* (1989) described their experience of using angiographic methods for control of bleeding: of 11 attempts, 10 were successfully localized and embolization was effective in 9.

Operation must be considered when non-surgical methods fail. Lesse *et al.* (1985) reported 394 patients with ES: ten were complicated with post-procedure bleeding, eight patients did not require blood transfusion, four settled with 2–4 units of blood each but six continued to bleed and required operation. There were no postoperative deaths. The remaining patient was an elderly lady with periampullary pancreatic tumour. Sphincterotomy was performed for relief of jaundice but she continued to bleed, with a fatal outcome. As in other situations of bleeding, timing of the operation can be a difficult decision: not to be too late, with the inherent risks of a seriously compromised patient, or too early, when there may still be a likelihood of spontaneous arrest. As an arbitrary measure, blood transfusion requirement of more than 4 units in 24–36 hours should be considered as an indication for operation. In the event of delayed bleeding, investigations should proceed along the lines of unknown upper gastrointestinal bleeding including endoscopy, before deciding to operate. At the time of operation, duodenum is fully mobilized and explored through a longitudinal incision. The ampulla is located; the bleeding site may be obvious or may be obscured by clots. If the sphincterotomy is small, it may be enlarged and the edges of cut margins sutured to convert the opening to a sphincteroplasty. Goodall (1985) pointed out that four out of six patients re-bled after operation, and recommended non-absorbable suture material. In our experience with four patients who required operation, the ampulla was sutured with a delayed absorbable material (polydioxanone) without any ill effects. Should the biliary tract contain residual stones (gallbladder or bile duct), provided the general condition of the patient is satisfactory, it would be appropriate to deal with it.

Perforation

Duodenal perforation is probably the most serious of all the post-sphincterotomy complications. Cotton *et al.* (1991), in an audit of over 12 000 ES, cited duodenal perforation in 1.3% of patients, of which 27% had surgical treatment with a mortality of 16%. In individual series, the incidence of duodenal perforation has ranged from 0.8–3% (Safrany, 1977; Lesse *et al.*, 1985) and the postoperative mortality has been as high as 35% (Safrany, 1978). The perforation usually involves the posterior duodenal wall and retroperitoneum but may occasionally be intraperitoneal.

There is no proof that the risk of perforation reduces with increasing experience. The risk is higher in patients with papillary stenosis than in patients with stones (Neoptolemos *et al.*, 1988) but there is no increased risk in patients with periampullary diverticula or previous Billroth II gastrectomy (Vaira *et al.*, 1989; Osnes *et al.*, 1986). Precut sphincterotomy where the ampulla is dissected prior to sphincterotomy is known to increase the risk of perforation (Cotton, 1989; Booth *et al.*, 1990).

The diagnosis of retroperitoneal perforation can be difficult (Lesse *et al.*, 1985) but the presence of air or contrast outside the confines of bile duct or duodenum on the abdominal radiograph should warn of the possibility. In a recent report, plain abdominal radiography showed free retroperitoneal or intraperitoneal gas in seven of eight patients (Chaudhary and Aranya, 1996). Other unusual manifestations of retroperitoneal perforation, such as appearance of a mass in the right iliac fossa 2 weeks after ES and bile staining of right flank along with scrotal swelling due to tracking of bile in the retroperitoneum, have been described (Lesse *et al.*, 1985). Patients in whom perforation is not obvious immediately will usually present with abdominal (right subcostal and back) pain, fever or features of ileus. It is important to differentiate retroperitoneal perforation from acute pancreatitis and early CT scanning is the best method of discrimination (Kuhlmann *et al.*, 1989).

There are no rigid guidelines for the management of perforation following ES. Recommendations vary from early operation in most cases to a policy of conservative management. Since the majority of perforations are small and confined, most gastro-enterologists endorse a non-operative expectant treatment. Such patients should be treated with intravenous fluids, antibiotics and nasogastric decompression and be very closely observed for features of sepsis or peritoneal irritation. Contrast radiology of the duodenum may demonstrate a free perforation, in which case operation is the best treatment. Sepsis-related complications are common, which may be because of impaired drainage of infected bile (due to calculus disease) into the duodenum. Therefore, if perforation is recognized at the time of sphincterotomy some endoscopists suggest the placement of a nasobiliary drain or insertion of a percutaneous transhepatic cannula to improve drainage and minimize retroperitoneal contamination (Bryne *et al.*, 1984).

Patients with obvious signs of sepsis or peritonitis are best managed by operative intervention. However, when features of sepsis are early or indefinite, the decision may not be easy or obvious, resulting in delay of treatment. A majority of the patients for ES are elderly and may not exhibit striking abdominal signs in spite of ongoing contamination. Delay in surgical treatment leads to increased mortality and morbidity from residual peritoneal sepsis.

When operation is undertaken early, the site of perforation may be obvious and is treated by suture repair. It is customary to divert the bile flow by T-tube drainage. Any periduodenal and retroperitoneal collection is drained at the same time. If stones are present in the biliary tree, they are dealt with appropriately (cholecystectomy, removal of duct calculi). When laparotomy is undertaken late, the site of perforation may not be obvious but considerable peritoneal contamination and organized sepsis are frequently present. Treatment is by thorough peritoneal debridement and drainage of the biliary tree and retroperitoneum. Occasionally, the duodenal defect may be extensive; in such a situation it may be appropriate to incorporate a method of pyloric exclusion (Graham *et al.*, 1979). In this operation the stomach is opened through the pyloric antrum close to the greater curve. The pyloric ring is closed from inside with an absorbable suture (polydioxanone) and a gastrojejunostomy is created at the site of gastrotomy. The absorbable suture will disintegrate in some weeks (or it can be removed endoscopically) and allow normal passage (p. 431).

Pancreatitis

Pancreatitis can occur after diagnostic ERCP and the risk is increased by sphincterotomy. Cotton *et al.* (1991) reported an overall incidence of 2.1% (1.3–3.1%) with a mortality of 10% and 6.4% required an operation. The diagnosis is usually obvious but if perforation is seriously considered, a CT scan will differentiate.

Rare complications

Impaction of the retrieval basket while attempting to remove stones from the common bile duct can occur infrequently. Sometimes it may be due to an inadequate sphincterotomy incision. The endoscope is removed leaving the basket *in situ*, and the patient is started on intravenous antibiotics. It is worth waiting for 24 hours, as some may disengage spontaneously. A plain radiograph of the abdomen taken 24 hours later will show any shift of the basket, in which case gentle traction may ease it out. If the impaction is static, laparotomy and open removal from the duodenum is undertaken. It may be necessary to lengthen the sphincterotomy incision, which is converted to a sphincteroplasty.

Gallstone ileus is a rare complication of endoscopic sphincterotomy especially when calculi more than 20 mm in size are released into the duodenum. The diagnosis may be elusive but awareness of the possibility will usually lead to appropriate treatment (p. 239).

REFERENCES

Bilbao, M. R., Dotter, C. T. and Lee, T. G. (1977) Complications of endoscopic retrograde cholangiopancreatography (ERCP). *Gastroenterology*, **70**, 314–320.

Billington, P. and Hargreaves, A. W. (1984) Spontaneous biliary peritonitis. *J. R. Coll. Surg. Edin.*, **29**, 184–185.

Booth, F. V., Doerr, R. J. and Khalafi, R. S. (1990) Surgical management of complications of endoscopic sphincterotomy with precut papillotomy. *Am. J. Surg.*, **159**, 132–136.

Bryne, P., Leung, J. W. C., Cotton, P. B. (1984) Retroperitoneal perforation during duodenoscopic sphincterotomy. *Radiology*, **150**, 383–384.

Chaudhary, A. and Aranya, R. C. (1996) Surgery in perforation after endoscopic sphincterotomy: sooner, later or not at all? *Ann. R. Coll. Surg. Engl.*, **78**, 206–208.

Chung, M. L., Chi, L. L., Edward, C. S. *et al.* (1996) Early versus delayed laparoscopic cholecystectomy for treatment of acute cholecystitis. *Ann. Surg.*, **223**, 37–42.

Classen, M. and Demling, L. (1974) Endoskopische Sphinkterotomie der Papilla Vateri und Steinnextraktion aus dem Ductus choledochus. *Dtsch. Med. Wschr.*, **99**, 496–497.

Cope, Z. (1970) A sign in gallbladder disease. *BMJ.*, **iii**, 147–148.

Corbett, C. R. R., Fyfe, N. C. M., Nichols, R. J. *et al.* (1986) Bile peritonitis after removal of T-tubes from common bile duct. *Br. J. Surg.*, **73**, 641–643.

Cotton, P. B. (1989) Precut papillotomy – a risky technique for experts only. *Gastrointest. Endosc.*, **35**, 578–579.

Cotton, P. B, Lehman, G., Vennes, J. *et al.* (1991) Endoscopic sphincterotomy complications and their management: an attempt at consensus. *Gastrointest. Endosc.*, **37**, 383–393.

Cox, M. R., Wilson, T. G., Luck, A. J. *et al.* (1993) Laparoscopic cholecystectomy for acute inflammation of the gallbladder. *Ann. Surg.*, **218**, 630–634.

Cushieri, A., Dubois, F., Mouiel, J. *et al.* (1991) The European experience with laparoscopic cholecystectomy. *Am. J. Surg.*, **161**, 385–387.

De Dombal, F. T. (1980) *Diagnosis of Acute Abdominal Pain*, Churchill Livingstone, Edinburgh, pp. 15–17.

Dunham, F., Marliere, P., Mortier, C. *et al.* (1985) Ultrasound guided percutaneous and transhepatic cholecystostomy: a complementary procedure to therapeutic endoscopy. *Endoscopy*, **17**, 153–156.

Dykes, E. H., Stewart, I., Gray, H. *et al.* (1984) Infusion cholecystography in the early diagnosis of acute gallbladder disease. *Br. J. Surg.*, **71**, 854–855.

Eggermont, A. M., Lameris, J. S. and Jeekil, J. (1985) Ultrasound guided percutaneous transhepatic cholecystostomy for acute acalculous cholecystitis. *Arch. Surg.*, **120**, 1354–1356.

Ellis, H. and Cronin, K. (1960) Bile peritonitis. *Br. J. Surg.*, **48**, 166–171.

Flancbaum, L., Majerus, T. C., Cox, E. F. (1985) Acute post-traumatic acalculous cholecystitis. *Am. J. Surg.*, **150**, 252–256.

Flowers, J. L., Bailey, R. W., Scovill, W. A. *et al.* (1991) The Baltimore experience with laparoscopic management of acute cholecystitis. *Am. J. Surg.*, **161**, 388–392.

Fowkes, F. G. R. and Gunn, A. A. (1980) The management of acute cholecystitis and its hospital cost. *Br. J. Surg.*, **67**, 613–617.

Fox, M. S., Wilk, P. J., Weissmann, H. S. *et al.* (1984) Acute acalculous cholecystitis. *Surg. Gynecol. Obstet.*, **159**, 13–16.

Freeman, M. L., Nelson, D. B., Sherman, S. *et al.* (1996) Complications of endoscopic biliary sphincterotomy. *N. Engl. J. Med.*, **335**, 909–918.

French, E. B. and Robb, W. A. T. (1963) Biliary and renal colic. *BMJ.*, **ii**, 135–138.

Gill, P. T., Dillon, E., Lesley, A. L. *et al.* (1985) Ultrasonography, HIDA scintigraphy or both in diagnosis of acute cholecystitis? *Br. J. Surg.*, **72**, 267–268.

Glenn, F. (1948) The surgical treatment of acute cholecystitis. *Surgery*, **23**, 397–404.

Glenn, F. and Heuer, G. J. (1946) The surgical treatment of acute cholecystitis. *Surg. Gynecol. Obstet.*, **83**, 50–54.

Glenn, F. and Thorbjarnarson, B. (1963) The surgical treatment of acute cholecystitis. *Surg. Gynecol. Obstet.*, **116**, 61–70.

Goodall, R. J. R. (1985) Bleeding after endoscopic sphincterotomy. *Ann. R. Coll. Surg. Engl.*, **67**, 87–88.

Gough, A. L., Edwards, A. N. and Keddie, N. C. (1976) Spontaneous perforation of common bile duct. *Br. J. Surg.*, **63**, 446–448.

Graham, J. M., Mattox, K. L., Vaughan, G. D. *et al.* (1979) Combined pancreaticoduodenal injuries. *J. Trauma*, **19**, 340–343.

Gunn, A. and Keddie, N. (1972) Some clinical observations on patients with gallstones. *Lancet*, **ii**, 239–241.

Herlin, P., Ericsson, M., Holmin, T. *et al.* (1982) Acute acalculous cholecystitis following trauma. *Br. J. Surg.*, **69**, 475–476.

Howard, R. J. (1981) Acute acalculous cholecystitis. *Am. J. Surg.*, **141**, 194–198.

Jarvinen, H. J. and Hastbacka, J. (1980) Early cholecystectomy for acute cholecystitis: a prospective randomized study. *Ann. Surg.*, **191**, 501–505.

Kuhlman, J. E., Fishman, E. K., Milligan, F. D. *et al.* (1989) Complications of endoscopic retrograde sphincterotomy: computer tomographic evaluation. *Gastrointest. Radiol.*, **14**, 127–132.

Kum, C. K., Goh, P. M. Y., Isaac, J. R. *et al.* (1994) Laparoscopic cholecystectomy for acute cholecystitis. *Br. J. Surg.*, **81**, 1651–1654.

Kune, G. A. and Sali, A. (1980) Biliary peritonitis, in *The Practice of Biliary Surgery*, Blackwell Scientific Publications, Oxford, p. 317.

Lai, E. C. S. (1990) Management of severe acute cholangitis. *Br. J. Surg.*, **77**, 604–605.

Lambert, M. E., Betts, C. D., Hill, J. *et al.* (1991) Endoscopic sphincterotomy: the whole truth. *Br. J. Surg.*, **78**, 473–476.

Lennon, F. and Green, W. E. R. (1983) Perforation of the gall bladder. *J. R. Coll. Surg. Edin.*, **28**, 169–173.

Lesse, T., Neoptolemos, J. P., Carr-Locke, D. L. (1985) Success, failures, early complications and their management following endoscopic sphincterotomy: results in 394 consecutive patients from a single centre. *Br. J. Surg.*, **72**, 215–219.

Levene, A. (1958) Acute torsion of the gallbladder. *Br. J. Surg.*, **45**, 338–340.

Lobingier, A. S. (1908) Gangrene of the gallbladder. *Ann. Surg.*, **48**, 72–73.

MacCallum, W. G. (1930) *William Stewart Halsted*, Johns Hopkins Press, Baltimore, MD, p. 44.

May, R. E. and Strong, R. (1971) Acute emphysematous cholecystitis. *Br. J. Surg.*, **58**, 453–458.

Melin, M., Sarr, M. G., Bender, C. E. *et al.* (1995) Percutaneous cholecystostomy: a valuable technique in high risk patients with presumed acute cholecystitis. *Br. J. Surg.*, **82**, 1274–1277.

Mitchell, A. and Morris, P. J. (1982a) Hospital admissions for acute cholecystitis: changes in the age and sex distribution in Oxford in the post-war period. *Br. J. Surg.*, **69**, 26–28.

Mitchell, A. and Morris, P. J. (1982b) Trends in management of acute cholecystitis. *BMJ.*, **284**, 27–30.

Morris, J. S., Gallo, G. A., Scheuer, P. J. *et al.* (1975) Percutaneous liver biopsy in patients with bile duct obstruction. *Gastroenterology*, **68**, 750–754.

Neoptolemos, J. P., Bailey, I. S. and Carr-Locke, D. L. (1988) Sphincter of Oddi dysfunction: results of treatment by endoscopic sphincterotomy. *Br. J. Surg.*, **75**, 454–459.

Osnes, M., Rosseland, A. R. and Aabakken, L. (1986) Endoscopic retrograde cholangiography and endoscopic papillotomy in patients with a previous Billroth II resection. *Gut*, **27**, 1193–1198.

Rattner, D. W., Ferguson, C. and Warshaw, A. L. (1993) Factors associated with successful laparoscopic cholecystectomy for acute cholecystitis. *Ann. Surg.*, **217**, 233–236.

Saaed, M., Kadir, S., Kaufman, S. L. *et al.* (1989) Bleeding following endoscopic sphincterotomy: angiographic management by transcatheter embolisation. *Gastrointest. Endosc.*, **35**, 300–303.

Safrany, L. (1977) Duodenoscopic sphincterotomy and gallstones removal. *Gastroenterology*, **72**, 41–42.

Safrany, L. (1978) Endoscopic treatment of biliary tract disease. *Lancet*, **ii**, 983–985.

Schofield, P. F., Hulton, N. R. and Baildam, A. D. (1986) Is it acute cholecystitis? *Ann. R. Coll. Surg. Engl.*, **68**, 14–16.

Scott, T. R., Bailey, R. W. and Zucker, K. A. (1992) Laparoscopic cholecystectomy: a review of 12,337 patients. *Surg. Laparosc. Endosc.*, **2**, 331–340.

Shemesh, E., Klein, E., Czeniak, A. *et al.* (1990) Endoscopic sphincterotomy in patients with gallbladder *in situ*: the influence of periampullary duodenal diverticula. *Surgery*, **107**, 163–166.

Sovia, M., Haveri, M., Taavitsainen, *et al.* (1986) The value of routine sonography in clinically suspected acute cholecystitis. *Scand. J. Gastroenterol.*, **21**, 70–74.

Vaira, D., Dowsett, J. F., Hatfield, A. R. W. *et al.* (1989) Is duodenal diverticula a risk factor for sphincterotomy? *Gut*, **30**, 939–942.

Verbanck, J. J., Demol, J. W., Ghilbert, G. L. *et al.* (1993) Ultrasound guided puncture for acute cholecystitis. *Lancet*, **341**, 1132–1133.

Wilson, W. A. (1958) Acute cholecystitis due to gas producing organisms. *Br. J. Surg.*, **45**, 333–337.

Wilson, R. G., Macintyre, I. M. C., Nixon, S. J. *et al.* (1992) Laparoscopic cholecystectomy as a safe and effective treatment for severe acute cholecystitis. *BMJ.*, **305**, 394–396.

Zucker, K. A., Flowers, J. L., Bailey, R. W. *et al.* (1993) Laparoscopic management of acute cholecystitis. *Am. J. Surg.*, **165**, 508–514.

10

Abdominal injuries

10.1 INTRODUCTION

Aristotle knew that the intestines could be ruptured by external violence that left no mark on the abdomen, but for centuries more attention was paid to penetrating injuries, which resulted from accidents, assaults and warfare; from these few recovered. In the American Civil War all abdominal wounds were treated conservatively and 90% died (Graham, 1958).

Surgeons began to operate electively in the abdomen in the last years of the 19th century but few would perform an emergency laparotomy for injury, and this view was confirmed when the policy of conservative management pursued in the Boer War of 1899–1901 was surprisingly successful. In the crowded streets and factories of cities there were many accidents but when Berry and Giuseppi (1908), working in London, reviewed 85 laparotomies for intestinal rupture they found that the mortality rate was 80%.

There seemed, therefore, little reason to change policy in the Army Medical Department when the First World War broke out in 1914. However, it was soon apparent that, in conditions very different from those in South Africa, few recovered from an abdominal wound. The policy had to be reconsidered and by 1915, with improved methods of resuscitation and blood transfusion, and with early laparotomy, the results were greatly improved. Since then, experience in each successive conflict has produced advances in treatment and in outcome (p. 421).

In the second half of this century the widespread use of weapons among the inhabitants of cities, and the great increase in the number and speed of road vehicles, has produced a range of injuries that has been called 'the neglected epidemic'; now, between 1 and 34 years of age, motor vehicle collisions are the leading cause of death in the USA (Baker, 1987). Many of these collisions are of great severity and in 1000 consecutive fatal accidents in England and Wales, 48% died before reaching hospital (Anderson *et al.*, 1988); abdominal injuries were prominent among those who died after admission and many of these deaths were due to failure to recognize their severity.

The relative incidence of closed and penetrating abdominal injuries varies from region to region, and nation to nation. In Europe and Australasia closed injuries are more common than penetrating wounds, although injury due to assault is steadily rising. If South Africa and the USA are compared, penetrating injuries after fights and assaults are twice as common as road

Emergency Abdominal Surgery. Edited by Peter F. Jones, Zygmunt H. Krukowski and George G. Youngson. Published in 1998 by Chapman & Hall, London. ISBN 0 412 81950 3.

accidents in South Africa, whereas the converse is the case in the USA (Muckart, 1991). In 1982 motor vehicles killed 45 000 Americans and guns killed 33 000 (Baker, 1987). However, among children with abdominal injuries Colombani *et al.* (1985) in Baltimore found that 94% were due to non-penetrating trauma, mostly sustained in road accidents, and overall 30% were due to a fall from a bicycle; in 2% the injury was due to abuse in the home.

10.2   CLOSED INJURIES

These are most often due to direct violence when, for instance, the rim of the steering wheel is driven into the abdomen in a head-on vehicle collision, or a crush injury of the chest drives a rib into the liver or spleen. Indirect violence, as occurs in deceleration after a fall from a height, can tear heavy organs such as liver, spleen or kidney, and a fracture of the pelvic ring can be complicated by injury to the bladder or urethra (p. 488). Some 50–60% of closed injuries are due to road accidents, and most victims are occupants of the vehicle, but 15% are on a motor cycle or pedal cycle and 15% are pedestrians. Other causes are falls, accidents at work or in the home, assaults and seat-belt injuries (p. 474; Cox, 1984).

For abdominal organs to be injured considerable force has to be applied and among 870 patients needing a laparotomy in Baltimore, 34% had fractures of the limbs, spine or pelvis, 18% had a head injury and 6% had major trauma to the thorax. In 23% the blood alcohol exceeded 100 mg/dl (Cox, 1984). These findings are all reminders that publicity and legislation must continue to effect reduction of speed and drink driving, and enforcement of use of seat-belts.

Organs affected

If attention is confined to patients needing a laparotomy, the spleen is most often injured (42%), followed by the liver (35%) and the intestines and their mesenteries (20%); retroperitoneal haemorrhage is the principal finding in 15% (Cox, 1984). However, if the diagnosis reached in every patient is considered, damage was limited to contusion of the abdominal wall in 40% and, because 'of the ease of detection of haematuria, injury to the kidney(s) is recorded in 30%. Overall, injury to organs requiring repair is relatively unusual – spleen 13%, liver 8%. Injury to the bowel is seen in less than 5% and the duodenum and pancreas are affected in only 1% of patients.

Diagnosis

Because it is known that the signs of blunt abdominal injury can be minimal, or slow to appear, many patients have to be admitted for observation and re-examination.

Many are confused or unconscious because of head injury or the effects of alcohol or drugs, and the consequent lack of sensible communication can increase the risk of overlooking another injury by three- or fourfold. It is particularly important to recognize that head injuries rarely cause a fall in blood pressure, and in the unconscious patient with signs of hypovolaemic shock the cause must be sought in the abdomen, chest, pelvis or fracture of the pelvis or a long bone. These sites must be carefully examined, including radiography, diagnostic peritoneal lavage and pleural tap. Muckart and Thomson (1991) have given some telling examples of the dangers of omission of any of these features of complete examination.

Other injuries may be so painful, and the conscious patient may be so distressed, that some abdominal discomfort may not be mentioned. This may be due to the characteristics of some injuries – especially rupture of the small bowel (p. 436) and delayed rupture of the spleen (p. 454) – that they cause few or no abdominal symptoms for some time after the event; even a tentative complaint of abdominal discomfort or shoulder-tip pain must be regarded with suspicion and calls for continued and repeated observation.

The details of the physical examination – which shares many of the features of penetrating injuries – are considered on p. 423. However, in a suspected closed injury, abdominal examination has to be particularly careful. There may be a useful hint of the force applied in the presence of bruising, or seat-belt tattooing, on the abdominal skin. Even slight abdominal tenderness, a suspicion of guarding, apparent absence of bowel sounds (p. 437), is enough to make a period of active observation (p. 50) essential.

REFERENCES

Anderson, I. D., Woodford, M., de Dombal, F. T. *et al.* (1988) Retrospective study of 1000 deaths from injury in England and Wales. *BMJ.*, **296**, 1305–1138.

Baker, S. P. (1987) Injuries: the neglected epidemic. *J. Trauma*, **27**, 343–348.

Berry, J. and Giuseppi, P. L. (1908) Traumatic rupture of the intestine. *Lancet*, **ii**, 1143–1145.

Colombani, P. M., Buck, J. R., Dudgeon, D. L. *et al.* (1985) One year experience in a regional paediatric trauma centre. *J. Pediatr. Surg.*, **20**, 8–13.

Cox, E. F. (1984) Blunt abdominal trauma: a 5 year analysis of 870 patients requiring celiotomy. *Ann. Surg.*, **199**, 467–474.

Graham, A. S. (1958) Penetrating wounds of the colon. *Surg. Clin. North Am.*, **38**, 1639.

Muckart, D. J. J. (1991) Trauma: the malignant epidemic. *S. Afr. J. Med.*, **79**, 93–95.

Muckart, D. J. J. and Thomson, S. R. (1991) Undetected injuries: a preventable cause of increased morbidity and mortality. *Am. J. Surg.*, **162**, 457–460.

10.3 BLAST INJURIES

Blast injuries occur when a shock pressure wave generated by high explosive travels through air or water. These injuries were recognized in the First World War, mainly in sailors thrown into the water when their ship was torpedoed, and then affected by depth charging. The effects of blast are more severe in underwater accidents than in air because water is incompressible and the effects spread further. Although it was significant in time of war, underwater blast is now unusual, but the wide use of antipersonnel mines and of bombs by terrorists means that blast injuries sustained in air are becoming more familiar.

The pressure wave striking the abdomen is transmitted through the muscles and solid viscera because they behave as liquids: kinetic energy is liberated at the interface where air and liquid meet, i.e. in the alveolae and in the intestinal wall. The characteristic lesions are multiple haemorrhages from rupture of alveolar or intestinal capillaries. Respiratory distress with coughing of bloody frothy sputum, and sometimes bloody diarrhoea, are consequently seen in blast injury (Mellor, 1988).

In February and March 1996 four military anti-tank mines were exploded in the streets of Tel Aviv and Jerusalem (Leibovici *et al.*, 1996). Two were set off in crowded buses and immediately killed half the occupants. In a closed space the pressure wave is exceptionally powerful and exerts great effect through the chest wall on the lungs. The alveolar membranes are severely damaged and the air-spaces become filled with blood and oedema fluid. Air can also enter the pulmonary veins and cause brain damage. In two other incidents the explosions took place in the open street, the pressure wave had a less concentrated effect, and only 8% of over 200 people affected were killed. Two of the survivors from the buses sustained blast perforations of the small bowel. Five others had a ruptured spleen but it was thought that they were sustained when the patients were thrown forcibly by the blast and landed awkwardly.

In another incident in Tel Aviv Paran *et al.* (1996) saw three patients with bowel injuries: one presented with signs of peritonism but the other two were asymptomatic for 24 and 48 hours before developing abdominal signs. At laparotomy these patients showed a subserosal haematoma in the terminal ileum, with a perforation at its margin. All had a resection and recovered.

The general experience is that the effects of bomb blast transmitted through air mainly affects the lungs and this is a consideration in the relatively few patients who present with abdominal signs and who require general anaesthesia for a laparotomy. In fact, it is more likely that they will need treatment for injuries sustained when they are thrown about by the blast wave, rather than primary blast injury of the abdomen.

REFERENCES

Leibovici, D., Gofrit, O. N., Stein, M. *et al.* (1996) Blast injury: bus versus open-air bombings. *J. Trauma*, **41**, 1030–1035.

Mellor, S. G. (1988) The pathogenesis of blast injury and its management. *Br. J. Hosp. Med.*, **39**, 536–539.

Paran, H., Neufeld, D., Shwartz, I. *et al.* (1996) Perforation of the terminal ileum induced by blast injury: delayed diagnosis or delayed perforation? *J. Trauma*, **40**, 472–475.

10.4　PENETRATING INJURIES

Until the second half of the 20th century experience of penetrating abdominal injuries was largely restricted to times of war. The change, during the First World War, from a conservative to an operative surgical approach resulted in a mortality rate of over 95% being halved to about 50%. When the Second World War broke out there had been considerable advances in the care of abdominal surgical patients, in intravenous fluid and electrolyte therapy, in blood transfusion and in anaesthesia. During the mobile war in the Western Desert it became clear that these advantages could be used to the best advantage if there was:

- speedy evacuation of the patient to a hospital where he could be operated upon and retained for 10–14 days;
- observance of the rule that the operation is an essential part of resuscitation, to be undertaken as soon as the maximum benefit of preoperative care has been obtained;
- continuation of intravenous fluids and nasogastric suction, with the patient remaining under the active supervision of the operating surgeon.

In subsequent wars in Korea and Vietnam it was possible to use helicopters for evacuation, with casualties reaching the hospital within an hour of wounding. Such speedy access to the full range of surgical care, along with the advent of antibiotics, brought major improvements in results: mortality in the Vietnam War was one-tenth of the rate of the Second World War and one-half of the death rate in the Korean War (Ornato *et al.*, 1985).

These major conflicts of the first part of the century have, to a considerable extent, given way to a different but still very grave source of penetrating abdominal wounding in the wide and increasing resort to guns and knives as weapons of assault in civilian life.

Motor vehicle collisions have now, in a number of countries, given way to assaults as the major source of abdominal trauma. This is the case in South Africa, where the weaponry has also changed, with a 30% reduction in stab wounds and an 800% increase in firearm injuries (Muckart *et al.*, 1995). These changes are due in part to the ready availability of handguns, in part to a greater tendency to settle scores with lethal weapons and in part to increasing gang warfare in big cities, often related to drug trafficking. This has produced a number of studies of the problem, especially from the USA and South Africa.

Pathology

The frequency of wounding of an abdominal organ by penetrating injury is roughly proportional to its size and extent of contact with the anterior abdominal wall, so the small intestine is the most consistently injured, irrespective of the nature of the weapon. In addition, stab wounds are most likely to enter the liver and the diaphragm, while gunshot injuries tend to damage the colon and major vessels (Feliciano and Rozycki, 1995).

Missile ballistics determine the extent of damage inflicted by firearms. **Weapons with high muzzle velocities** – greater than 600 m/s – cause three types of injury:

- the damage due to the passage of the missile itself;
- a secondary missile effect due to the energy of the missile accelerating the tissue in its path, so that this in turn acts as a missile, widening the area of damage;
- a cavitation effect, due to energy of the shock wave expanding outwards to produce a cavity, which then rapidly contracts, drawing foreign material into the wound.

Pressure effects can be exerted on tissues well away from the wound track, e.g. on the colon, which has an adequate but not rich blood supply.

When **shells** detonate they throw out multiple fragments, which travel at high speeds; because they are irregularly shaped they are soon slowed after piercing the skin. **Antipersonnel mines** explode at very close quarters and throw off innumerable small fragments at high speeds; they have no great bulk but their speed enables them to pepper the skin and penetrate to some depth, sometimes into the abdomen while leaving only a small entry wound; these can cause damage at several different sites.

Low-velocity missile wounds are usually due to attack from handguns, which have a muzzle velocity of 200–300 m/s. Range is, as always, an important factor: above 6 m the small individual pellets inflict scattered superficial wounds, but at a range of 1 m the effect is similar to a high-velocity missile (this is a significant factor in a suicide attempt). A bullet from a pistol at 50 m will make only a narrow track through the tissues, its speed will fall away and it may come to rest in the body.

From a practical point of view, the admitting surgeon may not know the speed of the missile. What is 'essential to understanding and properly treating the gunshot wound is objective evaluation of the wound itself' (Fackler, 1988).

Sharp implements. The effects of a stabbing are limited to the track of the knife. Depth of wounding varies widely, from a nick in the skin to penetration of viscera and vessels. Unlike gunshot wounds, 30–40% of stabbings involve the abdominal wall only, and these are detected by exploration which shows peritoneum to be intact. The position of the entry wound will indicate the organs likely to be injured, with stabs in the back liable to injure the kidneys, ureters, duodenum, liver, spleen and inferior vena cava; none of these retroperitoneal injuries will necessarily be detected by abdominal examination. An intravenous urogram or a CT scan is likely to be indicated, and active observation will play an important role in management.

In about 40% of stabbings signs of hypovolaemia, peritoneal irritation, evisceration or alimentary haemorrhage will show that laparotomy is urgently needed. If there are few signs but exploration of the wound shows that the peritoneum has been breached, management depends on experience: centres that see few such patients are likely to explore the abdomen, but centres that see many stab injuries are likely to practise selective observation (Huizinga *et al.*, 1987). Lambrianides and Rosin (1984) found that in 42 of 100 stabbings the entry wound was on the thorax and in 10 the blade had traversed the diaphragm and entered a viscus.

Impalement is an unusual but dramatic form of penetrating injury. It tends to occur after a fall from a height, so the rectum may be involved (p. 444).

REFERENCES

Fackler, M. L. (1988) Wound ballistics – a review of common misconceptions. *J.A.M.A.*, **259**, 2730–2736.

Feliciano, D. V. and Rozycki, G. S. (1995) The management of penetrating abdominal trauma. *Adv. Surg.*, **28**, 1–40.

Huizinga, W. K. J., Baker, L. W. and Mtshali, Z. (1987) Selective management of abdominal and thoracic stab wounds with established peritoneal penetration. *Am. J. Surg.*, **153**, 564–568.

Lambrianides, A. L. and Rosin, R. D. (1984) Penetrating stab injuries of the chest and abdomen. *Injury*, **15**, 300–303.

Muckart, D. J. J., Meumann, C. and Botha, J. B. D. (1995) The changing pattern of torso trauma in Kwa Zulu/Natal. *S. Afr. J. Med.*, **85**, 1172–1174.

Ornato, J. P., Caren, E. J., Nelson, M. M. *et al.* (1985) Impact of approved medical emergency services and emergency trauma care on the reduction of mortality in trauma. *J. Trauma*, **25**, 575–579.

10.5 GENERAL MANAGEMENT OF ABDOMINAL INJURIES

Patients with abdominal injuries present in widely different ways, ranging from those with obvious deep wounds who are in imminent danger of exsanguination and death, to the patient with a history of recent blunt trauma whose signs may only suggest an internal injury.

10.5.1 EXAMINATION AND ASSESSMENT

All these patients should be managed by Advanced Trauma Life Support (ATLS) principles (Alexander and Proctor, 1993). **A**irway, **B**reathing, **C**irculation, **D**isability and **E**xposure are the key sequential elements for a successful outcome of the primary survey. When there is sufficient personnel these elements are conducted in a horizontal manner. This allows rapid progression to the secondary survey, and identification and prioritization of each element of the injuries, and offers the best chance of uncomplicated survival.

In a few 'damage-control-type laparotomy' (p. 424) will be immediately required. In a significant number very early laparotomy (p. 425) to stop bleeding and to arrest and clear up faecal contamination will be needed. Decisions will be made, especially in suspected blunt injury, on **detailed examination of the abdomen**.

1. The whole appearance of the patient can provide vital information. There is a look of pallor, anxiety and stillness about a patient with an abdominal injury that is characteristic. Breathing may be shallow and quick because it is painful. In the early stages of hypovolaemic shock the forehead and nose are cool, and the collapsed veins on the back of the hand hanging over the side of the bed and delayed capillary return in the nail bed, are useful signs of peripheral vasoconstriction which precedes a fall in blood pressure, as is serial counting of the pulse rate.
2. Remembering the force exerted in these accidents, examination must include the thorax, the pelvis and the long bones, where injuries causing serious blood loss can profoundly influence outcome. It is necessary to uncover the whole patient and this may involve some cutting of clothing. Signs of bruising and clothing or seat-belt tattooing are good indicators of the forces applied. The foreskin needs to be retracted to look for urethral bleeding. At the same time, movement of the chest and the abdominal wall can be observed.
3. In the abdomen, the slightest degree of tenderness and guarding is significant. When the circumstances are suspicious the apparent absence of signs must lead to institution of the full regime of active observation (p. 50). Bowel sounds can be misleading, because they can be heard in some patients with internal haemorrhage. However, an abdomen that becomes and remains silent, especially if there is some tenderness, is very suggestive of perforation of bowel. In unconscious patients there must be a watch for a resentment of abdominal palpation and a clear sign of guarding is especially valuable.
4. Performance of a rectal examination provides the opportunity to examine the back of the chest and trunk, the buttocks and the perineum, before examining the rectum for evidence of tenderness or the feel of blood in the pouch of Douglas, or the presence of blood on the examining glove. The significance of blood at the urethral meatus, or a high-riding prostate, is considered on page p. 488.
5. A specimen of urine must be examined and appropriate action taken if there is haematuria (p. 486).
6. **Radiographic examination**
    (a) A *chest X-ray* can give vital information about a rupture of a diaphragm and confirm suspicions of haemo- and pneumothorax. Fracture of the upper three ribs, with a widened mediastinum, suggests possible aortic rupture.
    (b) A *plain supine abdominal X-ray* will give details of a fractured pelvis. Free gas is not often seen in a lateral decubitus film, but the picture of air around a retroperitoneal rupture of the duodenum is characteristic (p. 430).
    (c) An *intravenous urogram* will be of great value in a suspected injury of the urinary tract (p. 486).

The circumstances will indicate that treatment is required at three different levels.

10.5.2 'DAMAGE-CONTROL LAPAROTOMY'

In the gravely injured patient, with all the signs of hypovolaemic shock, the measures outlined in Chapter 1 will have been applied, including attention to ventilation and a haemo- or pneumothorax, and delivery of fluids through two 12 FG (or larger) cannulae in both forearms, connected to high-capacity giving sets and in-line heating sets.

When classical signs of hypovolaemic shock are present some 25% of circulating blood volume has already been lost: although laparotomy to secure haemostasis is urgently required, many of these patients will not withstand a long procedure, and they require 'damage-control-type laparotomy' (Rotondo, 1993). With a conventional approach these patients are liable to develop perioperative hypothermia, metabolic acidosis and coagulopathy, which, together, are likely to be fatal. Sharp and Locicero (1992) have identified the high-risk factors to be: age over 50; pH < 7.18; temperature < 33°C; prothrombin time > 16; and more than 10 units of packed red cells already transfused. In these circumstances a relatively short laparotomy with 'perihepatic and intra-abdominal packing, followed by planned reoperation, may be lifesaving' (Burch *et al.*, 1992).

A long midline incision is made: 'the patient will not die from a big incision, but may very likely succumb if some important injury is overlooked' (Turner, 1940). Extension into the thorax or mediastinum may be needed and the patient should be draped accordingly. For each 10 units of packed cells Sharp and Locicero (1992) recommend 2–4 units of fresh frozen plasma and 6–12 units of platelets to be given. The correct strategy is to recognize early during the laparotomy those patients who will benefit from an abbreviated operation, before temperature and pH fall to a critical level, and evidence of coagulopathy appears, with oozing from all surfaces and absence of clotting. The principles of damage-control laparotomy include the following.

- Repair only those vessels vital to life, ligate all others.
- Apply dry laparotomy packs to diffusely bleeding surfaces in the pelvis and retroperitoneal spaces. For the disrupted liver, packs are placed under the diaphragm to achieve tamponade when the incision is closed under some tension (see Figure 10.7).
- Ruptured intestine should be cleaned and ligated or stapled on each side of the perforation, to prevent contamination.
- Remove a seriously fractured and actively bleeding spleen or kidney.
- Rupture of the gallbladder or the urinary bladder should be closed with a single purse-string suture. Bile duct injuries are packed.
- If the pancreas is transected it should be ligated with umbilical tape.
- The abdominal packs achieve their full effect when the incision is closed, under tension, with towel clips applied to the skin edges, 1–2 cm apart. Occasionally the edges cannot be brought together, owing to oedema of the bowel and mesentery, and then a silo must be constructed – 3 litre dialysis fluid bags opened out and sterilized make an effective cover, and are sutured to the edges of the linea alba and peritoneum with continuous 1/0 or 2/0 monofilament nylon.

These patients require close and frequent supervision in the intensive care unit by both the surgeon and the intensivist. In patients with a sutured incision a careful watch must be kept over the first 48 hours for development of the 'abdominal compartment syndrome'. Pressure rises within the abdomen because of haemorrhage and/or increasing oedema of the bowel, which is due to a long period of exteriorization at the first operation, with stretching and compression of the mesenteric veins and consequent poor venous return.

The signs of this syndrome are a tense distended abdomen, oliguria (due to a direct effect on renal circulation) and hypoxia (from the pressure causing marked elevation of the diaphragm). If the bladder is drained, 50 ml of saline is injected into it and the catheter is connected to a water manometer, with zero at the symphysis pubis in the supine patient, the intraperitoneal pressure can be measured (Burch *et al.*, 1996). The normal range is 3–15 cm H_2O, 15–25 cm is worrying and at 25–35 cm decompression is urgently needed. Morris *et al.* (1996) warn that these patients should be preloaded (to prevent ischaemic–reperfusion injury) with an intravenous solution made up of 1 litre 0.45% physiological saline with 50 g mannitol and 50 mEq of sodium hydrogen carbonate; 2 litres of the solution are given.

The best preventative of the syndrome is readiness to use a silo closure at the first laparotomy. Patients who require decompression, with removal of packs, haemostasis and a silo closure, have twice the mortality of those who have the silo applied at the first operation.

The majority of deaths beyond 48 hours in these gravely injured patients arise from multiple organ failure, and this is most often due to residual sepsis in the abdomen or the layers of the incision. We favour a readiness to re-explore when complications are suspected, and find that with such a policy 20–30% of patients require another laparotomy, of which 80% are positive. We favour the use of polyglactin mesh to maintain 'closure' after repeated operations (Emmink *et al.*, 1993).

Stage two of this regime continues in the intensive care unit, where any evidence of hypothermia, acidosis or hypocoagulability is corrected and the patient is brought into a relatively stable stage.

The **third stage** of planned re-exploration usually takes place after 24–48 hours, although it may have to take place earlier if bleeding is not satisfactorily controlled. At this operation packs are cautiously removed and definitive repairs are performed. Ligated sections of bowel will be resected and an anastomosis made.

Cue *et al.* (1990) treated 35 such patients, of whom 31 needed perihepatic packing and four required packing to stem retroperitoneal bleeding. In 12 it proved impossible to arrest bleeding, but in eight with coagulopathy and 15 with persistent bleeding from the liver, packing secured haemostasis; this allowed these patients to be stabilized and to proceed to definitive repair.

10.5.3   EARLY LAPAROTOMY

Most patients with penetrating wounds and a minority with blunt injury are not *in extremis* but clearly require early laparotomy to arrest bleeding, control faecal contamination and to treat evisceration. In any infraumbilical injury the Lloyd-Davies lithotomy–Trendelenburg position is of particular value in allowing free access to the rectum, perineum and urethra. A long midline incision allows rapid entry to the abdomen and does not encroach on potential enterostomy sites.

The first step is to secure haemostasis and then proceed to a systematic laparotomy. The small bowel and its mesentery is thoroughly searched as it is brought out, loop by loop, and placed on and covered by wet packs. Blood is removed by scooping and by suction and a warm saline wash is given to clear the field. The whole colon is searched and this leads on to the rectum, the bladder and the pelvic organs. The spleen, stomach, liver and gallbladder and, most importantly, the diaphragm, are all reviewed. The retroperitoneal area requires detailed inspection because it is easy to miss an important injury (Maull and Enderson, 1991). There may be a hint from staining that the extraperitoneal duodenum or colon has been injured and the lateral paracolic gutter should then be opened up; Kocher's manoeuvre will expose the back of the duodenal loop and then the kidneys and ureters can be inspected.

In blunt injuries, especially from a steering wheel or bicycle handlebars, it is essential to examine the pancreas by opening the greater omentum below the gastroepiploic arch, and lifting the stomach and inserting retractors to allow inspection of the whole length of the pancreas. Drains will be appropriate in a variety of situations and are essential in thoracoabdominal injuries. Secure closure of the incision is achieved by mass suture with gauge 1 polydioxanone (PDS).

10.5.4 OBSERVATION AND INVESTIGATION

In about half the victims of stabbing and as many as two-thirds of patients who could have sustained a blunt injury, there will, under observation, be evidence of steady improvement and they can soon be discharged. It must always be remembered that 10–12 hours can pass before there is tenderness and guarding due to blunt intestinal injury.

The surgeon is very much aware, in both blunt and penetrating injuries, that bedside examination, however careful, has limitations, especially when an entry wound is consistent with a retroperitoneal injury and the patient is confused or comatose. Injury from a high-velocity missile, which causes a small entry wound on the chest, the thighs or buttocks, or the back of the trunk, can have penetrated an abdominal organ or vessel, which will need identification. Among these difficult patients, who remain fairly stable under observation but who have disquieting features including abdominal tenderness away from the entry wound, there are four main techniques of investigation.

Diagnostic peritoneal lavage (DPL)

This was introduced by Root in 1965. He passed a peritoneal dialysis catheter *via* a trocar into the pelvis and if non-clotting blood was not aspirated he irrigated the abdomen with 1000 ml of warm physiological saline, moved the patient from side to side and examined the fluid that was returned. If it was grossly blood-stained or contained more than 100 000 red cells/mm^3, the result was positive. Since then DPL has been widely used and one main conclusion is that if the result is negative this excludes significant intraperitoneal bleeding: it does not exclude intestinal or diaphragmatic penetration. The standard criteria for a positive result are a red cell count over 100 000/mm^3, white cell count over 500/mm^3, amylase over 200 u/100 ml, or visible intestinal content in the return. Purely visual estimation of red cell count is unreliable.

Problems associated with DPL include the following.

- A positive red cell count can result from injury during insertion of the trocar. To avoid this an open approach is used, with insertion of the dialysis catheter through peritoneum under vision.
- Lacerations of spleen and liver that do not require repair can cause significant bleeding. A stab wound of the diaphragm may cause no bleeding.

- Leakage from intestinal perforation can be delayed for up to 10 hours, so early DPL can produce a normal return.
- DPL cannot be repeated and does itself produce some peritoneal irritation for as much as 48 hours. Adding protein electrophoresis of lavage fluid gives a more accurate indication of significant peritoneal wounding.

The main conclusion to be drawn is that, although DPL is cheap and can be undertaken anywhere, the results have to be interpreted with great care in the light of repeated examination of the patient. Ultrasound is increasingly being preferred to the use of DPL.

Ultrasound

Ultrasound is safe and non-invasive and is increasingly being used with portable apparatus by emergency-room surgeons to provide a speedy survey of the injured abdomen. Its principal merit is reliable detection of an excess of fluid in the pericardial sac or the peritoneal cavity. Rozycki *et al.* (1993) reported on the examination of 476 patients by surgical staff after a period of training in ultrasonic technique. The examination covered the pericardium, the right and left upper abdominal quadrants and the pouch of Douglas. In 77% the result was a true negative and in 15% a true positive. There were 4% false-negative and 3.5% false-positive examinations, and these were mostly corrected by DPL and continued observation. The relative simplicity, speed and non-invasive character of ultrasound, its availability in A&E departments and its wide applicability, including pregnancy, mean that it can, used with discrimination, make a valuable contribution.

Computed tomography

CT scanning will also identify collections of fluid and will delineate accurately injuries of the spleen, liver and kidneys. Its disadvantages are that it can only be carried out by a radiologist in the radiology department, it separates the patient from nursing and medical staff for 10–15 minutes and so can only be used in stable patients, it is expensive and it exposes the patient to a very large dose of radiation. Neither ultrasound nor CT can demonstrate intestinal injuries reliably.

The main role of CT is likely to lie in assessing the extent of injury of a solid organ in a stable patient in whom a conservative line of management is being considered. It is very well suited to investigation of a retroperitoneal haematoma and in stable patients with a pelvic fracture it is the investigation of choice (Liu *et al.*, 1993). It is clearly the best method of assessing blunt trauma in children who are in a stable haemodynamic state (Richardson *et al.*, 1997).

Laparoscopy

Diagnostic laparoscopy using a 5 mm direct-viewpiece telescope with minimal or hand insufflation – mini-laparoscopy – can be carried out in the A&E department under local anaesthesia and sedation. It will detect haemorrhage, though not necessarily its source, and the presence of fibrin strongly suggests a bowel perforation; however, it is not possible to carry out a thorough search of the whole small bowel. It is uniquely successful in identifying rupture of the diaphragm but the dangers of insufflation producing tension pneumothorax must be remembered. The indications for diagnostic mini-laparoscopy, especially in blunt trauma, require better definition, because less invasive methods seem to be as accurate in determining the need for operation.

Conclusions

In the patient with equivocal findings, the results of continued observation and these investigations should combine to give an indication as to whether laparotomy is indicated or whether it is right to continue observation. Experience shows how difficult it can be to detect abdominal injury in some patients, especially in the retroperitoneal area, and Cuthbert Wallace's dictum is still relevant, that in this area of surgery it is safer when in continued doubt to explore rather than wait further on events. When this decision is taken after careful weighing of the evidence there is no discredit in finding no major injury; on other occasions a similar decision will reveal serious trouble.

REFERENCES

Alexander, R. H. and Proctor, H. J. (1993) *Advanced Trauma Life Support Program for Physicians*, 5th edn, American College of Surgeons, Chicago, IL.

Burch, J. M., Oritz, V. B., Richardson, R. J. *et al.* (1992) Abbreviated laparotomy and planned reoperation for critically injured patients. *Ann. Surg.*, **215**, 276–284.

Burch, J. M., Moore, E. E., Moore, F. A. *et al.* (1996) The abdominal compartment syndrome. *Surg. Clin. North Am.*, **76**, 833–842.

Cue, J. I., Cryer, H. G., Miller, F. B. *et al.* (1990) Packing and planned reexploration for hepatic and retroperitoneal haemorrhage: critical refinements of a useful technique. *J. Trauma*, **30**, 1007–1013.

Emmink, B., Thomson, S. R., Moodley, M. *et al.* (1993) Laparotomy closure using perisplenic polyglactin mesh. *J. R. Coll. Surg. Edin.*, **38**, 177–178.

Liu, M., Lee, C. H. and P'eng, F. K. (1993) Prospective comparison of diagnostic peritoneal lavage, computed tomographic scanning and ultrasonography for the diagnosis of blunt abdominal trauma. *J. Trauma*, **35**, 267–270.

Maull, K. I. and Enderson, B. L. (1991) Missed injuries: the trauma surgeons' nemesis. *Surg. Clin. North Am.*, **71**, 399–418.

Morris, J. A., Eddy, V. A. and Rutherford, E. J. (1996) The trauma celiotomy: the evolving concepts of damage control. *Curr. Probl. Surg.*, **33**, 611–700.

Richardson, M. C., Hollman, A. S. and Davis, C.F. (1997) Comparison of computed tomography and ultrasonographic imaging in the assessment of blunt abdominal trauma in childhood. *Br. J. Surg.*, **84**, 1144–1146.

Root, H. D., Hauser, C. W., McKinley, C. R. *et al.* (1965) Diagnostic peritoneal lavage. *Surgery*, **57**, 633–637.

Rotondo, M. (1993) 'Damage Control': an approach for improved survival in exsanguinating penetrating abdominal injury. *J. Trauma*, **35**, 375–383.

Rozycki, G. S., Ochsner, M. G., Jaffin, J. H. *et al.* (1993) Prospective evaluation of surgeons' use of ultrasound in the evaluation of trauma patients. *J. Trauma*, **34**, 516–527.

Sharp, K. W. and Locicero, R. J. (1992) Abdominal packing for surgically uncontrollable haemorrhage. *Ann. Surg.*, **215**, 467–475.

Turner, G. G. (1940) Some notes on abdominal injuries. *BMJ.*, **i**, 679–682.

10.6 GASTROINTESTINAL INJURIES

10.6.1 RUPTURE OF THE STOMACH

The mobile stomach is well protected by the rib cage, and it is exceptional for the stomach to be affected by blunt abdominal trauma. On the other hand, in 100 stabbing injuries seen at an accident department in West London, 44 required laparotomy and liver (18), stomach (14) and jejunum (14) were the viscera most often injured (Lambrianides and Rosin, 1984). Care must be exercised in searching the gastro-oesophageal region and both curvatures. The lesser sac will need to be opened, by dividing the gastrocolic omentum, to examine the posterior aspect of the stomach. The stomach is a particularly vascular organ and generally can be readily repaired by excision of the tear and suture.

The other ruptures of the stomach are usually described as 'spontaneous', although there is usually a precipitating factor. They are very unusual and most reports are of one or two cases: there were only 43 such reports in 1963 when Albo *et al.* found that most had recently ingested unusually large amounts of food or drink; some have been associated with gastric outlet obstruction. There are now five reports of rupture following the use of sodium bicarbonate to relieve indigestion: Mastrangelo and Moore (1984) saw a fit 31-year-old man who had taken half a teaspoonful of baking soda in water after eating a large meal. One minute later he experienced intense epigastric pain and on admission was collapsed with signs of peritonitis. Laparotomy revealed much gas and food along the lesser curvature, which was sutured; he made a slow recovery. All the reports emphasize the intensity of the pain, the rapid onset of hypotension, the characteristic linear tear along the lesser curvature and the high mortality: 34 out of 40 reported cases died.

REFERENCES

Albo, R., Lorimier, A. A. and Silen, W. (1963) Spontaneous rupture of the stomach in the adult. *Surgery*, **53**, 797.

Lambrianides, A. L. and Rosin, R. D. (1984) Penetrating stab injuries of the chest and abdomen. *Injury*, **15**, 300–304.

Mastrangelo, M. R. and Moore, E. W. (1984) Spontaneous rupture of the stomach in a healthy adult man after sodium bicarbonate ingestion. *Ann. Intern. Med.*, **101**, 649.

10.6.2 INJURIES OF THE DUODENUM AND PANCREAS

These are not common injuries: only five duodenal injuries were seen in the community hospital in Eindhoven, Holland in 15 years (Carol and Jakimovicz, 1982) and in Chicago University Hospital only 6% of 227 primary admissions for abdominal trauma were for pancreatic injuries (Henarezos *et al.*, 1983). However, when they do occur it is particularly important that these injuries should be recognized, and then treated correctly, because the complications can be severe (Campbell and Kennedy, 1980).

In civilian practice in Europe most injuries arise from motor vehicle accidents, whereas in South Africa 85% are due to penetrating injury (Madiba and Mokoena, 1995). Before seat-belts were generally worn it was the rim of the steering wheel that was forced into the epigastrium of the driver, compressing the head and neck of the pancreas, and sometimes the second part of the duodenum, against the lumbar spine. Poorly adjusted seat-belts, falls against railings and blows in the epigastrium continue to cause injuries in the area. In North America missile and stabbing attacks are a major cause of pancreaticoduodenal damage and in high-velocity gunshot wounds very severe and widespread effects are likely, with a particular risk of damage to great vessels (Weigelt, 1990). In Belfast, where penetrating wounds from street fighting were twice as common as blunt injuries, Campbell and Kennedy (1980) found that an average of three other organs were injured, major vessels, liver and kidneys being most affected. These had a predictably adverse effect on mortality.

Broadly, blunt injuries tend to produce extraperitoneal rupture of the duodenum and most intraperitoneal disruptions are due to penetrating injury. However, it is vital to inspect all aspects of the duodenum once injury is suspected. Some 80% of ruptures affect the second part. Some of these occur at the junction of duodenum with the pancreas and particular care is needed to identify them.

Pancreatic ruptures vary between a superficial crack in the capsule, without any involvement of ducts, and complete transection or disruption. If diagnosis is delayed, traumatic pancreatitis may supervene, bringing with it the threat of major secondary haemorrhage as autolysis of the pancreas proceeds; formation of a pancreatic abscess is a further possible serious complication.

Diagnosis

Because the posterior aspect of the duodenum and the whole of the pancreas are retroperitoneal the signs of closed injury may be few, and delayed. Abdominal pain may be felt and occasionally patients complain of pain referred to the testicle. Upper abdominal tenderness is likely. The only specific sign is that if the retroperitoneal duodenum is ruptured the plain abdominal radiograph may show, in about 50% of patients, the characteristic outlining of the right kidney by air (Sperling and Rigler, 1937).

There are no specific symptoms or signs of pancreatic injury, and if the pancreas alone is injured there is likely to be some delay before the signs indicate the need for exploratory laparotomy. Estimation of the serum amylase is not likely to be of much practical help: Cogbill *et al.* (1982) found that only two of 20 preoperative estimations were elevated in patients with pancreatic injury.

The important point to remember when there has clearly been a severe blow on the epigastrium is that the earlier pancreaticoduodenal injuries can be treated the better, because both cause leakage of active enzymes, and the risks of traumatic pancreatitis as a cause of secondary haemorrhage and fistula are considerable. Water-soluble contrast X-rays or contrast-enhanced CT can be helpful, provided the patient is in a stable haemodynamic state. Suspicion, and a readiness to explore the abdomen when in doubt, are the basis of early diagnosis of closed injuries.

Once the decision to perform laparotomy has been taken it is still necessary to take specific steps to visualize the duodenum and pancreas.

Much of the first and second parts of the duodenum can be seen by simple retraction and inspection. If there is any hint of bruising or bile-staining around the duodenum it is essential to perform Kocher's mobilization, incising the peritoneum lateral to the whole of the second and some of the third part of the duodenum. The loose areolar tissue behind the pancreas is gently divided so that the whole duodenal loop is hinged forward for inspection. The third part is still partially concealed by the hepatic flexure of the colon and this can be mobilized downwards and medially. Finally, the ligament of Treitz is divided to allow complete inspection of the duodenojenunal flexure and terminal portion of the third part.

Exposure of the duodenum also reveals both surfaces of the head of the pancreas, but the neck, body and tail are concealed in the lesser sac. It is particularly important to lift up the transverse colon and look at the root of the mesocolon, where there may be a tell-tale haematoma.

The best way to obtain a good view of the body of the pancreas is to divide the gastrocolic omentum transversely just below the gastroepiploic arch, dividing the omental branches as they are met. The lesser sac is then opened out, with retractors holding the stomach up and the mesocolon being drawn downwards. This may not immediately show a rupture because the pancreas may be surrounded by blood, and the capsule must be incised, and blood and clot sucked and mopped away, so that the actual surface of the pancreas can be seen.

In splenic injury it is always important to examine the tail of the pancreas for damage, as it may lie within the splenic hilum.

Management

Duodenum

Isolated duodenal tears can usually be repaired by excising the edges back to a healthy bleeding edge and effecting a closure with Gambee sutures of 2/0 or 3/0 braided nylon. Great care must be exercised over viability because the effects of crush injury or a missile may be widespread, and it is vital that the suture line should heal by first intention. Duodenal suture lines should invariably be drained.

Mann (1979) remarks that in a bruised duodenal wall it can be difficult to detect a tear, and suggests injection of some methylene blue down a nasoduodenal tube as a test of integrity.

When there is a severe degree of duodenal injury with loss of tissue, or severe bruising of the duodenal wall, then simple suture will not ensure against later breakdown.

There are two methods of dealing with this situation.

1. Moore and Moore (1984) have adopted the operation of **pyloric exclusion**. The duodenal wound is excised and sutured in the best manner that is appropriate; this may lead to some narrowing. Reinforcement with omentum may be used. A gastrotomy 4 cm long is then made in the distal greater curvature and through this the pylorus is grasped with Babcock forceps, brought into the wound and a purse-string suture of 0 polyglactin is inserted and tied so as to occlude the pylorus: absorption of this suture will take about 3 weeks. A side-to-side antecolic gastrojejunostomy is then made. Provided there is no distal jejunoileal damage it is very desirable to make a feeding jejunostomy as high in the jejunum as is feasible. We use a 5 FG infant feeding tube threaded 20 cm or so down the jejunum, which is brought out through a separate stab incision.

In this way the damaged area is rested for several weeks.

Moore and Moore (1984) have used this method on 13 occasions and found that it is safe and effective. They emphasize the need to provide sump drainage down to the duodenum, and although some fistulae were seen they all healed spontaneously. They have encountered no problem with stomal ulceration.

This method seems preferable to the more severe procedure of duodenal 'diverticulization' of Berne *et al.* (1974) in which the first part of the duodenum is divided, an antrectomy performed and a permanent gastrojejunostomy constructed. They introduce a suction drain into the duodenum, beside the repair, as well as draining the paraduodenal tissues.

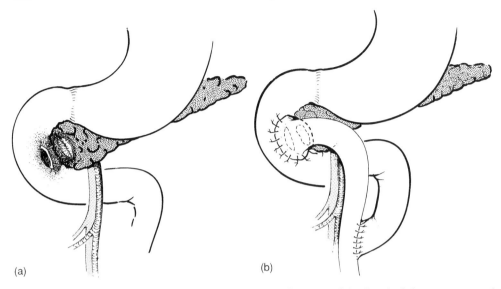

Figure 10.1 **(a)** A blunt injury has produced a deep fracture of the head of the pancreas and a tear of adjacent duodenum with surrounding bruising. **(b)** Repair by suturing the spatulated open end of a Roux loop on to surrounding pancreas and duodenum, using interrupted through-and-through non-absorbable sutures.

2. The other method of duodenal repair is to use jejunum, as a Roux-en-Y loop onlay or cap. If there is an appreciable defect in the duodenal wall, or if debridement back to healthy bleeding duodenum produces a sizeable defect, then this cannot be repaired by direct suture. In this situation it is a relatively straightforward procedure to construct a short Roux-en-Y loop from upper jejunum, and to suture the open end of the loop to the duodenal defect (Figure 10.1).

The other advantage of this repair is that it can also be used on adjacent pancreatic damage, which is very likely to be present if there is an appreciable duodenal defect. In this respect a Roux loop is much more adaptable than a jejunal patch, which is the other method of repairing duodenum. Occasionally, limited resection and end-to-end anastomosis is appropriate.

Mann (1979) describes a remarkable seat-belt injury which had completely divided the second part of the duodenum and disrupted the ampulla of Vater; much of the adjacent duodenum was necrotic and required excision of most of the second part. A 15 cm pedicled tube of jejunum was isolated, and the proximal end was anastomosed to the healthy first part of duodenum. The ampullary area was implanted into the side of the jejunal loop, which was joined distally to the side of upper jejunum. The young woman made a smooth recovery.

Pancreas
The **pancreas**, lying within the duodenal loop, is very likely to be damaged in crushing and penetrating injuries, as well as duodenum, and some of the methods already considered are applicable to pancreatic lesions. It is useful to separate lesions of the head and neck from those sited in the body and tail (Campbell and Kennedy, 1980).

The **body and tail** of pancreas are injured rather more often than the head. Fractures of the body are liable to open or divide pancreatic ducts and if they are left to drain there is a high incidence of complications, such as pancreatitis, fistula formation, secondary haemorrhage and sepsis. All these are serious conditions in patients usually with other injuries, and secondary operations are often unsatisfactory.

A reasonable approach is therefore to view all injuries to pancreas which lie to the left of the superior mesenteric artery with great care, and if the damage is more than superficial to consider **distal pancreatectomy**. It is very difficult to judge ductal integrity in the bruised tissue and the penalties for leaving it undiagnosed are severe.

Distal pancreatectomy is a relatively simple procedure and all reports show that it produces good results. It may or may not be feasible to preserve the spleen, but in an emergency it is usually necessary to remove it because the process of separating the splenic artery and vein is time-consuming.

The spleen is mobilized as in splenectomy (p. 451) by dividing the lienorenal ligament and the short gastric vessels. There is a good bloodless plane behind the body of the pancreas, which allows it to be lifted forward along with the spleen and splenic vessels. The peritoneum of lesser sac is divided over the vessels until the point of transection is reached, and here the splenic artery and veins are isolated and divided (Figure 10.2).

If the fracture of the body of pancreas is complete the specimen can now be removed, and attention turned to the torn proximal end of pancreas. The divided main duct may be visible and can be picked up and tied off with thread. Interrupted mattress or through-and-through non-absorbable sutures are inserted and tied to close off the divided surface of the pancreas; these can include bleeding points. The suture line usually heals well and, although it is essential to leave a tube drain down to this point, it is unusual to see a fistula form.

The procedure that must be avoided is suture of tears in the surface of the pancreas. The sutures do not, in any case, hold. If a duct is divided they are inappropriate and if ducts are intact they are unnecessary. If a tear of the pancreas is clearly superficial then the correct treatment is to leave a tube drain alongside it.

Injuries to the head of the pancreas are considerably more difficult to treat. Everyone is agreed that pancreaticoduodenectomy carries an almost prohibitive mortality and should only be used in exceptional circumstances. Campbell and Kennedy (1980) found that nearly all their cases could be satisfactorily treated by suturing the open end of a Roux loop, suitably enlarged by a Cheatle back-cut, over the damaged surface of pancreas (and if necessary adjacent duodenum) using interrupted through and through non-absorbable sutures. We have found this to be easier and more effective than anticipated (Figures 10.1 and 7.5).

If damage is concentrated around the neck, and if the pancreas and bile ducts within the duodenal loop are intact, it may be feasible to perform an extended distal pancreatectomy.

In all these severe injuries it is important to maintain nasogastric suction for some days and it is then that the value of a **feeding jejunostomy** becomes evident. This is easily and quickly established at the end of the operation (p. 431).

Closed-tube drainage down to duodenum and pancreas is essential and should be retained for 7–10 days.

Results

Campbell and Kennedy (1980) saw 12 deaths among their 39 patients, of which five were due to massive penetrating injuries that were not reparable. They felt that seven deaths were

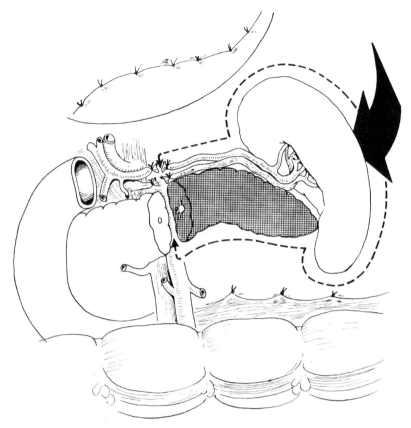

Figure 10.2 Distal pancreatectomy. The gastrocolic omentum has been divided and the stomach retracted upwards. The short gastric vessels are divided to reveal the splenic hilum. The large arrow shows the plane along which spleen and pancreas are mobilized from behind. The splenic artery and vein have been tied and divided at the level of the rupture of the pancreas. The dotted line encloses the tissue that is removed.

potentially preventable. In three cases there was delay in recognizing pancreatic injury and this proved to be a major adverse factor; in another three with injuries to the head of pancreas there was inadequate treatment by suture and drainage, which was followed by fatal pancreatitis and haemorrhage. The subject is well reviewed by Wilson and Moorehead (1991).

REFERENCES

Berne, C. J., Donovan, A. J., White, E. J. and Yellin, A. E. (1974) Duodenal 'diverticulization' for duodenal and pancreatic injury. *Am. J. Surg.*, **127**, 503–507.

Campbell, R. and Kennedy, T. (1980) The management of pancreatic and pancreatico-duodenal injuries. *Br. J. Surg.*, **50**, 845–850.

Carol, E. J. and Jakimovicz, J. J. (1982) Retroperitoneal rupture of the duodenum following blunt abdominal trauma. *Acta Chir. Scand.*, **148**, 541–544.

Cogbill, T. H., Moore, E. E. and Kashuk, J. L. (1982) Changing trends in the management of pancreatic trauma. *Arch. Surg.*, **117**, 722–728.

Henarezos, A., Cohen, D. M. and Moossa, A. R. (1983) Management of pancreatic trauma. *Ann. R. Coll. Surg. Engl.*, **65**, 297–300.

Madiba, T. E. and Mokoena, T. R. (1995) Favourable prognosis after surgical drainage of gunshot, stab or blunt trauma of the pancreas. *Br. J. Surg.*, **82**, 1236–1239.

Mann, A. (1979) Jejunal replacement of second part of duodenum following severe trauma. *Austr. N.Z. J. Surg.*, **49**, 92–95.

Moore, J. B. and Moore, E. E. (1984) Changing trends in the management of combined pancreatic and duodenal injuries. *World J. Surg.*, **8**, 791–797.

Sperling, L. and Rigler, L. G. (1937) Traumatic retroperitoneal rupture of the duodenum. *Radiology*, **29**, 521–524.

Weigelt, J. A. (1990) Duodenal injuries. *Surg. Clin. North Am.*, **70**, 529–539.

Wilson, R. H. and Moorehead, R. J. (1991) Current management of trauma to the pancreas. *Br. J. Surg.*, **78**, 1196–1202.

Intramural haematoma of the duodenum

This is a rare condition but it needs to be recognized. It is well described by Webb and Taylor (1967). As a result of blunt trauma to the upper abdomen, e.g. from a blow from a bicycle handlebar (the condition is most often seen in young people), a haematoma forms in the submucosal, intramuscular or subserosal plane of the second, third or fourth part of the duodenum. It can also occur after minor trauma in a patient with coagulation defect.

Some 24–48 hours elapse from the time of the injury (which may be forgotten) until bilious vomiting and right upper quadrant pain commence; the vomiting is repeated and distressing. There may be some tenderness over the duodenal loop. Sometimes the signs lead to laparotomy for suspected appendicitis, but sometimes the prominent vomiting, with few abdominal signs, is investigated with an opaque swallow, which shows hold-up in the duodenum, sometimes with a 'coiled-spring' appearance due to the oedematous folds of mucosa.

No nourishment can be retained so a laparotomy is done, when a black retroperitoneal mass is seen behind the transverse mesocolon, medial to the hepatic flexure. Exploration of the duodenal loop reveals a dark-blue swelling of the wall – when this is explored dark blood clot is evacuated.

Experience shows that this condition does not threaten viability, but the obstruction to the lumen can take 10–14 days to resolve. The hepatic flexure should be mobilized and the whole duodenal loop carefully examined, and Kocher's manoeuvre should be performed to check for any damage to the posterior wall. A gastrostomy will avoid prolonged use of a nasogastric tube, and a feeding jejunostomy is a sounder method of feeding than the intravenous route.

The serum amylase should be regularly checked because traumatic pancreatitis may complicate this injury.

Reference

Webb, A. J. and Taylor, J. J. (1967) Traumatic intramural haematoma of the duodenum. *Br. J. Surg.*, **54**, 50–56.

10.6.3   INJURIES OF THE JEJUNUM AND ILEUM

Much of the stomach, small bowel and colon lie beneath the anterior abdominal wall, and so are often involved in penetrating abdominal injuries. The pattern of injury is quite different in blunt trauma, with the solid organs being injured much more frequently than the hollow viscera – Dauterive *et al.* (1985) found that only 7% of laparotomies for blunt abdominal trauma were for intestinal injuries. The mechanism involved is most often a crushing force exerted on the bowel or mesentery, caught between the object hitting the abdominal wall and the spine. Some perforation of small bowel may be due to compression of a closed loop, causing a blow-out. In a deceleration accident the faeces-filled bowel may be torn away from the mesentery.

When Berry and Giuseppi studied **blunt intestinal injury** in London in 1908 they collected 132 patients and found that 51 were the result of vehicle accidents, 24 were crush injuries, and 39 were due to kicks and blows. In only 14 patients was the colon injured. When Dauterive *et al.* studied the subject in Baltimore in 1985, 90% of injuries were caused by cars (77%) or motor cycles (13%), and 5% were due to industrial accidents. A total of 60 patients sustained 83 major intestinal injuries, 64 involving small bowel and 19 the colon. Jejunum and ileum were equally liable to blunt injury, but the duodenum was more rarely affected.

An important finding was that 24 of the 64 small-bowel injuries involved the mesentery, resulting in devascularization of the bowel and the need for resection in 22.

The cause of **penetrating injuries** depends on the customs of the country (p. 420) but generally the alimentary tract is more liable to injury than the solid organs. However, in stab injuries there can be no certainty about the path of the injury, and in high-velocity missile injuries the secondary missile cavitation effects can cause severe damage to vessels, and therefore visceral circulation, well beyond the area of visible damage. Fragments of the missile may cause multiple injuries.

Clinical picture

As in most abdominal injuries, a great deal can be learnt from looking at the patient: stillness, pallor and anxiety are important physical signs. Breathing may be painful and shallow. It is fortunate that almost all patients with **closed intestinal injury** complain of immediate abdominal pain and continue to experience some discomfort. Berry and Giuseppi (1908) made a point of this, recording early onset of pain in 51 of 59 patients studied in detail; other writers on this subject make the same point and this is certainly confirmed by personal experience. Almost all patients vomit.

What is likely to be lacking at an early stage are abdominal signs to back up the symptoms and this lack can be misleading. **The importance of a complaint of abdominal pain after an injury cannot be overstressed**. This must always lead to retention of the patient for continued close observation. It is characteristic of patients with blunt intestinal injury that they have few or no signs of peritoneal irritation in the hours immediately after wounding, and there is a good pathological reason for this. A traumatic perforation is often small and the characteristic eversion of the mucosa, which produces a pouting rosette of tissue, effectively closes the perforation during the period of ileus that follows the injury. It is only as some peristaltic activity returns that intestinal juice emerges to produce the signs of parietal peritoneal irritation. Consequently, it is not unusual for patients to walk away from the scene of the accident and take themselves to an accident department, or to return home and only later suffer increasing abdominal pain. This is well seen in some seat-belt injuries of the intestines (p. 474).

Delayed onset of signs is also, perhaps surprisingly, a feature of some stab wounds. Donaldson *et al.* (1981) found that 64 out of 89 patients, at the time of their admission, showed no signs of surgical shock and had normal bowel sounds. Under observation 34 developed signs and came to laparotomy, when nine were found to have significant intraperitoneal bleeding and 13 had visceral perforations. The lesson must be that anyone who sustains an abdominal injury and thereafter complains of abdominal pain must be closely observed for several hours.

The significance of bowel sounds is, in the individual patient, difficult to assess. Clearly their presence does not exclude an intestinal perforation, at the early stage at which little or no leakage has occurred. However, although their absence does not necessarily indicate an injury, this sign should make the observer watchful. A youth, running across a road, collided with scaffolding and came into a casualty department complaining of abdominal pain. The abdomen was relaxed and not tender, but no bowel sounds were heard, and the casualty officer decided to detain him. Two hours later there was a little tenderness, which increased, and at laparotomy a jejunal perforation was sutured.

It is unusual to see free gas under the diaphragm in an erect X-ray. Fitzgerald *et al.* (1960) found free gas in only two of 15 patients with a perforation of the small bowel.

The whole history and the physical signs have to be carefully put together; active observation is likely to be the most useful investigation. Peritoneal lavage was positive in 57 of the 60 patients of Dauterive *et al.* (1985), and ultrasonography may show an excess of fluid in the abdomen. CT has limited value in hollow organ perforation.

In **blunt injury** the appearance of the perforations is very constant: an everted rosette of mucosa pouting through a split in the muscularis which is about 1 cm diameter. It should never be assumed that these are necessarily single, although they certainly can be, and the whole length of the intestine must be carefully searched. These injuries usually lie away from the mesentery and can be readily seen. If the viability of the surrounding bowel is assured these ruptures can be repaired with serosubmucosal sutures of 3/0 braided nylon or polyglactin. When there are multiple perforations it is usually possible to repair each one but it is worth considering a limited resection. Transections will require excision of the two ends back to bleeding tissue and end-to-end anastomosis.

Disinsertion of the small-bowel mesentery from the intestine often requires treatment by resection, because blood supply to the bowel wall is questionable. The injury necessary to produce disinsertion is necessarily violent, so damage to adjacent bowel is quite likely. The same considerations apply in wounds of the mesentery: the arterial pulsation beside the bowel must be studied, and it is sometimes helpful to test viability by making a short nick through serosa into longitudinal muscle to see if there is active bleeding.

Experimental work on rabbit ileum (Paterson-Brown *et al.*, 1990) suggested that if the length of mesenteric disinsertion is less than twice the circumference of the affected bowel the residual circulation should be adequate. Areas of contusion of the bowel wall in closed injuries can be hard to assess and the same investigation suggested that if the length of the contusion is less than the bowel circumference it should survive. These observations provide some facts on which to base a difficult assessment.

Wounds at the root of the small-bowel mesentery can produce serious effects. A case of massive haemoperitoneum was seen in a man who, crushed against a wall by a fork-lift, had a crack in the side of his superior mesenteric vein. It proved possible to suture this with a 5/0 arterial silk suture, and with a large blood transfusion he survived.

Missile injuries produce unpredictable damage and the spread of the effects of high-velocity missiles must always be remembered when deciding whether suture repair is safe: one must be sure of viability before closing perforations by simple suture. A second-look laparotomy in 24–48 hours can provide invaluable information.

REFERENCES

Berry, J. and Giuseppi, P. L. (1908) Traumatic rupture of the intestine. *Lancet*, **ii**, 1143.

Dauterive, A. H., Flancbaum, L. and Cox, E. F. (1985) Blunt intestinal trauma: a modern-day review. *Ann. Surg.*, **201**, 198–203.

Donaldson, L. A., Findlay, I. G. and Smith, A. (1981) A retrospective review of 89 stab wounds of the abdomen and chest. *Br. J. Surg.*, **68**, 793–796.

Fitzgerald, J. B., Crawford, E. S. and De Bakey, M. E. (1960) Surgical consideration of non-penetrating abdominal injuries: an analysis of 200 cases. *Am. J. Surg.*, **100**, 22.

Paterson-Brown, S., Francis, N., Whawell, S. *et al.* (1990) Prediction of the delayed complications of intestinal and mesenteric injuries following experimental blunt abdominal trauma. *Br. J. Surg.*, **77**, 648–651.

10.6.4   INJURIES OF THE COLON

In civilian practice in Western Europe and Scandinavia it is unusual to see injuries of the large bowel. Penetrating abdominal wounds are, for the most part, infrequent and only about 5% of large-bowel injuries are due to blunt trauma. With fewer major military engagements, those with the greatest experience of penetrating injuries are civilian surgeons working in trauma centres in the USA and South Africa (Edwards and Galbraith, 1997).

Modern methods of treatment have moved a long way from the uncoordinated treatment offered in the war of 1914–1918 and the official insistence during the Second World War that the injured colon should be exteriorized, or isolated by making a proximal colostomy, and that simple closure should never be practised in the field. At that time these rules produced a great improvement in results but by 1951, with further experience, Woodhall and Ochsner showed that there was a place in civilian practice for primary suture of colon wounds. Since then much further experience has accumulated and been analysed, and the major conclusion of this work is summarized by Thomson *et al.* (1996), based on experience of over 1000 colon injuries treated in Durban, that 'in civilian colon trauma the trend in management is moving away from exteriorization and towards intraperitoneal closure (IPC). This is because of the realization that outcome is determined by the severity of the injuries and the physiological effects of contamination, and not by the type of colon management.'

The experience of George *et al.* (1989) illustrates this conclusion. In 102 patients with penetrating intraperitoneal colon injuries the aim was to close the injury wherever possible, without regard to associated injuries or the amount of faecal contamination. In the event, a primary suture repair was done in 83, segmental resection with anastomosis in 12 and only in seven was resection with proximal end-colostomy deemed necessary. All the 83 repairs healed, and there was one suture-line failure in the anastomosis group. Whatever method of closure is used, some principles are always followed: a thorough search of the whole abdomen, remembering that missiles produce multiple fragments and there can be injuries in obscure sites, especially in retroperitoneal colon; coordinated antibiotic policy; control of faecal leakage and then thorough peritoneal debridement. For those who see relatively few colorectal wounds the priority will be to select methods that will best serve the patient, and these may be more cautious than those used by centres with wide experience, though these will demonstrate the possibilities.

To give an account of developments in this field it is useful to separate the treatment of stab wounds of the colon from those due to missile injury, and then consider wounds of the rectum and iatrogenic injuries.

Stab wounds of the colon

The force exerted by these wounds is localized to the actual track of the weapon, so the edges of a freshly incised wound of intestine can be expected to be viable. This makes primary suture of these wounds a sound undertaking, under strictly defined conditions. This is very relevant in the large cities of North America and Southern Africa, where stab wounds are common, there is great pressure on hospital beds and the patients are rarely in a social position to cope with a colostomy. In Durban in the 1980s between 80% and 90% of colon injuries were due to stabbing and a prospective study of over 1000 colon injuries was made (Thomson and Baker, 1991).

The policy was to perform two-layer closure of clean recent colon injuries but to practise mandatory exteriorization of the sutured colon whenever it was deemed too risky to leave the sutured wound within the abdomen. The suture line could then be watched and if it healed well the exteriorized colon could be returned to the abdomen after some days, so avoiding the 6–8-week wait required before a formal colostomy could be closed.

The **technique of primary suture**, and of **exteriorization of primarily sutured colon (EPSC)** can be considered together.

Whenever a colorectal injury is seen, which usually means that there is faecal contamination of the peritoneal cavity, it is reasonable to commence parenteral antibiotics (e.g. tetracycline or gentamicin, ampicillin and metronidazole).

As a first step after opening the abdomen it is useful to evacuate all faeces with liberal lavage with warm saline and then tetracycline solution. After the usual thorough search for other injuries, attention is turned to the colon. As in the duodenum, it is exceptionally important to remember that much of the ascending and descending colon is extraperitoneal, so a very careful search must be made for evidence of gas or blood under the peritoneum in anyone with a posterior or flank entry wound, or a penetrating renal injury. If there is one wound only on the front of the colon then it must be assumed there is another on the posterior retroperitoneal aspect and it must be sought, as in mobilizing ascending or descending colon in right or left hemicolectomy. Any necessary debridement of the colon wound is performed, and the edges of the colon injury must be seen to bleed freely. A single layer of interrupted serosubmucosal sutures of 3/0 braided nylon is used to repair the bowel. Defects in the mesenteric area must be closed by careful placement of two or three interrupted sutures, held long, and tied after all are inserted.

Once the closure has been performed and any necessary procedures on other organs completed, a further tetracycline lavage is performed. If the criteria indicate the need for exteriorization, then the affected area of colon must be mobilized so that it will easily reach the anterior abdominal wall. This is easy in transverse and sigmoid colon, but requires wide mobilization elsewhere. This is achieved by incising the peritoneum lateral to the colon and

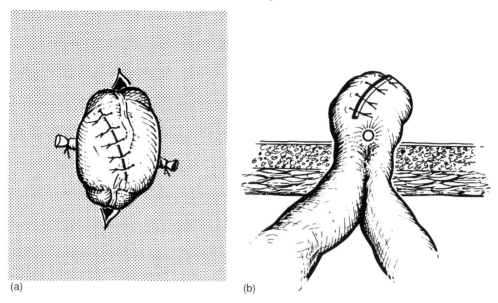

(a)   (b)

Figure 10.3 Exteriorization of primarily sutured colonic injury. **(a)** Appearance of the finished operation. **(b)** The route through the abdominal wall, with the loop supported by the catheter.

dissecting in the retroperitoneal space so that the colon, hinged on the mesocolon, can swing up and be passed easily through a suitably placed incision. This is sited away from the main vertical incision, so that a colostomy bag will easily fit over it and adhere to surrounding skin. The incision needs to be some 10 cm long and parallel with the line of the colon to be exteriorized, the muscles being incised in the line of the incision with cutting diathermy. At the midpoint of the colon wound a length of tubing is passed through the mesocolon and is used to draw the colon through the incision (Figure 10.3(a)).

The loop must lie comfortably, with a smooth curve (Figure 10.3(b)) so that flatus and faeces can easily pass through, and there must be no tension. It is important to tailor the length of the incision to the build of the patient so that the loop fits snugly in the incision: not too tight but not so loose that small bowel could herniate alongside it. The tubing is sutured to the skin on each side of the incision and cut short, to allow an adhesive colostomy bag to be placed over the colon: this protects the bowel, keeps it in a warm and moist atmosphere and allows immediate inspection of viability and of the progress of healing in the sutured wound. During the next few days flatus and sometimes faeces can pass through the loop and be passed *per rectum*.

If the colonic loop continues to look healthy and the wound to heal then it is possible to replace the loop in the abdomen some time between the fifth and tenth day. This depends on the recovery of the patient, and is performed under general anaesthesia. The colon can usually be freed from the skin and muscles by finger dissection. A thorough tetracycline lavage of the wound is performed, a drain is led down to the suture line *via* a stab wound, and the peritoneum and muscles are closed with interrupted polydioxanone. The skin is loosely approximated as in formal colostomy closure. If, during the days after colon repair, the suture line is seen to open and leaks faecal material, then the rest of the sutures are removed and the wound is opened up, so converting the exteriorization to a loop colostomy. This is managed in the usual way and closed later, generally after 6–8 weeks.

EPSC was given its first prospective trial by Kirkpatrick in 1977 and 42 of 61 patients healed satisfactorily. In Baker and Robbs's (1981) trial, 219 patients had primary intraperitoneal closure (IPC) of the colon wound and 163 were treated by EPSC; in 37 the suture line broke down while the colon was exteriorized and were converted to conventional loop colostomy but the remaining 119 (73%) healed and patients were spared the problems of a colostomy. They emphasize that whenever there was doubt EPSC was chosen.

Exteriorization, using EPSC, has particular merit in two situations:

- when repair is effected in the presence of general peritonitis;
- when there is extensive subserosal bruising in the colon, or there is a large mesenteric haematoma, even if the bowel itself appears viable.

Missile injuries

In the not so distant past most missile injuries were sustained in armed conflict, but changing customs and practices mean that now the casualties of war are as often civilians as combatants. In civilian life, other changing customs mean that, in the hospitals of many cities, missile wounds now greatly outnumber stab wounds of the colon (Muckart *et al.*, 1995).

It is reasonable to separate these two causes of injury. Missiles can cause more widespread damage than stabbings, both on account of their explosive force and the fact that exploding shells and mines produce multiple fragments. The other equally important reason is to adapt treatment to circumstances, which can vary greatly between front-line hospitals and well-equipped city trauma centres.

Reports from experienced teams in these centres, who may see several abdominal penetrating wounds each day, show what can safely be done when patients arrive swiftly and remain under the care of the operating surgeon until discharge. In recent prospective studies in the USA (George *et al.*, 1989; Chappius *et al.*, 1991) and South Africa (Demetriades *et al.*, 1992), in which more than 75% of injuries were due to missiles, the conclusion was that primary repair, or resection and anastomosis, should be considered for all civilians with penetrating colon wounds, and this decision was not dependent on associated risk factors (other injuries, faecal contamination or shock). It is repeatedly noted that, when other circumstances lead to death, it is not the colonic repair that has failed. In the study of Chappius *et al.* (1991) a prospective randomized study was made, without exclusions, in which stomal diversion was compared with primary repair in the treatment of intraperitoneal colon injury. The conclusion was that diversion was not safer than repair, and it carried the disadvantages of the presence of a stoma and the need for a later closure operation.

Thomson *et al.* (1996) considered the treatment of patients with multiple penetrating injuries. Among 668 patients, 71 had multiple wounds; 41 had IPC and 30 a colostomy or exteriorization procedure. The result was that the IPC had a rather better outcome than those who had a stoma.

The methods available are the same as those for stab wounds:

- primary repair with return to the abdominal cavity (IPC);
- resection and primary anastomosis;

- EPSC;
- exteriorization of an injury as a loop colostomy;
- Paul–Mickulicz resection, with double-barrelled colostomy;
- protective proximal colostomy above multiple repairs or resection and anastomosis.

The first two methods are favoured in experienced hands; the others may be used when circumstances are unfavourable, or judgement suggests that some protection is needed.

Morris and Sugrue (1991), working in a Red Cross hospital in Kabul, Afghanistan, under daily rocket attack, with very basic facilities, treated 70 patients with abdominal wounds. In 35 colon and rectum and in 33 small bowel was injured, and the methods used illustrate the way in which treatment is adapted to the circumstances, the facilities and the experience of the operating team. In the right colon, where exteriorization produces problems, they favoured hemicolectomy and anastomosis, and in some they extended this into the transverse colon. A few patients had primary repair. In the presence of severe contamination they chose resection, ileostomy and a distal mucous fistula. In the descending and sigmoid colon some primary repairs of small perforations were performed; otherwise, perforations were exteriorized as loop colostomies. Wounds low in the sigmoid, which cannot be exteriorized, were treated as rectal injuries.

The other factor that may have considerable influence is the presence of **associated injuries**. Ganchrow *et al.* (1970) in Vietnam saw 220 patients with colon and rectal wounds, and 191 (87%) had major associated injuries. Small bowel, liver, stomach, spleen and the thorax were most affected. The extent of these wounds must influence decisions on the treatment of the large-bowel injuries. They emphasized the importance of obtaining haemostasis before closure, and of providing drainage so that collections of blood could not provide a good culture medium for residual contaminants.

10.6.5   INJURIES OF THE RECTUM

The great majority of rectal wounds are due to penetrating injuries: they were the cause in 95 of the 100 consecutive patients with rectal wounds reported by Burch *et al.* (1989). Firearms had produced 82 injuries, sexual practices six, implements three and four were iatrogenic in origin. The five blunt injuries were due to falls and crush fractures of the pelvic ring.

It is useful to distinguish three varieties of injury.

(a) Intraperitoneal rectum

These are managed in the same way as injuries of distal sigmoid. They cannot be exteriorized, and after thorough cleaning they can usually be closed by suture and a proximal colostomy formed. The rectum is then washed out (see below). Occasionally, damage is so severe that it is best to perform a Hartmann-style resection.

(b) Extraperitoneal rectum

These tend to result from missile injuries of the buttocks, perineum, sacral region and the upper thigh, as well as the lower abdomen. There will be big differences in the degree of damage caused by high- and low-velocity missiles. With the close proximity of the urinary and genital tracts, the pelvic nerves and vessels and the bony pelvis, the likelihood of complex injuries is great. The rectum is a natural storage place for faeces, so faecal contamination can be severe.

Procedure
1. Gentle digital examination of the rectum is almost certain to reveal blood in the lumen, and a tear may be felt. There may be evident injury to the anal canal and it is then important to assess the state of the sphincters. The whole of the mucosa of the extraperitoneal rectum can be visualized by a gentle sigmoidoscopy. A tear was either felt or seen in 91 of the 100 patients of Burch *et al.* (1989). Injury to the bladder and urethra is very likely so a catheter should be gently passed: if there is any haematuria, and the state of the patient allows, a single-shot IVP and a cystogram can then be very helpful.
2. Once anaesthetized, movement should be kept to a minimum. It is best to excise posterior buttock and other wounds first and then place the patient in lithotomy–Trendelenburg position, so that there is easy access to the rectum, urethra and perineum without further change of position.
3. The next step is to open the abdomen, perform the usual thorough laparotomy and attend to other injuries. A penetrating wound of extraperitoneal rectum is likely to have caused bleeding, so there may be obvious blood beneath the pelvic peritoneum. A missile or impalement injury may well have emerged into the peritoneal cavity through a tear in the pelvic peritoneum.

    It is important to secure as good a view as possible of the rectum so dissection follows the lines of the abdominal phase of abdominoperineal excision. The pelvic peritoneum is opened beside the rectum, ureters are identified, the front of the rectum is separated from bladder or vagina, and the retrorectal space is opened up. In the course of this dissection, injury to the bladder may be found, and if the sacrum has been involved pieces of bone may have injured the rectum. After thorough saline lavage to clear out blood, faeces, pieces of bone and foreign bodies, tears of the rectum can be repaired using interrupted inverting sutures of polydioxanone. However, Thomson *et al.* (1992) do not generally do this unless the wound is extensive.

    In missile wounds the damage to the pelvis and sacrum may be considerable, with severe haemorrhage from branches of the internal iliac artery. Views differ on the value of ligating the internal iliac artery at its origin, but this will sometimes seem necessary.
4. All are agreed that a colostomy must be made above the rectum, and if there are no colon wounds this will be made in the usual way in the sigmoid colon. There is however no agreement over the need for complete separation of the two limbs of the colostomy. Lavenson and Cohen (1971), writing from experience of over 50 war injuries of the rectum, are emphatic on the need for a divided colostomy, and this may be a wise precaution in these circumstances, where nursing attention may be intermittent. Personal observation of a large number of loop colostomies made by the technique described on page p. 285, with full mucocutaneous suture, leads us to doubt whether there is spill of faeces into the distal stoma, and the work of Schofield *et al.* (1980) supports this belief. Utilizing the distal stoma, it seems sensible to empty the rectum of faeces by irrigation, although opinion on this varies. We run 1 in 200 aqueous cetrimide solution through a wide catheter, and pass a wide-bore proctoscope to assist drainage from the rectum. If

there is much faeces in the rectum it is better to dilate the anus and do a manual evacuation. Several litres of washout may be needed to clear the rectum. Sometimes this irrigation usefully reveals leakage through an unnoticed rectal wound, and this can be repaired. Lavenson and Cohen (1971) compared 16 patients who had no washout with ten patients whose rectum was thoroughly cleared of faeces by irrigation through the colostomy and found that seven fistulae developed in the 16 non-irrigated patients and only one in the ten who were irrigated. Of equal importance was the fact that no pelvic sepsis developed, whereas this was a serious problem in the 16 without irrigation, three developing gastric haemorrhage from stress ulcers, and two having osteomyelitis of the sacrum.

5. At one time there was complete agreement on the necessity of draining the perirectal space *via* the perineum, but experienced surgeons do not generally do this (Thomson *et al.*, 1992). If drainage is used the fingers of the right hand are passed down to a point beside the sacrococcygeal joint, and the skin is incised over this point. With an artery forceps and the fingers this incision, which traverses the glutei, levator ani and Waldeyer's fascia, is widened to 3–4 cm in length so that it will easily accommodate one or two wide, soft tube drains, with large side holes. These are drawn up to lie alongside the length of the rectum and securely tied in.

(c) Wounds of the perineum and anal canal

Both missile wounds and some traffic accidents can result in the most severe injuries to the anal canal and extraperitoneal rectum. The sphincteric ring may be disrupted, and in the most severe cases the rectum can be torn away from the anal canal. It is also important to remember that if a patient falls from a height on to the buttocks there may be serious pulping of the glutei, with or without anal injury. In these circumstances there is a real danger of a gas-forming anaerobic infection of the dead muscle, if this is not recognized and muscle excised (Walt, 1983). Unusual sexual practices can also lead to serious injuries to this region (p. 445).

Apart from mandatory proximal colostomy and thorough lavage to evacuate all faeces from the rectum and surrounding tissues, the procedure will have to be guided by the prevailing circumstances. Repair of the anal sphincter may well be appropriate, as may full-thickness sutures to reattach viable rectum to the anorectal ring. With debridement of all injured muscle, and provision of free drainage, these measures can greatly assist later repair.

Impalement is a specific form of anal injury that produces some dramatic results. Lear *et al.* (1981) describe a remarkable case that illustrates many principles of the care of these patients.

To escape from a burning building a woman jumped from a second-floor window and landed on a tree. She was impaled on a branch 5 cm in diameter which entered through the anal canal and emerged below the right nipple. She was rescued by sawing through the branch and brought to hospital with it *in situ*. A chest X-ray showed no pneumothorax so she was resuscitated, anaesthetized and placed in lithotomy–Trendelenburg position. At laparotomy the branch was found to enter the rectum, to have perforated small-bowel mesentery and torn the right lobe of the liver and the abdominal wall, and to emerge through the right breast. Another surgeon working in the perineum gradually withdrew the branch, allowing suture repair of the liver, right hemicolectomy for the devascularized ileocaecal angle and a defunctioning right iliac ileostomy. The perineal surgeon repaired the torn rectum and anal sphincter, and placed perineal drains. The patient eventually made a full recovery.

This and other reports emphasize the importance of leaving the impaling object *in situ* until the patient is anaesthetized, is under full antibiotic cover and a good stock of blood is available. The abdomen and/or chest is then opened and the object is slowly withdrawn, allowing each damaged structure to be identified and repaired.

Suction injuries are described in a remarkable paper (Cain *et al.*, 1983) in which five children between 18 months and 5 years of age, living in different areas of the USA, were described who sat on unprotected drains in swimming pools that had a continuous evacuation–filtration–return system of water purification. The suction on the outflow was so strong that the child's buttocks sealed the rim of the drain, rectal prolapse occurred and then a length of small bowel was sucked out through a rent in the anterior rectal wall. This resulted in a wide tearing of the bowel away from its mesentery. All five children had an extensive resection, and three were only surviving on home intravenous feeding, having between 0 and 14 cm of remaining small bowel.

Pneumatic injuries are generally due to practical jokes in which a compressed air hose is placed close to the anus. The force of the air readily penetrates through the clothing and the anal canal: the rectum generally resists rupture but the sigmoid is readily torn. This is an urgent case for laparotomy: the pneumoperitoneum can embarrass respiration through elevation of the diaphragm (Thomson *et al.*, 1994).

Sexual practices are responsible for a number of rectal injuries. **Retained foreign bodies**, inserted for erotic purposes, are fairly common problems. The history is often deliberately misleading, but digital and plain X-ray examination usually reveals the nature of the objects, which are very various: vegetables (such as courgettes), vibrators, tools, poles, pens and pencils may be found. A difficult extraction arose when a young man complained of constipation, examination showed a large mass above the pelvic diaphragm, and X-ray revealed a tin some 16×5 cm. Eventually, under general anaesthesia, the anal canal was progressively dilated and the fingers were introduced, but no hold was obtained. We then borrowed a pair of Kielland's forceps and, with a firm grip on the lower end and strong pressure on the upper end of the tin from the abdomen, we delivered a long, round tin wrapped around by several nappies.

Fortunately, many such objects can be removed in the emergency department, but it must be a rule that these patients are then sigmoidoscoped by a surgeon, and admitted for observation if there is any doubt about a rectal tear.

Homosexual practices lead to a number of injuries of the sphincters and rectum, of which the introduction of the fist is the most dangerous. Barone *et al.* (1983) saw 67 such injuries in men in New York over 3 years. There were 55 non-perforating lacerations of rectal mucosa, of which three required blood transfusion and transanal suture. Two men had suffered disruption of the sphincters, which were sutured. There were ten transmural rectal perforations, all of which showed signs of peritonitis, and required laparotomy and colostomy. One patient died from Fournier's gangrene.

Perineal injuries in children are a mixture of accidents and the results of sexual molestation. Jones and Bass (1991) reported 463 children under the age of 13 seen over 12 years in Cape Town: 143 (31%) had fallen astride, mostly on to bicycle crossbars and fences, and a surprising 58 (12%) had suffered impalement. Among girls, 76 had suffered rape and 50 other sexual attacks. In 87% the injury was minor, but 126 girls needed examination under anaesthesia, 17 had tears extending into the vaginal vault and 29 had anorectal injuries requiring repair of the rectum and anal musculature: 14 required a protective colostomy.

10.6.6   IATROGENIC INJURIES

Although there are a number of different causes of these injuries, they are quite uncommon. However, when they occur the effects can be serious, so these injuries need to be known, so that preventive measures can be taken and speedy recognition and treatment provided.

Endoscopic injuries

The **sigmoidoscope** was for a long time the only instrument likely to produce a tear because of undue pressure exerted on the rectal wall by the rigid instrument. Gabriel (1963) reported only two perforations at St Mark's Hospital in 20 years, and he calculated that 8000–10 000 sigmoidoscopies were performed each year.

Colonoscopy also has a safe record. Macrae *et al.* (1983) reviewed the first 5000 examinations at the same hospital and four perforations occurred, all successfully repaired. These occurred when the method was being learned. In a small tear occurring in clean prepared bowel, conservative treatment may be very carefully used, with close observation (Thomson *et al.*, 1994).

The main danger arises when **diathermy division of the stalk of a polyp** is undertaken through either a sigmoidoscope or a colonoscope. If the loop is tightened too far down the stalk of the polyp then the diathermy current may damage the muscle coat of the bowel, or in an extreme case actually cut through it. Prevention depends on accurate placement of the loop around the stalk, clear of both polyp and bowel wall, and then the risk appears to be very slight. In the course of performing some 300 such polypectomies we have seen this happen once, and then the signs of pelvic peritonitis appeared within about 4 hours; laparotomy, excision and suture of the defect on the anterior rectal wall, with sigmoid colostomy, were followed by a quick recovery. If there is doubt an erect chest X-ray is likely to show free gas under the diaphragm. Damore *et al.* (1996) review the subject. However, the situation could be much more serious if the injury was to the extraperitoneal rectum, where symptoms would develop more slowly.

Macrae *et al.* (1983) saw two such perforations in the course of 1795 snare polypectomies: one was recognized and repaired, but in the other it was 7 days before the patient returned to St Mark's with signs of peritonism and a 2 cm defect was sutured.

Haemorrhage after snare polypectomy is either primary or secondary. Macrae *et al.* (1983) saw 42 primary haemorrhagic episodes, of which 29 were minor, but in 13 between 1 and 5 units of blood had to be transfused and three required laparotomy, colotomy and oversewing of the bleeding point. Six patients had a secondary haemorrhage 5–14 days later. We have only had to operate on one such patient, who was bleeding so fast after snare polypectomy that transfusions into both arms were barely keeping pace with her loss and she suffered a cardiac arrest in the anaesthetic room. Fortunately, she was resuscitated and a rapid sigmoid colotomy and oversewing of the arterial bleeding point was followed by a complete recovery.

Although **explosive injuries** are very unusual, considering the number of diathermy snare polypectomies that are carried out, they did cause very serious damage when mannitol solutions were being used for bowel preparation. Modern methods using polyethylene glycol seem to be safe.

Gynaecological operations are carried out close to the rectum, and not infrequently pelvic viscera are adherent to it. If there is any doubt about rectal integrity the rectum should be irrigated with 1 in 200 aqueous cetrimide solution, which will demonstrate any leak or mucosal bulge.

A pelvic haematoma can collect after hysterectomy, and become infected and cause bacteraemia. It is wise to evacuate the infected area at laparotomy and irrigate the rectum; if there is any hint of a leak proximal colostomy is needed.

Other injuries

Perforation during barium enema examination. Although this is most unusual, it is unpredictable and when it occurs calls for prompt action. Nahrwold *et al.* (1971) found that infusion of 200 ml of sterile barium sulphate into the peritoneum of dogs was invariably fatal, with intense serosal inflammation and marked ascites. Removal of the barium did not help, but rapid infusion of Ringer's lactate allowed eight of 11 dogs to survive.

Harned *et al.* (1982) questioned 50 radiologists who had performed 106 000 barium enemas: they had seen 18 perforations and all the patients had recovered. They had also seen 11 perforations when a barium enema was done soon after a biopsy had been taken through a rigid sigmoidoscope, so it is clearly unwise to allow this to occur.

These perforations are seen at once by the radiologist and speedy action needs to be taken by the surgeon, with a fast intravenous infusion, systemic antibiotics and immediate laparotomy.

The jaws of colonoscopic biopsy forceps – only 2–3 mm long – do not seem to offer any danger of causing a perforation.

Perforation due to enemas has become almost unheard of since Higginson's syringes, with their hard nozzle, have been discarded.

Rectal thermometers have occasionally caused a tear, usually in babies. The strict rule must be that they are not introduced more than 2 cm.

Colostomy irrigation has produced a number of perforations in the past. It is now becoming a popular method of securing a predictable evacuation, but the new cone-shaped nozzle makes it very unlikely that any damage can occur.

In the only example we have seen the catheter had breached the colon subcutaneously, producing a sizeable abscess beside the colostomy. The stoma was encircled, colon mobilized and a cuff containing the perforation removed. The abscess was drained laterally and the colon edge sewn afresh to the skin.

10.6.7 BLUNT COLORECTAL INJURIES

Blunt trauma causes only about 5% of colorectal injuries and, because considerable force is needed, nearly all are due to motor vehicle collisions. There are often other serious injuries, and diagnosis can be difficult. The site affected is often a tear in the mesentery, and if bleeding is not enough to cause general and abdominal signs then the slow onset of ischaemia in the colon may not be noticed. A young man was admitted after a severe blow on the left costal margin. We suspected a ruptured spleen but the signs were not convincing until, on the fifth day, he became very tender; laparotomy revealed 10 cm of gangrenous colon due to avulsion of 15 cm of the transverse mesocolon. With resection and a double-barrelled colostomy he quickly recovered.

This delay in diagnosis comes out clearly among the 19 patients reported by Howel *et al.* (1976). Nine patients had obvious signs and were promptly operated upon. In eight more than 48 hours elapsed before the abdominal signs indicated the need for laparotomy, and in five the diagnosis depended on repeat peritoneal lavage being positive.

This report also emphasizes the high incidence of retroperitoneal injury in these patients, probably as a result of steering wheel and seat-belt injury being a common association. Four had pancreatic and two duodenal injuries. This finding rather supports the view that most cases of blunt intestinal injuries are due to compression between the anterior force and the spine or pelvis. It is also an important reminder to search the retroperitoneum in blunt injuries.

An important type of blunt rectal injury is associated with **crush injuries of the pelvis** (Froman and Stein, 1967). They examined 75 patients and found rectal injuries in 12. Some had linear lacerations of the rectum or of the anal canal running up into the rectum, some associated with rupture of the posterior urethra. Nine required repair with defunctioning colostomy. In three patients the rectum and anal canal, with the sphincters, had been torn away from perianal skin and had retracted upwards. It was possible to excise the wound, draw down the anal canal and reattach it to surrounding skin. Remarkably, all three had full sphincter control after their colostomies had been closed.

REFERENCES

Baker, L. W. and Robbs, J. V. (1982) Selective management of penetrating injuries of the colon. *S. Afr. J. Surg.*, **20**, 275–282.

Barone, J. R., Yee, J. and Nealon, T. F. (1983) Management of foreign bodies and trauma of the rectum. *Surg. Gynecol. Obstet.*, **156**, 453.

Burch, J. M., Feliciano, D. V. and Mattox, K. L. (1989) Colostomy and drainage for civilian rectal injuries: is that all? *Ann. Surg.*, **209**, 600–610.

Cain, W. S., Howell, C. G., Zeigler, M. M. *et al.* (1983) Rectosigmoid perforation and intestinal evisceration from transanal suction. *J. Pediatr. Surg.*, **18**, 10.

Chappius, C. W., Frey, D. J., Dietzen, C. D. *et al.* (1991) Management of penetrating colon injuries. *Ann. Surg.*, **213**, 492–498.

Damore, L. J., Rantis, P. C., Vernava, A. M. *et al.* (1996) Colonoscopic perforations: etiology, diagnosis and management. *Dis. Colon Rectum*, **39**, 1308–1314.

Demetriades, D., Pantanowitz, D. and Charalambides, D. (1992) Gunshot wounds of the colon: role of primary repair. *Ann. R. Coll. Surg. Engl.*, **74**, 381–384.

Edwards, D. P. and Galbraith, K. A. (1997) Colostomy in conflict: military colonic surgery. *Ann. R. Coll. Surg. Engl.*, **79**, 243–244.

Froman, C. and Stein, A. (1967) Complicated crushing injuries of the pelvis. *J. Bone Jt Surg.*, **49B**, 24–32.

Gabriel, W. B. (1963) *The Principles and Practice of Rectal Surgery*, H. K. Lewis, London, p. 398.

Ganchrow, M. I., Lavenson, G. S. and McNamara, J. J. (1970) Surgical management of trauma injuries of the colon and rectum. *Arch. Surg.*, **100**, 515–520.

George, S. M., Fabian, T. C., Voeller, G. R. *et al.* (1989) Primary repair of colon wounds. *Ann. Surg.*, **209**, 728–734.

Harned, R. K., Consigny, P. M. and Cooper, N. B. *et al.* (1982) Barium enema examination following biopsy of the rectum or colon. *Radiology*, **145**, 11–16.

Howell, H. S., Bartizal, J. F. and Freeart, R. J. (1976) Blunt trauma involving the colon and rectum. *J. Trauma*, **16**, 624–632.

Jones, L. W. and Bass, D. H. (1991) Perineal wounds in children. *Br. J. Surg.*, **78**, 1105–1107.

Kirkpatrick, J. R. (1977) The exteriorization anastomosis: its role in surgery of the colon. *Surgery*, **82**, 362–365.

Lear, G. H., De, K. R. and Birt, St J. (1981) Impalement injury by a tree branch from rectum to right nipple. *Injury*, **12**, 495–498.

Lavenson, G. S. and Cohen, A. (1971) Management of rectal injuries. *Am. J. Surg.*, **122**, 226–230.

Macrae, F. S., Tan, K. G. and Williams, C. B. (1983) Towards safer colonoscopy: a report on the complications of 5000 diagnostic or therapeutic colonoscopies. *Gut*, **24**, 376–383.

Morris, D. S. and Sugrue, W. J. (1991) Abdominal injuries in the war wounded of Afghanistan: report from the Red Cross Hospital in Kabul. *Br. J. Surg.*, **78**, 1301–1304.

Muckart, D. J. J., Meumann, C. and Botha, J. B. C. (1995) The changing pattern of penetrating torso trauma in Kwa Zulu/Natal. *S. Afr. Med. J.*, **85**, 1172–1174.

Nahrwold, D. L., Isch, J. H., Benner, D. A. and Miller, R. E. (1971) Effect of fluid administration and operation on the mortality rate in barium peritonitis. *Surgery*, **70**, 778–781.

Schofield, P. F., Cade, D. and Lambert, M. (1980) Dependent proximal loop colostomy: does it defunction the distal colon? *Br. J. Surg.*, **67**, 201–202.

Thomson, S. R. and Baker, L. W. (1991) The current status of the management of civilian injuries of the colon, in *Surgery Annual 23 (Pt 1)*, (ed. L. Nyhus), Appleton & Lange, Norwalk, CT, pp. 203–224.

Thomson, S. R., Stupp, C. and Baker, L. W. (1992) Management of civilian rectal injuries. *Trauma Emerg. Med.*, **9**, 590–594.

Thomson, S. R., Fraser, M., Stupp, C. H. *et al.* (1994) Iatrogenic and accidental colon injuries – what to do? *Dis. Colon Rectum*, **37**, 496–502.

Thomson, S. R., Baker, A. and Baker, L. W. (1996) Prospective audit of multiple penetrating injuries to the colon: further support for primary closure. *J. R. Coll. Surg. Edin.*, **41**, 20–24.

Walt, A. J. (1983) Management of injuries of the colon and rectum, in *Advances in Surgery 16*, (ed. L. D. Maclean), Year Book Medical Publishers, Chicago, IL, p. 277.

Woodhall, J. P. and Ochsner, A. (1951) The management of perforating wounds of the colon and rectum in civilian practice. *Surgery*, **29**, 305–320.

10.7   INJURIES OF THE SPLEEN

For many years the spleen was regarded as an expendable organ. Some 4% of circulating blood volume passes through it each minute, so blood loss can be severe, and splenectomy seemed to be a quick and safe method of securing haemostasis. However, for some 30 years it has been recognized that the spleen is an important constituent of the reticuloendothelial system. It is active in trapping encapsulated organisms, and it produces antibodies, and opsonins, which promote the phagocytosis of encapsulated bacteria. It plays a major role in the maturation of reticulocytes and lymphocytes and the regulation of platelets. This recognition has had a major impact on the management of the injured spleen.

The spleen is the intraperitoneal organ most injured in blunt abdominal trauma, and 50–60% of splenic injuries are due to motor vehicle collisions in the UK (Sargison *et al.*, 1968), Scandinavia (Bergqvist *et al.*, 1980) and North America (Livingstone *et al.*, 1982). Other causes are sporting injuries (5–10%), falls (5–10%), accidents at home, school or work (5–10%) and accidents on the farm (3–4%).

Among children 30% of injuries result from bicycle accidents (Bergqvist *et al.*, 1985). The spleen can be injured by quite a minor mishap, and often it is the only viscus injured – among 267 patients with a ruptured spleen only 26 had other abdominal injuries, including nine involving the diaphragm (Hunter *et al.*, 1984).

Rupture of the spleen is one of the best-known accidents but it is not often encountered by individual surgeons. Sargison *et al.* (1968) in Aberdeen found an annual incidence of about 1 per 100 000 population, so the average district hospital will admit only two or three splenic injuries each year.

The **mechanisms of injury** include the following.

- Many spleens are mobile, and are injured when tossed about in an accident, with sharp traction on an adhesion to the pulp.
- Direct trauma can occur, especially when an overlying rib fracture penetrates the spleen.
- Rarely, in a deceleration accident the spleen can be torn from its pedicle.
- **Subcapsular rupture** is likely to be followed by delayed rupture (p. 454).

Clinical picture

Symptoms. In a typical case the patient is knocked down by a car and suffers concussion and perhaps a fracture. Abdominal pain may not at first be very noticeable, localized to the left upper quadrant but spreading over the abdomen. Kehr's sign (really a symptom) of pain felt in the lateral part of the left supraclavicular fossa is highly significant, but absent in 20–30% of patients.

Other injuries are common. In 267 patients studied by Hunter (1984) 137 had been concussed, 121 had traumatized chests, 48 fractures of long bones and 20 fractures of the pelvis; these injuries can easily overshadow the abdominal situation and it must be actively and thoughtfully assessed.

Signs. The appearance of the patient – one of pallor with a look of anxiety – can be most significant, even while the hands and forehead are still warm and dry. Hunter (1984) found that 30% of their 267 patients maintained a tachycardia over 100/min and a systolic pressure below 100 mmHg in spite of resuscitation, and needed prompt operative haemostasis: 50% responded to resuscitation and 20% did not show signs of hypovolaemia.

It must be stressed that maintained hypotension in a concussed patient must not be explained as a consequence of head injury, and a source of haemorrhage must be sought in the chest, abdomen or fracture sites.

Abdominal tenderness is nearly always present – three-quarters of patients will show tenderness, and usually guarding, in the left upper quadrant. Many show generalized tenderness. The semi-conscious patient will often stir and groan when the left upper quadrant is palpated. A most significant sign occurs when pressure over this area makes the patient complain briskly of left shoulder-tip pain (Kehr's sign). On a number of occasions this sign has been elicited from an abdomen showing only modest tenderness, and made us think seriously about rupture of the spleen.

The urine must be examined because the commonest associated injury is renal contusion.

Management

Bearing in mind the effects of splenectomy, which will be detailed later, there will be a strong bias, especially in children, to avoid this operation. In penetrating injuries it will usually be necessary to explore the abdomen. In closed injuries, two distinct situations are faced.

1. The patient shows clear signs of hypovolaemia at the time of admission, and hypotension and tachycardia continue in spite of vigorous resuscitation
In these circumstances operative arrest of the source of bleeding is clearly an essential element in resuscitation.

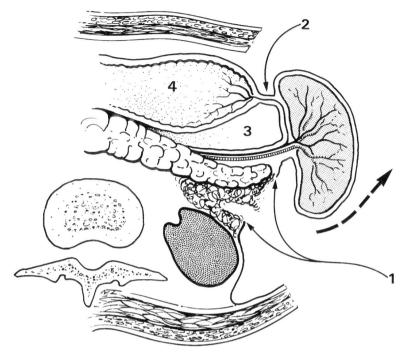

Figure 10.4 Splenectomy. A transverse section through spleen, pancreas and left kidney. The lienorenal ligament has been divided (1) to allow the spleen to swing forward. The gastrosplenic ligament (2) contains the short gastric vessels: when divided this gives access to the lesser sac (3). When the stomach (4) is drawn medially, the body and tail of the pancreas can be seen, the pedicle of the spleen isolated and splenic artery and vein, or their branches, ligated and divided.

Because the whole abdomen must be explored to find all possible injuries, a long midline incision is used. When the peritoneum is opened in this situation a daunting flow of blood can occur, because the tense abdominal muscles to some extent tamponade the flow of blood from the torn splenic pulp. The likely injuries causing speedy intra-abdominal haemorrhage involve the spleen, the liver and the small-bowel mesentery or the mesocolon, and these areas are carefully inspected and palpated in turn. A splenic rupture can often be felt, and visualization is eased by standing on the right, getting the assistant to retract the costal margin and using a strong sucker to clear the field. If the spleen is bleeding fast the next step is to bring it up into the wound. The surgeon's left hand is used to draw the posterior rim of the spleen medially, the right hand can then, with long scissors, divide the lienorenal ligament of peritoneum close to the spleen. If this cut is carried right round the length of the posterior border the spleen will begin to come up into the wound. Occasionally with fast haemorrhage and a poor view the lienorenal attachment can be broken with one's fingertips. The next step is to gain access to the splenic hilum and to do this the gastrosplenic ligament must be swiftly opened up, drawing the greater curvature of the stomach medially with tissue forceps and quickly ligating and dividing the short gastric vessels. This gives access to the lesser sac, and reveals the tail of the pancreas and the splenic pedicle (Figure 10.4); the splenic artery can be occluded by the left thumb and index finger, and the situation reviewed.

Generally, if bleeding has been as fierce as described, there will be a tear of a main branch of the splenic artery, in the hilum, and splenectomy will be needed. However, a careful review of the splenic injury along the lines indicated below is advisable, especially if the patient is a child in whom splenorrhaphy is particularly desirable. Splenectomy is also generally undertaken for the injured spleen, as part of damage control, and when there is severe or continued occult bleeding from intra-abdominal retroperitoneal and extra-abdominal sites.

If splenectomy is decided upon, the anatomy of the splenic pedicle must be carefully studied. Sometimes it is easy to separate the artery from the vein, and then the artery should be ligated first, then the vein. Some care should be taken to avoid tearing the vein because the bleeding is worryingly profuse. It is much safer to pass a strong ligature on an aneurysm needle and tie it, rather than clamping the vessels with artery forceps which can be pulled off. In other individuals the tail of the pancreas comes very close to the hilum of the spleen and this dissection of artery and vein can be difficult: they may have to be ligated with a single tie of strong thread. Every effort should be made to avoid damage to the tail of pancreas and sometimes it pays to tie off the two or three main branches of the artery and vein within the hilum. Finally, strands joining the lower pole to the region of the splenic flexure need division. Once the spleen is out it is important to check all possible bleeding points and the stumps of the artery and vein, particularly if removed in haste. The greater curvature can be torn in the rush to remove a pulped spleen. Therefore the stomach must be checked and the tear repaired. If there is any doubt about the integrity of the pancreatic tail, a closed drainage system should be left down to the splenic pedicle for 3–4 days.

The effects of splenectomy   This is an appropriate place to consider the effects of those unavoidable splenectomies. Viewed superficially these appear to be negligible, but doubts began to appear in 1952 when King and Shumaker reported on the after-effects of the operation in 100 patients: of five infants who had splenectomy for haemolytic anaemia in the first 6 months of life, all had a severe infection within 3 years of the operation, and in two this proved fatal. By 1962 Horan and Colebatch in Melbourne had studied 142 children for at least 2 years after splenectomy: 17 children had suffered a major acute illness, with fever and prostration, and five of the children had died in uncontrollable bacteraemic shock. In over half, *Streptococcus pneumoniae* was cultured, in others *Neisseria meningitidis* and *Haemophilus influenzae*. This grave syndrome was named 'overwhelming post-splenectomy infection' (OP-SI). In 1972 Eraklis and Filler reviewed 1386 splenectomized children in North America and found that 34 (2.4%) had died from OP-SI, but only three had had the spleen removed for trauma. Splenectomy for haematological disease in the first year of life carries a risk of OP-SI as high as 20%, and the risk remains three to five times greater for those under 5 compared to over-5-year-olds (Horan and Colebatch, 1962).

These papers, and the many written since, have aroused a very proper respect for the functions of the spleen. Some conclusion on the balance to be drawn between the value of these functions and the safe treatment of the injured spleen can be based on the reviews of Walker (1976) and Holdsworth *et al.* (1991).

- Walker (1976) studied the 821 children who had a splenectomy in England and Wales during 1960–1964. Among the 389 children who had the spleen removed for accidental injury, the risk of OP-SI was only 0.5%.

- Many reports show that the dangerous time to remove the spleen is during the first 5 years of life – especially during infancy, when the risk of subsequent serious infection is about 15%.

It seems, therefore, that so far as the surgery of the traumatized spleen is concerned, the risk of later OP-SI is low, and it is unusual for very young children to injure their spleen. These facts do not diminish the case for avoiding splenectomy wherever it is correct to do so, but they provide a useful background against which to decide whether, on balance, it would be in the interests of the individual patient to remove a badly damaged spleen.

2. The patient who remains normotensive, or who is resuscitated quickly and remains stable

At this stage the diagnosis of ruptured spleen is provisional, based at first on the clinical picture. Statistically the spleen (along with the kidney) is the organ most likely to be affected in a closed injury, and in a stable patient a CT scan will provide precise information (Mirvis *et al.*, 1989). There is a sound case for conservative management of some splenic injuries – in 47% of 413 children having a splenectomy for a ruptured spleen, the spleen was no longer bleeding at the time of removal, and could be expected to heal (Wahlby and Domellof, 1981).

However, there is no certainty about how a damaged spleen will behave, and there may be other injuries – especially rupture of the small intestine – that will only slowly produce clear signs of parietal peritoneal irritation (p. 436), so safe conservative management depends on a high standard of active observation.

In 1971 Douglas and Simpson in Toronto started treating children with a suspected ruptured spleen on a selective basis. Those actively bleeding were taken to theatre but in others enough blood was transfused to maintain a stable circulation and they were kept on strict bed rest for 7 days. In 1984 Filler reported on 128 patients so managed and only 37 had required laparotomy, the others making a good recovery. These 91 patients had had their splenic injury confirmed by ultrasonography – now a CT scan would generally be used, both for diagnosis and for supervision of healing.

There are uncertainties in the outcome of conservative treatment. Mahon and Sutton (1985) treated 52 adults with a closed injury and considered that 11 were in a stable state and suitable for observation. Over the space of 45 days, five showed sudden deterioration (one on the 12th and one on the 18th day) and three became increasingly uncomfortable and anaemic; all eight required splenectomy. Non-operative management must not be taken to lengths that are more dangerous than the small risk of later OP-SI. The current view is that conservative management should only continue if blood transfusion is not required. This is because the risk of acquiring a transmissible disease, e.g. hepatitis, is greater than the risk of OP-SI (Jalovec *et al.*, 1993). Conservative management is a more worrying method than having free recourse to splenectomy, but it is now clear that, even if laparotomy is necessary, it may be possible to repair the spleen. Dretzka was the first to do this in 1930.

Splenic preservation   In all except minor iatrogenic tears it is essential to mobilize the spleen completely, so that the whole surface can be seen. It is most important not to damage capsule in doing this because intact capsule is essential for holding structures. The procedure of dividing the lienorenal ligament has already been described, but it must be done more delicately than when quickly mobilizing a severely ruptured spleen.

Morgenstern (1985) recommends opening the gastrocolic omentum first, to expose the splenic artery. The apex of one of its loops is isolated and a nylon tape is passed around it twice and drawn up to stop flow: in this way bleeding is lessened and it is much easier to assess damage to the spleen. Several methods of splenic repair are available and are reviewed by Wilson and Moorehead (1992) and Schweizer *et al.* (1992).

Local haemostasis. In small tears (such as happen during gastrectomy) that result in a raw bleeding surface, it is often possible to obtain haemostasis by local tamponade. Microfibrillar collagen, if available, can be sprinkled on gelfoam strips or squares, carefully keeping it dry, and if applied to the bleeding surface and held firmly in place for some minutes there is a good chance of arrest of bleeding. The same treatment can be applied to a subcapsular haematoma: this is unroofed, clot is removed and the collagen applied.

Suture repair. Localized cracks in the splenic pulp can often be closed by a series of 2/0 or 0 chromic catgut mattress sutures, passed on curved atraumatic needles. Fortunately the splenic capsule is (like the liver) toughest and thickest during childhood and will often hold stitches well, though they are more likely to cut out in adults. Tying these sutures over Teflon buttresses, or over a roll of omentum, may diminish the tendency to cutting-out. Slim *et al.* (1979) in Beirut operated on 84 patients with splenic injuries. A total of 62 needed splenectomy, but suture repair was performed on 22; 17 had relatively superficial lacerations, but in five they were deep, with almost complete separation of the two halves. Nevertheless chromic catgut sutures passed on liver needles drew the halves together and all healed, as judged by later scans. All these repairs need drainage for about 7 days and the great majority heal well, but postoperative vigilance is important because the occasional repair breaks down with late bleeding after 6–7 days (Oakes, 1981).

Mesh splenorrhaphy has gained growing acceptance for burst injuries (Buntain and Lynn, 1979). It holds the segments of spleen together with a ladder or mesh of polyglycolic acid wrapped firmly round it (Figure 10.5).

In deeper fractures towards one pole there may be obvious spurting vessels, which can be picked up and tied off. Beyond these the splenic pulp may be discoloured and obviously devascularized. It may be possible to isolate the segmental vessel in the hilum, tie it and then amputate by finger fracture the affected pole of the spleen. The superior polar branch of the splenic artery is usually readily identified in the hilum, although the greatest care has to be exercised to avoid damage to the adjacent splenic vein. The raw surface that is left may be reasonably dry, or it may be feasible to insert polydiaxonone sutures through pledgets to buttress the suture and prevent it from cutting through the parenchyma (Figure 10.6).

Alternatively, Hoivik and Solheim (1983) have shown that if the short gastric and left gastroepiploic vessels are intact the main splenic artery can be ligated above the pancreas: anastomotic channels from these vessels join the splenic artery distal to the ligature and allow perfusion of the spleen. Scintiscans made 4–5 months later showed normal splenic perfusion in the five patients so treated. It is now very unusual for a patient to die from an isolated injury. Mortality in most series is 10–15%, because of the effects of other injuries, especially to the head and thorax.

10.7.1 DELAYED RUPTURE

Although this is a well-known syndrome it still generally presents in an unexpected way, and two of our patients illustrate this.

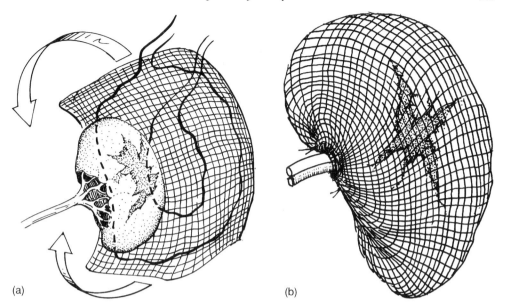

(a) (b)

Figure 10.5 Mesh splenorrhaphy. **(a)** A square of polyglycolic acid or polyglactin mesh is cut to size which will wrap around the spleen, and two long "0' sutures of the same material are placed as shown. The spleen is wrapped in the mesh and the suture near the periphery is drawn up so as to bunch the mesh bag and the splenic pedicle. **(b)** The second suture is then tightened near the widest point of the spleen, to apply compression to the area of rupture. Tension is adjusted to achieve haemostasis while avoiding any risk of ischaemia.

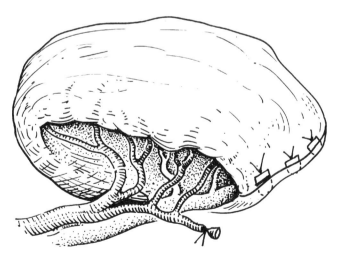

Figure 10.6 Detachment of the one pole of the spleen has been treated by ligation of the polar artery, and suture of repair of the raw surface, with the knots of these sutures reinforced by tying them over pledgets and a wrap of polyglactin mesh.

A middle-aged lady with a dyspeptic history was seized with sudden onset of upper abdominal pain. She came in, mildly shocked, with generalized abdominal tenderness and rigidity. A perforated peptic ulcer was diagnosed, but at laparotomy blood welled out of the incision and a ruptured spleen was removed. Later she recalled that 36 hours previously she had stumbled while walking to her family doctor for her usual alkaline mixture. We then remembered that she had complained of marked left shoulder-tip pain. Foster (1970) reported that some 70% of patients with delayed rupture experience left shoulder pain when bleeding commences.

A young man sustained complex fractures of the left radius and ulna and was awaiting open reduction on the third day after the accident when he complained of abdominal pain. The orthopaedic resident asked for a surgical opinion. Pain was localized in the left abdomen, where there was slight tenderness and guarding. However, palpation beneath the left costal margin produced sharp pain in the left shoulder, not previously noticed. A rupture of the spleen was suspected and confirmed at operation, when a steady oozing of blood was continuing. The few signs would not have been acted on without the rather striking production of Kehr's sign on pressure over the splenic area (p. 450).

McIndoe gave the first detailed account of delayed rupture in 1932. He emphasized the fact that patients lived a normal life, and did not think about the accident, for a period of days. There was often a dull ache in the splenic area. The length of the latent period was generally between 2 and 6 days, but it can be as long as 3 weeks. It seems likely that bleeding is confined within a subcapsular haematoma until the moment the capsule gives way. The onset of bleeding is marked by sharp aggravation of pain, usually referred to the left shoulder, and it soon spreads over the abdomen. The bleeding can be rapid and lead quickly to circulatory collapse.

10.7.2 SPONTANEOUS RUPTURE

Spontaneous rupture is most likely to be seen in countries where malaria, kala-azar and typhoid fever are common. Glandular fever may be complicated by spontaneous rupture: the patient of Rawsthorne *et al.* (1970) had an influenzal illness for 10 days and then awoke in the night with severe left shoulder pain which spread down to the left upper abdomen. The spleen was three times the normal size, with a tear in the upper pole.

In Papua New Guinea, a malarious area, Hamilton and Pikacha (1982) saw 62 patients with rupture of the spleen without any history of major trauma. Of these, 19 died before any treatment could begin, 20 needed laparotomy, with three having splenorrhaphy, and 23 were observed; they all had an intravenous infusion running for 1 week, with blood available, and were closely watched for a further week, and all settled uneventfully.

10.7.3 IATROGENIC RUPTURE

Iatrogenic rupture is sometimes very difficult to avoid during a difficult operation in the left upper quadrant. This used to be treated by splenectomy but now it is often possible to employ one of the methods of splenic repair.

REFERENCES

Bergqvist, D., Hedelin, H. and Lindblad, B. (1980) Traumatic splenic rupture during 30 years. *Acta Chir. Scand.*, **146**, 41–45.

Bergqvist, D., Hedelin, H., Lindblad, B. and Matsch, T. (1985) Abdominal injuries in children: an analysis of 348 cases. *Injury*, **16**, 217–220.

Buntain, W. L. and Lynn, H. B. (1979) Splenorrhaphy: changing concepts for the traumatized spleen. *Surgery*, **86**, 748–760.

Douglas, G. J. and Simpson, J. S. (1971) The conservative management of splenic trauma. *J. Pediatr. Surg.*, **6**, 565–570.

Dretzka, L. (1930) Rupture of the spleen. *Surg. Gynecol. Obstet.*, **51**, 258–261.

Eraklis, A. J. and Filler, R. M. (1972) Splenectomy in childhood: a review of 1413 cases. *J. Pediatr. Surg.*, **7**, 382–388.

Filler, R. M. (1984) Experience with the management of splenic injuries. *Austr. N.Z. J. Surg.*, **54**, 443–445.

Foster, R. P. (1970) Delayed haemorrhage from the ruptured spleen. *Br. J. Surg.*, **57**, 189–192.

Hamilton, P. R. and Pikacha, D. (1982) Ruptured spleen in a malarious area. *Austr. N.Z. J. Surg.*, **52**, 310–313.

Hoivik, B. and Solheim, K. (1983) Splenic injury ligation in splenic injuries. *Injury*, **15**, 1–5.

Holdsworth, R. J., Irving, A. D. and Cuschieri, A. (1991) Post splenectomy sepsis and its mortality rate: actual versus perceived risks. *Br. J. Surg.*, **78**, 1031–1038.

Horan, M. and Colebatch, J. H. (1962) Relation between splenectomy and subsequent infection: a clinical study. *Arch. Dis. Child.*, **37**, 398–414.

Hunter, R. A., Kiroff, G. and Jamieson, G. G. (1984) The injured spleen: should consideration be given to conservative management? *Austr. N.Z. J. Surg.*, **54**, 129–135.

Jalovec, L. M., Boe, B. S. and Wyffels, P. L. (1993) The advantage of early operation with splenorrhaphy versus non-operative management for blunt splenic injury. *Am. Surgeon*, **59**, 698–704.

King, H. and Shumacker, H. B. (1952) Splenic studies: 1. Susceptibility to infection after splenectomy performed in infancy. *Ann. Surg.*, **136**, 239–242.

Livingstone, C. D., Sirinek, K. R., Levine, B. A. and Aust, J. B. (1982) Traumatic splenic injury. *Arch. Surg.*, **117**, 670–677.

McIndoe, A. H. (1932) Delayed haemorrhage following traumatic rupture of the spleen. *Br. J. Surg.*, **20**, 249–268.

Mahon, P. A. and Sutton, J. E. (1985) Non operative management of adult splenic injury due to blunt trauma: a warning. *Am. J. Surg.*, **149**, 716–721.

Mirvis, S. E., Whitley, N. O. and Gens, D. R. (1989) Blunt splenic trauma in adults: CT-based classification and correlation with prognosis and treatment. *Radiology*, **171**, 33–39.

Morgenstern, L. (1985) Conservative surgery of the spleen, in *Current Operative Surgery*, (eds A. Cuschieri and T. P. J. Hennessy), Baillière Tindall, London, p. 74.

Oakes, D. D. (1981) Splenic trauma. *Curr. Probl. Surg.*, **18**, 342–401.

Rawsthorne, G. B., Cole, T. P. and Kyle, J. (1970) Spontaneous rupture of the spleen in infectious mononucleosis. *Br. J. Surg.*, **57**, 396–398.

Sargison, K. D., Cole, T. P. and Kyle, J. (1968) Traumatic rupture of the spleen. *Br. J. Surg.*, **55**, 506–508.

Schweizer, W., Bohlen, L., Dennison, A. *et al.* (1992) Prospective study in adults of splenic preservation after traumatic rupture. *Br. J. Surg.*, **79**, 1330–1333.

Slim, M. S., Najjar, N. E. and Mishalany, H. G. (1979) Preservation of the injured spleen. *Br. J. Surg.*, **66**, 671–672.

Wahlby, L. and Domellof, L. (1981) Splenectomy after blunt abdominal trauma. *Acta Chir. Scand.*, **147**, 131–135.

Walker, W. (1976) Splenectomy in childhood: a review in England and Wales 1960–4. *Br. J. Surg.*, **63**, 36–43.

Wilson, R. H. and Moorehead, R. J. (1992) Management of splenic trauma. *Injury*, **23**, 5–9.

10.8 INJURIES OF THE LIVER

The liver is both large and solid, and is at risk both in blunt crushing or deceleration accidents and in penetrating abdominal or thoracoabdominal wounds. The hepatic parenchyma is fairly fragile and, once the capsule is broken, it can easily fracture, particularly in older patients. The hepatic vessels and ducts are held firmly within the parenchyma, so when a fracture occurs these hollow structures are also easily torn; severe bleeding can therefore follow and is the principal cause of death in liver injuries.

Pringle (1908) noticed that the crushing injuries of liver that he treated in Glasgow Royal Infirmary were more often fatal than the penetrating stabbing accidents. One reason for this is that forces that are sufficient to fracture the liver are also likely to damage other organs: among 20 consecutive hepatic injuries seen by Blumgart and Vajrabukka (1972) only in two were injuries restricted to the liver. Ten had concussion, nine had fractures of long bones and/or pelvis, and eight had chest injuries, of whom seven required assisted ventilation. In penetrating wounds, while stab injuries are not usually serious unless they penetrate major vessels, missile wounds can cause major damage, especially shotgun and high-velocity gun injuries.

The causes of liver injury vary with the social customs of the country concerned. In Western Europe and Australasia about 70% of injuries are non-penetrating, and most of these are due to motor vehicle accidents (Little and Fliescher, 1980). Adult patients are mostly seated in cars travelling at high speed or on motorcycles, but children are often on pedal cycles. A few occupations, such as coal mining, are particularly likely to produce crush injury of the trunk, and children's games cause a number of accidents through falls from a height. In countries where offensive weapons are most often carried the position is reversed and Walt (1978) in Detroit, reporting 331 hepatic injuries, found that only 12% were due to blunt trauma: 60% were gunshot wounds and 28% were stabbing injuries. In South Africa, of 429 injuries undergoing laparotomy over a 10-year period, 47% were due to stabs, 21% to firearms and 31% followed blunt injury (Krige *et al.*, 1997).

The cause of the injury makes a great difference to the final outcome. The mortality figures in Walt's study were 1.1% in 91 stabbings but 15% in 186 gunshot wounds. In shotgun injuries mortality was 23%, similar to the blunt injury mortality of 20%, but the cause of death differed: in shotgun wounding death was usually due to the liver wound, but in many blunt injuries the major cause of death was often the effects of the violence on the brain, heart, lungs or skeleton. Krige *et al.* (1997) reported mortality rates of 2%, 11% and 27% respectively for stabs, firearm and blunt trauma.

Patterns of injury can be broadly classified as due to deceleration or to direct violence (Walt, 1969). The heavy liver is held in position by suspensory ligaments and in sudden deceleration shearing forces develop, especially around the falciform ligament, so it is not unusual to find longitudinal splits parallel to the ligament, 10–15 cm long and several centimetres deep. Hardy (1972) studied the patterns of injury in 50 patients who died from blunt hepatic trauma. He found that in 44 the major wound was in the postero-superior segment of the right lobe, where there was a ragged, fissured bursting injury 10–15 cm in diameter. He concluded that the liver had been crushed between sternum and vertebral column, possibly by the steering wheel, and that this produced such a rise of pressure within the inelastic hepatic capsule that it burst 'like a paper bag'. Only in seven patients were the hepatic vessels directly injured.

Spontaneous rupture of the liver is occasionally seen. There is a tendency for this to occur in late pregnancy. There is also an association, though very rare, between vascular fragile benign hepatic adenomas and long-term use of oral contraceptives. Baum *et al.* (1973) described seven such young women, four of whom presented in a state of collapse with a haemoperitoneum due to rupture of an adenoma. All had a partial hepatectomy, three on the right lobe and one on the left, and one died from exsanguination.

Diagnosis

There are no specific signals of closed injury to the liver, and they are diagnosed on suspicion. There may be difficulty in breathing because of fractured ribs, or haemo- or pneumothorax. Bruising may indicate where force was applied. Other injuries may be more obvious – impaired consciousness from head injury, or the pain and disability of fractures. Blumgart and Vajrabukka (1972) emphasize that in fractures of the pelvis transfusion and pelvic immobilization should lead to improvement in general condition, and if this does not occur abdominal bleeding may be continuing.

Non-operative management

Improvements in imaging with ultrasound, and particularly CT, allow grading of the less severe injuries and detection of other intra-abdominal damage, and these observations provide a sound basis for decisions on management. In patients who are haemodynamically stable CT scanning can detect subcapsular and intrahepatic haematomas (Reed *et al.*, 1992) and serial scanning shows whether these are stationary and, later, resolving. CT with contrast enhancement remains the best available technique for staging liver injuries. CT is not so accurate at grading severe injuries, but haemodynamic instability usually indicates the need for laparotomy.

The accuracy of CT scanning, and advances in paediatric resuscitation have led, as in the management of splenic injuries, to an extended trial of non-operative management in children, and this has proved to be safe in those who remain stable after resuscitation. The subject is reviewed by Losty *et al.* (1997).

Operative techniques

Minor injuries

Fortunately two-thirds to three-quarters of liver injuries come into this category. Many have stopped bleeding by the time they are found and it is important not to disturb these more than is necessary, otherwise clot may be dislodged and bleeding will recur. Most quiescent, superficial cracks can be left alone if they are dry. Alternatively, provided an 0 or 1 chromic catgut suture can be passed beneath the fissure on a 50 mm or 75 mm curved atraumatic needle without leaving any dead space, it is possible to close these wounds. If these sutures are gently tied, any bleeding should be controlled. In a friable liver it is helpful to tie the sutures over absorbable oxfibrin buffers. In the deeper parallel-sided fissures that may occur, e.g. beside the falciform ligament, which are still bleeding, it is sometimes helpful to pass deep catgut sutures on an 85 mm liver needle and tie these over a pedicled strip of great omentum. Access to some cracks and fissures on the posterior and superior aspects of the liver is restricted and if they are dry it is right simply to provide drainage to the area: some argument continues over this but provided a soft silicone tube drain is led into a sterile closed bag *via* a stab wound there is no evidence that this promotes sepsis, and it can be invaluable later as a check on further leakage of bile or blood. Nine out of ten of Walt's (1978) series of 277 penetrating liver injuries were dealt with in this way, as were 82% of a mixed group of 446 injuries from Cape Town, with negligible morbidity or mortality.

Major injuries

Because these are so much in the minority it is hard for the surgeon to obtain experience in the difficult surgical decisions and procedures that will be required to salvage these patients. Even in the surgical unit of Calne *et al.* (1982), with specific hepatic interests, only two or three cases were seen each year. Any hospital with an accident unit can be faced with such an injury and it is wise to have a plan of procedure worked out.

Calne *et al.* (1982) outline some important principles:

> The objective should be to do the minimum necessary to stop bleeding by suture, arterial ligation, resection, debridement and packing, before resorting to lobectomy. If the patient's haemodynamic state can be restored to normal, there is a much better chance of saving him, and further surgery can be done, as necessary, as a semi-elective procedure later. Control of bleeding by packing may be easy and life-saving.

It is important to remember that haemorrhage is likely to increase as soon as the abdomen is opened (Pringle, 1908). This is true for both the primary operation and the secondary operation when caval and hepatic venous trauma has been previously packed. The presence of clots tends to indicate the sector of the abdomen in which to search. The examination of the liver is not easy, because of its position and the bare extraperitoneal surface. If there is free bleeding from an obvious rupture it is useful to apply Pringle's (1908) manoeuvre of digital compression of the hepatic artery and portal vein between the left index finger in the foramen of Winslow and the thumb applied to the front of the free edge of lesser omentum. An angled vascular clamp can be applied subsequently. Usually it is best to release the artery and vein once firm pressure on a pack in the wound is established and when other intra-abdominal bleeding sources have been identified and controlled. Access through a midline incision frequently proves to be sufficient but median sternotomy greatly improves access without necessarily entering either pleural cavity. When the pack is removed all bleeding may have ceased and it is useful to know that in over 300 wounds so treated Lucas and Ledgerwood (1976) saw no case of recurrent bleeding.

However, as pressure on the artery and vein is released and the pack removed, visible bleeding points may be identified, and these may be under-run and tied off, with removal of fragments of liver that are obviously not viable – 'resectional debridement'. It is helpful to use ligaclips for bleeding points lying deep in fissure fractures but if there is any problem controlling arterial bleeding from the depths, finger fracture of the parenchyma with inflow control and suture ligation of the identified bleeding points is the safest option.

Walt (1978) found that this was required in about 5% of their patients. If the area remains reasonably dry, without evidence of any serious deeper fissuring, the operation can be concluded, with good drainage to this raw area. Rarely in a narrow deep split of the right lobe liver with profuse arterial bleeding, controlled by Pringle's manoeuvre, ligation of the hepatic lobar artery must be considered. Lucas and Ledgerwood (1976) used hepatic artery ligation alone, successfully, on nine occasions in their series of 312 injuries. Dr Mays (Aaron *et al.*, 1975) has been a most consistent advocate, arguing that a collateral circulation from the other lobar artery develops after ligation, to supplement the 50–70% of hepatic oxygenation that comes from the portal circulation. The liver wound should be packed and the retractors rearranged to give a good view of the porta hepatis. The peritoneum over the porta is incised and the common bile duct and the common hepatic artery dissected out. The right lobar branch of the hepatic artery usually passes behind the bile duct. If possible it is desirable to ligate the right artery distal to the origin of the cystic artery, but this may not be feasible, and then cholecystectomy is needed.

The finding of a subcapsular haematoma suggests that a substantial area of underlying parenchyma has been fractured, and the only safe treatment is to unroof it and assess the damage. Treatment is then as for open rupture of the liver.

When bleeding continues in spite of these measures, as it does in some 5–10% of patients, control of the haemorrhage is paramount. Surgery for major hepatic trauma has a mortality rate quoted between 36% and 76% (Yellin *et al.*, 1971), which is most often due to exsanguination, and the mechanism is most likely to be blunt trauma. The decision to continue with definitive surgical arrest of bleeding, or to adopt a 'damage-control' approach, is one that must be carefully taken. For the surgeon without special facilities it is best to practise specific haemostatic packing, and then to transfer the patient; if working in isolation, the time gained by temporary packing and attention to resuscitation and the care of other injuries may be life-saving. Madding and Kennedy (1971) made it clear that retention of packs in the liver for more than 2–3 days results in high mortality from sepsis, but temporary packing gives time for the patient to stabilize, and for correction of hypocoagulable states and deranged physiology.

Before inserting the packs the liver must be fully mobilized. The first assistant compresses the liver to minimize bleeding. The surgeon frees the injured lobe from its peritoneal attachments by dividing the falciform ligament along the diaphragm until the suprahepatic portion of the inferior vena cava is reached. The triangular ligament and the two leaves of the coronary ligament are divided to expose the bare area until the borders of the retrohepatic inferior vena cava are reached. The results from Cambridge (Calne *et al.*, 1982) and the Hammersmith Hospital units (Smadja *et al.*, 1982) show that it is better for the surgeon inexperienced in hepatic surgery to pack, close the abdomen and arrange urgent transfer to a unit with such experience. The technique of packing is well described by the Cape Town Group (Krige *et al.*, 1992). The packs are layered predominantly postero-superiorly to allow compression by the natural rib cage with some subhepatic packs to provide counter-compression (Figure 10.7).

Though the tamponade may be greater when fascial closure is obtained this can result in abdominal compartment syndrome and IVC obstruction. Packing can still be used effectively if an abdominal containment procedure has been employed.

In major parenchymatous 'burst injuries' the technique of mesh hepatorrhaphy has been adapted from the well-described technique for splenic conservation. The advantages of the prosthetic mesh over the perihepatic packing in appropriately selected cases are in expert hands appealing. Effective haemostasis is achieved both in animal models and humans (Reed *et al.*, 1992; Stevens *et al.*, 1991) and re-laparotomy to remove the packs, with the risk of re-bleeding, is avoided. The risk of development of abdominal compartment syndrome is minimized as there are no packs to take up the valuable intra-abdominal space. The risk of intra-abdominal sepsis is reduced. In addition the mesh does not interfere with postoperative radiological studies and, if re-look laparotomy is required, reoperation is unlikely to interfere with the hepatic haemostasis.

Of the two techniques described, the 'pita pocket' and the 'purse-string', the former in the authors' opinion is the most reliable and is described in detail. After full mobilization of the liver the pita-pocketed technique can be applied (Figure 10.8).

It uses two flat sheets of prosthetic mesh whose two adjacent edges are held together by a running absorbable suture, forming the pocket. The liver is slipped into the pocket so that

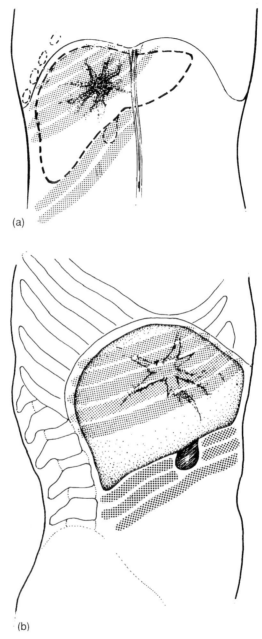

(a)

(b)

Figure 10.7 Perihepatic packing. Dry laparotomy packs with radio-opaque markers are layered into the posterior, superior and lateral aspects of the right lobe, but are not placed within the fissures of the liver. This achieves tamponade between the ribcage plus the diaphragm and liver. Further packs are placed below the liver and then the abdomen is closed.

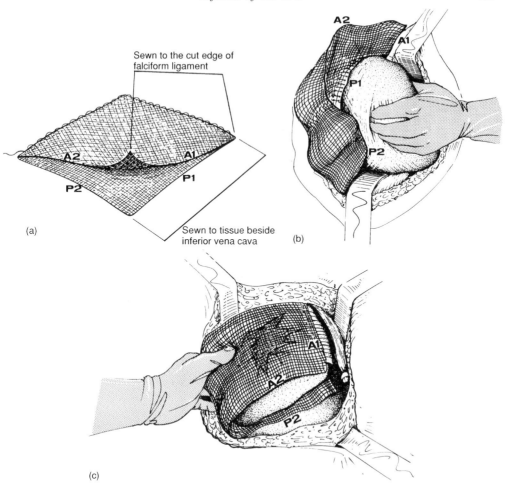

Figure 10.8 Compression of the right lobe of the liver by the "pita pocket' technique (adapted and redrawn from Reed *et al.*, 1992). (**a**) Two square meshes of polyglycolic acid or polyglactin mesh are sewn together on two adjacent sides. (**b**) The mobilized liver is rolled forward and the posterior side of P1 of the pocket is sewn to tissue beside the inferior vena cava. The pocket is brought round to envelope the right lobe. (**c**) The anterior side A1 can now be attached to the edge of the divided falciform ligament, which remains attached to the liver. This leaves the sides A2 and P2 ready to be sewn firmly together, under tension, with a continuous suture to apply compression.

the two open sides of the pocket are positioned medially and inferiorly. The posterior medial flap is sutured to the adventitial tissue lateral to the vena cava. A running absorbable suture is then used to attach the superior medial free border to the falciform ligament. Finally a running absorbable suture is used to bring together the two free inferior borders of the pocket. In placing this final suture it is important to ensure that sufficient compression is generated to produce compressive haemostasis. Throughout the procedure, the important role of the first assistant in maintaining compressive haemostasis cannot be overemphasized.

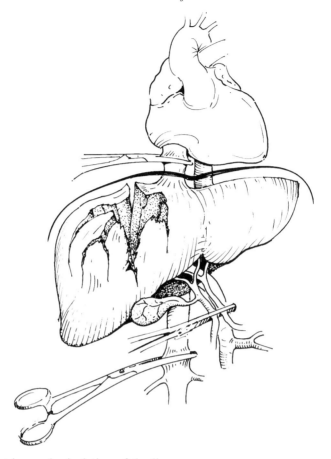

Figure 10.9 Total vascular isolation of the liver.

Cholecystectomy was initially recommended for fear of pressure necrosis and perforation of the gallbladder. These worries seem unfounded and cholecystectomy is rarely necessary. Perihepatic drains are left *in situ*. When mesh hepatorrhaphy is used correctly for hepatic parenchymal bleeding and not for juxtacaval and hepatic vein lacerations, the mortality rate is a commendable 25% (Reed *et al.*, 1992; Stevens *et al.*, 1991). Intraoperatively, the surgeon actually sees that haemostasis is achieved, unlike in perihepatic packing. What is important with this technique and perihepatic packing is early recognition of the severity of the injury and prompt application of the mesh (or packing) before the patient's condition (acidosis, coagulopathy and hypothermia) deteriorates.

If packing has been used transfer to a major specialized unit should be the next step. If it is not a feasible solution then the surgeon working in isolation can retain the packs for 2–3 days to allow the patient to stabilize before reoperation. At this stage an experienced operating and theatre team must be geared to proceed to hepatic resection or venous repair if this is necessary. This is despite the fact that in the majority of patients the wound remains dry when this delayed removal of packs takes place. We believe that atriocaval shunting in the acute phase is fraught with problems (Burch *et al.*, 1988) and has no real place in this scenario, or at the removal of packs stage, when total vascular isolation is a less complex option that can be highly effective (Krige *et al.*, 1990; Yellin *et al.*, 1971). This procedure usually follows packing of the liver for severe retroperitoneal bleeding from the inferior vena cava. Good retraction is required. With the juxtahepatic packs still *in situ* the infrahepatic IVC is mobilized and encircled with care to avoid damage to lumbar veins. The suprahepatic IVC is easiest to isolate in the pericardium through a window in the diaphragm. Clamps are then applied first across the portal triad, the infrahepatic IVC and then the suprahepatic IVC (Figure 10.9).

The remaining packs are then removed and complete mobilization of all the ligaments of the liver and its bare area can now be achieved in a dry field. The torn veins can now be seen and repaired with fine vascular sutures (6/0 Prolene) and the clamps removed, firstly from the infrahepatic IVC to get air and clots out of the system, then the portal triad clamp, and lastly the intrapericardial IVC. Alternatively, a liver resection can be undertaken.

REFERENCES

Aaron, S., Fulton, R. L. and Mays, E. T. (1975) Selective ligation of the hepatic artery for trauma of the liver. *Surg. Gynecol. Obstet.*, **141**, 187–189.

Baum, J. K., Holtz, F., Bookstein, J. J. *et al.* (1973) Possible association between benign hepatomas and oral contraceptives. *Lancet*, **ii**, 926–929.

Blumgart, L. H. and Vajrabukka, T. (1972) Injuries to the liver: analysis of 20 cases. *BMJ.*, **i**, 158–164.

Burch, J. M., Feliciano, D. V. and Mattox, K. L. (1988) The atriocaval shunt: facts and fiction. *Ann. Surg.*, **207**, 555–568.

Calne, R. Y., Wells, P. C. and Forty, J. (1982) Twenty six cases of liver trauma. *Br. J. Surg.*, **69**, 365–368.

Hardy, K. J. (1972) Patterns of liver injury after fatal blunt trauma. *Surg. Gynecol. Obstet.*, **134**, 39–43.

Krige, J. E. J., Worthley, C. S. and Terblanche, J. (1990) Severe juxtahepatic venous injury: survival after prolonged vascular isolation without shunting. *HPB Surg.*, **3**, 39–45.

Krige, J. E. J., Bornman, P. C. and Terblanche, J. (1992) Therapeutic perihepatic packing in complex liver trauma. *Br. J. Surg.*, **79**, 43–46.

Krige, J. E. J., Bornman, P. C. and Terblanche, J. (1997) Liver trauma in 446 patients. *S. Afr. J. Surg.*, **35**(1), 10–15.

Little, J. M. and Fliescher, G. (1980) Liver injuries in Sydney: a 20 year experience. *Austr. N.Z. J. Surg.*, **50**, 495–500.

Losty, P. D., Okoye, B. O., Walter, D. P. *et al.* (1997) Management of blunt liver trauma in children. *Br. J. Surg.*, **84**, 1006–1008.

Lucas, C. E. and Ledgerwood, A. M. (1976) Prospective evaluation of haemostatic techniques for liver injuries. *J. Trauma*, **16**, 442–446.

Madding, G. F. and Kennedy, P. A. (1971) *Trauma to the Liver*, 2nd edn, W. B. Saunders, Philadelphia, PA.

Pringle, J. H. (1908) Notes on the arrest of hepatic haemorrhage due to trauma. *Ann. Surg.*, **48**, 541–549.

Reed, R. L., Merrel, R. C. and Meyers, R. C. (1992) Continuing evolution in the approach to severe liver trauma. *Ann. Surg.*, **216**, 524–538.

Smadja, C., Traynor, O. and Blumgart, L. H. (1982) Delayed hepatic resection for major liver injury. *Br. J. Surg.*, **69**, 361–364.

Stevens, S. L., Maull, K. I., Enderson, B. L. and Meadors, J. N. (1991) Total mesh wrapping for parenchymal liver injuries: a combined clinical and experimental study. *J. Trauma*, **31**, 1103–1109.

Walt, A. J. (1969) The surgical management of hepatic trauma and its complications. *Ann. R. Coll. Surg. Engl.*, **45**, 319–339.

Walt, A. J. (1978) The mythology of hepatic trauma – or Babel revisited. *Am. J. Surg.*, **135**, 12–18.

Yellin, A. E., Chaffee, C. B. and Donovan, A. J. (1971) Vascular isolation in the treatment of juxtahepatic venous injuries. *Arch. Surg.*, **102**, 566–573.

Penetrating injuries

The principles of treatment are the same. Stab wounds that have stopped bleeding can usually
be left alone, with a drain left beside them. If bleeding continues, either cautious extension
will be needed, to allow oversewing of the point, or pressure is applied through packing.
Gunshot wounds are likely to cause more extensive wounding, and require treatment as for
a serious crush injury.

Bluett *et al.* (1984) reviewed 102 penetrating injuries, 47 due to stabbings and 55 due to
shooting incidents. Stab injuries were mostly left to heal, with a strong emphasis on closed
drainage to the site of injury. In through-and-through wounds that were bleeding briskly they
evolved a useful method which they believe saved a number of resections. A 22 FG Jacques
catheter is passed along the track of the wound to emerge at the end nearest to the abdominal
wall. To the eyes of the catheter are tied three or four Penrose drains and these are drawn
through the liver wound to emerge on the farther side: the catheter is cut away. The drains
are brought out through a stab wound. Bluett *et al.* found that this tampon stopped bleeding
in 13 stab and missile tracks. After 7–8 days the drains are slightly shortened, but they were
not removed, on average, for 30 days. Several of the tracks leaked bile for some weeks but
all eventually healed.

Although 30% of the stabbed patients and 50% of those injured by missiles were shocked
on arrival, no one required hepatic artery ligation. Suture, ligation of bleeding points,
debridement, tamponade and six lobectomies secured haemostasis; three patients with major
missile injuries of the vena cava were the only fatalities in the whole series.

Reference

Bluett, M. K., Woltering, E. and Adkins, R. E. (1984) Management of penetrating hepatic injury: a review of 102
    consecutive patients. *Am. Surgeon*, **50**, 132–142.

10.8.1   TRAUMATIC HAEMOBILIA

This is a fairly unusual event, but injury of one kind or another is the cause of most cases.
Sandblom pointed out in 1948 that there was a recognizable diagnostic triad:

● an injury to the liver in the preceding days or weeks;
● haematemesis and/or melaena;
● biliary colic, sometimes accompanied by jaundice.

The injury may be accidental or iatrogenic. The **accidental injuries** are mostly blunt
traffic accidents, although penetrating injuries may also produce the essential lesion, which
is a cavity in the liver parenchyma into which bleeding occurs.

This may be a slow collection or it may be a sudden bursting of an arterial or arteriolar
aneurysm. It is a particular hazard in a deep liver wound that is superficially closed by suture,
leaving a deep unclosed cavity. At some stage blood is suddenly discharged from the cavity
down an open biliary passage, through the ampulla of Vater into the duodenum, whence it is
either vomited or passed as melaena. The volume and speed of bleeding varies greatly, but
in some cases is sufficient to cause acute hypovolaemia.

The other major cause of such bleeding is **iatrogenic injury** to a hepatic artery, either by needle biopsy or by percutaneous transhepatic cholangiography (PTC). Occasionally, the injury is overvigorous operative exploration of the intrahepatic bile ducts, seeking for a retained stone.

Caret *et al.* (1984) calculate that haemobilia complicates about 2% of accidental injuries and about 4% of PTC examinations: it is rare after fine needle biopsy. The commonest time for it to occur is about 4 days after needling of the liver and about 3 weeks after blunt injury.

The major differential diagnosis after abdominal injury is stress ulceration, which is not unexpected after a major hepatic rupture. The occurrence of biliary colic may be a helpful point. Gastroduodenoscopy is essential to exclude stress ulceration, and the diagnosis may be clinched by seeing fresh blood in the duodenum, emanating from the ampulla of Vater. Diagnosis often hinges on the combination of circumstances and is clinched by selective hepatic arteriography. In 56 arteriograms (Caret *et al.*, 1984) an arterial lesion was seen in 53, although the final proof, contrast medium in the biliary tree, was only seen in three. If coeliac axis catheterization is negative it must be remembered that the right hepatic artery is a branch of the superior mesenteric artery in 5–8% of individuals, and this was demonstrated in two of the 56 patients just quoted.

With the skill of the interventional radiologist it is generally possible to embolize the appropriate artery with gelatin sponge (Corr *et al.*, 1992). The need to perform hepatic resection has now more of less ceased, although if embolization fails it may be necessary to undertake selective hepatic arterial ligation.

In a case in which very brisk haemobilia followed a needle liver biopsy we experienced considerable difficulty in establishing the diagnosis because a small duodenal ulcer was thought to be the source of bleeding. When bleeding recurred a second endoscopy fortunately showed blood issuing from the ampulla of Vater. However, although arteriography demonstrated an arterial aneurysm it was not possible to embolize the artery, because it arose from the superior mesenteric artery. Vigorous bleeding continued, and it was therefore necessary to expose the superior mesenteric artery and ligate the branch running to the right lobe of the liver. Recovery was uneventful.

REFERENCES

Caret, P., Baumer, R., Roche, A. *et al.* (1984) Hepatic haemobilia of traumatic or iatrogenic origin. *World J. Surg.*, **8**, 2–6.

Corr, P., Beningfield, S. J., Krige, J. E. J. (1992) Selective hepatic artery embolisation in liver injury. *Injury*, **23**, 347–349.

Sandblom, P. (1948) Haemorrhage into the biliary tract following trauma – 'traumatic haemobilia'. *Surgery*, **24**, 571.

10.8.2   INJURY TO THE EXTRAHEPATIC BILIARY TREE

Injuries to the extrahepatic biliary tree are fortunately rare with major centres encountering fewer than ten per year (Bade *et al.*, 1989; Posner and Moore, 1985). Though first described by Drysdale (1861) following blunt trauma, they are currently more commonly due to penetrating trauma (Feliciano *et al.*, 1985; Bade *et al.*, 1989). Gallbladder injury is four times commoner than ductal injury (Bade *et al.*, 1989; Posner and Moore, 1985). The injury is usually diagnosed at laparotomy. In ductal injury vascular structures in the free edge of the hepaticoduodenal ligament may often be injured and control of brisk haemorrhage takes priority and will dictate the outcome (Feliciano *et al.*, 1985). The whole area may be a haemorrhagic, contused mess and the clue to the diagnosis is bile staining. This is particularly true if the injury is to the hilum or the intrapancreatic portion of the bile duct. In this setting when operative and patient conditions are unfavourable it is better to create a controlled fistula by intubating the biliary tract and placing a drain adjacent to the injury site and returning at a later date for definitive restoration of bilioenteric continuity. If a tangential injury involves less than one-third of the circumference then repair can be effected with a T-tube inserted through an untraumatized part of the duct to both stent and decompress the repair (Feliciano *et al.*, 1985; Bade *et al.*, 1989). If there is a complete transection and the patient is stable then choledochojejunal anastomosis is the preferred reconstruction (Posner and Moore 1985; Bisuttil *et al.*, 1980). The duct is small and persons with experience in the technique should be present. The duct can be spatulated somewhat and an interrupted technique using 4/0 polydioxanone employed. All the anterior ductal sutures are placed first from serosa to lumen with the needles remaining attached and clipped sequentially. All the posterior sutures are now placed through both the duct and the inferior edge of the jejunotomy. The jejunum is then parachuted down to lie tension-free against the duct and the sutures are tied with the knots on the inside. The anterior ductal sutures are then placed through the superior edge of the jejunotomy to complete the anastomosis, which is drained with a soft Silastic tube drain.

REFERENCES

Bade, P. G., Thomson, S. R., Hirshberg, A. and Robbs, J. V. (1989) Surgical options in traumatic injury to the extrahepatic biliary tract. *Br. J. Surg.*, **76**, 256–258.

Bisuttil, N. W., Kitahama, A., Cerise, E. *et al.* (1980) Management of blunt and penetrating injuries to the porta hepatis. *Ann. Surg.*, **191**, 641–648.

Drysdale, T. M. (1861) Case of rupture of the common duct of the liver. Formation of a cyst containing bile. Death occurring on the fifty-third day. *Am. J. Med. Sci.*, **12**, 399–404.

Feliciano, D. V., Bitondo, C. G., Burch, J. M. *et al.* (1985) Management of traumatic injuries to the extra hepatic biliary ducts. *Am. J. Surg.*, **150**, 705–709.

Posner, M. C. and Moore, E. E. (1985) Extrahepatic biliary tract injury: operative management plan. *J. Trauma*, **25**(9), 833–837.

10.9   RETROPERITONEAL HAEMORRHAGE

Appreciable bleeding can occur into the retroperitoneal space in injuries to the kidney, duodenum and pancreas, but voluminous retroperitoneal haemorrhage is more likely to accompany rupture of an abdominal aortic aneurysm, or to complicate the commonest cause of all, double or diametric fractures of the pelvic ring, which cause some 50–60% of retroperitoneal haematomas. In these, diastasis or fracture of the pubic arch, with a fracture running close to the sacroiliac joint, allows distortion of the ring, and this is very likely to tear branches of the internal iliac vessels, which lie beside the posterior fracture. The haemorrhage from such a tear can be fierce and continuing, with the extensive retroperitoneal space accommodating as much as 4 litres of blood.

Most retroperitoneal haematomas are due to vehicle collisions or falls, so other injuries, especially to the head, are likely. When these are added to the effects of substantial loss of blood the effects can be grave. In San Francisco Selivanov *et al.* (1984) studied 81 patients with retroperitoneal haematoma and found a mortality of 20%: 15 of the 16 deaths followed blunt injuries and 11 were associated with fractures of the pelvis. Some 30% of the 81 haematomas were due to gunshot or stabbing injuries and these mostly affected the retroperitoneal viscera or the great vessels.

The clinical evidence for closed retroperitoneal haemorrhage is non-specific, and is likely to be dominated in many cases by the signs of hypovolaemic shock and fracture of the pelvic bones, such as external rotation of a leg and swelling of the thigh. Abdominal tenderness is variable but there is likely to be some distension. This is likely to be augmented by the paralytic ileus that is a common complication of retroperitoneal haematoma (p. 258). Hurt *et al.* (1983) showed that ileus was particularly likely to complicate diametric pelvic fractures with large haematomas, and these episodes were likely to continue for 6–7 days. Rectal examination may show a boggy mass surrounding the rectum. It is not unusual for blood to leak through into the peritoneum, so there may be signs of guarding and a positive peritoneal lavage. Bleeding from a pelvic ring fracture can be limited by the use of the military antishock trousers (MAST) for emergency control of this type of bleeding. The envelope is applied around the whole of the body below the nipple line and inflated to a pressure of 30 cm H_2O. It can be left on for 24–36 hours and sometimes when it is released there is no recurrence of bleeding (Dove *et al.*, 1981). The difficulty of using the suit is that access to the urethra, rectum and abdomen is denied to the surgeon during the period of inflation, and this can be particularly worrying when repeated observation of the abdomen is required. An additional problem is that most patients need respiratory assistance during the period of inflation.

An alternative method of arresting haemorrhage is to block the responsible vessels. Attempts in the past to do this by surgical ligation were generally unsatisfactory, but much better results have been obtained by selective arterial catheterization and angiography, followed by therapeutic embolization (Matalon *et al.*, 1979).

In **penetrating wounds** the haematoma is usually discovered in the course of laparotomy, and Costa and Robbs (1985) studied 106 such patients with stab or handgun wounds of the abdomen. Central haematomas are explored because either great vessels or pancreas/duodenum are so likely to be injured. In 15 of 23 such injuries the aorta or IVC was directly repaired, and duodenum was sutured in five. The expanding central retroperitoneal haematoma is a very serious challenge, because it has to be explored and is likely, once uncovered, to allow severe bleeding from the aorta or vena cava. Inflow control of the aorta at the hiatus and precise digital pressure are needed when the haematoma is opened. Access can then be improved by mobilizing the splenic or hepatic flexures and the duodenum, and with more adjacent proximal and distal control the repair of the vessel can be achieved. In 22 expanding haematomas, the inferior vena cava was injured in nine, the aorta in five and the portal vein in two patients.

Pelvic haematomas generally show signs of active bleeding from iliac vessels and need exploration and repair. The treatment of flank haematomas is more debatable. In flank wounds with ongoing haematuria Costa and Robbs (1985) used intravenous urography and renal angiography, and in all 15 patients a specific lesion was shown and definitive surgery carried out. However, the angiogram may show that selective embolization is appropriate. If a flank haematoma is stable and the urogram shows no major disruption of the kidney their advice is to leave the haematoma undisturbed: in 58 such patients none came to harm.

In **closed injuries** treatment is directed to the cause of the bleeding, a rupture of the kidney, duodenum, pancreas or aortic aneurysm being dealt with along the usual lines. The paralytic ileus that often complicates convalescence can be slow to relent, and parenteral feeding is then important.

At the other end of the scale of bleeding, it must be constantly remembered, when performing a laparotomy for abdominal trauma, that the signs of retroperitoneal perforation of the duodenum, or rupture of the pancreas, may be few (p. 430). There may appear at first to be nothing amiss, until the small bowel is brought out of the abdomen and a methodical search is made. The unusual but important sign of blood lying under the peritoneum at the root of the transverse mesocolon is characteristic of an occult rupture of the body of the pancreas.

REFERENCES

Costa, M. and Robbs, J. V. (1985) Management of retroperitoneal haematoma following penetrating trauma. *Br. J. Surg.*, **76**, 662–664.

Dove, A. F., Poon, W. S. and Weston, P. A. M. (1981) Haemorrhage from pelvic fractures: dangers and treatment. *Injury*, **13**, 375–381.

Hurt, A. V., Ochsner, J. L. and Schiller, W. R. (1983) Prolonged ileus after severe pelvic fracture. *Am. J. Surg.*, **146**, 755–757.

Matalon, T. S. A., Athanasoulis, C. A., Margolies, M. N. *et al.* (1979) Hemorrhage with pelvic fractures: efficacy of transcatheter embolization. *A.J.R.*, **133**, 859–864.

Selivanov, V., Chi, H. S., Alverdy, J. C. *et al.* (1984) Mortality in retroperitoneal haematoma. *J. Trauma*, **24**, 1022–1027.

10.10   THORACOABDOMINAL INJURIES

The liver, stomach and spleen lie within the thoracic cage, so any penetrating wound of the lower chest may traverse the diaphragm and injure these or other abdominal viscera. Some 10–15% of lower thoracic stab wounds and 30–40% of missile injuries to the chest enter the abdomen. Penetration of the thorax from an abdominal wound occurs but is very much less common. In 90% of thoracoabdominal penetrations, the entry wound lies below the fourth rib anteriorly and the tip of the scapula posteriorly. All stab wounds will occur in this area and the majority of these will be in the left lower chest, which is where a right-handed assailant is most likely to land the blow. However in missile injuries, especially those from a high-velocity weapon, the entry wound may be anywhere in the chest, neck or shoulder. On the right side, missiles tend to arrest within the liver, but on the left they are liable to travel on, involving stomach and colon, and a much higher risk of bacterial contamination (Huizinga *et al.*, 1987).

Diagnosis

Any penetrating injury of the thorax is likely to cause a haemo- and/or pneumothorax, and these injuries may initially dominate the clinical picture and call for urgent action. Occasionally, omentum has visibly prolapsed through the entry wound. If there is an exit as well as an entry wound of a missile it is usually possible to decide on the viscera likely to have been injured during its passage. When there is abdominal visceral injury there are usually signs of abdominal tenderness and guarding. Sandrasagra (1977) studied 23 thoraco-abdominal wounds among 100 consecutive patients with penetrating chest wounds. He found signs of peritoneal irritation in 15 but in eight there were no abdominal signs: in five of the eight injury was limited to the diaphragm and the liver and in three the visceral injuries were confined to the lesser sac. Absence of bowel sounds over a period of 2 minutes is likely to be significant. Radiography of the chest and abdomen may reveal retained foreign bodies. Talbert *et al.* (1980) found that when there was doubt about the direction taken by a missile, and few abdominal signs, peritoneal lavage was helpful in identifying patients with abdominal injuries, and laparoscopy can also provide information (Sosa *et al.*, 1992).

10.10.1 TRAUMATIC RUPTURE OF THE DIAPHRAGM

Faced with a patient with an abdominal injury it must be remembered that one of the possible effects is a rupture of the diaphragm. The surgeon must consider this possibility during examination and endeavour to prevent late complications by reaching a diagnosis at the time of injury. It is not a common injury, and signs can be few, so it is very liable to be overlooked.

In civilian practice the incidence of penetrating and closed injuries will depend on the country in which the report is written. In Johannesburg, Adamthwaite (1984) reported 34 cases, and more than half (19) were due to stab wounds. In the UK, penetrating wounds of the diaphragm are rare, and nearly all are due to blunt injury. These closed injuries are generally the more serious because the causative injury is generally severe. Hence associated injuries to the head, pelvis and long bones, which in themselves carry a serious prognosis, are common. In addition the tear of the diaphragm tends to be long, so allowing herniation of viscera and consequent cardiorespiratory embarrassment.

Closed diaphragmatic rupture

Bowditch (1853) reviewed 68 cases and emphasized the signs of absent breath sounds in the affected hemithorax, and the mediastinal shift. Bryan (1921) in a Hunterian Lecture described a girl of 5, run over by a taxicab, with a tear of the left diaphragm through which stomach and colon had entered the left pleural sac, causing complete collapse of the left lung and marked mediastinal shift to the right. This case illustrates some characteristic features: the severe crushing road traffic injury, the preponderance of left-sided injuries and the severe effects on heart and lungs. Harley (1977) made a study of 58 personally treated patients; 34 were involved in a road accident. A few others had been crushed between objects or fallen from a height, while 12 were coal miners injured underground. There were serious concomitant injuries in 45 (77%). Almost all the tears were radial in direction, in the left half of the diaphragm. The mechanism of the rupture is not certain, although it seems to involve a sudden rise of intra-abdominal pressure, acting on the diaphragm which is unprotected and has negative intrathoracic pressure acting on its upper surface. It may be necessary for the glottis to be open at the moment of impact (Harley, 1977). This theory would explain why the presence of the liver largely protects the right hemidiaphragm and the majority of diaphragmatic ruptures affect the left side. Once a tear has occurred, this negative pressure will encourage herniation of abdominal viscera into the chest.

Clinical features

Rupture of the diaphragm usually occurs when a severe force is exerted on the abdomen so patients are often shocked and have other serious injuries. In the 47 patients seen by Lucido and Wall (1963), 21 had a ruptured spleen, 15 had a fractured pelvis, eight had a fractured femur and 11 had severe head injuries. Other reports make the same point (Guth *et al.*, 1995). In particular, there is an association between fracture of the pelvis and rupture of the diaphragm. There are therefore likely to be signs arising from other injuries in ill patients, so it is not difficult to miss the presence of diaphragmatic rupture at the time of injury. In patients whose rupture is recognized, dyspnoea, tachycardia, cyanosis and hiccup are generally seen and examination will show absence of breath sounds, mediastinal shift and poor movement of the affected chest. Most patients are hypotensive.

Chest radiography can often establish the diagnosis beyond reasonable doubt. It should be a rule to take an X-ray of the chest in all patients who sustain an injury to the trunk. It is usually abnormal or atypical but can be completely normal (Guth *et al.*, 1995). Several radiological appearances are suggestive of herniation.

- A high arched shadow crossing the left pleural space. This shadow is thrown by the fundus of the herniated stomach but it can look very like an elevated left diaphragm and is liable to be reported as such. Beware of this conclusion, especially when it is combined with mediastinal shift. Nearly all so-called eventrations after injury are in fact diaphragmatic ruptures.
- Shift of the mediastinum to the right.
- There may be considerable opacification of the left hemithorax by blood, especially at the base, when it may be confused with a high diaphragm. Careful inspection may show gas-filled spaces, which will indicate the presence of herniated loops of large intestine. Sometimes the outline of the spleen can be seen above the diaphragm.
- In right-sided rupture the hemidiaphragm appears to be very high: this is the shadow of the liver, which has prolapsed into the chest through a large rent in the dome.

The experience of Ebert *et al.* (1967) shows that these signs need to be looked for. In 29 patients, 12 had a negative chest X-ray while in ten radiographic signs were present but went unrecognized. There should be no hesitation over having a further chest film after 2–3 days, when there may be clear signs of herniation (Salleh, 1973).

Passage of a nasogastric tube can be very helpful. It may obstruct at the lower end of the oesophagus because the stomach has rotated up into the chest or it may enter the herniated stomach and be seen in the thorax in the X-ray. An injection of gastrografin may clarify the situation. If this happens the tube may allow valuable decompression of the air under tension in the stomach, which will greatly ease respiration. This can be quite an important part of treatment before induction of anaesthesia.

The delayed presentation of a traumatic diaphragmatic hernia can present considerable problems because it will, by definition, occur in a person who has been well, and has forgotten about the injury that caused the undiagnosed hernia.

Guth *et al.* (1995) reported 57 patients with a diaphragmatic hernia due to blunt abdominal trauma. In 50 the diagnosis was made within 24 hours. In 29 left-sided tears the chest X-ray was diagnostic; in 21 the tear was discovered when the severity of injury to other viscera made it necessary to undertake emergency laparotomy or thoracotomy. In seven patients diagnosis was delayed between 2 days and 3 months, when new symptoms required further investigation. Delay in diagnosis can be much more prolonged and is considered in Chapter 5.

Evidence is accumulating that the more liberal use of thoracoscopy (Spann *et al.*, 1995) and laparoscopy (Sosa *et al.*, 1993; Simon and Ivatury, 1995) will reduce the incidence of delayed herniation and the morbidity of a formal cavity exploration.

Treatment

In penetrating injuries haemo- and/or pneumothorax will require immediate attention. It must generally be assumed that a missile that could have entered the abdomen will have caused visceral damage. However, if X-rays show a bullet lodged in the liver this may be best left alone, with a drain to remove any leakage of bile. It is usually best to excise and close the thoracic wound, with intercostal drainage, and then make a thorough search of the abdomen at laparotomy.

In blunt injuries of the left diaphragm the patient may be acutely ill, with herniated viscera in the chest and mediastinal displacement. In close cooperation with the anaesthetist the abdomen is opened and the viscera are reduced and suitably repaired; colon, spleen and stomach are those most often displaced. Intercostal drainage is established, the thorax washed out and the diaphragmatic rent repaired with non-absorbable sutures. A period in intensive care is likely to be needed.

REFERENCES

Adamthwaite, D. N. (1984) Diaphragmatic hernia presenting itself as a surgical emergency. *Injury*, **15**, 367–369.

Bowditch, H. I. (1853) Diaphragmatic hernia. *Buffalo Med. J.*, **9**, 65.

Bryan, C. W. G. (1921) Injuries of the diaphragm: with special reference to abdomino-thoracic wounds. *Br. J. Surg.*, **9**, 117–147.

Ebert, P. A., Gaerter, R. A. and Zuidema, G. D. (1967) Traumatic diaphragmatic hernia. *Surg. Gynecol. Obstet.*, **125**, 59–65.

Guth, A. A., Pachter, H. L. and Kim, U. (1995) Pitfalls in the diagnosis of blunt diaphragmatic injury. *Am. J. Surg.*, **170**, 5–9.

Harley, H. R. S. (1977) Traumatic diaphragmatic hernia due to blunt injury, in *Trauma of the Chest*, (eds W. G. Williams and R. E. Smith), John Wright, Bristol, p. 80.

Huizinga, W. K. J., Mtshali, Z. and Baker, L. W. (1987) Selective management of abdominal and thoracic stab wounds with established peritoneal penetration. The eviscerated omentum. *Am. J. Surg.*, **153**, 564–568.

Lucido, J. L. and Wall, C. A. (1963) Rupture of the diaphragm due to blunt trauma. *Arch. Surg.*, **86**, 989–999.

Salleh, H. B. M. (1973) Diaphragmatic rupture due to blunt trauma. *Br. J. Surg.*, **60**, 430–433.

Sandrasagra, F. A. (1977) Penetrating thoraco-abdominal injuries. *Br. J. Surg.*, **64**, 638–640.

Simon, R. J. and Ivatury, R. R. (1995) Current concepts in the use of cavitary endoscopy in the evaluation and treatment of blunt and penetrating truncal injuries (review). *Surg. Clin. North Am.*, **75**, 157–174.

Sosa, J. L., Sims, D., Martin, L. and Zepp, R. (1992) Laparoscopic evaluation of tangential gunshot wounds. *Arch. Surg.*, **127**, 109–110.

Sosa, J. L., Markley, M., Sleeman, D. *et al.* (1993) Laparoscopy in abdominal gunshot wounds. *Surg. Laparosc. Endosc.*, **3**, 417–419.

Spann, J. C., Nwariaku, F. E. and Wait, M. (1995) Evaluation of video assisted thoracoscopic surgery in the diagnosis of diaphragmatic injuries. *Am. J. Surg.*, **170**(6), 628–630.

Talbert, J., Graenberg, J. C., Sy, G. and Brown, R. S. (1980) Peritoneal lavage in penetrating thoracic trauma. *J. Trauma*, **20**, 979–981.

10.11   SEAT-BELT INJURIES

The use of lap–shoulder seat belts by the drivers and front-seat passengers of motor vehicles has reduced the risk of death in a collision by 43% (Evans, 1987). However, the pressure exerted by the belt at the moment of impact on the chest and abdomen can be great: if the belt is loose or the subject is sitting awkwardly, the lap belt can exert pressure not on the iliac crests as intended but on any part of the alimentary tract lying between the abdominal wall and the lumbar spine. As a consequence, perforation of the small bowel and tears of the mesentery are particularly likely to occur; occasionally the colon is involved.

Ryan and Ragazzon (1979) compared abdominal injuries seen in the 6 years before and the 6 years after the wearing of seat-belts became compulsory in Victoria, Australia. Injuries to the kidneys and spleen remained at the same level, but injuries to the liver were halved, while intestinal injuries doubled. There was a noticeable increase in diaphragmatic injuries, and this was attributed to the sharp increase in intra-abdominal pressure that occurs when the lap belt is driven into the abdomen.

The important practical result of these intestinal injuries is that they do not immediately produce symptoms. In common with all blunt injuries of the intestines, leakage is generally delayed, so there may be few signs, and these patients may be allowed home from the accident department. A serious view must be taken of any hint of abdominal pain or tenderness and a very careful search made for tattoo marks on the skin of the chest or abdomen caused by the pressure of the belt (Pedersen and Jansen, 1979).

When signs of peritoneal irritation indicate the need for laparotomy, it must be remembered that great force was applied over the whole length of the belt, so more than one loop of bowel and its mesentery may be affected: close attention must be paid to the quality of the mesenteric circulation when repairing or resecting the bowel.

REFERENCES

Evans, L. (1987) Fatality risk reduction from seat-belt use. *J. Trauma*, **27**, 746–749.

Pedersen, S. and Jansen, U. (1979) Intestinal lesions caused by incorrectly placed seat-belts. *Acta Chir. Scand.*, **145**, 15–18.

Ryan, P. and Ragazzon, R. (1979) Abdominal injuries in survivors of road trauma before and since seat-belt legislation in Victoria. *Austr. N.Z. J. Surg.*, **49**, 200–202.

10.12   CONCLUSIONS

In summary it is important to be aware of the mechanism and pattern of injury encountered. This will dictate the injuries suspected and subsequently found. Effective resuscitation on well-founded principles is an absolute prerequisite for success. Laparotomy may well be necessary as an integral part of resuscitation. The patient must be viewed as a whole and not as a set of individual injuries being treated by different surgeons. In certain patients with massive injuries the damage control approach has much to commend it and requires senior personnel to be present to make the critical decisions involved. The operative solution for individual organ injuries requires a sound anatomical knowledge, surgical judgement and technical expertise for a successful outcome. These are skills not idly acquired.

Understanding the pathophysiological sequelae of the injury and its treatment is essential in the postoperative phase when major organ support systems are utilized. The need to return to the abdomen in selected cases must be remembered and is a sign of surgical maturity not inadequacy. Adopting these approaches at the various phases in management will result in the optimal outcome not only for the simple injuries but for those who have been most severely traumatized.

11

Urological emergencies

11.1 INTRODUCTION

In family practice, and in Accident and Emergency departments, urinary tract emergencies are often seen. Some patients merit elective review at a urological clinic, but a number have to be admitted because of the severity of their complaint. In many hospitals these patients come under the care of general surgeons. The aim of this chapter is to review the major urological emergencies and to suggest guidance on management that can be safely followed by the emergency surgeon. This has become even more important as the shortened training programme and the early specialization of surgical trainees in the UK and throughout the world has meant that the experience of these trainees in urological procedures has been reduced considerably. Expedient care provides much for these patients. It is recognized, however, that the preliminary treatment may require subsequent definitive specialist attention.

11.2 ACUTE URINARY TRACT INFECTION

Acute urinary tract infection (UTI) presents as acute cystitis and is readily recognized and treated on an outpatient basis. The infections that the general surgeon may meet as emergencies are likely to offer more difficulty in diagnosis, and require prompt treatment.

An ill, febrile, fretful, restless infant who has refused feeds and vomits, may well have an acute UTI. Too young to complain, and without noticeable urinary complaints – being still in nappies – it is essential to include urinalysis in the examination. A clean-catch specimen is needed, or failing this a catheter specimen obtained *via* the urethra or by suprapubic puncture. Microscopy will show more than ten pus cells per high power field, and culture more than 10^5 bacteria/ml. Following control of the sepsis, full urological investigation is needed because a significant congenital abnormality is likely to be found in 35–40% (McKerrow *et al.*, 1984). In older children and in pregnant women an attack of acute pyelitis is likely to present with shivering, malaise, pain in the back and loin, dysuria and a fever of 39–40°C. If there is obstruction to drainage from the kidney, there may be tenderness and even some guarding over the kidney and ureter. This can raise suspicions of appendicitis or,

Emergency Abdominal Surgery. Edited by Peter F. Jones, Zygmunt H. Krukowski and George G. Youngson. Published in 1998 by Chapman & Hall, London. ISBN 0 412 81950 3.

on the left, diverticulitis. The urine will usually show evidence of infection, but if there is ureteric obstruction this may be absent. An urgent ultrasound scan may be very helpful. Serious damage can occur in the infected and obstructed kidney, and if pyonephrosis is present, relief of the obstruction is needed. It may be possible to pass a ureteric stent to achieve decompression (p. 499), or a percutaneous nephrostomy may be required.

In 75–80% of acute UTI the responsible organism is *E. coli*. If S. *faecalis, Pseudomonas* or *Proteus* is grown this suggests a more chronic infection due to stones, a neoplasm, or urinary stasis. Prompt antibiotic treatment of any acute UTI needs to be based on the likely sensitivity of the infecting organism. These sensitivities will vary from hospital to hospital. For the seriously ill patient the intravenous route may be appropriate. In the latter group gentamicin, cefotaxime or ciprofloxacin are useful first-line antibiotics, although sensitivities must be checked as soon as possible.

REFERENCE

McKerrow, W., Davidson-Lamb, N. and Jones, P. F. (1984) Urinary tract infection in children. *BMJ.*, **289**, 299–303.

11.3   ACUTE OBSTRUCTION OF THE RENAL PELVIS AND URETER

Acute obstruction of the ureter by a calculus is a regular cause of admission to a surgical unit. Most other causes of obstruction are unusual. Congenital narrowing of the pelviureteric junction can become a complete obstruction and in older patients a renal neoplasm may present with clot colic.

11.3.1   RENAL AND URETERIC CALCULI

Urinary calculi are two or three times more common in men than women, and most patients are between 30 and 60 years of age. In the older man pain in the loin and flank may well be due to a leaking abdominal aortic aneurysm and failure to consider this may have dire consequences (p. 519).

'Renal colic' is a convenient but inaccurate term. Oxalate stones, which account for 75–80% of all cases, are rough and irregular and usually impact in the ureter – at the pelviureteric junction, the pelvic brim or the ureterovesical junction. The result is the sharp onset of severe, agonizing, pain which is felt in the loin, flank, iliac fossa or referred into the scrotum or vulva, depending on the point of impaction. Pallor and sweating are noticeable, as is the restless change of position as the patient seeks relief – a very different picture to the stillness of the patient with peritonitis. These patients may be nauseated and vomit. Haematuria is noticeable in about one-third, but microscopic haematuria is usually present. Abdominal signs are not impressive, though there may be some tenderness over the kidney or ureter. This will be more marked if the urine is infected and there is a measure of obstruction.

The patient will describe the pain as the worst they have ever had and therefore the early administration of an analgesic is essential. Diclofenac sodium is the drug of choice but an opiate may be needed. Not only is there no advantage in attempting to force a diuresis by administering a high volume of fluids, it may be harmful (O'Flynn, 1980). Anticholinergic drugs are not helpful.

An intravenous urogram (IVU) is the investigation of choice. Only 7–10% of stones are non-opaque, and the plain film will often reveal a stone, although a small one may be lost over the shadow of the pelvic bones. In an emergency IVU, films are exposed at 5 and 30 minutes, when a nephrogram is often seen. A film taken at 3–4 hours is likely to show a dilated pelvis, or the ureter outlined down to the impacted stone – when the stone is small this may be the only way of identifying it. Further films, taken with the patient prone at 12–24 hours after injection, will show the degree of hold-up above the calculus.

Many stones pass spontaneously given time, and a useful guide is the diameter, measured on a plain X-ray. Sandegard (1956) studied 324 patients and found that in 90% the stone was less than 6 mm in width; 80–90% of small stones (less than 4 mm) and about half the stones 4–6 mm in width passed spontaneously within 6 weeks of diagnosis. Stones of all sizes which are retained in the upper half of the ureter often cause some obstruction to urine flow, but this is rarely complete, and a balance has to be struck between unduly early intervention and harmful delay. Provided there is no infection of the urine that is held back above a stone it is reasonable to await events, except in stones clearly too large to pass into the bladder. The patient is allowed home and advised to pass urine into a suitable container until the stone is seen to pass.

If no stone is recovered, and attacks of ureteric pain continue, a repeat X-ray is performed in 7–10 days. If there has been further descent it is reasonable to wait, especially for stones less than 6 mm in width. If the stone is stationary in the upper half of the ureter a further IVU is indicated, with a single film at 30 minutes to assess drainage and function. If this is satisfactory, observation should continue. Intervention has to be considered if pain is severe, or if there is increasing obstruction judged by loss of function. There are now a variety of extraction techniques available that have greatly reduced the indications for open operation – percutaneous nephrostomy, extracorporeal short-wave lithotripsy, and lithotripsy *via* the ureteroscope. These all require expert application.

For the surgeon who must treat these patients without urological assistance or access to the above techniques, there are various indications for intervention.

- If a small stone, up to 5 mm diameter, becomes stuck, simply passing a ureteric catheter beyond the calculus and retaining for 24 hours has proved useful in the past (O'Flynn, 1980). One could also use a ureteric stent, which will not only relieve the obstruction but may also dislodge the stone. A Dormier basket must only be used in the lower third of the ureter by an experienced operator as it can cause severe damage to the ureter.
- When a larger stone is stationary in the ureter and there is continuing pain, ureterolithotomy is indicated. Two rules must be observed.
  - The opacity must be confirmed to be a ureteric calculus. This is reasonably certain if the IVU shows the dilated ureter ending at the opacity. If this proof is lacking the presence of a stone must be confirmed by passing a ureteric catheter and injecting 2–3 ml of 45% Hypaque or a non-ionic contrast material to outline the ureter.
  - *En route* to the theatre a plain abdominal X-ray must be obtained because calculi have a surprising tendency to migrate on the day appointed for the operation, and the latest information must be available before making the incision. The techniques of ureterolithotomy are described in urological texts.

- There is some urgency when the kidney fails to opacify on the IVU, is tender and the patient becomes feverish and unwell. The distended and infected renal pelvis must be decompressed to forestall damage to the kidney. After removal of the calculus, a ureteric stent should be passed through the ureterotomy up into the renal pelvis and down into the bladder to ensure that there is no other obstruction and to splint the ureter. It can be retrieved subsequently.
- Occasionally no radio-opaque calculus is demonstrated. This may be because the stone is radiolucent, and then the IVU usually shows hold-up in the ureteric phase. The obstruction may not be due to a stone. Congenital pelviureteric junction narrowing can cause obstruction, or it can occur in pregnancy, with functional obstruction of the right ureter at the pelvic brim.
- In older patients, with clot obstruction, a neoplasm of the kidney, renal pelvis, or ureter has to be considered.

REFERENCES

O'Flynn, J. D. (1980) The treatment of ureteric stones: report on 1120 patients. *Br. J. Urol.*, **52**, 436–438.
Sandegard, E. (1956) Prognosis of stone in the ureter. *Acta Chir. Scand. Suppl.*, **21**.

11.3.2 CALCULOUS ANURIA

This is rare and is usually due to calculous obstruction of the only functioning kidney. In this urgent situation drainage must be established by inserting either a nephrostomy or ureteric stent. If the stone is easily removable this can be combined with urinary drainage.

11.3.3 SPONTANEOUS RUPTURE OF THE KIDNEY AND URETER

This is a rare event, although Kettlewell *et al.* (1973) describe 16 patients seen over 18 months. The rupture may occur in the renal parenchyma or the pelvis, and is usually due to impaction of a calculus (Shaw, 1957). Such extravasation should be treated by decompression of the upper urinary tract with a ureteric stent. The stone can then be treated on its own merit.

While some of these patients present with classical renal/ureteric colic, others present with an acute abdomen and, on the right side, are explored as a case of acute appendicitis. The caecum is found to be floating forward on a retroperitoneal collection of urine. Unless a stone can be felt in the ureter it is wise to drain the retroperitoneal space and await the result of an IVU. If possible the IVU should be carried out at the time of the laparotomy as it may be prudent to relieve the ureteric obstruction under the same anaesthetic.

REFERENCES

Kettlewell, M., Walker, M., Dudley, N. *et al.* (1973) Spontaneous extravasation of urine secondary to ureteric obstruction. *Br. J. Urol.*, **45**, 8–14.
Shaw, R. E. (1957) Spontaneous rupture of the kidney. *Br. J. Surg.*, **45**, 68–72.

11.4 ACUTE RETENTION OF URINE

Good management of this common condition calls for medical as well as surgical skills. The great majority of patients have bladder outlet obstruction due to benign hyperplasia or carcinoma of the prostate. It is, however, important to recognize other causes of retention. It can be caused by malignant spinal cord compression due to metastatic carcinoma, and recognition allows prompt spinal decompression. Paraplegia may be avoided if the diagnosis is made in time. Patients with bladder outflow obstruction give a characteristic history but often have chronic respiratory and cardiac disease, which affects selection of treatment. Faecal impaction is a cause of retention in long-stay patients and children with encopresis. Neurological examination in a young adult may identify signs of multiple sclerosis. Few women are affected: retroversion of a large fibroid or gravid uterus may obstruct the bladder and large ovarian cysts have been confused with a distended bladder. Patients with oliguria or anuria may be referred with an inaccurate diagnosis of retention and an ultrasound scan is valuable in showing an empty bladder. Urethral stricture is now an uncommon cause of retention.

11.4.1 PROSTATIC OBSTRUCTION

Most patients arrive in distress and need urgent relief from their acute retention. A well-directed history and examination should define the likely cause, and in prostatic obstruction catheterization should be promptly carried out. A rectal examination carried out prior to relieving the retention is unlikely to be of value as the distended bladder will push the prostate down.

Catheterization of the bladder is usually a straightforward procedure but can be extremely difficult and hazardous for the patient. It should be performed carefully, bearing mind that urinary tract infection is the commonest nosocomial infection. If, as is usual, it is decided to pass a urethral catheter, it must be remembered that the urethra is a delicate structure easily injured by the use of undue force, for which the long-term penalty – for the patient – is a stricture.

After 48 hours it is reasonable to remove the catheter and many manage to micturate satisfactorily. An outpatient appointment is then made for the urological clinic. Those who cannot pass have to be re-catheterized and then referred to a urologist. Occasionally, passage of a catheter in the presence of infected urine precipitates an episode of bacteraemia and endotoxaemia. This is a serious event and needs vigorous treatment with intravenous fluids and antibiotics effective against the likely organisms such as the coliforms and enterococci. Appropriate antibiotics include cefotaxime, co-amoxiclav, ciprofloxacin and gentamicin.

If an inexperienced operator has one unsuccessful attempt to pass a catheter then more senior help should be sought. Success in catheterization depends considerably on experience and one further attempt by the senior doctor can be made. If this fails, and especially if there is any blood on the catheter tip, it is right to proceed to closed suprapubic catheterization (p. 482). This gives the patient speedy relief, allows the uraemic patient time to recover and minimizes the risk of injury to the urethra.

In patients with chronic retention without renal impairment it may not be necessary to pass a catheter as many of these patients can pass urine by 'overflow'. These patients should be referred to the urologist, who will have the opportunity to operate on an patient with an uninfected lower urinary tract. A catheter should be passed if there is renal impairment, or if the patient is uncomfortable, or distressed by overflow incontinence. It is now accepted that there is no need to decompress the bladder slowly.

11.4.2   CLOT RETENTION

The patient is likely to be particularly uncomfortable, pale and hypovolaemic with an unusually tense bladder. There may be some blood at the external meatus; if a catheter is passed little urine drains, and there is blood clot in the eye of the catheter. Sometimes this can be treated by passing a three-way catheter and using irrigation, but it may be necessary to give a general anaesthetic, pass a wide cystoscope and suck out the clot with a 50 ml syringe. Further investigation will be required. Most cases are due to bleeding from a vascular, hyperplastic prostate rather than from a malignant neoplasm.

11.4.3   FAILURE TO PASS A CATHETER

This arises in several situations.

11.4.3.1   Meatal stenosis

This is immediately evident at the first attempt. In an older patient acute retention should be relieved by inserting a suprapubic catheter under local anaesthesia. This allows time for a general assessment and recognition of other problems, e.g. prostatic obstruction. In a young, fit patient it is reasonable to give a general anaesthetic and dilate up the meatus with graduated straight metal bougies. The bladder is then emptied with a catheter. The patient should then be reviewed at a urological outpatient clinic. If the stenosis is recurring a meatotomy will be needed.

11.4.3.2   Urethral stricture

This condition, once common, is now unusual. Some date from an accident and it is salutary to recognize that most strictures are now iatrogenic in origin. If the patient is not aware of having a stricture, a catheter is likely to be passed, and will be held up, usually in the bulb. Irregularity or a fold in the urethra can cause this and it is worthwhile for an experienced operator to attempt very gentle passage of an 18 FG urethral sound (e.g. Clutton's). This may negotiate a fold or the external sphincter, and can be followed by a Foley catheter. If it does not pass or the operator is at all worried then suprapubic catheterization is needed. A urologist can then carry out a urethroscopy and dilate the stricture or perform a urethrotomy.

11.4.3.3   Impacted urethral calculus

This is a rare event, which may follow an episode of ureteric colic or may be due to a stone originating in the bladder. The patient experiences acute pain in the urethra and sudden arrest of the urinary stream. The stone tends to impact in the penile urethra and so may be palpable. In the presence of acute retention it is wiser to insert a suprapubic catheter. The patient can then undergo a urethroscopy on the urology list, when it may be possible to break up the stone with a pneumatic lithotripter. If this fails and the stone is in the penile urethra, it should be removed through a short central incision and the urethra closed with one or two sutures. After 72 hours the suprapubic catheter can be clamped and the patient allowed to pass urine normally. There are rarely any long-term sequelae.

11.4.3.4 Phimosis

This is an unusual cause of actual retention, but sometimes a boy is seen with ballooning of the preputial space, and a thin stream of urine is spraying out from a minute opening in the foreskin. The treatment is circumcision.

In the adult, balanitis xerotica obliterans can cause extreme narrowing of the preputial orifice. The emergency treatment is either a dorsal slit or a circumcision. The former can be performed under a local anaesthetic.

11.4.3.5 Paraphimosis

This is a painful accident that is liable to befall any uncircumcised male with a degree of phimosis. The preputial meatus is relatively inelastic so, when an erection occurs or the foreskin is drawn back, the soft glans penis emerges through the preputial opening with difficulty. When the opening is fairly small there will be some obstruction to venous return from the glans, and it immediately becomes cyanosed and shiny. If the prepuce is not speedily brought forward the oedema of the glans will increase and it will become irreducible. A paraphimosis then exists. This must be promptly treated both because it is painful and because damage can occur to the unreduced glans.

Manipulation and cold compression can often effect reduction. The oedema can be reduced by compressing the glans between the surgeon's palms for several minutes. Then the operator sits facing the patient, with two thumbs compressing the glans and the index and middle fingers hooked behind the foreskin. With forbearance on the part of the patient, and some patience, this is often successful.

However, paraphimosis is an embarrassing complaint and this leads to delay before the patient seeks advice. By then, and especially in boys, manipulation may not be practicable or tolerated. Under a general anaesthetic reduction can usually be achieved. These patients should be advised to have a circumcision which can, if appropriate, be carried out during the same admission. If there is reflex retention of urine the bladder should be emptied with a catheter, which is then removed.

11.4.4 SUPRAPUBIC CATHETERIZATION

A large, tense bladder can usually be seen and felt but if, as in an obese patient, there is doubt, it must be visualized by ultrasound. It is nearly always possible to perform closed catheterization but this is only safe if the bladder is full. Even with a previous lower abdominal incision it is possible and safe to carry out the procedure if the fundus of the bladder lies at the umbilicus.

This operation must not be performed by a novice except under expert supervision, and only an experienced surgeon should operate on an obese patient.

The patient lies flat and the suprapubic area is shaved, cleaned and isolated with sterile towels. The operator is gowned and scrubbed. The skin 2 fingerbreadths above the symphysis pubis is infiltrated with lignocaine and adrenaline, and this is carried down to and through the linea alba, which can be felt as a point of resistance. Allow 5 minutes for this to take effect.

An appropriate trocar and catheter is used. First, pass a spinal needle mounted on a 5 ml syringe vertically down the anaesthetized track into the bladder, and aspirate urine – this confirms that the bladder can be safely entered along this track. Incise the skin at this point and advance the scalpel down to and just through the linea alba. Hold the trocar and catheter vertically – it should not be directed downwards – and pass it in a controlled manner down the incised track and onwards into the bladder. The trocar is removed and the catheter is immediately spigoted, so that while the bladder is distended the catheter can be advanced and the balloon inflated. The catheter is attached to the drainage system, and as the bladder empties the balloon may descend and draw the catheter further in. When the bladder is empty, advance the catheter another 2–3 cm before fixing at skin level. These precautions are important to ensure that the catheter cannot escape from the bladder.

Open suprapubic cystostomy is now rarely required. The main exception arises when the urethra is ruptured, the bladder must be drained and is likely to be impalpable. It then has to be located through a Pfannenstiel incision. The rectus muscles are separated and the bladder is located behind the symphysis pubis. The front of the bladder is cleared by sweeping fat and the peritoneal fold upwards with a swab. The detrusor fibres and blood vessels should then be seen, and two stay sutures are inserted. A needle mounted on a syringe is inserted between them and urine is aspirated to confirm identification of the bladder. A stab incision is made in the skin and rectus sheath above the incision, and a 22 FG or 24 FG plastic Foley catheter is passed through it. With the sucker working an incision is made between the stay sutures and the catheter is inserted into the bladder and the balloon inflated. If necessary this incision is narrowed around the catheter with an absorbable suture. The catheter is attached to the drainage system, the bladder is emptied and the catheter secured with a strong suture to the skin at a suitable level, and the incision is closed.

11.5 SCROTAL EMERGENCIES

11.5.1 TRAUMA

There is usually a history of injury. There may be visible bruising or a laceration. If the testicle is acutely tense and tender a haematocele must be suspected, and explored. Lacerations will require exploration, excision and suture. The value of ultrasound scanning in testicular trauma is controversial.

Scrotal haematomata can follow any elective operation such as procedures on epididymal cysts, hydroceles or vasectomies. Their occurrence can lead to significant morbidity with fibrosis and scrotal thickening. Haemostasis at the initial operation should therefore be meticulous. If a haematoma does develop then the blood collects in the scrotal wall and exploration, unless the haematoma is expanding, is rarely of value.

Occasionally a blow on the scrotum leads to examination and a symptomless swelling of the testicle is found. This may be the manner in which a neoplasm is discovered.

11.5.2 ACUTE EPIDIDYMITIS, EPIDIDYMO-ORCHITIS AND TORSION

Judged on physical signs alone, these three conditions cannot be reliably differentiated. Age gives some indication because 75% of torsions occur in the first 20 years of life, especially between 10 and 20, compared to only 27% of cases of epididymitis/epididymo-orchitis. Fewer than 3% of torsions occur over the age of 30 (Goulborne *et al.*, 1984). In torsion the other testis usually shows a horizontal lie, and the torted testicle lies high in the scrotum. In early epididymitis the lower pole is first affected and is distinctly palpable apart from the testis, and the cord is thickened. In epididymo-orchitis both the testicle and epididymis are swollen and extremely tender. The patient may be pyrexial and the urine infected. These distinctions are rarely clear-cut, and many testicles have been lost from holding to a diagnosis of infection for too long: the only safe course when in doubt is to explore the scrotum without delay (p. 133). Ultrasound scanning may be of value in determining whether an abscess is present and to differentiate between a infective process and a malignant tumour.

Patients with epididymitis/epididymo-orchitis usually respond quickly to antibiotic treatment, extra fluids and bed rest unless an abscess has formed. Antibiotics active against urinary tract organisms should used.

11.5.3 IDIOPATHIC SCROTAL GANGRENE

This uncommon condition is an anaerobic necrotizing cellulitis of the scrotal and perineal coverings. Although Fournier first described the condition in healthy young men in 1884, it is now seen more frequently in the elderly and a similar condition occasionally affects the perivulval tissues in women. We have seen it in a young man during treatment of major trauma with high-dose inotropes who developed classical Fournier's gangrene with sloughing of the entire scrotal skin due to intense vasospasm. There is a strong association with diabetes mellitus, and it may follow scrotal or urethral injury and abdominal surgery.

The patient is suddenly taken with severe pain in the scrotum; within hours it is red and swollen and in 24–48 hours the patient is acutely ill and patches of gangrene appear, accompanied by a faeculent odour. There may be crepitus in the tissues. There is a remarkable localization to the scrotum and, in preantibiotic days, the whole scrotal skin would slough away, leaving the testes viable and exposed. Culture of the pus shows a polymicrobial flora – anaerobic haemolytic streptococci with *E. coli*, staphylococci and *Bacteroides* spp., and microscopy shows an obliterative endarteritis (Hejase *et al.*, 1996).

Treatment must be commenced immediately: diabetes is often out of control, and septicaemia is a real threat so systematic treatment with metronidazole, ampicillin and gentamicin is started. As soon as possible the sensitivities are reviewed. Local treatment requires thorough debridement of all dead tissue, which often means removal of the scrotal skin. Hejase *et al.* (1996) treated 38 patients and found that 25 were diabetic. In 33 the penile skin was also affected, and 23 required a suprapubic cystostomy. Honey dressings were found to be very effective in cleaning the wound and encouraging granulations over the exposed testes, which survive through the testicular circulation. When ready, the area can be covered with skin grafts, and the final results are generally good.

REFERENCES

Goulbourne, I. A., Nixon, S. J. and Macintyre, I. M. C. (1984) Computer-aided diagnosis in acute testicular pain. *Br. J. Surg.*, **71**, 528–531.

Hejase, M. J., Simonin, J. E., Bihrie, R. *et al.* (1996) Genital Fournier's gangrene: experience with 38 patients. *Urology*, **47**, 734–739.

11.6   INJURIES OF THE URINARY TRACT

11.6.1   PENILE INJURIES

Lacerations of the penis should be repaired by suturing or by a circumcision. The most common cause is the trouser zip, although other rarer causes have been reported.

11.6.2   RENAL INJURIES

Blunt abdominal trauma injures the kidney more often than any other viscus, while the ureter is the most rarely injured structure. Bass *et al.* (1991) in Cape Town found that the kidney was affected in 56% of 587 children admitted after blunt abdominal injury and in Leeds, among 265 patients of all ages, 40% had a renal injury (Wilson, 1963). It may be that this high frequency is related to the ease with which haematuria can be detected, and in fact most kidney injuries are not serious. The incidence of penetrating injury varies considerably – it is relatively unusual in Western Europe but in Detroit, among 102 patients with a major renal injury, 67 were due to gunshot, 20 to stab wounds and only 15 to blunt injury (Hai *et al.*, 1977). Penetrating injuries are considered in Chapter 10, p. 468.

Pathology

- Most injuries are contusions. The parenchyma is broken, with some interstitial haemorrhage, but the capsule is intact. The IVU may show some impairment of concentration but no deformity. These injuries heal naturally.
- Capsular rupture implies that a perirenal haematoma forms, but it is limited and is absorbed. These two types account for 80–85% of injuries.
- Parenchymal rupture means that a deeper tear has involved one or more calyces, so extravasation of urine occurs. Severity varies from a localized injury, which can heal, to a serious disruption that causes an increasing perirenal haematoma, or bleeding into the collecting system, with brisk haemorrhage down the ureter.
- Vascular injury is most likely to result from a deceleration accident – in a fall from a height the momentum in the solid kidney exerts sufficient traction on the vascular pedicle to cause intimal damage or, rarely, disruption of a vessel. Both these types of injury can require urgent surgical intervention.

Clinical picture

About 80% of adult patients are males, and 75% are below the age of 30, but in children the sexes are about equal in number (Bass *et al.*, 1991). Road accidents, sports (especially rugby football) and accidental falls at work and play account for most blunt injuries (Slade, 1971).

Haematuria is nearly always present, and in 70–80% it is macroscopic. However, the intensity of haematuria does not relate directly to the severity of the accident, and in patients with a severe vascular injury there may be no blood in the urine. In severe injuries there may be bruising over the flank, swelling and tenderness over the kidney, and evidence of serious blood loss.

Management

In assessing whether there is any evidence that the kidneys have been damaged following abdominal trauma there are two investigations that are of value in the Emergency Department. The first is ultrasound scanning and the second a high-dose IVU. In a patient with macroscopic haematuria an IVU should be carried out. If the patient has microscopic haematuria and is stable with no abdominal signs further investigations of the urinary tract are not required. In patients with macroscopic haematuria or with signs of intra- or extraperitoneal injury then an ultrasound scan as well as an IVU will be of value to assess the kidneys and other abdominal organs. One should remember that renal damage may be associated with liver or splenic injury. If an infusion IVU is carried out in the Emergency Department then a film after 10–20 minutes should be taken. This can be of value in three ways:

- It provides evidence of the function of the contralateral kidney. This can be of great significance if a major problem arises in the injured kidney. Slade (1971) found that five of 140 patients had little or no function in the contralateral kidney.
- Definite information is obtained on the injured kidney, and this can be important because a serious injury does not always produce immediate signs of bleeding in the loin.
- The injured kidney may already have been abnormal. In 140 renal injuries, Slade (1971) found 11 ipsilateral and two contralateral congenital hydronephroses, and in nine of the 11 the injury had disturbed drainage through the pelviureteric junction. A boy in our care stumbled in the playground, hitting his right flank, and came in 12 hours later having passed no urine. The bladder was empty and the right flank felt full. The IVU showed no evidence of a left kidney and faint signs of a large right hydronephrosis. Urgent exploration revealed a haematoma around the narrow pelviureteric junction. A pyeloplasty, with pyelostomy, was performed, after which he remained well.

After admission all these patients are kept in bed with frequent recordings. Each specimen of urine passed is examined for the presence or absence of blood. Regular examination of the patient should continue, remembering the delay that can occur before a secondary haemorrhage occurs. Evidence of other intra-abdominal damage may also become apparent (p. 423).

If the patient remains stable but there is evidence on the IVU of significant renal damage a contrast-enhanced CT gives a clearer demonstration of parenchymal damage. It must be remembered this exposes the patient to irradiation equivalent to some 400 chest X-rays. Most of these patients settle but when there is major disruption there is a danger of secondary haemorrhage at 7–10 days, and this can present considerable operative problems. When active bleeding from the kidney demands operative intervention there is a good case for approaching across the peritoneum, because this gives direct access to the vessels – this is important in both primary and secondary haemorrhage. Access to the right kidney is obtained by performing Kocher's mobilization of the duodenal loop. To approach the left kidney either the duodenojejunal flexure is widely mobilized and reflected to the right and the dissection is carried up beneath the transverse mesocolon, or the splenic flexure is reflected to the right thus exposing the kidney. Sometimes a partial nephrectomy can be performed, with suture of the defect in the renal pelvis and drainage *via* a ureteric stent. It is in these urgent situations that the information from the IVU performed in the Emergency Department can be so valuable.

Fowler *et al.* (1982) saw 201 patients with a renal injury and 174 were considered to have an insignificant injury on the basis of the admission IVU; these all settled. In 27 there were parenchymal injuries and nine settled under observation; eight showed displaced calyces and on exploration these were repaired by suture or partial nephrectomy. Eight had an injury to the vascular pedicle but only one kidney was salvaged.

There is now a distinct bias toward the conservative management of renal injuries and scepticism about the value of emergency angiography. When there is parenchymal rupture a close watch must be kept, at first for secondary haemorrhage and later for urinary leakage from a ruptured calyx, producing a perirenal collection: this may require drainage under ultrasound guidance. Later there should be a regular watch for the onset of hypertension.

REFERENCES

Bass, D. H., Semple, P. L. and Cywes, S. (1991) Investigation and management of blunt renal injuries in children: 11 years' experience. *J. Pediatr. Surg.*, **26**, 196–200.

Fowler, J. W., Smith, M. F. and Buist, T. A. S. (1982) The assessment and management of severe renal trauma. *Br. J. Urol.*, **54**, 329–333.

Hai, M. H., Pontes, J. E. and Pierce, J. M. (1977) Surgical management of major renal trauma: a review of 102 cases treated by conservative surgery. *J. Urol.*, **118**, 7–9.

Slade, N. (1971) Management of closed renal injuries. *Br. J. Urol.*, **43**, 639–645.

Wilson, D. H. (1963) Incidence, aetiology, diagnosis and prognosis of close abdominal injuries. *Br. J. Surg.*, **50**, 381–389.

11.6.3   INJURIES OF THE RENAL PELVIS AND URETER

These are very uncommon and are not, in blunt injuries, readily diagnosed because haematuria is unusual. The few reported cases have mostly occurred in children after a road accident, and have involved disruption of the pelviureteric junction. Diagnosis has generally had to wait for the collection of enough extravasated urine to produce a mass in the loin. Reconnection of the ureter to the pelvis can be difficult on account of extensive fibrosis.

The ureter is occasionally injured in penetrating wounds, but more often the injury occurs during an intra-abdominal operation. Damage within the pelvis should be treated by reimplantation into the bladder. The value of the relatively simple operation of transureteroureterostomy should be remembered as a valuable method of preserving the function of a kidney when the damage occurs above the pelvic brim.

11.6.4   INJURY TO THE LOWER URINARY TRACT

The bladder and the posterior urethra are liable to be injured in similar accidents, and may present in rather similar ways. They are all potentially serious but are not often seen, so the experience of individual surgeons is limited.

Traumatic **intraperitoneal rupture of the bladder** is classically associated with a forceful blow on the overfilled bladder. This may occur in a fall, or from the pressure exerted by a car seat-belt in a deceleration accident. Possible difficulties in diagnosis are illustrated by a 10-year-old girl who fell from a horse. She complained of lower abdominal pain and could not pass urine. When a catheter was passed a quantity of normal-looking urine was drained. Next day the abdomen was tender and guarded, and laparotomy revealed a long transverse tear in the dome of the bladder, with the catheter tip lying in urine that had collected in the pouch of Douglas.

Flancbaum *et al.* (1988) reported 29 patients who were involved in major incidents (85% were road accidents): 65% were in shock, 97% had haematuria, and at laparotomy 21 had an intraperitoneal rupture of the bladder. They emphasize that in these high-energy accidents the bladder does not have to be full to suffer disruption from hydraulic pressure waves.

In the unusual event of **spontaneous rupture of the bladder** the presentation can be obscure. Weakness of the bladder wall may be due to the presence of a neoplasm or the scar of a cystostomy. Pressure may rise because of postoperative or postpartum retention of urine. A woman of 29 presented 3 days after a normal vaginal delivery. She had not passed urine since the delivery, and complained of malaise, vomiting and a swollen abdomen. The abdomen was generally tender, with signs of free fluid. The serum creatinine was 538 mmol/l: a catheter yielded only 10 ml of urine. At laparotomy 6 litres of urine was aspirated and a 1 cm tear at the apex of the bladder was repaired (Roberts *et al.*, 1996). Heyns and Rimington (1987) emphasize that these patients can present with the signs of renal failure due to self-dialysis through the peritoneal membrane.

Traumatic extraperitoneal rupture of the bladder is generally due to a fracture of the pelvic ring involving the superior pubic ramus, in which a spicule of bone penetrates the anterior wall of the bladder. This injury is likely to be overshadowed by the other effects of a major accident: the breach is small and likely to heal with catheter drainage of the bladder.

Rupture of the posterior urethra is associated with a major pelvic fracture involving the pelvic ring, but it only rarely complicates these fractures. Glass *et al.* (1978) reviewed 333 consecutive fractures of the pelvis and only 19 produced a ruptured urethra. The problem lies in the fact that the bladder and prostate are displaced because the puboprostatic ligaments are disrupted, allowing the membranes to be stretched and either partially or completely divided. In the latter case bladder and prostate ride high in the pelvis, above blood clot and bony fragments, and there is wide separation of the two ends of the urethra.

Unlike the bladder injuries, blood is usually visible at the external urinary meatus, and in complete rupture rectal examination may reveal a high and mobile prostate.

Some of the patients from all four of these groups will have received a major injury and treatment will concentrate on resuscitation and repair of viscera. An urgent IVU should be done as soon as practicable to provide a check on the kidneys and to show the size and position of the bladder, and any sign of extravasation. The next step should be urethrography. Taking full precautions to avoid introduction of infection, a soft 12 FG Foley catheter is passed for 3–4 cm; 5–10 ml of 10% water-soluble contrast medium is injected and antero-posterior X-rays are taken. If there is no sign of extravasation from the urethra the catheter is gently advanced onwards into the bladder; if urine drains a cystogram is obtained and the balloon is inflated. It should be remembered that the extravasation may only be seen on the film taken following drainage of the contrast. If no abnormality is found the catheter can be left on closed drainage.

Intraperitoneal ruptures of the bladder can be extensive and require repair in two layers with absorbable sutures. It is usually best to drain the bladder through a suprapubic catheter. After 10 days the catheter can be spigoted, and removed when normal micturition is resumed.

If the urethrogram shows extravasation from the membranous urethra the catheter is withdrawn and an open suprapubic cystostomy is established (p. 482). If specialist urological advice is available it should be sought forthwith so that one expert individual can supervise treatment from the start. There are urologists who advise delaying any operative procedure, those who favour immediate repair, and those who prefer to bring the ends of the ruptured urethra together and use definitive measures at a later date.

For the surgeon who cannot transfer the patient to an expert, the balance of opinion would favour a procedure to bring the ends of the urethra together, and this should be done as soon as the patient is fit. The retropubic space is exposed through a Pfannenstiel or vertical incision and blood clot and bony fragments cleared, the cavity irrigated and bleeding points sealed. A 14 FG Foley catheter is passed up the urethra, through its open end, and held. An 18 FG or 20 FG Foley catheter is introduced through a stab wound into the bladder and passed down the prostatic urethra. The ends of the catheters are aligned and firmly tied together, and then the well-lubricated catheters are drawn up into the bladder, where the two balloons are inflated. This procedure will need to be coordinated with the orthopaedic surgeon, who will be wishing to reduce and fix the pelvic fractures. Finally traction is exerted and maintained on the urethral catheter, bringing the apex of the prostate down to the triangular ligament and aligning and approximating the two ends of the urethra. This needs to be maintained by elastic traction. The suprapubic catheter is placed on closed drainage.

This procedure gives time for the patient to recover and for plans to be made for further treatment of the injuries. Clark (1985) give a good description of this operation, as he does of other urological techniques mentioned in this chapter.

Rupture of the anterior urethra is a distinct entity and results from a blow in the perineum which crushes the bulb of the urethra against the pubic arch. Loose manhole covers are now a rare cause of an unusual injury, but falls on to the crossbar of a bicycle or the back of a chair, or a kick during an assault occur. Heddle and Robb (1974) saw six patients in 4 months who had been driving go-karts with a dangerous narrow vertical support for the steering wheel which had been driven into the perineum in sudden stops. Another unusual cause is pressure from the ring of a Thomas splint (Logie and Garvie, 1977).

The history, and the presence of blood at the external urinary meatus with a perineal haematoma, are characteristic. Occasionally, bleeding from the meatus can be profuse and the perineum has to be explored to secure haemostasis.

If a urethral injury is suspected the first step is to perform a urethrogram which will show whether there is any breach of the urethral mucosa.

1. The urethrogram is normal but there is bleeding from the meatus. If there is any difficulty in passing urine it is wise to insert a suprapubic catheter and rest the urethra for 10 days. The perineal haematoma is left alone unless it is exceptionally tense.

2. The urethrogram shows some extravasation, but there is also filling of the bladder. This suggests a partial tear and it is wise to provide rest for the urethra with a suprapubic catheter.

3. The urethrogram shows only extravasation in the perineum. If transfer to a urologist is not possible the patient should be placed in lithotomy–Trendelenburg position and the abdomen and perineum thoroughly cleaned and shaved. An open suprapubic cystostomy is established. The perineum is then explored through a curved transverse incision well in front of the anus, and the two ends of the urethra are sought with the aid of catheters passed from the bladder and down the urethra. The aim is to tidy the wound, secure haemostasis and restore end-to-end continuity of the urethra by suture of the roof only. A silicone stent can be left in the urethra, emerging at the meatus and through the abdominal wall, and the perineal wound is closed. The cystostomy can be retained until the integrity of the new urethra has been tested.

REFERENCES

Clark, P. (1985) *Operations in Urology*, Churchill Livingstone, Edinburgh, p. 97.

Flancbaum, L., Morgan, A. S., Fleisher, M. *et al.* (1988) Blunt bladder trauma: manifestation of severe injury. *Urology*, **31**, 220–222.

Glass, R. E., Flynn, J. T., King, J. B. *et al.* (1978) Urethral injury and fractured pelvis. *Br. J. Urol.*, **50**, 578–582.

Heddle, R. M. and Robb, W. A. T. (1974) Go-kart injuries of the urethra. *J. R. Coll. Surg. Edin.*, **19**, 310.

Heyns, C. F. and Rimington, P. D. (1987) Intraperitoneal rupture of the bladder causing biochemical features of renal failure. *Br. J. Urol.*, **60**, 617–622.

Logie, J. R. C. and Garvie, W. H. H. (1977) Urethral injury following use of a Thomas splint. *Br. J. Urol.*, **49**, 522–523.

Roberts, C., Oligbo, N. and Swinhoe, J. (1996) Spontaneous bladder rupture following normal vaginal delivery. *Br. J. Obstet. Gynaecol.*, **103**, 381–382.

12

The acute abdomen in pregnancy and the puerperium

12.1 INTRODUCTION

Many younger women seek medical advice because of an attack of acute abdominal pain, but relatively few are, at the same time, pregnant. Because both the pregnancy and the source of the pain can contribute to the whole clinical picture, this is a situation that calls for carefully judged diagnostic and therapeutic decisions. In some of these patients these decisions are made under pressure, because the severity of the haemorrhage or sepsis that prevails offers an urgent threat to mother and baby.

Because they see relatively few of these patients, obstetricians and surgeons do not have the chance to build up personal experience, so it is important to study the literature and to take every opportunity to consult together over the care of these patients.

12.2 EMERGENCIES ARISING FROM THE PRESENCE OF A PREGNANCY

12.2.1 EARLY IN PREGNANCY

12.2.1.1 Ectopic pregnancy

Although the majority of patients with an extrauterine pregnancy (EP) are treated by gynaecologists, an important minority are first seen by general surgeons, and among them will be patients with severe internal haemorrhage. The incidence of EP has been rising. During 1970–1978 in the USA incidence doubled from 4.5 to 9.4 per 1000 pregnancies (Stabile and Grudzinskas, 1990); in Turku, Finland, the annual number treated trebled between 1966 and 1985 (Markinen *et al.*, 1989); and in Aberdeen the numbers increased from 3.0 to 8.7 per 1000 maternities between 1950 and 1984 (Flett *et al.*, 1988). This rise may be partly an artefact due to better ascertainment with wider use of laparoscopy, but there is almost certainly a true rise in incidence associated with the use of intrauterine contraceptive devices, a higher incidence of pelvic inflammatory disease and, paradoxically, the wide use of laparoscopic sterilization (Flett *et al.*, 1988). Elsewhere, incidence is much higher – in South Korea, Kim *et al.* (1987) found an incidence of 1 in 24 full-term deliveries.

Emergency Abdominal Surgery. Edited by Peter F. Jones, Zygmunt H. Krukowski and George G. Youngson. Published in 1998 by Chapman & Hall, London. ISBN 0 412 81950 3.

With earlier diagnosis fewer of these conceptions reach the stage of sudden rupture and mortality remains low: about three deaths are seen annually in the UK, where about 10 000 cases are now treated each year (Report on Confidential Enquiries, 1996). The estimated case fatality rate fell from 0.4/1000 in 1988–1990 to 0.3/1000 in 1991–1993. Ectopic pregnancy is responsible for about 4% of maternal deaths and the Confidential Enquiry has, over the years, repeatedly commented on the need for awareness of EP as the cause of acute lower abdominal pain, and for expert management by surgeons and anaesthetists of hypovolaemia and its consequences. Many cases of tubal rupture only survive because such facilities and expertise are kept in a state of readiness.

Pathology

The fertilized ovum can embed and develop in several extrauterine sites, including very rarely the ovary and the abdominal cavity, but the great majority occur in the fallopian tubes. Implantation in the fallopian tubes takes place through the invasive action of the trophoblast. Muscle and blood vessels are invaded, as in the uterus, but with none of the protection afforded by the thick uterine wall. A tubal pregnancy is highly unstable and the likely outcome is either a tubal abortion or tubal rupture.

In **tubal abortion** the ovum is extruded through the fimbriated end, accompanied by a variable amount of bleeding. When this bleeding is slow, it accumulates to produce a **pelvic haematocele**. In **tubal rupture** the embedding of the ovum continues through the wall until the chorionic villi break through on the peritoneal surface, when rapid and serious haemorrhage can occur; before this occurs bleeding can be successively faster and slower, giving repeated episodes of pain.

The nearer implantation is to the uterus, the higher is the incidence of rupture (Figure 12.1).

When implantation occurs in the isthmus tubal rupture is very likely, and, because the tube is thinnest at this point, bleeding occurs early. In the unusual interstitial pregnancy the

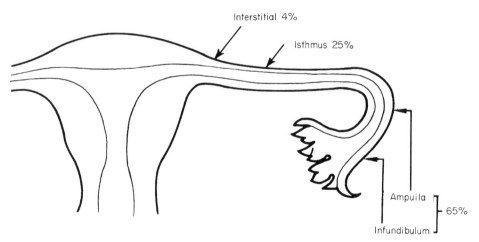

Figure 12.1 The site of implantation of tubal ectopic pregnancies, with their relative frequency. About 10% of distal implantations become tubal abortions.

embryo embeds within the uterine cornu, so erosion of the muscle takes longer and haemorrhage occurs late; it tends to be very brisk.

The vaginal bleeding that occurs in EP is withdrawal bleeding, due to the death of the placenta and cessation of hormonal production. It takes time for the uterine decidua to loosen so the blood is dark and comes late, in contradistinction to bleeding in a miscarriage, which is fresh in colour and often copious.

Clinical picture

The general surgeon's picture of an EP is likely to be the memory of a healthy young woman who is suddenly taken with severe generalized abdominal pain and suffers rapid circulatory collapse. In Southampton in 1988–1990 these patients constituted 21% of 147 tubal pregnancies treated (Norman, 1991).

Sudden abdominal pain and collapse is characteristic of rupture of a pregnancy in the isthmus. Pain is severe and generalized over the abdomen, and is often felt in the shoulder-tips. Rupture can occur as early as the fourth week, so there may be no history of a missed period and there may not, at first, be vaginal bleeding. This picture, with rapid onset of the signs of hypovolaemia and a positive pregnancy test, make a characteristic picture, and the need for urgent treatment is unmistakable.

Symptomatic ambulant group. Because these patients present in a much less dramatic way they may not receive so much attention. However, they account for some 75% of ectopic pregnancies and they carry a potentially dangerous condition. The main complaints are of lower abdominal pain, often unilateral, and of episodes of faintness – this is a very characteristic symptom. The patient may remark that the last period was scanty, or that there has been some vaginal staining, or a period may have been missed, but a few consider the last period to have been normal. As in all cases of abdominal pain in woman of childbearing age, the first step is to determine whether the patient is truly pregnant, and it must be remembered that for some this possibility will be a delicate matter. Some care and understanding must be devoted to taking the history (p. 508).

To decide this matter a slide test is made on the urine, which will detect beta-hCG at a concentration of 25–50 IU/l. In a trial of 130 women who attended an A&E department in Glasgow with abdominal pain or abnormal vaginal bleeding, the urine of all 12 with an EP gave a positive result, and none of the 51 women who had a negative result proved to be pregnant (Kingdom *et al.*, 1991). It is important not to be misled by a history of previous sterilization. In 155 ectopic pregnancies seen in Aberdeen during 1975–1982, 30 (19%) had been sterilized, almost all by laparoscopic techniques (Flett *et al.*, 1988).

On examination, the lower abdomen is tender, and this may be general or localized, with some guarding and pain on percussion. On vaginal examination movement of the cervix is clearly painful. Great care must be exercised over seeking an adnexal mass, lest a tubal pregnancy be ruptured. Other possibilities at this stage are acute appendicitis or some ovarian pathology occurring at an early stage of a normal pregnancy. The next step in this suspicious situation, in hospital practice, is to consult a gynaecologist, who is likely to perform transvaginal pelvic ultrasonography. This should show clearly whether the pregnancy is intra- or extrauterine. If the uterus does not show a gestation sac, and the history does not suggest a spontaneous miscarriage, then there is a strong likelihood that there is an EP. Another suggestive feature would be failure of the serum hCG (on a quantitative estimation) to double in 48 hours (Check *et al.*, 1982). If the pregnancy is a very early one ultrasound may not be conclusive and the matter can be settled by proceeding to diagnostic laparoscopy, which will usually yield a precise diagnosis. If the lone surgeon is not in a position to use a laparoscope then laparotomy is indicated, and salpingectomy will be indicated if a tubal pregnancy is found.

The importance of gynaecological input, if at all possible, must be emphasized, since the management of unruptured ectopic pregnancy has changed a great deal in recent years. Firstly, surgery can usually be laparoscopic (Magos *et al.*, 1989). Secondly, it is now normal practice to conserve the fallopian tube if it is not bleeding too much after linear salpingostomy (removing the gestation sac from the tube), or the patient can be treated medically with methotrexate. Both methods require follow up with hCG monitoring but can result in a persisting ectopic pregnancy in 5–15% of cases (Seifer *et al.*, 1990; Stovall, 1995). Some of these persisting pregnancies may present as an emergency with rupture.

Pelvic haematocele. This is not an emergency, although overenergetic pelvic examination can make it into one. Frequency of micturition and rectal tenesmus are characteristic of the presence of a sizeable pelvic haematoma.

Occasionally the pregnancy develops **on the ovary**, when the presentation is similar to a tubal pregnancy. Very rarely an **abdominal pregnancy** develops, and can grow to some size. If this situation is encountered the fetus is removed, but it is vital not to disturb the placenta. The cord is tied and divided and the placenta is left to atrophy.

Management

The general surgeon is most likely to be operating on the acute emergency with active bleeding. The general principles of treatment of hypovolaemia will be applied (p. 9). There is danger in spending time on replacing lost blood because a basic treatment of hypovolaemic shock is to secure haemostasis. While a theatre is made ready and an experienced anaesthetist is found, first-line resuscitation with intravenous fluids and oxygen by mask proceeds. Without waiting for cross-matched blood, the abdomen is opened through a midline incision, the uterus is grasped and drawn upwards, the bleeding tube is identified and brought up into the wound, and two curved clamps are applied as in Figure 12.2. This should arrest bleeding, allow time to evacuate the blood and clot, and give a few minutes for rapid transfusion to proceed and for the circulation to stabilize.

This is one of the situations in which autotransfusion can be very helpful, especially if bank blood is lacking or there is no donor known to be HIV-negative, or the patient is a Jehovah's Witness. It is particularly valuable in developing countries and Jongen (1997) found it to be life-saving in 28 women who arrived at a hospital in Tanzania in severe hypovolaemic shock. Blood is scooped out of the abdomen with a sterile steel soup ladle, filtered through six layers of gauze into a 540 ml blood donor set or bottle and immediately returned to the circulation. (Blood must not be used if it is haemolysed, if there is any suspicion of bacterial contamination or if the presence of the fetus suggests rupture of the amniotic sac, which could release thromboplastin, which may cause DIC.)

There is usually no need to remove the ovary. The tube is removed between the two curved clamps and the two pedicles are under-run and tied off with strong thread or catgut. Any bleeders within the broad ligament must be secured. Severe haemorrhage can occur in interstitial rupture, which leaves a raw crater at the cornu of the uterus. Deep through-and-through absorbable sutures on a curved, round-bodied needle should be inserted and firmly tied to under-run all bleeding points. If rupture should occur into the broad ligament the area

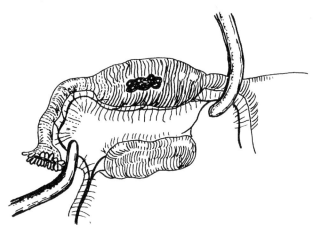

Figure 12.2 Arrest of bleeding from a ruptured tubal pregnancy. Placing the forceps in these positions stops the main inflow from the ovarian and uterine arteries. The medial forceps is placed on the tube at the point of junction with the uterus.

must be carefully inspected when blood pressure has returned to normal: bleeding points are best under-run.

The diagnosis of the unruptured or leaking EP is usually made at laparoscopy. Before this examination the gynaecologist will have discussed the possible diagnoses with the patient, and will know whether she is keen to have the tube conserved, if this is possible. About one-third of patients with an EP do not have a living child and so many will welcome this opportunity, while recognizing the risk of suffering another EP.

Culdocentesis has been largely superseded by laparoscopy, but it is still helpful where endoscopy is not available. Lucas and Hassim (1970) in Zambia needled the pouch of Douglas in 155 possible ectopic pregnancies. Aspiration of dark, non-clotting blood predicted an EP in 93 of 100 subsequently proven cases.

Outcome

A small number of patients bleed so fiercely that they do not reach hospital. Hospital mortality is now very low, but the Confidential Enquiries for 1991–1993 considered that all of the eight deaths reported were associated with substandard clinical management, mainly delay in diagnosis and inexpert resuscitation (Report on Confidential Enquiries, 1996).

12.2.1.2 Abortion and septic abortion

A spontaneous abortion during the first half of pregnancy produces some fresh vaginal bleeding, which at first constitutes a threatened miscarriage. If bleeding continues, accompanied by uterine pain, loss of the fetus becomes inevitable. This clinical picture is not often confused with an EP, and these patients are unlikely to appear in surgical wards.

A septic abortion is now rarely seen in a setting in which termination of pregnancy is legal. This is a virulent form of pelvic peritonitis, with possible gas-forming anaerobic infection of the myometrium. These patients are often bacteraemic and require urgent resuscitation and intensive care. After taking swabs for bacteriology from the offensive lochia, parenteral penicillin is started in large doses. A transvaginal scan will show whether there are retained products of conception; evacuation will then be necessary when antibiotic cover is in place.

12.2.1.3 Acute retention of urine due to a retroverted gravid uterus

This occurs about the 14th week of pregnancy. A period of dysuria precedes retention, which is of the overflow type. Treatment is urgently needed: the bladder is catheterized and placed on closed drainage. A urinary antiseptic and high fluid intake is prescribed. If the patient lies prone as much as is possible disimpaction of the uterus usually follows. If it does not, gynaecological advice will be needed.

REFERENCES

Check, J., Weiss, I. M. and Lurie, D. (1992) Analysis of serum human chorionic gonadotrophin levels in normal singleton, multiple and abnormal pregnancies. *Hum. Reprod.*, **7**, 1176–1180.

Flett, G. M. M., Urquhart, D. R., Fraser, C. *et al.* (1988) Ectopic pregnancy in Aberdeen, 1950–1985. *Br. J. Obstet. Gynaecol.*, **95**, 740–746.

Jongen, V. H. W. M. (1997) Autotransfusion and ectopic pregnancy: an experience from Tanzania. *Trop. Doct.*, **27**, 78–79.

Kim, D. S., Chung, S. R., Park, M. I. *et al.* (1987) Comparative review of diagnostic accuracy in tubal pregnancy: a 14 year survey of 1040 cases. *Obstet. Gynecol.*, **70**, 547–554.

Kingdom, J. C. P., Kelly, T., MacLean, A. B. *et al.* (1991) Rapid one step urine test for human chorionic gonadotrophin in suspected complications of early pregnancy. *BMJ.*, **302**, 1308–1311.

Lucas, C. and Hassim, A. M. (1970) Place of culdocentesis in diagnosis of ectopic pregnancy. *BMJ.*, **i**, 200–202.

Magos, A. L., Baumann, R. and Turnbull, A. C. (1989) Managing gynaecological emergencies with laparoscopy. *BMJ.*, **299**, 371–374.

Makinen, J. I., Errkola, R. U. and Laippala, P. J. (1989) Causes of the increase in the incidence of ectopic pregnancy. *Am. J. Obstet. Gynecol.*, **160**, 642–646.

Norman, S. G. (1991) An audit of the management of ectopic pregnancy. *Br. J. Obstet. Gynaecol.*, **98**, 1267–1272.

Report on Confidential Enquiries (1996) Report on Confidential Enquiries into Maternal Deaths in the United Kingdom 1991–93, HMSO, London.

Seifer, D. B., Gutman, J. N., Doyle, M. B. *et al.* (1990) Persistent ectopic pregnancy following laparoscopic linear salpingostomy. *Obstet. Gynecol.*, **76**, 1121–1125.

Stabile, I. and Grudzinskas, J. G. (1990) Ectopic pregnancy: a review of incidence, aetiology and diagnostic aspects. *Obstet. Gynecol. Surv.*, **45**, 335–347.

Stovall, T. G. (1995) Medical management should be routinely used as primary therapy for ectopic pregnancy. *Clin. Obstet. Gynecol.*, **38**, 3546–3552.

12.2.2 LATE IN PREGNANCY

12.2.2.1 Accidental antepartum haemorrhage (abruptio placentae)

In this condition there is haemorrhagic separation of the normally sited placenta from the uterine wall. It can vary from a minor bleed to complete separation. A large volume of blood may remain trapped in the uterus, but usually there is some vaginal loss. It occurs in late pregnancy, usually in a multigravida, with a frequency of about 1 in 100 pregnancies (Hurd *et al.*, 1983). Typically there is a sudden onset of severe lower abdominal pain, rapid onset of shock, a very hard, tender uterus and no sign of life in the fetus. When there is no vaginal loss the patient may present problems to the surgeon, because the whole abdomen can be tender and guarded. The suddenness of onset of pain and shock is unlike most causes of general peritonitis, except perhaps perforation of a viscus, but diagnosis is difficult and calls for urgent consultation with an obstetrician.

The first priority is accurate replacement of the blood loss, and as soon as this is underway, ultrasonography of the uterus should provide valuable positive or negative information. When confirmed, the main aim is to empty the uterus, but the outlook for the fetus is always grave. If the fetus is alive, emergency caesarean section will be required.

12.2.2.2 Rupture of the uterus

This rare condition (1 in 1000–2000 pregnancies) presents a similar picture, with the essential feature that there is usually, at least in developed countries, the abdominal scar of a previous caesarean section. Some mothers complain of 'something giving way' and fetal parts may be palpable: ultrasonography can be very helpful. From a practical point of view, the picture of abruptio placentae, uterine rupture, intraperitoneal haemorrhage (p. 499) and perforation of a viscus, can be very difficult to distinguish. The only safe course is to be ready to embark on emergency laparotomy unless there are the clearest signs of abruptio placentae.

12.2.2.3 Red degeneration of a fibroid

With the regular use of antenatal ultrasonography, the presence of a uterine fibroid is usually known fairly early in pregnancy. As pregnancy proceeds fibroids soften and become more vascular, and may be the site of thrombosis, venous engorgement and local inflammation reaction. This produces local tenderness which can, if suitably sited, give a fair imitation of acute appendicitis. Alders' sign (1951) may then be helpful. The site of maximal tenderness is marked and the patient is asked to roll on to her left side. If the site of tenderness moves to the left it probably arises from an abnormality of the uterus or adnexae; if it remains unmoved the source lies outside the uterus, e.g. in the appendix. Treatment is conservative unless there are grave doubts about the diagnosis. The uterine blood flow increases many times during pregnancy so removal of a fibroid should not be attempted.

12.2.2.4 Pre-eclampsia

The first symptom of this serious complaint of the second half of pregnancy, which can progress with great speed, may be epigastric pain. In pre-eclampsia the portal sinusoids are dilated, fibrin thrombi form and there is periportal necrosis, which can cause microscopic haemorrhage, and then subcapsular haemorrhage – the source of the pain. To identify these patients, the blood pressure must be measured and urinalysis performed in any pregnant woman presenting with upper abdominal pain, especially in the later stages (Barry *et al.*, 1994).

REFERENCES

Alders, N. (1951) A sign of differentiating uterine from extrauterine complications of pregnancy and the puerperium. *BMJ.*, **ii**, 1194.

Barry, C., Fox, R. and Sirrat, G. (1994) Upper abdominal pain in pregnancy may indicate pre-eclampsia. *BMJ.*, **308**, 1562–1563.

Hurd, W. W., Miodovnik, M., Hertzberg, V. *et al.* (1983) Selective management of abruptio placentae: a prospective study. *Obstet. Gynecol.*, **61**, 467–473.

12.3 EMERGENCIES CONNECTED WITH PREGNANCY

12.3.1 ACUTE PYELITIS AND PYELONEPHRITIS

The basic pathology is the dilatation and loss of tone that naturally occurs in the renal pelves and ureters during pregnancy. These effects are partly hormonal and partly mechanical resulting from pressure exerted by the uterus on the ureters at the pelvic brim (Baird, 1935). Urinary stasis is maximal at midterm, after which hypertrophy of the ureteric musculature improves propulsion. Symptomless bacteriuria occurs in 10–12% of pregnant women, but only some 10% will develop a symptomatic infection. The risk of a clinical infection is considerably greater in women with a past history of infection, and they require supervision (Chng and Hall, 1982).

Acute pyelonephritis occurs in only 1–2% of pregnancies. It has a fairly sudden onset with loin pain, vomiting and a high fever, sometimes with rigors. Tenderness is usually maximal in the loin but there may be tenderness over the dilated ureter. It is this that can raise doubts about appendicitis, but high fever and a rigor are quite exceptional in appendicitis. This doubt must be resolved because the appropriate treatments are totally different. It cannot be too strongly emphasized that a most critical view of the nature of the urinary deposit must be taken in all cases of abdominal pain in pregnancy. If necessary, a catheter specimen should be taken. If a shaken unspun specimen shows many pus cells and the shimmer of motile bacilli under the high power microscope, and the clinical picture is typical, then a diagnosis of true urinary tract infection can be made and treatment promptly started (p. 476).

If acute pyelitis or pyelonephritis seems the likely diagnosis but the urine contains few pus cells, then there are two possibilities.

1. The patient does not have pyelitis. It is not uncommon for a few pus cells to be found in the urine during a pregnancy, and this is not necessarily abnormal. Too often the report of 'a few pus cells' has been given too much attention, and the diagnosis of appendicitis or intestinal obstruction has been unduly delayed. Such delay was responsible for two deaths, in patients with acute appendicitis, recorded in the current Confidential Enquiries (Report on Confidential Enquiries, 1996).

2. The ureteric obstruction at the pelvic brim, which has predisposed to the infection, is preventing infected urine from reaching the bladder. On a few occasions we have found it valuable to perform ureteric catheterization under local analgesia. It provides a sample of ureteric urine and may relieve the pain of the distended ureter. Baird (1935) also found that severe ureteric pain can occur in pregnancy in the absence of infection, as a result of obstruction at the pelvic brim. If this is suspected, with pain and tenderness felt well back in the loin, an ultrasound scan should be helpful in diagnosis, and we have seen ureteric catheterization provide dramatic relief of pain. Over a period of 6 years Eckford

and Gingell (1991) saw ten women with this picture, and they obtained immediate relief, with a free flow of urine, by passing a double-pigtail silicone-elastomer ureteric stent: this was left *in situ* until after delivery.

12.3.2 TORSION OF AN OVARIAN CYST

Ovarian cysts are not uncommon, and are liable to undergo torsion if based on a narrow pedicle. Cysts are generally identified at the first ultrasonic scan of a pregnancy and the usual practice is to remove them during the second trimester. This prevents later torsion and any problems during the delivery. Most of these cysts are dermoids or cystadenomas, and a few are corpus luteum cysts; a very small minority are carcinomas (p. 510).

12.3.3 HAEMATOMA OF THE RECTUS ABDOMINIS

A haematoma within the rectus abdominis can look very much like an intraperitoneal emergency. It is due to rupture of a branch of the inferior epigastric artery, usually within the muscle, causing some disruption. Bleeding usually extends behind the muscle and can extend widely towards the loin, because there is no posterior rectus sheath below the arcuate line. A haematoma is usually associated with pregnancy, but is seen in men as well as women. Coughing and multiparity are frequent features, and rupture seems to be most common in late pregnancy, rather than during labour.

Diagnosis can be difficult. There is a readily visible acutely tender swelling, strictly unilateral, which feels very superficial. If it is recognized that it is also rather fixed, and the rest of the abdomen is soft and painless, the diagnosis may be suggested.

Treatment will usually be conservative and the gradual appearance of bruising, or Cullen's sign, will confirm the diagnosis. However, occasionally haemorrhage is profuse and Thomas's (1945) patient presented with signs of internal haemorrhage, clot was removed from the front of the peritoneum and back into the loin, and a bleeding branch of the inferior epigastric artery was secured.

12.3.4 INTRAPERITONEAL HAEMORRHAGE

This is a collection of relatively rare conditions, all of which present with sudden severe bleeding into the peritoneal cavity in the later months of pregnancy or early in the puerperium.

12.3.4.1 Aneurysms of the aorta and its branches

Cases of dissecting aneurysm of the thoracic and abdominal aorta are described, particularly in Marfan's syndrome (Pretre and Segesser, 1997). Women with this syndrome should normally have been assessed prior to pregnancy and advised against pregnancy if they are at high risk of aortic dissection (because of an aortic root more than 40 mm across, or a family history of dissection; Oakley, 1997). However because Marfan's syndrome is not always easy to diagnose and because women may not always take advice, it is necessary to be alert to the possibility of aortic dissection as a cause of acute abdominal or chest pain during pregnancy or shortly after delivery (Lipscomb *et al.*, 1997). Some of the best-known examples of rupture of an aneurysm occur in the splenic artery (O'Grady *et al.*, 1977). These are unusual in being twice as common among women as in men, with a tendency to rupture in the third trimester. The bleeding initially distends the lesser sac, producing severe upper abdominal pain; the patient soon shows signs of hypovolaemia and there is acute tenderness, sometimes with a palpable mass, in the epigastrium. Then, after a period of hours and even days, there is sudden circulatory collapse and diffuse severe abdominal pain and tenderness as the blood and clot bursts through the confining lesser omentum or gastrosplenic ligament. This picture of a double, spaced-out, rupture is described by Abramovich *et al.* (1969) and O'Grady *et al.* (1977), following a normal delivery. Rupture of the middle colic artery and of the veins over the adrenal are also described, and general surgical principles will be applied in securing haemostasis.

12.3.4.2   Rupture of uterine veins

These patients are in the later stages of a normal pregnancy when they are seized with severe lower abdominal pain, with acute tenderness over one lower quadrant, and they develop signs of internal haemorrhage. Immediate recourse to laparotomy, with caesarean section, reveals a bleeding leash of veins or a tear on the surface of the uterus or broad ligament. Marrow (1960) described two such patients, with survival of mother and baby.

12.3.4.3   Rupture of the liver and spleen

Rupture of the liver is fortunately a rare complication of pre-eclampsia (p. 497). These patients are generally multipara over the age of 30, who are suddenly seized with severe pain in the right upper quadrant, spreading to the back and shoulder. Their previous hypertensive state may, for a time, disguise the severity of the bleeding, but the cold, sweating patient with tachycardia and air hunger gives the lie to this. Bis and Waxman (1976) reviewed 91 patients and found that all presented in the second half of pregnancy, 40% in the last 3 weeks and 12% in the 24 hours after delivery.

Everything depends on expert management of the blood loss and urgent laparotomy. This will at first be exploratory, to determine the site of the bleeding to be in the liver. Pringle's manoeuvre (1904; p. 460) is helpful in producing a drier field, and giving time for a caesarean section. There are problems in securing haemostasis because the friable liver will not usually hold sutures. Bleeding vessels should be under-run and once the haematoma is evacuated, firm packing and drainage seems to have been the method most often used (p. 461).

Spontaneous rupture of the spleen occasionally occurs near term and has been successfully treated by splenectomy (Henderson and Keeping, 1979).

12.3.4.4   Torsion of the uterus

This is a very rare but serious problem that mimics intraperitoneal haemorrhage because blood is trapped in the uterus and is not available to the circulation. When the torsion is released overloading of the circulation may be a problem.

The greatest care must be taken over the patient in the later stages of pregnancy who develops acute distress, with diffuse abdominal pain and tenderness. Unless there is the clearest possible evidence of abruptio placentae there should be a strong bias towards speedy resuscitation and laparotomy, because precise diagnosis is rarely possible. The cause may be one of the conditions already described, or one of the gastrointestinal emergencies described in the next section. Early laparotomy is most likely to secure a live mother and baby. The closest collaboration of obstetrician and surgeon is needed.

REFERENCES

Abramovich, D. R., Francis, W. and Helsby, C. R. (1969) Two cases of ruptured aneurysm of splanchnic arteries in pregnancy. *J. Obstet. Gynaecol. Br. Cwlth*, **76**, 1037–1039.

Baird, D. (1935) The upper urinary tract in pregnancy and the puerperium, with special reference to pyelitis of pregnancy. *J. Obstet. Gynaecol. Br. Emp.*, **42**, 577–595; 733–794.

Bis, K. A. and Waxman, B. (1976) Rupture of the liver associated with pregnancy: a review of the literature and report of 2 cases. *Obstet. Gynecol. Surv.*, **31**, 763–773.

Chng, P. K. and Hall, M. H. (1982) Antenatal prediction of urinary tract infection in pregnancy. *Br. J. Obstet. Gynaecol.*, **89**, 8–11.

Eckford, S. D. and Gingell, J. C. (1991) Ureteric obstruction in pregnancy – diagnosis and management. *Br. J. Obstet. Gynaecol.*, **98**, 1137–1140.

Henderson, P. R. and Keeping, J. D. (1979) Spontaneous rupture of the spleen in late pregnancy. *Austr. N.Z. J. Obstet. Gynaecol.*, **19**, 116–118.

Lipscomb, K. J., Smith, K. C., Clark, B. *et al.* (1997) Outcome of pregnancy in women with Marfan's syndrome. *Br. J. Obstet. Gynaecol.*, **104**, 201–206

Marrow, A. E. (1960) Rupture of varicose veins of the uterus associated with pregnancy. *J. Obstet. Gynaecol. Br. Emp.*, **67**, 792–795.

Oakley, C. M. (1997) Management of pre-existing disorder in pregnancy: heart disease. *Prescribers Journal*, **37**, 102–111.

O'Grady, J. P., Day, E. J., Toole, A. L. *et al.* (1977) Splenic artery aneurysm rupture in pregnancy. *Obstet. Gynecol.*, **50**, 627–630.

Pretre, R. and Segesser, L. K. B. (1997) Aortic dissection. *Lancet*, **3491**, 461–4.

Pringle, J. H. (1904) Notes on the arrest of hepatic haemorrhage due to trauma. *Ann. Surg.*, **48**, 541–549.

Report on Confidential Enquiries (1996) Report on Confidential Enquiries into Maternal Deaths in the United Kingdom 1991–93, HMSO, London.

Thomas, R. C. (1945) Rupture of the rectus abdominis muscle during pregnancy. *J. Obstet. Gynaecol. Br. Emp.*, **52**, 580–583.

12.4 GASTROINTESTINAL EMERGENCIES ARISING DURING PREGNANCY

Alimentary tract emergencies that arise in the course of a pregnancy share with other conditions discussed in this chapter the fact that they are fairly uncommon, but can be difficult to diagnose and to treat successfully. In Melbourne, O'Neill (1969) found that 158 non-obstetric abdominal emergencies had been treated over 14 years in the Women's Hospital, while 91 500 women had been delivered. Acute appendicitis accounted for some 40% of these patients, with intestinal obstruction and biliary tract disease each contributing about 15%.

12.4.1 ACUTE APPENDICITIS

The incidence of acute appendicitis in pregnancy in Europe and North America is about 1 in 1500–2000 deliveries; among 100 women with appendicitis only one or two will be pregnant. About 50% of cases are seen in the second trimester, about 30% in the first and 20% in the third, including the occasional difficult case that presents during labour or the puerperium (Finch and Lee, 1974).

In the first trimester the picture is complicated in two different ways.

- In the first weeks of pregnancy the patient presents with the symptoms and signs of acute appendicitis at a time when she does not realize she is pregnant. Because an ectopic pregnancy can produce a similar picture it is essential to resolve this differential diagnosis; if the pregnancy test is positive the patient is placed in the 'symptomatic ambulant' group of potential ectopic pregnancies and investigated (p. 56).
- In the second half of the trimester nausea and vomiting are often experienced, sometimes with abdominal discomfort, and these complaints may be accepted as part of a normal pregnancy. However, at this stage the symptoms and signs of acute appendicitis are not modified and diagnosis should proceed in the normal way.

As pregnancy advances diagnosis becomes more difficult. The growing uterus stretches the abdominal wall, so the valuable sign of muscle guarding is weakened, while the caecum is displaced upwards and outwards. Baer *et al.* in 1932 made investigations that would now be quite unethical when they gave barium meals to 78 women, at various stages of pregnancy, and plotted the site of the caput caeci. The displacement thus demonstrated explains why pain and tenderness is felt at waist level under the ribs, and out towards the flank, in later pregnancy. Movements of the baby may aggravate the pain. About one-third of patients notice a shift of pain and nausea and vomiting are common.

Temperature is not much raised, but notice must be taken of a pulse rate over 100/min. Tenderness over the appendix is consistently found but may not be well localized. Guarding and percussion tenderness are not the reliable signs we normally depend on to detect peritoneal irritation. Pelvic examination is not likely to be helpful on account of the elevation of the appendix. The white cell count can be as high as $15 \times 10^9/l$ in a normal pregnancy.

One feature that figures in all reports is the delay that occurs before these patients reach hospital. Tamir *et al.* (1990) found a mean delay of 60 hours among 54 patients, of whom 26 had a gangrenous and 23 a perforated appendix. They also found that 13 of these patients had a urinary infection: the problems of interpreting the urinary deposit are considered on page p. 498. As the uterus rises the site of tenderness may be high enough to suggest a diagnosis of acute cholecystitis, and then ultrasonography can be helpful.

It must always be remembered that in later pregnancy acute appendicitis occurs in the free peritoneal cavity, beyond the reach of the omentum, and fibrinous adhesions do not readily form because of the adjacent Braxton Hicks contractions of the uterus, so early removal is important. Exploration may have to be decided on with less clear-cut evidence than would normally be expected; Parker's (1954) thoughtful paper brings this out clearly.

Scott-Combes *et al.* (1992) suggest that fine catheter peritoneal cytology can be helpful. A woman with a 32 weeks' pregnancy presented with signs that suggested acute appendicitis, but a low white cell count. A catheter was introduced at the point of maximum tenderness and the aspirate showed only 10% of neutrophils (p. 46), so the patient was observed and the episode settled, and they record another similar experience. This investigation should be remembered, because many papers show that patients who do not have appendicitis can still present suspicious signs and there is a high negative exploration rate; however, these explorations rarely affect the fetus (Tamir *et al.*, 1990). Nothing disturbs the fetus more than appendicitis progressing to perforation as it lies alongside the uterus.

Technique

The patient should be secured around the hips and the table tilted towards the left – this improves exposure and the return through the inferior vena cava. A muscle-splitting incision is made over the site of maximum tenderness. If labour soon ensues the fibres of this incision will tend to approximate, and it should not give undue discomfort. The aim is to avoid contact with the uterus and particular care is exercised over placement of retractors.

A major problem arises when appendicitis with peritonitis occurs in the last weeks of a pregnancy. Operation is quite likely to be followed by a stillbirth and the rapid descent of the uterus does not assist resolution of the peritonitis. If there is a great concern to deliver a healthy baby, e.g. in an elderly primipara, there is a case to be made for performing a lower-segment caesarean section, then proceeding to appendicectomy and thorough peritoneal toilet, backed up by a full course of systemic antibiotics (p. 143–50). We have experience of this course proving to be successful, and O'Neill (1969) quotes three such operations, with good results; the closest collaboration is needed between obstetrician and surgeon.

Many of these patients are dehydrated after a day or two of vomiting, but correction requires close attention – they are very sensitive to fluid overload and Confidential Enquiries for 1988–1990 draws special attention to the risks of ARDS in the puerperium.

Outcome

Maternal death is now rare and some 90% of babies are delivered safely.

12.4.2 INTESTINAL OBSTRUCTION

The incidence of intestinal obstruction during pregnancy is about half that of appendicitis, but they share the problem that their principal symptoms of pain and vomiting are also experienced during a normal pregnancy. However, acute onset of central colicky abdominal pain and the vomiting of bile should arouse suspicion. **Adhesions** cause about one-half of these cases, many dating from the time when a girl was explored for suspected appendicitis; they offer a real threat of strangulation. **Volvulus** is relatively common during pregnancy, accounting for 30% of all obstructions, which is about ten times the normal incidence. An important cause in the puerperium is **acute functional colonic obstruction**. **External hernias** rarely entrap bowel because their internal openings are covered by the uterus; however, the existence of a **diaphragmatic hernia** may well be revealed during pregnancy.

A recent review of 66 pregnant patients with an **adhesive obstruction** found that 98% complained of abdominal pain, 82% had vomited but only 30% were constipated (Perdue *et al.*, 1992). Close attention needs to be paid to the details of the history. In particular, epigastric or periumbilical pain that continues – whether as attacks of colic or a steady pain – for more than 6 hours, without any signs developing in the uterus, is not likely to be due to a complication of the pregnancy. Occasionally pain is felt in the back. It is always significant if vomit is bile-stained or brown and offensive. Occasionally, bowels move after the onset of the pain, but constipation is more usual.

Near to term the intermittent nature of uterine contractions, with palpable hardening, must not be confused with intestinal colic. Auscultation over a period can be helpful, especially when tell-tale splashing sounds build up as the patient grimaces over the next painful spasms. Abdominal distension can be concealed because the bowel tends to be pushed back into the flanks by the large uterus. Tenderness can be difficult to assess, but must always arouse a suspicion of strangulation (p. 189). Over 80% of patients show signs of intestinal obstruction in plain abdominal films (Perdue *et al.*, 1992; Connolly *et al.*, 1995), and here concern about possible harm to the fetus must be kept in proportion. Taking one supine and one erect abdominal plain film involves a radiation exposure of 0.1 rad, yet the risk of causing a malformation during the early pregnancy is only 1 in 1000 after exposure to 10 times that dose – 1.0 rad – and the effect of fetal irradiation on possible later neoplastic disease remains undecided (Mole, 1979). The diagnostic value to mother and child of these X-rays must, on balance, outweigh these very slight risks. In a small number of cases, including some strangulating obstructions, plain films may not reveal any abnormality, and full attention must always be given to the symptoms and signs. A chest X-ray will be needed to confirm diaphragmatic herniation.

In some 25% of adhesive obstructions a resection of ischaemic bowel is required, and this is understandable because there is an average delay of 48 hours before these patients are admitted, and another 48 hours elapse before they come to laparotomy (Perdue *et al.*, 1992; Connolly *et al.*, 1995).

Volvulus is the other major intestinal accident and is mostly seen in late pregnancy and the puerperium. Sigmoid colon and caecum are roughly equally affected and usually show typical appearances on X-ray (p. 291–8). A small-bowel volvulus may hang suspended from an adhesion or from a persistent vitellointestinal duct. Occasionally, malrotation of the midgut is the basis, with the midgut suspended on a single dorsal mesentery with a very narrow base; these patients may have had previous attacks of abdominal colic. Goodwin (1968) underlines the need to pay close attention to these patients – they present with severe continuous epigastric pain and vomiting, but in the early curable stages there are disquietingly few abdominal signs (p. 209).

A young woman, at 29 weeks, had some colicky abdominal pain which settled in the back. Soon the back became very sore and vomiting persisted. There was a little upper abdominal fullness and tenderness and definite release pain. Because of this, and the original complaint of colic, laparotomy was performed and revealed a volvulus of the midgut: only 2 feet of jejunum was viable. A jejunocolic anastomosis was made and slowly the patient became able to maintain weight on a controlled diet (Davidson, 1976).

The changes in intra-abdominal pressure that occur during pregnancy and delivery will occasionally reveal the presence of a **diaphragmatic hernia**. Any suggestion of dyspnoea or chest pain in a patient with obstructive symptoms is a signal for clinical and radiographic examination of the chest; there may be few abdominal signs (p. 177).

Goldthorp (1966) found that, among 150 obstructions during pregnancy, 5% were due to **colorectal carcinoma**. In the earlier stages of pregnancy the obstruction can be dealt with in the appropriate manner (Chapter 7) and once the fetus is viable it will often be appropriate to perform caesarean section before resection.

Acute functional colonic obstruction is a well recognized complication of the puerperium, especially after caesarean section (p. 303).

These patients require a very thoughtful assessment, and often reassessment, of a picture that is often confusing. Many patients are dehydrated when finally admitted and they need skilful restoration of fluid and electrolyte balance, which is of special importance in maintaining the placental circulation.

12.4.3   PEPTIC ULCERATION

The large majority of women who suffer from a peptic ulcer when they become pregnant find that symptoms tend to improve (Clark, 1953). This is probably because they take more rest and study their diet more than usual. The major complications of perforation and haemorrhage are quite unusual. Perforation has generally presented in a typical manner, and prompt operation has allowed survival of mother and child (Jones *et al.*, 1969). Diagnosis is more difficult in the puerperium (p. 506). Major haemorrhage has demonstrated the remarkable ability of the mother to withstand blood loss, which contrasts with the sensitivity of the fetal circulation to haemorrhage (Becker-Andersen and Husfeldt, 1971). Endoscopic treatment may be used (p. 355), but if operation is needed for severe bleeding a caesarean section may be needed to secure access, and this can offer the best chance for the baby (Jones *et al.*, 1969).

12.4.4   ACUTE PANCREATITIS

Among 282 women with acute pancreatitis, seven were pregnant at the time of the attack and 12 cases occurred within 3 months of delivery (McKay *et al.*, 1980). This group of patients is notably young and most have gallstones. Alcohol-induced pancreatitis is very unusual. Most settle on a conservative regime and a number go on to have a cholecystectomy during the second trimester. Hyperemesis gravidarum was suspected in 14 of 52 patients seen by Corlett and Mishell (1972) because they had repeated vomiting and little or no pain, so it is important to estimate the serum amylase. It is also vital to remember other causes of a raised amylase – one of these patients was found to have a small-bowel strangulation after 3 days of observation for presumed pancreatitis (p. 383).

12.4.5   ACUTE CHOLECYSTITIS

This is an unusual complication of pregnancy but when it occurs the clinical picture is usually recognizable and can be confirmed by ultrasonography. Most attacks subside with conservative treatment (Woodhouse and Haylen, 1985). If there are recurrent attacks then cholecystectomy is best undertaken during the second trimester, because there is a distinct risk of miscarriage if operation is carried out in the first trimester. Elerding (1993) suggests that the laparoscopic approach can be selectively used.

12.4.6   INFLAMMATORY BOWEL DISEASE

If a pregnancy starts when the disease is quiescent about two-thirds of patients will go through to a normal delivery. Sulphasalazine and corticosteroids can be taken as needed. Relapses are a little more frequent in Crohn's disease (Willoughby and Truelove, 1980; Miller, 1986). Among the minority who experience a relapse, most can be maintained on medical treatment until the fetus is viable. In a few control is not achieved and then toxic megacolon is a distinct risk. This may call for colectomy during pregnancy (Cooksey *et al.*, 1985) or, more often, in the puerperium (Anderson *et al.*, 1987); subtotal colectomy and ileostomy is the most appropriate operation. Hill *et al.* (1997) record six patients with peritonitis due to perforated Crohn's disease during pregnancy and the puerperium; they emphasize the importance of making a stoma after emergency resection and peritoneal toilet, leaving anastomosis to a later occasion. Kelly *et al.* (1994) describe a patient with very active proctocolitis who needed an episiotomy for delivery of a 3.2 kg baby. Copious diarrhoea and incontinence led to a spreading infection of the sutured episiotomy and eventually rectal excision was required for incontinence and rectal haemorrhage. They suggest that timely caesarean section may be correct for a full-term baby when colitis is very active, followed by resection which would permit later pouch construction.

12.5 EMERGENCIES IN THE PUERPERIUM

This is a particularly dangerous time for an abdominal emergency to arise, because the symptoms are so likely to be given an obstetric explanation, such as 'after pains' (uterine contractions). In fact, anything more than intermittent lower abdominal discomfort and windy pains should be considered abnormal: careful analysis of the site, degree and character of abdominal pain is vital.

Recurring spasms of central colicky abdominal pain, with bile-stained vomiting, must suggest intestinal obstruction; many more cases of obstruction arise in the week after delivery than in any other week of a pregnancy, and this is clearly related to the changed positions of viscera (Morris, 1965). A loop of bowel can be caught when an adhesive band changes position and tension, volvuli can occur, and the strains of labour may precipitate strangulation of bowel in a diaphragmatic hernia. Acute functional colonic obstruction is liable to follow a caesarean section (p. 303). Radiology can be used normally, and can give vital information.

A striking feature of the puerperium is the inability of the abdominal wall, after a long period of stretching, to respond to parietal peritoneal irritation with guarding or rigidity. In the presence of general peritonitis the abdomen may be distended and diffusely tender, but there is little guarding and this can lead to underestimation of the true state of affairs (Munro and Jones, 1975). Rupture of abdominal viscera may be precipitated and rupture of the liver and splenic artery aneurysm are reported (p. 499); also, rarely, spontaneous rupture of the bladder (Roberts *et al.*, 1996), which presents as increasing ascites with signs of renal failure.

One difficulty is that the medical and nursing staff of a maternity hospital necessarily work a shift system, which means that it is difficult for changing staff to detect a deteriorating situation. Everyone must be alert to pick up a departure from the normal course of the puerperium: one clinician must then be responsible for thoughtful assessment and reassessment of the situation.

REFERENCES

Anderson, J. B., Turner, G. M. and Williamson, R. C. N. (1987) Fulminant ulcerative colitis in late pregnancy and the puerperium. *J. R. Soc. Med.*, **80**, 492–494.

Baer, J. L., Reis, R. A. and Arens, R. A. (1932) Appendicitis in pregnancy. *J.A.M.A.*, **98**, 1359–1364.

Becker-Andersen, H. and Husfeldt, V. (1971) Peptic ulcer in pregnancy. *Acta Obstet. Gynaecol. Scand.*, **50**, 391–395.

Clark, D. H. (1953) Peptic ulcer in women. *BMJ.*, **i**, 1254–1256.

Connolly, M. M., Unti, J. A. and Nora, P. F. (1995) Bowel obstruction in pregnancy. *Surg. Clin. North Am.*, **75**, 101–113.

Cooksey, G., Gunn, A. and Wotherspoon, W. C. (1985) Surgery for acute ulcerative colitis and toxic megacolon during pregnancy. *Br. J. Surg.*, **72**, 647.

Corlett, R. C. and Mishell, D. R. (1972) Pancreatitis in pregnancy. *Am. J. Obstet. Gynecol.*, **113**, 281–290.

Davidson, A. I. (1976) Intestinal obstruction in pregnancy. Report to Surgical Staff Meeting, Aberdeen Royal Infirmary, May 1976.

Elerding, S. C. (1993) Laparoscopic cholecystectomy in pregnancy. *Am. J. Surg.*, **165**, 625–627.

Finch, D. R. A. and Lee, E. (1974) Acute appendicitis complicating pregnancy in the Oxford region. *Br. J. Surg.*, **61**, 129–132.

Goldthorp, W. O. (1966) Intestinal obstruction during pregnancy and the puerperium. *Br. J. Clin. Pract.*, **20**, 367–376.

Goodwin, D. P. (1968) Volvulus of the small intestine in labour. *Br. J. Surg.*, **55**, 469–470.

Hill, J., Clark, A. and Scott, N. A. (1997) Surgical treatment of acute manifestations of Crohn's disease during pregnancy. *J. R. Soc. Med.*, **90**, 64–66.

Jones, P. F., McEwan, A. B. and Bernard, P. M. (1969) Haemorrhage and perforation complicating peptic ulcer in pregnancy. *Lancet*, **ii**, 350–352.

Kelly, M. J., Hunt, T. M., Wicks, A. C. B. *et al.* (1994) Fulminant ulcerative colitis and parturition: a need to alter current management? *Br. J. Obstet. Gynaecol.*, **101**, 166–167.

McKay, A. J., O'Neill, J. and Imrie, C. W. (1980) Pancreatitis, pregnancy and gallstones. *Br. J. Obstet. Gynaecol.*, **87**, 47–50.

Miller, J. P. (1986) Inflammatory bowel disease in pregnancy: a review. *J. R. Soc. Med.*, **79**, 221–225.

Mole, R. H. (1979) Radiation effects on prenatal development and their radiological significance. *Br. J. Radiol.*, **52**, 89–101.

Morris, E. D. (1965) Intestinal obstruction and pregnancy. *J. Obstet. Gynaecol. Br. Emp.*, **72**, 36–44.

Munro, A. and Jones, P. F. (1975) Abdominal surgical emergencies in the puerperium. *BMJ.*, **iv**, 691–694.

O'Neill, J. P (1969) Surgical conditions complicating pregnancy. *Austr. N.Z. Obstet. Gynaecol.*, **9**, 94–99, 249–252.

Parker, R. B. (1954) Acute appendicitis in late pregnancy. *Lancet*, **i**, 1252–1257.

Perdue, P. W., Johnson, H. W. and Stafford, P. W. (1992) Intestinal obstruction complicating pregnancy. *Am. J. Surg.*, **164**, 384–388.

Roberts, C., Oligbo, N. and Swinhoe, J. (1996) Spontaneous bladder rupture following normal vaginal delivery. *Br. J. Obstet. Gynaecol.*, **103**, 381–382.

Scott-Combes, D. M., Vipond, M. N. and Thompson, J. N. (1992) Acute right iliac fossa pain in pregnancy: the role of fine catheter peritoneal cytology. *Br. J. Surg.*, **79**, 1105.

Tamir, I. L., Bongard, F. S. and Klein, S. R. (1990) Acute appendicitis in the pregnant patient. *Am. J. Surg.*, **160**, 571–576.

Willoughby, C. P. and Truelove, S. C. (1980) Ulcerative colitis and pregnancy. *Gut*, **21**, 469–474.

Woodhouse, D. R. and Haylen, B. (1985) Gall bladder disease complicating pregnancy. *Austr. N.Z. J. Obstet. Gynaecol.*, **25**, 233–237.

13

Gynaecological disorders

13.1 INTRODUCTION

Because acute abdominal pain is common in young women, they are often seen as an emergency by the general surgeon. The common causes (appendicitis, pelvic inflammatory disease and ectopic pregnancy) often present in an atypical fashion, so it is not surprising that general practitioners may sometimes refer to the 'wrong' ward. It is incumbent on the receiving specialist to make a careful assessment as to whether to continue management or to refer on. The approximate proportion of young women with acute abdominal pain who had acute appendicitis was described by Walmsley *et al.* (1977) as 21%, not too different from the 33% recorded by Salkey (1993) and in both series there were almost as many women with gynaecological conditions. It might be thought that the preoperative assessment is not too important since the diagnosis will readily become apparent at laparoscopy or laparotomy, but this would be disregarding the fact that many gynaecological (and some surgical) conditions do not require emergency surgery, and some may not even need surgery.

An emergency consultation concerning an abdominal problem in a woman of any age requires attention to the gynaecological history and examination, without which the diagnosis may be missed and the management inappropriate.

13.1.1 HISTORY

The history should encompass menstruation, sexual activity and contraception and should be obtained in the privacy of a single room, or at least out of earshot of other patients.

The key elements of the menstrual history are the date of the last menstrual period (LMP), whether the woman is actually menstruating at the time of presentation, whether the menstrual periods are usually painful, and the association of any previous episodes of the presenting complaint with menstruation. If the first day of a woman's LMP is more than 14 days ago, or if the LMP was not normal when it came (e.g. flow less than normal, or at a time when it was not expected) the possibility that the woman may be pregnant must always be considered. Remember that women may report any vaginal bleeding that they experience as a period, even if it is not a true period. If she is menstruating at the time of presentation, there

Emergency Abdominal Surgery. Edited by Peter F. Jones, Zygmunt H. Krukowski and George G. Youngson. Published in 1998 by Chapman & Hall, London. ISBN 0 412 81950 3.

is a possibility that abdominal pain is an unusually severe episode of dysmenorrhoea, though this would be more likely if dysmenorrhoea was something she had experienced before. Severe pain around the time of menstruation would also be compatible with rupture of an endometrioma.

The relevance of sexual activity is that it may help in assessing the likelihood of pregnancy, of sexually transmitted disease or of ectopic pregnancy, where recent-onset dyspareunia is a key feature. The doctor needs to be sensitive to the fact that although most women will regard an enquiry as to whether they are sexually active, when the last occasion of coitus took place and whether intercourse was painful, as a straightforward matter, some will regard the question as intrusive or offensive, and may have good reasons to give misleading information (e.g. an adolescent whose mother or father is present). Confidentiality is essential, and may need enquiry in the absence of accompanying relatives or partner.

Contraception is important because pregnancy is obviously more likely in a woman who is actively trying to become pregnant, or who is using contraception intermittently or not at all, or who is using a relatively ineffective method of contraception. Some methods of contraception, such as the progesterone-only pill, which is usually taken continuously, and the intrauterine contraceptive device, or previous female sterilization, may be associated with a high relative rate of ectopic pregnancy (i.e. if contraception fails the resulting pregnancy is more like to be a tubal one).

A history of involuntary infertility may of course be caused by anovulation, or impaired fertility in the male, but might be associated with chronic pelvic infection or endometriosis, which could be relevant to the acute onset problem. The history should therefore include any investigation that may have been done, and any treatment such as ovulation induction or assisted reproduction. Vaginal discharge should be enquired about: some white or mucusy discharge is quite normal but an offensive or itchy discharge is suggestive of infection. Urethritis or discharge in the sexual partner could also be important.

13.1.2 PELVIC EXAMINATION

Where a woman presents with lower abdominal or pelvic pain or where abdominal examination suggests a mass arising from the pelvis or pelvic tenderness, a gentle bimanual vaginal examination is essential to assess the size and mobility of the uterus and adnexae, the presence of masses in the pouch of Douglas, the presence or absence of uterine or adnexal tenderness or cervical excitation tenderness (where a small amount of movement in the cervix produces a larger amount of movement of the uterine fundus and adnexae and is therefore helpful in the diagnosis of, e.g. ectopic pregnancy). The bladder should be emptied prior to examination.

It is obviously preferable that this examination should be done by an experienced gynaecologist, but if this is impossible, it should not be omitted, unless the woman is virgo intacta and/or does not permit examination. In the event of difficulty in performing vaginal examination, a bimanual rectal examination (with the patient supine) may give some useful information. A gynaecologist would normally also wish to do a speculum examination to assess the cervix and the presence of vaginal discharge, to watch for the presence of retained products of conception or fibroid polyps and to take appropriate high vaginal and cervical swabs.

The gynaecological assessment will usually include a measurement of the beta-hCG, even if the menstrual history is not suggestive of pregnancy, and a transvaginal ultrasound, which can usually be done on the ward by the gynaecologist. A clear view of the uterus, tubes and ovaries can be obtained without requiring a full bladder, and in some cases (e.g. intra- or extrauterine pregnancy) a definite diagnosis can be made. This may reduce reliance on diagnostic laparoscopy, which still has a mortality (16 per 10 000 in Finland, according to Virtanen and Makinen, 1995) and morbidity (2.7 per 1000 in Holland; Jansen *et al.*, 1997). Some interventions, such as aspiration of cysts or abscesses, can be done under scan control.

13.2   OVARIAN CYSTS

It is in the emergency situation that a surgeon is most likely to have to undertake initial management or surgery for women who prove to have ovarian cysts, benign or malignant. For example, in North-west England in 1991/2 (Woodman *et al.*, 1997) 28% of emergency admissions with ovarian cancer were operated upon by surgeons, compared to 13% of elective admissions. In Scotland in 1987 (Junor *et al.*, 1994) 35% of women with ovarian cancer were first seen by a surgeon, but only 10% were operated upon by surgeons.

Careful preoperative assessment will allow appropriate referral to gynaecologists of most cases, and advice and/or referral during surgery may also be possible. If the surgeon has to operate, it can be difficult to assess how conservative to be.

13.2.1   FUNCTIONAL CYSTS

Follicular or corpus luteum cysts are common in the reproductive age-group and usually asymptomatic. They are less common in women taking the combined oral contraceptive pill, as that suppresses ovulation. They may however present with acute pain and tenderness when rupture and haemorrhage occur, or when the ovary (and often the tube) undergoes torsion. If preoperative assessment shows an adnexal mass, transvaginal ultrasound will usually be helpful in determining whether it is ovarian or tubal; if an ovarian cyst is unilocular, has no solid components and is less than 5 cm in diameter, it is likely to be functional. Rupture of such a cyst can usually be treated conservatively if the pain and tenderness improve after a few hours and surgery is required only if significant haemorrhage has occurred. Surgery should be as conservative as possible, confined to oversewing the bleeding area. If a cyst is seen at laparoscopy or laparotomy but looks functional (thin-walled and translucent) aspiration is not helpful, as it does not prevent recurrence, but a follow-up scan is indicated to make sure that the diagnosis is correct.

If torsion of an ovarian cyst occurs, the patient is more likely to be systemically unwell with persisting tachycardia and pyrexia. The pain is of sudden onset, severe, unilateral and colicky. Because torsion occurs in cysts with a long pedicle, the palpable abdominal mass may lie surprisingly high, with its lower pole easily felt and some side-to-side mobility. Apart from the pain experienced by the woman, the condition is serious as it may lead to loss of the ovary and tube, and thrombosis of the ovarian vein may occur and extend centrally. If the condition is diagnosed early, it may be possible to undo the torsion and conserve the ovary and tube if they look viable, but excision of the tube and ovary are often required if they have undergone several revolutions and are not viable. The infundibulopelvic ligament must be clamped, together with the tube and ovarian ligament at the uterine cornua.

Bilateral multiple functional cysts occasionally occur through ovarian hyperstimulation and if the cysts have grown rapidly, they may present as an emergency with pain. Ovarian hyperstimulation is a rare but extremely morbid condition, associated with ascites and thromboembolism. It is almost always the result of ovulation induction, usually with gonadotrophins but occasionally with clomiphene citrate, but can be idiopathic (Edi-Osagie and Hopkins, 1997) or, in a less severe form, associated with trophoblastic disease. Where there has been ovulation induction, the problem usually presents in a conception cycle. From the surgical point of view, the importance of being aware of the condition is that although the cysts are large and may cause considerable pain, the treatment is supportive, not surgical (Jenkins *et al.*, 1995) and should be undertaken by a specialist in reproductive medicine. Polycystic ovary syndrome may predispose to this complication of ovulation induction, but does not itself present as an emergency.

Endometriomas ('chocolate cysts') are considered under endometriosis.

13.2.2 BENIGN NEOPLASMS

Benign ovarian neoplasms are not likely to present to the surgeon as an emergency unless they undergo rupture or torsion. Diagnostic and surgical problems may arise if the cyst is adherent to adjacent structures such as bowel or bladder, or if it extends retroperitoneally, as often happens in cysts occurring after hysterectomy. (The ureters are then at risk during surgery).

Dermoid cysts are commonest in young women, and are always benign. Teeth and bone may show up on X-ray and solid components on scan. They can be very large and are often bilateral. Although referred to as cysts, dermoids feel heavy, doughy and solid, and are opaque on inspection, with a smooth white capsule. Because they are benign and usually in a young woman, every effort should be made to do a cystectomy, conserving as much normal ovary as possible. It is preferable, however, not to spill any of the cyst contents into the peritoneal cavity as they can be irritant. If spillage occurs, the contents are easily recognized as sebaceous.

Other common benign neoplasms are serous cystadenomas and mucinous cystadenomas. Both can be multilocular, but a serous cystadenoma appears to contain yellow fluid whereas the contents of a mucinous cyst look bluish. Ideally, of course, surgery should be performed in the light of scan information on whether the cyst has features suggestive of malignancy, and after full discussion with the woman of her reproductive wishes; but in an emergency, it is better in a premenopausal woman to remove the cyst alone if that is feasible, or the affected ovary if the cyst has replaced the ovary, provided that the cyst is contained within the capsule without excrescences. In a postmenopausal woman, however, the presence of a benign neoplasm, even if unilateral, would be a good indication to remove both ovaries. Particular care should be taken not to spill the contents of a mucinous cystadenoma lest this results in a pseudomyxoma peritonei.

It is not of course always possible to be sure at operation what the histology will be, and it does not necessarily reflect badly upon the emergency surgeon if subsequent repeat laparotomy proves necessary. This is certainly preferable to unnecessary radical emergency surgery.

13.2.3 OVARIAN CARCINOMA

Because ovarian cancer presents late and may mimic other conditions the general surgeon may, when undertaking emergency surgery for conditions such as intestinal obstruction, discover that the primary pathology is ovarian cancer. This is usually characterized by unilateral or bilateral ovarian tumours with external excrescences, often adherent to and invading adjacent organs, often with widespread peritoneal and omental deposits and ascites. The ovarian primary may not be the largest tumour. Three recent British reviews of ovarian cancer, encompassing 2307 women who had surgery, have compared the nature of the surgery performed and the women's survival if operated upon by a surgeon compared to when the operation was done by a gynaecologist (Junor *et al.*, 1994; Kehoe *et al.*, 1994; Woodman *et al.*, 1997). These cases occurred in the late 1980s and early 1990s. Much of the surgery was elective, of course, and not relevant to the topic of emergency surgery, but surgeons were especially likely to have been involved in the emergency cases. Unfortunately, they were less likely to have examined women vaginally prior to abdominal surgery, less likely to have performed radical surgery, more likely to have considered the case inoperable and more likely to leave residual tumour (> 2 cm). Crude survival rates are worse for women operated upon by surgeons; this is of course partly explained by case mix, as surgeons tend to be operating on older women with more advanced disease, but, after adjustment for such factors, all the studies show a significantly higher risk for operation by a surgeon.

It is to be hoped that the excess mortality could be avoided by more extensive preoperative assessment, including gynaecological consultation, and/or by seeking the collaboration of a gynaecologist, preferably an oncologist, when the diagnosis only becomes clear at operation. Even if this is impossible, postoperative referral to a multidisciplinary team for chemotherapy and/or further surgery is essential.

13.3 TORSION OF THE FALLOPIAN TUBE

Torsion of the fallopian tube alone is much less common than torsion of the ovary and tube together. Although an ultrasound scan may assist with diagnosis, Ferrera *et al.* (1995) describe how the finding of a tubal swelling on scan may be misinterpreted as pelvic sepsis. The diagnosis is most likely to be made at laparoscopy/laparotomy for suspected torsion of an ovarian cyst, since the pain is of sudden onset, colicky and unilateral. If the tube is salvageable and unusually mobile, it may be anchored by suturing the mesosalpinx to the back of the broad ligament. If gangrenous, it must be excised as in salpingectomy for ectopic pregnancy (p. 494).

13.4 CRYPTOMENORRHOEA

Young women who have not yet menstruated but who have secondary sex characters (breast development, pubic and axillary hair) may very occasionally present with abdominal swelling and pain (usually with a history of recurring pain at approximately monthly intervals) with or without urinary retention (Nisanian, 1993). The diagnosis is usually very simply made by inspection of the vulva with the thighs abducted, when a bulging bluish membrane is evident, this being a literally intact hymen. The abdominal swelling is a haematocolpos, with or without haematometra and haematosalpinges. In the unlikely event of a gynaecologist not being available the surgical management is simple – under general anaesthesia a cruciate incision should be made in the hymen and the altered blood allowed to drain. Abdominal surgery is not required. Complicated cases (with reduplication of the genital tract) must always be referred to a gynaecologist for assessment.

13.5 RUPTURE OF THE GRAAFIAN FOLLICLE

Rupture of the graafian follicle occurs at ovulation. This is 14 days before the start of the next menstrual period which is usually 14 days after the start of the last menstrual period in a 28-day cycle. It may, if accompanied by bleeding into the peritoneal cavity, cause pain (*'Mittelschmerz'*), which will settle within a few hours as the blood is diluted by peritoneal fluid. Surgery is hardly ever needed but it may enter into the differential diagnosis of other conditions.

13.6 ENDOMETRIOSIS

The prevalence of endometriosis is difficult to establish accurately because of variation in ascertainment. It can be asymptomatic even when disease is extensive. Series based on findings at operation are likely to overestimate the incidence. On the other hand, histological evidence of endometriosis can be found in lesions that do not look to the inexperienced naked eye like endometriosis. A recent study (Vessey *et al.*, 1993) showed an incidence of around 0.5–0.8 per 1000 women years in women aged 35–49 (the peak age). Although endometriosis is associated with infertility, partly because of tubal distortion but also because of various cytotoxic factors in the peritoneal fluid (Rock and Markham, 1992), it is found in both nulliparous and parous women. It is less common in current oral contraceptive users and in the 2 years after a delivery.

The key diagnostic feature is that the presentation is likely to be during the first few days of a menstrual period, and that there may be a history of secondary dysmenorrhoea (acquired period pain) and dyspareunia.

Endometriosis is thought to arise either from retrograde menstruation through the fallopian tubes, from coelomic metaplasia or from activation of embryonic cell-rests. The latter two theories would explain how endometriosis may be found anywhere in the peritoneal cavity, for example in the large or small bowel or even in the urinary tract.

13.6.1 ENDOMETRIOMAS

Endometriosis is most common in the pelvic peritoneum, the uterosacral ligaments and the ovaries. Endometriomas may form in the ovaries, due to recurrent retention of menstrual blood in an enclosed cyst (often referred to as a 'chocolate cyst' because of the dark colour of the altered blood). If such a cyst ruptures, acute pain will result from spillage of the contents and may present to the surgeon. The condition is most likely to be mistaken as pelvic appendicitis, as there will be marked tenderness on rectal examination. The cyst must be removed and peritoneal lavage performed. It is unlikely however, that the lesion will be an isolated one, and, since the condition can be treated medically or surgically, and does not always require treatment (West, 1993), the opinion of a gynaecologist should be sought as to whether more needs to be done. Surgery may be difficult because of adhesions and should normally be done electively after full discussion with the woman.

13.6.2   OBSTRUCTION OF THE LARGE BOWEL

Obstruction occurs because of fibrosis, when there is endometriosis in the bowel wall adjacent to the ovaries, or in the rectovaginal septum, but is rare because of the wide lumen of the large bowel. The fibrotic lump can be mistaken for a stenosing carcinoma. The histology should be established prior to definitive surgery, which may require gynaecological input.

13.6.3   OBSTRUCTION OF THE SMALL BOWEL

This is a very rare problem as endometrial deposits in the small bowel are much less common than in the large bowel. They presumably arise from metaplasia (Ridley, 1968) and in many cases are present when there is no sign of pelvic endometriosis. Deposits are most likely to cause obstruction when they are in the terminal ileum because of its narrow lumen. At operation, especially if there are no endometriotic deposits seen in the pelvis, it may be difficult to differentiate between endometriosis and other conditions such as carcinoid and Crohn's disease and this situation is discussed on p. 233.

13.7   ACUTE PELVIC INFLAMMATORY DISEASE (PID)

This is an infective condition affecting the endometrium, fallopian tubes and sometimes the ovaries as well. In principle the infection ascends through the cervix from the lower genital tract. The condition can be chronic and asymptomatic, but the general surgeon is likely to see only those women who have acute severe disease. The incidence seems to be increasing but the epidemiology and natural history of the condition are not clearly established because of variation in severity and ascertainment, but it is generally agreed that the 'gold standard' for ascertainment would be a diagnosis at laparoscopy (Jacobson and Westrom, 1969) or plasma cell endometritis (Korn *et al.*, 1995).

Early diagnosis is worthwhile not just to avert the severe illness that can occur but also to prevent the adverse effects upon female fertility (especially tubal function, hence predisposing to ectopic pregnancy).

13.7.1   HISTORY

The presenting history of severe PID is of acute or acute-on-chronic pelvic pain, usually with dyspareunia and vaginal discharge. It is less common in oral contraceptive users and commoner in IUCD users but only in the early months after insertion. When associated with IUCD use it can occasionally be fatal (Smith *et al.*, 1983). Rather surprisingly, considering its aetiology, it has been reported in women with prior sterilization (Reedy *et al.*, 1994). There is usually a marked pyrexia and perhaps rigors.

13.7.2 EXAMINATION

The USA Center for Disease Control and Prevention (1993) suggested as minimal criteria for diagnosis the following:

- abdominal tenderness;
- cervical motion tenderness;
- adnexal tenderness.

Unfortunately, however, this triad has a sensitivity of only 33%, specificity of 88% and positive predictive value of 71% (Korn *et al.*, 1995) and thus many cases would be misdiagnosed. In clinical practice, an important feature that distinguishes pelvic inflammatory disease from, for instance, appendicitis or complications of an ovarian cyst, is that salpingitis is virtually always bilateral.

A number of studies have tried to improve the positive predictive value of the CDC criteria by evaluating other features such as vaginal pus, raised erythrocyte sedimentation rate (ESR), C-reactive protein or white cell count in the blood, but with limited success (Korn *et al.*, 1995; Peipert *et al.*, 1996; Miettinen *et al.*, 1993). Transvaginal ultrasound may be helpful in establishing at least a working diagnosis, and can be used as a guide to aspiration of pyosalpinges or tubo-ovarian abscesses (Aboulghar *et al.*, 1995; Teisala *et al.*, 1990).

13.7.3 MANAGEMENT

If the woman has only a low-grade pyrexia and is not acutely ill, treatment with intravenous antibiotics may be appropriate but with careful surveillance in case the diagnosis is wrong. If an IUCD is present, it should be removed forthwith. If she does not settle quickly, laparoscopy is essential.

Laparoscopy is usually advisable in a more severe case but may be superseded by transvaginal ultrasound, since that can be used without general anaesthesia to aspirate pus and, if indicated, to instil antibiotics into the abscess cavity. However, if appropriate expertise is not available, laparoscopy/laparotomy is essential. Rupture of an abscess into the peritoneal cavity will present as an acute emergency and laparotomy and drainage is essential, together with resuscitation and intravenous antibiotic therapy.

The choice of antibiotic requires local knowledge of the likely organisms. A recent study from Finland (Heinonen and Mietlinen, 1994) showed that the most common organisms in both mild and severe cases were *C. trachomatis*, followed by *N. gonorrhoeae* then *E. coli* and *H. influenzae*. In severe cases with tubo-ovarian abscess, multiple organisms were invariably involved, with anaerobes as well, and antibiotic therapy must take this into account. A rare organism in the peritoneal cavity is *S. pneumoniae* which seems to be more common in the presence of an IUCD (Gruer *et al.*, 1983). Peritonitis is then characterized by a large amount of peritoneal fluid. Another rare organism that has been reported to cause tubo-ovarian sepsis in the presence of an IUCD is *Actinomyces* (Muller-Holzner *et al.*, 1990), especially with long-term use; however, the presentation is chronic rather than acute.

The preferred antibiotic for the treatment of gonorrhoea is amoxycillin, which must be given intravenously in severe cases. The addition of probenecid will prolong the action of the drug by reducing renal excretion. If the woman is allergic to penicillin, spectinomycin or ciprofloxacin can be alternatives. If there is a poor response to therapy, a second-generation cephalosporin such as cefuroxime can be tried, or gentamicin. If *Chlamydia* infection has been diagnosed, treatment is with tetracycline or erythromycin. The possibility of an anaerobic infection can be covered by giving metronidazole in addition.

REFERENCES

Aboulghar, M. A., Mansour, R. T. and Serour, G. I. (1995) Ultrasonographically guided transvaginal aspiration of tubo-ovarian abscesses and pyosalpinges: an optional treatment for acute pelvic inflammatory disease. *Am. J. Obstet. Gynecol.*, **172**, 1501–1503.

Center for Disease Control and Prevention (1993) Sexually transmitted diseases: treatment guidelines. *M.M.W.R.*, **42**(No. Rr-14), 75–78.

Edi-Osagie, E. C. O. and Hopkins, R. E. (1997) Recurrent idiopathic ovarian hyperstimulation syndrome in pregnancy. *Br. J. Obstet. Gynaecol.*, **104**, 952–954.

Ferrera, P. C., Kass, L. E. and Verdile, V. P. (1995) Torsion of the fallopian tube. *Am. J. Emerg. Med.*, **13**, 312–314.

Gruer, L., Collingham, K. E. and Edwards, C. W. (1983) Pneumococcal peritonitis associated with an IUCD. *Lancet*, **ii**, 677.

Heinonen, P. K. and Miettinen, A. (1994) Laparoscopic study on the microbiology and severity of acute pelvic inflammatory disease. *Eur. J. Obstet. Gynecol. Reprod. Med.*, **57**, 85–89.

Jacobson, L. and Westrom, L. (1969) Objectivized diagnosis of acute pelvic inflammatory disease. *Am. J. Obstet. Gynecol.*, **105**, 1088–1098.

Jansen, F. W., Kapiteyn, K., Trimbos-Kemper, T. *et al.* (1997) Complications of laparoscopy: prospective multicentre observational study. *Br. J. Obstet. Gynaecol.*, **104**, 595–600.

Jenkins, J. M., Mathur, R. S. and Cooke, I. D. (1995) The Management of Severe Ovarian Hyperstimulation. *Br. J. Obstet. Gynaecol.*, **102**, 2–5.

Junor, E. J., Hole, D. J. and Gillis, C. R. (1994) Management of ovarian cancer: referral to a multidisciplinary team matters. *Br. J. Cancer*, **70**, 363–370.

Kehoe, S., Powell, J., Wilson, S. *et al.* (1994) The influence of the operating surgeon's specialisation on patient survival in ovarian cancer. *Br. J. Cancer*, **70**, 1014–1017.

Korn, A. P., Hessol, N., Padian, N. *et al.* (1995) Commonly used diagnostic criteria for pelvic inflammatory disease have poor sensitivity for plasma cell endometritis. *Sex. Transm. Dis.*, **22**, 335–341.

Miettinen, A. K., Heinonen, P. K., Laippala, P. *et al.* (1993) Test performance of erythocyte sedimentation rate and c-reactive protein in assessing the severity of acute pelvic inflammatory disease. *Am. J. Obstet. Gynecol.*, **169**, 1143–1149.

Muller-Holzner, E., Geschwendtner, A., Abfalter, E. *et al.* (1990) Actinomycosis and long-term use of intrauterine devices. *Lancet*, **336**, 939.

Nisanian, A. C. (1993) Haematocolpometra presenting as urinary retention. *J. Reprod. Med.*, **38**, 57–59.

Peipert, J. F., Boardman, L., Hogan, J. W. *et al.* (1996) Laboratory evaluation of acute upper genital tract infection. *Obstet. Gynecol.*, **87**, 730–736.

Reedy, M. B., Galan, H. L. and Patterson, K. M. (1994) Acute pelvic inflammatory disease after tubal sterilisation. *J. Reprod. Med.*, **39**, 752–754.

Ridley, J. H. (1968) Histogenesis of endometriosis. *Obstet. Gynecol. Surv.*, **23**, 1.

Rock, J. A. and Markham, S. M. (1992) Pathogenesis of endometriosis. *Lancet*, **340**, 1264–1267.

Salkey, B. (1993) Diagnostic laparoscopy. *Surg. Laparosc. Endosc.*, **3**, 132–134.

Smith, P. A., Ellis, C. J., Sparks, R. A. *et al.* (1983) Deaths associated with intrauterine contraceptive devices in the United Kingdom between 1973 and 1983. *BMJ.*, **238**, 1537–1538.

Tersala, K., Heinenen, P. K. and Punnonen, R. (1990) Transvaginal ultrasound in the diagnosis and treatment of tubo-ovarian abscess. *Br. J. Obstet. Gynaecol.*, **97**, 178–180.

Vessey, M. P., Villard-Mackintosh, L. and Painter, R. (1993) Epidemiology of endometriosis in women attending family planning clinics. *BMJ.*, **306**, 182–184.

Virtanen, H. S. and Makinen, J. I. (1995) Mortality after gynaecologic operation in Finland 1985–1991. *Br. J. Obstet. Gynaecol.*, **102**, 54–57.

Walmsley, G. L., Wilson, D. H., Gunn, A. A. *et al.* (1977) Computer-aided diagnosis of lower abdominal pain in women. *Br. J. Surg.*, **64**, 538.

West, C. P. (1993) Endometriosis. *BMJ.*, **306**, 158–159.

Woodman, C., Baghdady, A., Collins, C. *et al.* (1997) What changes in the organisation of cancer services will improve the outcome for women with ovarian cancer? *Br. J. Obstet. Gynaecol.*, **104**, 135–139.

14

Vascular emergencies

14.1 INTRODUCTION

Atherosclerosis, which can cause stenosis, occlusion or dilatation and rupture of arteries, produces abdominal emergencies that are more acute and life-threatening than those resulting from inflammation or a neoplasm. In this chapter the common vascular causes of the acute abdomen, such as ruptured and symptomatic aortic aneurysms and mesenteric ischaemia, are dealt with, but rarer and often misdiagnosed conditions, such as aortoenteric fistulas, visceral artery aneurysms, aortic dissections and mesenteric venous thromboses are also discussed. All these conditions have the common feature that without rapid diagnosis, often made on clinical grounds alone, and equally urgent treatment, death of the organ and indeed the patient is usually inevitable. The mortality in patients with a vascular abdominal emergency exceeds 50% and a heightened awareness of these conditions and the urgency required offers the only prospect of improvement in this grave outlook.

14.2 ABDOMINAL AORTIC ANEURYSM

14.2.1 RUPTURED ABDOMINAL AORTIC ANEURYSM

The incidence of aortic aneurysm and subsequent rupture has been increasing in the Western world for the last 30 years and now ranks as the 13th most common cause of death, responsible for 15 000 deaths per year in the USA (Reilly and Tilson, 1989). The true incidence of aortic aneurysm rupture is not known but Bengtsson and Bergquist (1993), reporting from Southern Sweden (where the post-mortem examination rate is constant at 85% over the last 16-year period) found an incidence of 5.6 per 100 000 inhabitants. Other population-based studies from the UK, USA and Scandinavia found incidences between 2.9 and 14.1 per 100 000 inhabitants. A report from a Minnesota community showed a sevenfold increase in incidence between 1957 and 1980 (Melton et al., 1984). There are three contributory reasons for the increased prevalence: improved diagnosis, more people reaching an age at which aneurysmal disease is common, and an increased incidence within this older population (Fawkes et al., 1989: Bengtsson et al., 1992).

Emergency Abdominal Surgery. Edited by Peter F. Jones, Zygmunt H. Krukowski and George G. Youngson. Published in 1998 by Chapman & Hall, London. ISBN 0 412 81950 3.

Although the exact mortality from ruptured aortic aneurysm is uncertain, population-based studies reveal a total mortality of between 77% and 94%. Rupture can complicate aneurysms of any size, with the risk being greatest in larger and expanding aneurysms. A linear relationship exists between initial size at diagnosis (diameter and length), the rate of expansion of diameter and rupture of aneurysms (Bengtsson *et al.*, 1993). Interestingly, in spite of an increased awareness, with earlier diagnosis and intervention for this condition, overall mortality rates have been consistent across all affected age ranges, at a time when mortality from stroke and coronary artery disease has declined dramatically (Lilienfield *et al.*, 1987).

14.2.2 PRESENTATION

Patients with ruptured aortic aneurysm present to the surgeon, either from the Emergency Department or from general practitioners directly to the Surgical Unit, in a state of collapse, often semiconscious or unconscious, with severe backache and associated abdominal pain that may mimic acute renal or ureteric pain. The onset of collapse and pain is often acute, with no antecedent history, and there really are no other conditions that present in this dramatic fashion. Any patient presenting with such a history should have the diagnosis of ruptured aortic aneurysm made forthwith and be immediately transferred to the operating theatre for resuscitation and surgery. The diagnosis should be made on the history alone in most patients and only rarely are supplementary investigations indicated. Failure to make the diagnosis at this stage and act promptly may result in the demise of the patient. When these patients are *in extremis* the history is only obtainable from the family or the referring doctors.

The patient's pallor and pain are the striking features. Blood pressure may be very low or unrecordable but it should be remembered that patients with aortic aneurysm are often hypertensive prior to rupture and a near-normal blood pressure may represent relative hypotension. When available, previous hospital or primary care records should indicate the patient's usual blood pressure. Examination of the abdomen may be difficult because of obesity, but a pulsating mass, often eccentric and extending down towards the iliac fossa, is typically present. Tenderness is always present in the conscious patient. Even in patients with a small, contained rupture who are haemodynamically stable, tenderness around the aneurysm is indicative of impending major rupture and should stimulate the surgical team into urgent action, although further investigation by ultrasound and/or CT scan may be appropriate if there is doubt about the diagnosis.

14.2.3 MANAGEMENT

Once the diagnosis is made, the patient should be taken immediately to theatre where a vascular surgical and anaesthetic team should attend. Rapid infusion of intravenous fluids to restore the blood pressure towards normal, away from the operating theatre, is likely to have disastrous consequences with death of the patient. The 'tearing force' that led to the rupture is strikingly reduced as long as the blood pressure is low and attempting to restore this 'tearing force' at the same time as the clotting factors are diluted by electrolyte solutions and plasma volume expanders is dangerous and inappropriate. Resuscitation should only start when the surgical team is available and ready in theatre to seal the hole in the aorta by surgical intervention. When resuscitation has to start away from the hospital, fluid replacement should be the minimum required to secure a recordable blood pressure.

Once in theatre the patient is draped for a long midline incision with access to both femoral arteries should distal anastomosis prove necessary. Peripheral venous access with at least two large-bore cannulas to allow rapid blood transfusion must be established and arterial and central venous catheters inserted subsequently as appropriate. At least 6 units of grouped and cross-matched blood must be ordered but Group O-negative blood may have to be used pending delivery. A urinary catheter should be in position by the time the operation starts.

When the abdomen is entered the diagnosis is immediately confirmed by the presence of a large retroperitoneal haematoma. Some free blood or blood-stained fluid is usually present in the peritoneal cavity, even when the rupture is retroperitoneal. The duodenojejunal junction is mobilized by dividing the haemorrhagic peritoneum to the left of the duodenojejunal junction and retracting the duodenum and small bowel towards the right side protected by a pack. The colon is retracted upwards and to the left, again with a gauze pack using deep Dyball or Deaver retractors initially, to help to retract the wound edges and abdominal contents, until the neck of the aneurysm has been controlled. Self-retaining retractors, such as an Omnitract, may be inserted but this is usually done once the clamp has been applied to the aorta.

The priority is to control the neck of the aneurysm, which is approached by blunt dissection with the fingers of the right hand, long Lloyd-Davies scissors or even the sucker. The left renal vein is often the only recognizable landmark in a haemorrhagic landscape in which the anatomy is difficult to define. The pulse in the aorta above the aneurysm is often hard to locate because of the relatively strong pulsation in the aneurysm and surrounding haematoma. If, as often happens at this stage, the patient is or becomes pulseless, opening the aneurysm and inserting a finger into the proximal aorta may be the quickest way to identify the neck of the aneurysm and apply a clamp to the proximal aorta. An aortic occlusion catheter or a Foley urinary catheter may be used to occlude the proximal aorta but it is our choice to occlude the aorta just above the aneurysm with side-to-side compression using a soft, straight vascular clamp such as a hydragrip Fogarty clamp. The aorta may be approached and a clamp applied as it passes through the diaphragm above the origin of the coeliac axis but this manoeuvre is seldom required. The left renal vein is at times stretched over the aneurysm and haematoma. It can be divided close to the vena cava, thereby maintaining venous drainage through the suprarenal and gonadal veins. This improves access to the proximal aneurysm by improving exposure of the aorta up to the renal arteries. It may also prevent accidental damage to the renal vein and facilitate the performance of the proximal anastomosis.

Once the proximal clamp is on the aorta the aneurysm is rapidly freed down to the iliac vessels and opened. If the iliac vessels are not aneurysmal they are controlled by applying angled vascular clamps. No attempt should be made to mobilize the iliac arteries because this often leads to damage of the iliac veins and side-to-side clamping is the easier and safer option. When the iliac arteries are aneurysmal it is necessary to isolate the common or even the internal and external iliac arteries distal to the affected segments. It is usually possible to anastomose the distal limbs of the bifurcation graft to the distal common iliac arteries but not infrequently the aneurysm extends on one or both sides into the internal iliac arteries, which makes it necessary to ligate the affected internal iliac artery and make the distal anastomosis to the external iliac artery or even the common femoral after opening the groins. Should the aneurysmal disease extend into both internal iliac arteries some vascular surgeons would argue that it is necessary to revascularize one internal iliac to preserve adequate flow to the pelvis and gluteal regions but little evidence exists in the literature that this is necessary and it is our preference to simply ligate the internal iliac arteries.

Prior to insertion of the graft the content of the aneurysm is removed, any bleeding lumbar vessels are secured with 2/0 Nurolon stitches and the inferior mesenteric artery, if patent, may be ligated or reimplanted into the graft once this is in place. The patent inferior mesenteric artery should be prepared with a patch of the aortic wall and back bleeding controlled with a clamp until the sigmoid colon can be carefully inspected once the aortic graft is in place. If there is any doubt about the integrity of vascular supply of the colon, the inferior mesenteric artery should be implanted into the graft.

An occasional finding when opening the aneurysm is the appearance of dark venous blood flowing into the aorta from an aortocaval fistula due to the rupture of the aneurysm into the adherent cava. This has been reported in 4% of ruptured aneurysms (Baker *et al.*, 1972). Spontaneous fistula formation to the left renal vein has also been reported but only in patients with an abnormal retro-aortic renal vein (Brener *et al.*, 1974; Merrill and Ernst, 1981). This bleeding is usually fairly easily controlled by compression of the vena cava above and below the tear using swabs on sticks or finger pressure and closing the defect in the aortic wall with for instance a 3/0 Prolene suture. That will close the vena cava which is adherent to the aortic wall.

The graft used should be either a bifurcation or a straight tube graft of Dacron or PTFE (polytetrafluoroethylene). Most vascular surgeons will probably choose a graft sealed with collagen, gelatin or albumin for the ruptured aneurysm repair, although a woven Dacron graft is a cheaper alternative. Grafts with a diameter of 16–20 mm are most commonly used and 3/0 or 4/0 Prolene sutures used for the anastomoses. When the suture lines are haemostatic the aneurysmal wall is used to cover the graft in a double-breasted fashion so that there are two layers of aortic wall between the duodenojejunal junction and the graft. It may also be possible to interpose peritoneum from the left side of the abdomen between the duodenum and the aneurysmal wall and graft anastomosis to pre-empt the risk of an aortoduodenal fistula.

During the operation good communication and cooperation between the anaesthetic and surgical teams is essential. The application and removal of clamps should be a mutual decision. Similarly, the surgical team needs to be notified of changing cardiac performance, CVP and blood pressure. Thus familiar and regular interaction between the anaesthetic and surgical team is essential. Postoperatively most patients with ruptured aortic aneurysm require elective ventilation and nursing in an intensive care unit.

The mortality rate from ruptured aneurysm differs markedly in reported series because of significant variation in the patient referral and selection patterns. Tertiary referral centres tend to operate on a selected group of patients who have survived initial rupture and tolerated resuscitation and long travelling time, and mortality rates less than 30% have been reported (Darke and Eadie, 1973). Indeed, a rate of 15% in a series of 61 consecutive patients is recorded (Lawrie *et al.*, 1979) but a more typical result from a regional vascular unit would be a mortality rate of about 50% (Samy *et al.*, 1995; Sayer *et al.*, 1997).

14.2.4 ACUTE SYMPTOMATIC AORTIC ANEURYSM

It is not unusual for a patient presenting with upper abdominal pain or flank pain, who on clinical examination and on further investigation is found to have an aortic aneurysm, to present to a general surgical unit. There may or may not be tenderness over the aneurysm and no other cause of the pain may be found. These patients are stable and the ultrasound and CT scans confirm that the aneurysm is intact. Any such patient should be regarded as having a symptomatic aortic aneurysm until proven otherwise and the aneurysm should be repaired urgently. At operation the reason for the symptoms is usually not obvious, but their disappearance after repair indicates a causal relationship between the aneurysm and the pain. Sometimes the duodenum may be quite adherent and stretching of the bowel wall maybe a mechanism for the pain. These patients are difficult to distinguish from those with contained rupture despite all modern investigative methods and they should therefore be operated upon urgently. The indications for surgery are therefore greater in these symptomatic patients than in those with asymptomatic elective aneurysms and the mortality is consequently higher (Sayer *et al.*, 1997).

Inflammatory aortic aneurysm is one specific type of symptomatic aneurysm, which accounts for up to 10% of all patients with aortic aneurysms; these typically present with backache, abdominal pain, weight loss and a high erythrocyte sedimentation rate. The diagnosis is usually made preoperatively by CT scan and ultrasonography (Crawford *et al.*, 1985; Bower *et al.*, 1989). The aetiology of the fibrous, thickened aneurysmal wall is not understood but the condition may be related to retroperitoneal fibrosis. It often involves the ureters, leading to obstructive uropathy, and may present with massive gastrointestinal haemorrhage due to spontaneous aortoenteric fistula formation.

14.2.5 THE INCIDENTAL AORTIC ANEURYSM

The first knowledge of the presence of an aortic aneurysm in a patient is occasionally at the time of laparotomy for another surgical condition. A large aneurysm carries a real risk of rupture in the postoperative period, after, for instance, colectomy for an obstructing colonic cancer. There is no evidence to support a policy of combined aneurysm repair with any bowel surgery, either elective or emergency (Lobbato *et al.*, 1985). However, the bigger the aneurysm the more likely that postoperative rupture may occur. We have had, on one occasion, to operate upon a ruptured aneurysm 4 days after emergency colectomy for rectosigmoid cancer. The conventional attitude is to deal with the emergency gastrointestinal problem, particularly when this is bleeding or an obstructing cancer, and return to deal with the aneurysm at a later date. A particular difficulty arises in the patient who has symptoms and signs that could originate from either gastrointestinal pathology or the coincidental aneurysm.

Such a patient presented as an emergency from abroad, generally unwell, with abdominal pain and a large aneurysm. At laparotomy he had a rectosigmoid inflammatory mass due to a ruptured diverticulum, chronic cholecystitis with a large gallstone partially extruding through the gallbladder, as well as a large abdominal aortic aneurysm with an unhealthy-looking wall. This situation was managed by resection of the aneurysm, cholecystectomy and anterior resection without any postoperative problems. When aneurysm surgery is performed in a potentially contaminated peritoneal cavity, our policy is to deal with the aneurysm first and close the retroperitoneal tissues carefully before proceeding with subsequent surgery. The aortic graft should be a gelatin-, albumen- or collagen-coated graft impregnated with rifampicin, and appropriate antibiotics should also be administered. It should be emphasized again that it is only under exceptional circumstances that it is justified to perform such combined procedures.

14.3 AORTOENTERIC FISTULAS

14.3.1 PRIMARY AORTOENTERIC FISTULAS

Aortoenteric fistulas may occur either as primary fistulas in patients with aortic aneurysm or as a secondary event in patients who have had previous aortic graft insertion for aneurysmal or occlusive disease. Primary aortoenteric fistula is an unusual presentation of aortic aneurysmal disease, seen by the author in only three patients, all of whom had inflammatory aortic aneurysms. A literature review in 1984 found 18 reported cases, mostly associated with aortic aneurysms, but infected aneurysms, cancer, bacterial aortitis and peptic ulcer accounted for some of the cases (Sweeney and Gadacz, 1984; Bower *et al.*, 1989). The fistula usually develops between the distal duodenum or proximal jejunum and the aorta, and presents with gastrointestinal haemorrhage. It is common for the first bleed to result in moderate haematemesis and/or melaena, following which gastroscopy may reveal no cause unless careful examination of the distal duodenum is undertaken. If no aortic aneurysm can be palpated the patient might well develop massive gastrointestinal bleeding either before or after discharge from hospital. This may lead to rapid death but can also result in surgery being undertaken by an unsuspecting gastrointestinal surgeon rather than a vascular surgeon. The aorta will need to be controlled above and below the fistula and thereafter the aortic wall should be left attached to the duodenum and the defect in it closed by inserting interrupted PDS sutures through the thickened aortic wall, with an omental patch covering the repair.

The vascular repair is achieved by closing the proximal aorta and iliac arteries, and reconstituting the blood supply to the lower limbs with axillofemoral bypass or *in situ* aortic reconstruction. If the graft is inserted *in situ* this should be a rifampicin-impregnated, collagen-, gelatin- or albumen-coated Dacron graft. It is common to keep such patients on long-term antibiotic therapy. Each individual unit sees few of these patients, and consequently experience is limited. No comparative studies are thus available to support the use of either procedure in preference, although the *in situ* procedure seems to be favoured at the present time.

14.3.2 SECONDARY AORTOENTERIC FISTULA

One of the most challenging surgical emergencies encountered is an aortoenteric fistula with gastrointestinal haemorrhage following previous aortic surgery for aneurysmal or occlusive disease. The condition is notoriously difficult to diagnose and to treat, but must always be considered in any patient with previous aortic surgery who presents with gastrointestinal haemorrhage or anaemia (p. 347).

A considerable number of people in any modern society now have prosthetic aortic grafts in place and as a result aortoenteric fistulae are not unusual and will occur more commonly in the future. As many as 4% of such patients may be affected (Peck and Eidemiller, 1992) but the more commonly recognized figure is about 1%. The different incidences reported may depend on the length of follow-up, since fistulas have been reported to occur even 27 years after the primary operation (Shindo *et al.*, 1993)

The mechanism of the formation of the fistula is uncertain in most cases. Infection may be introduced with the original operation, but in other instances, bacteraemia following graft insertion may lead to infection. It is also possible that false aneurysm formation around one anastomosis may cause pressure damage to surrounding bowel wall and the creation of a fistula with secondary infection. In a series of prosthetic graft infections from St Mary's Hospital, 28 patients out of 50 had an aortoenteric fistula, 16 communicating with the duodenum, ten with the remaining small bowel and two with the colon (Hannon *et al.*, 1996).

The diagnosis should be suspected in a patient with massive gastrointestinal haemorrhage who has had previous aortic surgery. In the event of massive bleeding there is seldom time for any diagnostic procedure except for laparotomy, although endoscopy, angiography, CT scans and barium studies have all been used with varying degrees of benefit (Van Baalen *et al.*, 1996). In the St Mary's series, no fistula was diagnosed by endoscopy but an indium-labelled white cell scan was performed in 19 patients and 15 scans were positive.

Systemic signs of infection such as elevated ESR, white cell count, anaemia and fever are present in approximately 50% and about 25% of patients have a positive culture of *E. coli*, with a similar percentage having cultures of *Staphylococcus aureus* from their graft.

The treatment options, when faced with this surgical challenge, are either local reconstruction with removal of the old graft, repair of the fistula and insertion of a new graft in the anatomically correct position, or closure of the aortic stump with extra-anatomic reconstruction. This is achieved most commonly by bilateral axillofemoral bypass. Local irrigation of the graft with antibiotics has also been tried by various groups, but is generally unsuccessful. Ten patients in the St Mary's series were treated by local techniques but either died from complications or required graft excision for recurrent graft infection and extra-anatomic reconstruction. Our own experience has been similar. Two patients died of recurrent graft infection, one 3½ years after the original operation. Another two patients survived up to 11 years after removal of the graft and bilateral axillofemoral reconstruction.

The use of antibiotic-impregnated graft has been supported by Strachan and colleagues (1991) and by Naylor and co-workers (1995). Grafts sealed with collagen, gelatin and albumin all bond with rifampicin but the bonding only lasts for a short time and its value remains unproven. Because the mortality from infected aortic graft has been reported to be as high as 77% (O'Hara *et al.*, 1986) and the morbidity due to amputation alone ranging from 11–57% (Champion *et al.*, 1982; Szilagyi *et al.*, 1972), it seems prudent to use every possible measure to reduce the potential morbidity and mortality of this complication.

REFERENCES

Baker, W. H., Shanzer, L. A. and Ehrenhaft, J. L. (1972) Aortocaval fistula as a complication of abdominal aortic aneurysms. *Surgery*, **72**, 933–938.

Bengtsson, H. and Bergquist, D. (1993) Ruptured abdominal aortic aneurysm: a presentation based study. *J. Vasc. Surg.*, **18**, 74–80.

Bengtsson, H., Bergquist, D. and Sternby, N. (1992) Increasing prevalence of abdominal aortic aneurysms: a necropsy study. *Eur. J. Surg.*, **158**, 19–23.

Bengtsson, H., Bergquist, D., Ekberg, A. *et al.* (1993) Expansion pattern and risk of rupture of abdominal aortic aneurysms that were not operated on. *Eur. J. Surg.*, **159**, 461–467.

Bower, T., Cherry, K. J. and Pairolero, P. C. (1989) Unusual manifestations of abdominal aortic aneurysms. *Surg. Clin. North Am.*, **69**(4), 745–754.

Brener, B. J., Darling, R. C., Frederick, P. L. *et al.* (1974) Major venous anomalies complicating abdominal aortic surgery. *Arch. Surg.*, **108**, 159–165.

Champion, M. C., Sullivan, S. N., Coles, J. C. *et al.* (1982) Aortoenteric fistula: Incidence, presentation, recognition and management. *Ann. Surg.*, **195**, 314–317.

Crawford, J. L., Stowe, C. L., Safi, H. J. *et al.* (1985) Inflammatory aneurysms of the aorta. *J. Vasc. Surg.*, **2**, 113–124.

Darke, S. G. and Eadie, D. D. G. (1973) Abdominal aortic aneurysmectomy: a review of 60 consecutive cases contrasting elective and emergency surgery. *J. Cardiovasc. Surg.*, **14**, 484–491.

Fawkes, F. G. R., MacIntyre, C. C. A. and Ruckley, C. V. (1989) Increasing incidence of aortic aneurysms in England and Wales. *BMJ.*, **298**, 33–35.

Hannon, R. J., Wolfe, J. H. N. and Mansfield, A. O. (1996) Aortic prosthetic infection: 50 patients treated by radical or local surgery. *Br. J. Surg.*, **83**, 654–658.

Lawrie, G. M., Morris, G. C. Jr, Crawford, E. S. *et al.* (1979) Improved results of operation for ruptured abdominal aortic aneurysms. *Surgery*, **85**, 483–488.

Lilienfeld, D., Gunderson, P., Sprafka, J. *et al.* (1987) The epidemiology of abdominal aortic aneurysms: mortality trends in the United States 1951–1980. *Arteriosclerosis*, **7**, 637–643.

Lobbato, V. J., Rothenberg, R. E., La Raja, R. D. *et al.* (1985) Coexistence of abdominal aortic aneurysm and carcinoma of the colon: a dilemma. *J. Vasc. Surg.*, **2**, 724–726.

Melton, L., Bickerstaff, L., Hollier, L. *et al.* (1984) Changing incidence of abdominal aortic aneurysms: a population-based study. *Am. J. Epidemiol.*, **120**, 379–386.

Merrill, W. H. and Ernst, C. B. (1981) Aorto-left renal vein fistula: hemodynamic monitoring and timing of operation. *Surgery*, **89**, 678–682.

Naylor, A. R., Clark, S., London, N. J. M. *et al.* (1995) Treatment of major aortic graft infection: preliminary experience with total graft excision and in situ replacement with a rifampicin bonded prosthesis. *Eur. J. Vasc. Surg.*, **9**, 252–256.

O'Hara, P. J., Hertzer, N. R., Beven, E. G. and Krajewski, L. P. (1986) Surgical management of infected abdominal aortic grafts: review of a 25 year experience. *J. Vasc. Surg.*, **3**, 725–731.

Peck, J. J. and Eidemiller, L. R. (1992) Aortoenteric fistulas. *Arch. Surg.*, **127**, 1191–1193.

Reilly, J. M. and Tilson, M. D. (1989) Incidence and etiology of abdominal aortic aneurysms. *Surg. Clin. North Am.*, **69**(4), 705–711.

Samy, A. K., Wilson, B. J., Engeset, J. *et al.* (1995) Abdominal aortic aneurysm: a 12 year experience in the Grampian Region, Scotland. *J. R. Coll. Surg. Edin.*, **40**, 180–184.

Sayer, R. D., Thomson, M. M., Nasim, A. *et al.* (1997) Surgical management of 671 abdominal aortic aneurysms: a 13 year review from a single centre. *Eur. J. Vasc. Endovasc. Surg.* **13**; 322–327.

Shindo, S., Tada, Y., Sato, O. *et al.* (1993) A case of aortocolic fistula occurring 27 years after aortofemoral bypass surgery, treated successfully by surgical management. *Surg. Today*, **23**, 993–997.

Strachan, C. J. L., Newsom, S. W. B. and Ashton, T. R. (1991) The clinical use of an antibiotic-bonded graft. *Eur. J. Vasc. Surg.*, **5**, 627–632.

Sweeney, M. S. and Gadacz, R. (1984) Primary aortoduodenal fistula: manifestation, diagnosis and treatment. *Surgery*, **96**, 492–497.

Szilagyi, D. E., Smith, R. F., Elliott, J. P. and Vandrecic, M. P. (1972) Infection in arterial reconstruction with synthetic grafts. *Ann. Surg.*, **176**, 321–333.

Van Baalen, J. M., Kluit, A. B., Maas, J. *et al.* (1996) Diagnosis and therapy of aortic prosthetic fistulas: trends over a 30-year experience. *Br. J. Surg.*, **83**, 1729–1734.

14.4   MESENTERIC ISCHAEMIA

The increasing frequency of mesenteric ischaemia as a presenting clinical problem is the consequence of an ageing population surviving the effects of generalized atherosclerosis through improvements in the medical care of other manifestations of this disease process. This has allowed patients to survive their original disease only to suffer acute mesenteric ischaemia.

The incidence of mesenteric ischaemia is not well recorded but, in a large American metropolitan area, mesenteric ischaemia was responsible for 0.1% of all hospital admissions (Kaleya *et al.*, 1992). It may present in acute or chronic forms and be of arterial or venous origin. Superior mesenteric emboli are responsible for 40–50% of episodes with acute ischaemia. Superior mesenteric artery thrombosis accounts for about 25% and between 20% and 50% of these patients have had a history of abdominal pain with or without weight loss in the weeks or months before the acute episode (Dunphy, 1936; Mavor *et al.*, 1962). Non-occlusive mesenteric ischaemia (NOMI) was first recognized by Ende in 1958 as a cause of bowel infarction in patients with cardiac failure and now causes 20–30% of episodes of acute mesenteric ischaemia and is frequently seen in patients in intensive therapy units who require vasoactive medication for hypovolaemia or cardiac failure (Ende, 1958). Mesenteric venous thrombosis was formerly a common cause of acute mesenteric ischaemia but now accounts for no more than 5% of all patients (Boley *et al.*, 1977).

The chronic form of mesenteric ischaemia does not threaten bowel viability but the blood supply is inadequate for normal intestinal function. In the acute form, intestinal viability is immediately threatened and unless rapid therapeutic measures are instigated bowel infarction ensues. The mortality rate is influenced by the cause of the acute ischaemia. Acute mesenteric arterial thrombosis carries the highest mortality (95%), and 50% of patients with embolic occlusion die, as do 30% of those with mesenteric venous thrombosis. Non-occlusive mesenteric ischaemia is associated with 67% mortality (Inderbitzi *et al.*, 1992), with many of those who survive being subsequently dependent upon parenteral nutrition.

The prognosis for this condition can only be improved by early diagnosis and treatment before bowel infarction has occurred.

14.4.1 ACUTE MESENTERIC ISCHAEMIA

For almost 40 years it has been recognized that light-microscopic changes occur in acute ischaemic bowel within 5–10 minutes of the onset of ischaemia (Khanna, 1959). In a condition in which early diagnosis is so important, it is vital to recognize the distinctive clinical picture of acute mesenteric arterial occlusion. 'Any person beyond the age of 50 years with known cardiovascular disease, who develops sudden severe abdominal pain of more than 2–3 hours duration, without abdominal rigidity and without significant tenderness, should be suspected of S.M.A. occlusion' (Klass, 1965). It is the disparity between the severe, distressing pain and the soft and barely tender abdomen that is so striking. The explanation for this is that, although intestinal mucosa is quickly affected by ischaemia, it takes some hours for changes to occur in the muscular coat and spread to the peritoneum. Consequently signs of peritoneal irritation are only manifest as tenderness and guarding after 6–8 hours, by which time the bowel is not likely to be salvageable.

In a typical case, the pain is of instantaneous onset and immediately becomes severe and diffuse. In a short time it is agonizing, and has a steady continuing character, but there may also be periodic exacerbations, which are hard to bear and in which the patient may sweat. Patients who have previously experienced an acute coronary occlusion usually consider the pain of mesenteric obstruction to be much more severe. By the time the diagnosis can be confirmed by clinical findings and modern investigative methods, such as ultrasound, abdominal X-ray, bowel contrast radiology, CT and MRI, as well as haematological and biochemical laboratory tests, bowel infarction has occurred. The only investigations justified at this early stage are a plain abdominal X-ray to exclude other pathology such as perforated bowel, and angiography, which may, in addition to confirming the diagnosis, allow therapy to be started. The argument against angiography is that it may introduce critical delay to surgical correction of mesenteric acute occlusion.

14.4.2   ACUTE MESENTERIC EMBOLISM

Superior mesenteric artery embolic occlusion is claimed to account for 40–50% of acute mesenteric ischaemic accidents. The origin is most commonly cardiac from thrombus in the left ventricle following myocardial infarction, or the atrium in patients with atrial fibrillation. About 30% of the patients have emboli to other sites at the same time and 5% of all peripheral emboli lodge in the superior mesenteric artery (Batellier and Kieny, 1990). When the diagnosis is made the clinicians must have the conviction to arrange for the patient to be transferred to the operating theatre immediately for mesenteric embolectomy. This condition is at least as urgent an emergency as ruptured aortic aneurysm and it is essential that clinicians of all disciplines learn to recognize and appreciate the urgency of this diagnosis, if the disastrous consequences are to be averted. Only on two occasions in almost 30 years of vascular surgical practice has the author been presented with patients with superior mesenteric embolism early enough to allow mesenteric embolectomy and complete preservation of bowel viability.

Mesenteric embolectomy is performed through a full-length midline laparotomy. The diagnosis is then confirmed by examination of the ischaemic small bowel and noting the absence of a pulse in the superior mesenteric artery. The superior mesenteric artery should be approached proximally by retracting the transverse colon proximally and anteriorly and the small bowel caudally. The inferior leaf of the transverse mesocolon is incised and the proximal superior mesenteric artery is dissected free between the fourth portion of the duodenum and the pancreas. A segment of superior mesenteric artery sufficiently long to allow an arteriotomy is prepared, usually on either side of the midcolic artery, and either a transverse or a longitudinal arteriotomy is performed. A size 3 or 4 embolectomy catheter is used to extract the embolus and the artery is repaired, usually without a venous patch. Full anticoagulant treatment should be initiated as soon as the diagnosis is made, as in any other patients with thromboembolic disease.

When there is uncertainty about the diagnosis, or the patient's general condition is so poor after a major myocardial infarct that surgical treatment is strongly contraindicated, angiography with a view to thrombolytic therapy and/or vasodilator treatment should be urgently arranged. No trials are available to compare thrombolytic and operative treatment but several case reports have demonstrated the usefulness of streptokinase, urokinase and recombinant tissue plasminogen activator in such patients (McBride and Gaines, 1994; Schoenbaum *et al.*, 1992). The Montefiore Medical Center in New York reports routine angiography on all patients with mesenteric ischaemia and uses catheter infusion of papaverine up to 30–60 mg/h in a concentration of 1 mg/ml pre- and postoperatively in their patients (Kaleya *et al.*, 1992)

14.4.3   SUPERIOR MESENTERIC ARTERY THROMBOSIS

Thrombosis of the superior mesenteric artery tends to occur in patients with a combination of severe generalized atherosclerosis involving the ostium of that artery and hypovolaemia, dehydration, hypotension or cardiac failure, but it may also be seen in patients with prothrombotic disorders such as SLE, aortic and visceral artery aneurysms and aortic dissection. The underlying disease may preclude aggressive surgical treatment. These patients should therefore have urgent angiography with a view to confirming the diagnosis and initiating transcatheter therapeutic measures such as angioplasty, thrombolysis and vasodilator treatment, with papaverine if possible.

Up to 50% of patients in this group may have had symptoms of chronic intestinal ischaemia prior to the sudden acute event, which is precipitated by occlusion of the essential collateral supply to the superior mesenteric artery. If the angiography suggests that the mesenteric artery is patent distally and vasodilator treatment is impossible because the mesenteric circulation cannot be cannulated, urgent revascularization of the superior mesenteric artery should be considered. Extensive bowel infarction will often be found at laparotomy and extensive resection is required. If the patient survives, long-term parenteral nutrition is often necessary.

14.4.4   NON-OCCLUSIVE MESENTERIC ISCHAEMIA

Most patients with mesenteric ischaemia suffer acute abdominal pain but up to 25%, particularly those with non-occlusive mesenteric ischaemia (NOMI) may experience little or no pain. Some of these patients may have developed intestinal ischaemia when ventilated or under the influence of sedative and analgesic drugs in an intensive care unit environment, and unexplained deterioration in a patient's condition, in conjunction with indicators of concomitant sepsis, should point to the diagnosis of mesenteric ischaemia as a possible cause. The diagnosis in these patients may only be entertained when the peritonitis and/or generalized septic state is present but even at this stage the diagnosis is largely made on clinical suspicion. Despite the wide range of laboratory and imaging investigations available, none are particularly helpful except angiography, although in acute mesenteric vein thrombosis, computed tomography may be the investigation of choice (Kim *et al.*, 1993). Magnetic resonance imaging (MRI) has been shown in animal experiments to distinguish between ischaemic and non-ischaemic tissue 1 hour after superior mesenteric artery ligation but its place in clinical practice is uncertain (Wilkerson *et al.*, 1990).

NOMI is thought to result from splanchnic vasoconstriction caused by vasoactive drugs or as a consequence of hypotension secondary to cardiac failure, dysrhythmias or hypovolaemia, and may persist after the primary cause has been corrected. It is therefore seen in patients who have suffered myocardial infarction, congestive cardiac failure, hepatic disease, renal failure, and particularly in patients on haemodialysis or following major cardiac and abdominal operations.

The angiogram shows spasm in the main jejunal and ileal branches of the superior mesenteric artery and the arcades, and the treatment is papaverine infusion until abdominal signs disappear and repeat angiography shows the mesenteric circulation to have returned to normal (Kaleya *et al.*, 1992).

Despite the accumulation of substantial knowledge about the pathogenesis of the local and systemic effects of ischaemia/reperfusion injury in mesenteric ischaemia, no clear therapeutic measures have been forwarded that improve the outlook for these patients (Bradbury *et al.*, 1995). For the ill and deteriorating patient in an intensive care unit, worsening abdominal signs are an indication for laparotomy and bowel resection in the attempt to save life; however, the patient's best opportunity for survival is provided by the alert surgeon, willing to commit to laparotomy on the basis of suspicion of the diagnosis, clinical experience and the summation of laboratory evidence.

14.4.5   ACUTE MESENTERIC VEIN THROMBOSIS

Acute mesenteric vein thrombosis was previously regarded as a common cause of mesenteric ischaemia and bowel infarction (Cokkinis, 1926). With the development of modern diagnostic methods such as ultrasound, angiography and CT it is now realized that venous thrombosis is often secondary to arterial occlusion and occurs when the bowel infarcts. These same modern diagnostic methods allow the true venous thrombosis to be detected as a separate clinical problem, but these account for less than 10% of mesenteric infarcts (Boley *et al.*, 1992). Experimental studies have shown that acute venous occlusion causes large fluid loss into the bowel wall and peritoneal cavity with resulting hypovolaemia, haemoconcentration, cardiovascular collapse with the development of a hypercoagulable state and subsequent propagation of venous thrombus with ultimately arterial thrombosis. It can therefore obviously be difficult at surgery or pathological examination to decide whether the arterial or the venous thrombosis was the primary pathology.

Acute mesenteric venous thrombosis is classified as primary or secondary. Primary disease is usually caused by hypercoagulable states such as may occur for instance after splenectomy, in polycythaemia rubra vera or in patients with antithrombin-III, protein-S and protein-C deficiencies, or even in young women on the contraceptive pill. Patients with secondary disease usually have carcinomatosis, intra-abdominal sepsis, portal hypertension or inflammatory bowel disease (Bradbury *et al.*, 1995).

The diagnosis of mesenteric venous thrombosis as a cause of the acute abdomen is difficult to make. CT may be the investigation of choice and is claimed to establish the diagnosis in 90% of patients (Harward *et al.*, 1989). Ultrasonography occasionally shows the thrombus and diminished venous flow in the superior mesenteric vein. Angiography by showing arterial spasm and sluggish flow may suggest the presence of venous obstruction and has been reported to demonstrate the clot in the superior mesenteric or portal vein (Clavien *et al.*, 1988).

The acute abdomen caused by mesenteric vein thrombosis demands emergency laparotomy and bowel resection when infarction has occurred. When the diagnosis is made full anticoagulation with heparin should be initiated and continued after the removal of the necrotic bowel. When the intestine is judged to be viable venous thrombectomy is occasionally successful (Bergentz *et al.*, 1974).

14.5   VISCERAL ARTERY ANEURYSMS

Most visceral artery aneurysms are diagnosed as incidental findings in patients undergoing angiographic examination but some present as emergencies following rupture, with a shocked, hypovolaemic patient with signs of intraperitoneal bleeding. Almost 3000 such cases have been documented in the world literature, 22% presented as emergencies and 40% of these died (Stanley, 1981). The vessels involved in order of frequency are the splenic artery in 60%, hepatic 20%, superior mesenteric 5.5%, coeliac axis 4% and all other intraperitoneal arteries in about 10% (p. 499).

Our own experience is limited to treating three female patients with visceral artery aneurysms. One presented shortly after giving birth to her fourth child, with severe abdominal pain and collapse with a large swelling in the right hypochondrium that was strikingly mobile and pulsatile. At surgery she had an 11 cm diameter spherical splenic artery aneurysm. Another patient of 73 years of age presented to a general surgical unit with severe abdominal pain and collapse, and preoperative abdominal scan showed an aneurysm of $7 \times 7 \times 8$ cm in diameter which was interpreted as a ruptured abdominal aortic aneurysm. At laparotomy the infrarenal aorta was normal and the ruptured aneurysm was anterior to the aorta and originated from the main hepatic artery. Both these large aneurysms were managed by clamping of the aorta at the diaphragmatic hiatus and opening of the aneurysm anteriorly where surrounding tissue had been pushed away by pressure from the aneurysm. Control of bleeding was simply by finger pressure on the lumen at one side of the aneurysm and a Fogarty catheter with a three-way tap acting as an occlusion catheter in the other end of the open artery. The proximal and distal arteries were then closed with continuous 3/0 Prolene sutures. The collateral flow to the spleen in the first patient and to the liver in the second was entirely satisfactory and both patients made straightforward recovery with no evidence of hepatic or splenic dysfunction thereafter. The third patient was a 68-year-old female who presented to a medical ward with abdominal pain, recurrent episodes of collapse with unrecordable blood pressure, and episodes of unconsciousness. On examination she had signs of peritoneal irritation and intraperitoneal free fluid. She was therefore immediately subjected to laparotomy, which confirmed the presence of blood in the peritoneal cavity with a large amount of clot in the lesser sac and a sausage-shaped mass in the free edge of the lesser omentum. The cause of the bleeding was rupture of an aneurysm of the left hepatic artery. This was treated by simply applying steel clips to the hepatic artery proximal and distal to the aneurysm. The patient had no further problems with liver circulation or liver function and lived to the age of 89.

Visceral artery aneurysms are therefore most likely to present to general surgeons rather than vascular surgeons and present as an acute emergency with sudden blood loss (p. 499). In our experience they have been fairly easy aneurysms to deal with but may not be so for a general surgeon without vascular surgical expertise. Where such a situation is encountered, the vascular surgical team should be engaged in the repair, which may involve repair with vein or prosthetic grafts.

14.6   AORTIC DISSECTION

Aortic dissection is a disease primarily of the thoracic aorta, most commonly in the ascending aorta. About 30% of all cases start in the descending thoracic aorta. The condition accounts for 0.3% of all deaths in Sweden (Svensjo *et al.*, 1996) and between 0.5% and 2.7% in the USA (Lilienfeld *et al.*, 1987). Some 90% of patients have a classical severe tearing chest pain: this is felt anteriorly with ascending dissection and between the shoulder blades with descending dissection. Most patients, accordingly, present to thoracic units.

A few patients, however, may have a silent dissection and present with acute abdominal pain due to occlusion of the coeliac, mesenteric or renal arteries and thus present to the abdominal surgeon with abdominal pain and signs suggesting visceral ischaemia. The general surgeon must be wary of the sequence of mesenteric ischaemia followed by haematuria then limb ischaemia, as indicative of downward extension of a thoracic aortic dissection progressively compromising the ostia of the feeding arteries. Dissection starting in the abdominal aorta is extremely rare but we have reported this (Youngson *et al.*, 1983).

When such a patient is encountered at laparotomy with intra-abdominal ischaemia, urgent surgery has to re-establish blood flow in the visceral arteries and this is most commonly done by fenestration of the aortic membrane. The infrarenal aorta is freed, as is the aorta at the diaphragmatic hiatus. The infrarenal aorta is clamped proximally and distally, usually with soft vascular clamps, and opened through its unaffected area, which is usually anteriorly on the right side. The false channel is bluish in colour and usually postero-laterally on the left. By applying a second soft clamp at the diaphragmatic hiatus, as much as possible of the aortic membrane, the detached intima and part of media is removed proximally. The membrane is split further proximally with a long pair of scissors, which are slid upwards to above the level of the coeliac artery. When the distal aorta is healthy the aortotomy may be closed in the normal way but when the dissection continues down to and beyond the bifurcation it may be necessary to insert a tube or bifurcation graft. Alternatively it may be possible to glue the aortic wall layers using gelatin/resorsin/formol (GRF) tissue adhesive so that perfusion of the true lumen only occurs when the aorta is closed. Compression of the aortic layers during the setting time of the adhesive may be best assured by inserting an appropriately sized Hegar dilator into the aorta (Borst *et al.*, 1994).

Whenever aortic dissection is encountered as an acute abdominal emergency it would seem prudent for the general surgeon to call upon the vascular and cardiovascular expertise within the hospital to help and advise on appropriate treatment, as the condition is rare and carries a high mortality. Few general surgeons will encounter this difficult problem more than once or twice in a lifetime of surgical practice, and aortic reconstruction, the mainstay of operative treatment, is now commonly done by cardiothoracic surgeons with the patient on cardiodistal bypass.

REFERENCES

Batellier, J. and Kieny, R. (1990) Superior mesenteric artery embolism: eighty-two cases. *Ann. Vasc. Surg.*, **4**, 112–116.

Bergentz, S., Ericsson, B., Hedner, U. *et al.* (1974) Thrombosis in the superior mesenteric and portal veins: report of a case treated with thrombectomy. *Surgery*, **76**, 286–290.

Boley, S. J., Sprayregen, S., Siegelman, S. S. *et al.* (1977) Initial results from an aggressive roentgenological and surgical approach to acute mesenteric ischaemia. *Surgery*, **82**, 848–855.

Boley, S. J., Kaleya, R. N. and Brandt, L. J.. (1992) Mesenteric venous thrombosis. *Surg. Clin. North Am.*; 72(1): 183–203.

Borst, H. G., Laas, J. and Buhner, B. (1994) Efficient gluing in aortic dissection. *Eur. J. Cardiothorac. Surg*, **8**, 160–161.

Bradbury, A. W., Brittenden, J., McBride, K. *et al.* (1995) Mesenteric ischaemia: a multidisciplinary approach. *Br. J. Surg.*, **82**, 1446–1459.

Clavien, P. A., Durig, M. and Harder, F. (1988) Venous mesenteric infarction: a particular entity. *Br. J. Surg.*, **75**, 252–255.

Cokkinis, A. J. (1926) *Mesenteric Vascular Occlusion*, Baillière Tindall, London.

Dunphy, J. E. (1936) Abdominal pain of vascular origin. *Am. J. Med. Sci.*, **192**, 109–113.

Ende, N. (1958) Infarction of the bowel in cardiac failure. *N. Engl. J. Med.*, **258**, 879–881.

Harward, T. R. S., Green, D., Bergan, J. J. *et al.* (1989) Mesenteric venous thrombosis. *J. Vasc. Surg.*, **9**, 328–333.

Inderbitzi, R., Wagner, H. E., Seiler, C. *et al.* (1992) Acute mesenteric ischaemia. *Eur. J. Surg.*, **158**, 123–126.

Kaleya, R. N., Sammartano, R. J. and Boley, S. J.. (1992) Aggressive approach to acute mesenteric ischaemia. *Surg. Clin. North Am.*, **72**(1), 183–203.

Khanna, S. D. (1959) An experimental study of mesenteric occlusion. *J. Pathol. Bacteriol.*, **77**, 575–590.

Kim, J. Y., Ha, H. K., Byun, J. Y. *et al.* (1993) Intestinal infarction secondary to mesenteric venous thrombosis. CT-pathologic correlation. *J. Comp. Assist. Tomogr.*, **17**, 382–385.

Klass, A. A. (1965) The treatment of superior mesenteric artery occlusion: a reappraisal. *Can. Med. Assoc. J.*, **93**, 309–312.

Lilienfeld, D., Gunderson, P., Sprafka, J. *et al.* (1987) The epidemiology of abdominal aortic aneurysms: mortality trends in the United States 1951–1980. *Arteriosclerosis*, **7**, 637–643.

McBride, K. D. and Gaines, P. A. (1994) Thrombolysis of a partially occluding superior mesenteric artery thromboembolus by infusion of Streptokinase. *Cardiovasc. Intervent. Radiol.*, **17**, 164–166.

Mavor, G. E., Lyall, A. D., Chrystal, K. M. R. *et al.* (1962) Mesenteric infarction as a vascular emergency: the clinical problems. *Br. J. Surg.*, **50**, 219–225.

Schoenbaum, S. W., Pena, C., Koeningsberg, P. *et al.* (1992) Superior mesenteric artery embolism: treatment with intra-arterial urokinase. *J. Vasc. Intervent. Radiol.*, **3**, 485–490.

Stanley, J. C. (1981) Abdominal visceral aneurysms, in *Vascular Emergencies*, (ed. G. Haimovic), Appleton-Century-Crofts, New York, pp. 387–396.

Svensjo, S., Bengtsson, H. and Bergquist, D. (1996) Thoracic and thoraco-abdominal aortic aneurysm and dissection: an investigation based on autopsy. *Br. J. Surg.*, **83**, 68–71.

Wilkerson, D. K., Mezrich, R., Drake, C. *et al.* (1990) Magnetic resonance imaging of acute occlusive intestinal ischaemia. *J. Vasc. Surg.*, **11**, 567–571.

Youngson, G. G., Engeset, J., Hussey, J. and Smith, G. (1983) Dissecting aneurysms of the infra-renal aorta. *Surgery*, **94**, 521–523.

15

Medical aspects of the acute abdomen

15.1 INTRODUCTION

Among all the patients admitted as an emergency to a general surgical ward with acute abdominal pain, fewer than one-half require an operation. The emergency surgeon has therefore to cultivate both a watchful eye for the true surgical emergency and a readiness to wait, observe and investigate so that the many in whom an operation would be inappropriate can be recognized and suitably treated. Many, who prove under observation to have the NSAP syndrome, will settle. Others with, for instance, acute pancreatitis will require expert management but rarely need operation. Some 10–15% will have a 'medical' condition that is presenting with acute abdominal symptoms; in many of these patients an operation is strongly contraindicated, and this chapter aims to survey the many illnesses that can present in this way.

The surgeon must also be prepared for those patients with a chronic medical illness who are overtaken by a surgical emergency. Often, urgent treatment of the chronic complaint is needed, e.g. in diabetes mellitus, before it is safe to proceed with an operation, and these situations are considered.

15.2 INTRATHORACIC DISEASE

15.2.1 CARDIOVASCULAR SYSTEM

Congestive cardiac failure can present with acute pain in the epigastrium and under the right costal margin. Demonstration of a tender palpable liver associated with jugular venous engorgement should make this condition clear.

An inferior **myocardial infarct** often presents with severe epigastric pain, but there is no tenderness. Early ECG changes may be few and urgent estimation of cardiac enzymes is needed.

In **pericarditis**, if the diaphragmatic area is affected, there can be epigastric pain, tenderness and guarding. Patients with a viral pericarditis (e.g. Coxsackie B infection) are often young; an ECG is essential for diagnosis. The friction rub is often evanescent.

Emergency Abdominal Surgery. Edited by Peter F. Jones, Zygmunt H. Krukowski and George G. Youngson. Published in 1998 by Chapman & Hall, London. ISBN 0 412 81950 3.

Surgery in patients with cardiovascular disease

A recent myocardial infarct offers a considerable risk, which begins to diminish after 3 months. Unstable angina is a contraindication to any but essential surgery, with perioperative complications in up to 28% of patients. Known coronary artery disease, diabetes mellitus and hypertension are important risk factors.

When operation is necessary, the anaesthetist should be involved in all preparations. A pulmonary artery catheter and transoesophageal echocardiography may be helpful. Patients on maintenance therapy should remain on it, including beta blockade, which has been shown to reduce intraoperative and later ischaemic episodes. Intravenous or percutaneous nitrates may be useful for those at risk of silent intraoperative ischaemia.

Prophylaxis against **endocarditis**, with gentamicin and ampicillin, is necessary before oral, oesophageal, bronchial and abdominal procedures for patients with any prosthetic cardiac valves and previous endocarditis.

Pacemakers. Patients with second- or third-degree heart block (complete) who do not have a permanent pacing system should have a temporary pacing system inserted prior to surgery. The surgeon should establish whether his patient is pacemaker-dependent before surgery, since the pacing function can be affected by electromagnetic interference such as that generated by diathermy. Diathermy devices should be placed as remotely as possible from the pacing system to avoid damage to or inadvertent reprogramming of the generator.

15.2.2 RESPIRATORY TRACT

Pneumonic consolidation, with or without pleurisy, especially if basal and close to the diaphragm, can cause acute abdominal pain, which may be worse on coughing. Dyspnoea, fever, cough and headache in an ill patient with abdominal pain will suggest a respiratory infection – or pulmonary embolism – but the chest X-ray may be normal. A pleural rub may be heard. This can be a difficult differential diagnosis, and unless the abdominal signs are very pressing the effect of medical treatment should be awaited. This is a situation in which fine catheter aspiration cytology at the site of maximum tenderness can be helpful (p. 46).

Emergency surgery in chronic respiratory disease

The history and often the general appearance and breathing of the patient will indicate the problem. Details of treatment by mouth and by inhaler are particularly important. (A dose of inhaled corticosteroids of over 2000 mg/d will cause some adrenal suppression, and this becomes of major significance to surgeon and anaesthetist if the patient is on oral corticosteroids.) Peri- and postoperative i.v. hydrocortisone, 50 mg 2–4 times in 24 hours, will be needed.

Patients with asthma or chronic obstructive pulmonary disease (COPD) require at least an estimate of peak expiratory flow rate (PEFR). A level under 50% of predicted flow indicates significant airflow obstruction and if it is below 33% blood gases should be measured. The presence of hypercapnia ($P_a\text{CO}_2 > 45$ mmHg or 6.7 kPa) means that general anaesthesia carries a high risk and postoperative ventilation will be needed. This is clearly a situation that requires very early consultation with the anaesthetist.

If the patient is expectorating green sputum it should be cultured and an empirical choice of antibiotic started forthwith – intravenous co-amoxiclav 1.2 g t.i.d. or cefuroxime 750 mg– 1.5 g t.i.d.

Postoperatively effective pain control and physiotherapy will be of special importance – every effort must be made to overcome the difficulty in coughing and restricted diaphragmatic movement.

15.2.3 BORNHOLM DISEASE

Otherwise known as epidemic pleurodynia, and first described in 1934 on the Danish island of Bornholm, this illness chiefly affects children and young adults. There are features of a viral infection – malaise, headache, high fever – with sharp pleural pain of sudden onset. This can be referred into the abdomen in the epigastrium and around the umbilicus. Nausea and vomiting are unusual and the abdominal signs are slight in comparison with the degree of pain.

15.2.4 SPINAL DISEASES

These can cause root pain in the distribution of the lower thoracic nerves, which is felt in the abdomen. Vertebral collapse can be due to osteoporosis or metastatic deposits or, rarely, osteomyelitis. Acute discitis in children may present with pain under the ribs and in the epigastrium (Leahy *et al.*, 1984) and spinal X-rays and a bone scan are wise investigations in obscure abdominal pain.

Oesophageal rupture (p. 155), strangulated diaphragmatic hernia (p. 178) and dissecting aneurysm of the aorta (p. 530) are other sources of acute abdominal pain.

15.3 ABDOMINAL DISEASE

15.3.1 ACUTE TONSILLITIS WITH MESENTERIC ADENITIS

Acute tonsillitis is a familiar cause of abdominal pain in general practice and these children rarely reach hospital. There can be some tenderness in the RLQ and this is presumably due to concurrent mesenteric adenitis, which settles quickly as the tonsillitis resolves.

15.3.2 LIVER DISEASE

Stretching of the liver capsule is usually considered to be the source of hepatic pain. The pain felt during the incubation period of **acute viral hepatitis** is a regular cause of emergency admission to a surgical ward, especially in children. At this stage jaundice is not noticeable and the pain, anorexia and nausea, and area of tenderness, can suggest a high retrocolic appendicitis – which is a very much commoner condition. With careful palpation an enlarged and tender liver may make the diagnosis plain. The alkaline phosphatase and transaminases are usually abnormal when the bilirubin is still within normal limits.

Acute alcoholic hepatitis must be remembered. The pain and tenderness are quite marked and, with the evident jaundice, can suggest biliary tract disease, but ascites, splenomegaly and mental confusion are often present. An ultrasound scan can be very helpful.

15.3.3   FAMILIAL MEDITERRANEAN FEVER

This condition was first described in 1945 as 'benign paroxysmal peritonitis' or recurrent polyserositis. It is inherited as an autosomal recessive trait, largely confined to inhabitants of eastern Mediterranean countries – Jews, Arabs and Turks – and in 90% of patients has appeared by the age of 20. In attacks there is sudden onset of severe abdominal pain and vomiting, and considerable abdominal tenderness and guarding, suggestive of peritonitis. About half these patients complain of pleuritic pain and arthralgia.

In 22 of 74 patients seen by Heller *et al.* (1958) in Tel Aviv a laparotomy had been performed, but now the disease is better recognized it is known that the attack eases in 6–12 hours. Relapses cannot be predicted and they continue throughout life, but colchicine (1.0–1.5 mg daily) seems to have a useful preventative effect.

15.3.4   CURTIS–FITZ-HUGH SYNDROME

It has been recognized for many years that there is a connection between genital tract infection in women and adhesions on the anterior surface of the liver. Stejano first noted it in Montevideo in 1920, Curtis reported on it in 1930, and in 1934 Fitz-Hugh described three women who presented with seemingly typical acute cholecystitis who in fact had gonococcal salpingitis and fine string-like adhesions between the liver and the anterior abdominal wall.

Wood *et al.* (1982) saw nine women between 18 and 49 years of age, admitted as cases of acute cholecystitis, all with typical signs under the right costal margin, yet in eight the ultrasonic scan was normal. All had signs of pelvic infection and all had positive serology for *Chlamydia trachomatis*. Laparoscopy in five showed signs of salpingitis and the typical fine Curtis–Fitz-Hugh adhesions over the liver. The reason for this association between two widely separate sites remains obscure.

It is common for women of this age-group to present with the picture of acute cholecystitis. Shanahan *et al.* (1988) found that, among 18 women between 15 and 35 years old who presented in this way, ultrasonography and cholecystography was negative in 10. They then made a prospective study of this age-group, and in seven of 15 consecutive admissions biliary tract investigations were negative. None had pelvic symptoms but all seven had positive results on screening for *C. trachomatis* infection and were treated with tetracycline.

It is clear from these findings that when younger women appear on admission to have acute cholecystitis, but this is not confirmed, the possibility of the Curtis–Fitz-Hugh syndrome must be investigated and treated.

15.4   ENDOCRINE DISORDERS

15.4.1   DIABETES MELLITUS AND THE ACUTE ABDOMEN

(a) 'The acute diabetic abdomen'

Diabetic ketoacidosis is defined as the occurrence of hyperglycaemia in the presence of a plasma bicarbonate of less than 17 mmol/l, with ketonuria, in an insulin-dependent diabetic (IDDM). One of its recognized features is that about 10% of these patients complain of acute abdominal pain, which is sufficiently severe for them to be sent into hospital with a diagnosis of acute appendicitis or intestinal obstruction. It is vital that a correct diagnosis is made in these gravely ill patients.

Here the history, as so often in emergency surgery, is very important. The patient, who is often a child or adolescent, has been unwell for some days, complaining of lassitude, thirst, anorexia and urinary frequency. In the last 24 hours the patient has begun to vomit and complain of diffuse abdominal pain. The striking feature at the bedside of these patients is how ill and dehydrated they look, with deep rapid acidotic breathing and mental confusion. There is acetone in the breath, and the pulse is thin and fast. The abdomen is scaphoid, and there is general tenderness, but little guarding, although tenderness may be localized over the RLQ.

Valerio (1976) gives a good description of three children between 5 and 10 years old whom he saw in the space of 4 months. Each child had been unwell for a week with thirst and loss of appetite, with more recent onset of abdominal pain. This is not the history of acute appendicitis of 24–48 hours duration: these patients have become notably dehydrated and the deep ketotic breathing is very different from the short, quick breaths taken with the tight painful abdomen of general peritonitis. This picture should prompt an immediate blood sugar estimation, because a urine specimen can be hard to obtain.

Active treatment, conducted in consultation with a specialist in diabetic medicine, is needed. A fast intravenous infusion of physiological saline and soluble insulin, with potassium added once the circulation improves, results in disappearance of the abdominal signs in 3–6 hours.

The reason for the abdominal pain remains unexplained. In some children the abdominal signs suggest appendicitis, but fortunately it is clear that the ketoacidosis must be treated first, and this gives time for the signs to settle. Campbell *et al.* (1975) reported 46 patients with significant abdominal pain among 211 cases of severe diabetic metabolic decompensation and found that, in those patients with a plasma bicarbonate above 10 mmol/l, the cause of pain was usually organic, e.g. appendicitis or pyelonephritis. Under close observation the signs in these patients did not improve.

(b) Acute abdominal disease or injury in a diabetic patient

A diabetic who is well controlled complains of the acute onset of abdominal pain and vomiting. Because eating has stopped an insulin injection has probably been omitted. Here the presentation is of, for instance, acute appendicitis in a relatively well patient.

A patient who has taken insulin or sulphonylurea drugs several hours before admission is liable to be hypoglycaemic, and the blood sugar should be promptly measured and appropriate intravenous fluids given. If possible a specialist in diabetic medicine should advise on management.

A useful fluid and insulin regime

If the blood glucose is over 15 mmol/l use physiological saline until the ward glucose is less than 15 mmol/l. Then commence 4% dextrose/0.18 saline with 13.5 mmol/l KCl in 500 ml. Infuse at a rate of 100 ml/h *via* an infusion pump. Continue this until the patient is eating again. Continuous 4% dextrose/0.18% saline is a more rational regime than alternating dextrose and saline and provides smoother blood glucose control. Check laboratory electrolytes, urea and glucose postoperatively and then daily. Adjust the addition of potassium to the infusion to maintain the serum potassium between 3.5 and 5 mmol/l.

Insulin infusion can be given *via* the syringe driver piggybacked on to the dextrose/saline infusion. Insulin concentration is 50 units of soluble insulin in 50 ml physiological saline. Initially, check the bedside glucose using sticks or a meter on an hourly basis and aim to keep the blood glucose between 5 and 10 mmol/l (Table 15.1).

If the blood glucose does not respond it is important to check the syringe pump and the infusion lines.

Table 15.1 Regime for insulin infusion in response to blood glucose

Sliding scale (as a guideline)	Insulin infusion rate (units/h)	
Ward blood glucose (mmol/l)	IDDM	NIDDM
<4	0.5	0
4–7	1	1
7–10	2	2
10–14	3	3
>14	4	4

When the patient is able to eat, the usual dose of subcutaneous insulin should be prescribed 30 minutes prior to eating and the insulin infusion discontinued 30 minutes after the subcutaneous injection. NIDDM patients should have their usual hypoglycaemic agents reinstituted at this stage. If intravenous fluids are required for a prolonged period postoperatively, the frequency of ward blood glucose testing can be reduced when an appropriate insulin infusion rate, e.g. 1 u/h, has been identified.

Aim to optimize blood glucose control in the peri- and postoperative period to help wound healing and reduce infection. Patients are often experts with respect to their own diabetes and their opinion on the postoperative insulin regime should be respected – they are often correct.

15.4.2 ACUTE ADRENAL INSUFFICIENCY

With the decline in tuberculosis as a cause, acute Addison's disease has become a rare condition, but these patients can present with acute abdominal pain and vomiting, and are sent into a surgical receiving ward. Autoimmune disease now accounts for two-thirds of cases. Others are due to metastatic deposits and infarction.

We admitted a previously healthy man of 39 who for 4 days had been feeling weak and complaining of increasing pain in the right lower chest and epigastrium. Nausea and vomiting were persistent over the 4 days. The pain was maximal in the right upper quadrant and was aggravated by movement. On the day of admission he felt cold and shivery and the pain was worse. He was described as 'tanned', was slightly confused and was distressed by the pain. The blood pressure was 80/40. The right side of the abdomen was tender with slight guarding, maximal under the right costal margin. The bowel sounds were active. Acute pancreatitis was considered to be a possible diagnosis and he was given intravenous saline and plasma. The serum amylase was normal but the sodium was 121 mmol/l and potassium 7.0 mmol/l. Adrenal failure was then suspected and he was given hydrocortisone intravenously and calcium resonium. The serum sodium remained at 121 for 24 hours but the following day he was mentally alert and pain-free. Subsequent tests suggested that he had autoimmune adrenalitis and 4 years later he remained well but continued to require twice-daily corticosteroids.

Clark *et al.* (1974) reported 34 patients with acute haemorrhage into the adrenal gland, 32 found at autopsy and two at operation. They particularly emphasize the continuous, localized, upper abdominal pain of increasing severity, localized under the costal margin. This is a difficult diagnosis but in our case the striking hyponatraemia and hyperkalaemia suggested the wisdom of commencing hydrocortisone.

15.5 METABOLIC DISORDERS

15.5.1 ACUTE INTERMITTENT PORPHYRIA

The porphyrin molecule is widely distributed in nature, combining with magnesium to form chlorophyll and with iron to form haem. Inborn disorders of haem/porphyrin metabolism are rare (1 in 50 000 prevalence in the UK). When the acute syndrome occurs it has major neurovisceral effects, which include abdominal pain and vomiting, and porphyrin is always present in the urine in these attacks, where it can be recognized by its tendency to redden on standing.

Goldberg (1959) gradually collected 50 patients in the Glasgow area, the majority being young women. Some 90% present with attacks of abdominal pain and vomiting, which can be severe: the pain can be either constant or colicky. Some two-thirds complain of weakness, especially in the arms, and many show signs of depression and psychological disturbance.

Attacks can be precipitated by taking a number of drugs, such as barbiturates, sulphonamides and some anaesthetics, and alcohol and the onset of menstruation are also associated with attacks. True abdominal signs are not so marked as the degree of pain. Treatment is supportive, with rest and intravenous fluids; chlorpromazine is helpful.

15.5.2 HAEMOCHROMATOSIS

This is a rare hereditary defect of iron metabolism whose mechanism is poorly understood. Excessive quantities are deposited in vital organs including the liver (which is consistently enlarged), the heart and the pancreas. Many patients suffer from diabetes mellitus, there is slate-grey pigmentation of the skin and they are subject to cardiac failure and joint pains. Together with a positive family history, these patients are likely to be identified. About one-quarter suffer from attacks of abdominal pain, which can be severe, with tenderness suggestive of appendicitis or cholecystitis. Identification of these patients is certainly important because in some the signs have led to a laparotomy, and this is dangerous because they are liable, after operation, to go into irreversible circulatory collapse, which may be due to Gram-negative septicaemia (MacSween, 1966).

15.6 DISORDERS OF THE BLOOD

Several disorders of the blood can present with acute abdominal symptoms, either because of abdominal bleeding within the abdomen, or because there is interference with the blood supply to abdominal viscera. Then it must be recognized that the prior existence of a haematological disease can seriously complicate operative management when a surgical emergency arises.

15.6.1 SICKLE CELL ANAEMIA

This is a hereditary type of chronic haemolytic anaemia in which erythrocytes, in conditions of hypoxaemia, become sickle-shaped, more rigid and less deformable; as a consequence they tend to aggregate and so block the microcirculation. This results in the acute and painful vaso-occlusive crisis typical of this disease. Sickle-cell carriers are found in 1 in 4 West Africans and in 1 in 10 Afro-Caribbeans. The number of patients in the UK was estimated to be 5000 in 1993 (Davies and Oni, 1997).

These occlusive crises can present with acute abdominal pain, with some tenderness and guarding. Mild jaundice and a palpable liver and spleen will suggest the diagnosis in a Negro patient, but there is a risk of intestinal infarction, and many have hyposplenism (due to multiple infarcts) and may consequently suffer from peritonitis. Leucocytosis up to 20 000/mm^3, but a differential count only 60–65% of neutrophils, is characteristic of a crisis. There is a tendency to arthritis and leg ulcers.

Diagnosis depends on recognizing the likelihood of sickling in a patient, and finding a severe chronic anaemia and a positive sickle test. The main task is then to watch the patient closely to decide whether this is an occlusive crisis or a surgical emergency in a sickle-cell patient.

If operation is indicated it is vital to maintain good oxygenation, transfusion of packed cells to maintain the haemoglobin over 120 g/l, and hydration to improve the microcirculation.

Sickle-cell families are familiar with crises and many are managed at home. Community services provide advice on analgesia – which is an important part of management of a crisis – along with extra fluids and rest. If paracetamol or codeine phosphate is not adequate, and abdominal pain continues, there must be medical assessment (Davies and Oni, 1997).

15.6.2 BLEEDING DISORDERS

Disorders of coagulation are numerous. They include the hereditary defects in coagulation factors and platelet formation, and acquired states such as liver failure, malabsorption, malignancy, and drug-induced disease. However, few cause abdominal symptoms, with the two exceptions of haemophilia and related syndromes, and overdosage with anticoagulants, which can cause much anxiety. In caring for these patients, the closest cooperation with a haematologist and the blood transfusion service is vital.

15.6.2.1 Haemophilia

Defects of **primary haemostasis** (adherence and aggregation of platelets) occur in von Willebrand's disease. The von Willebrand's (vW) factor acts as a 'glue' to bind platelets to damaged epithelium and also as a 'bodyguard' to protect factor VIII from proteolytic destruction. Both sexes are equally affected and there is a propensity to bleeding into mucous membranes, but severe, life-threatening haemorrhage is rare. Desmopressin is the drug of first choice, either intranasally or intravenously.

Defects of **secondary haemostasis** (consolidation of the haemostatic plug with fibrin mesh) occur in the haemophilias – A and B (Christmas disease) – with deficiency of factor VIII and factor IX respectively. These are essential to the intrinsic coagulation cascade (Rizza, 1994). Both are X-linked, female carriers with one normal gene showing partial deficiency. Severe haemophilia (in affected males) causes widespread spontaneous haemorrhage into joints, muscles, abdominal viscera and elsewhere and is associated with factor VIII levels less than 1 IU/dl (i.e. less than 1% of normal). Moderate disease with haemorrhage after minor trauma has factor VIII levels of about 1–5 IU/dl. Mild disease (with levels from 5–40 IU/dl) gives little rise to disease but creates problems during surgery. Haemophilia A has a prevalence of 1 in 10 000 to 1 in 20 000 with some 5500 registered patients in the UK. Christmas disease is less common, with only some 1100 registered patients. Since the disease is manifest early in life the surgeon will at least know the background problem when first asked to see the patient.

Anscombe (1970) showed, in a survey over 10 years at the Manchester Haemophilia Centre, that over 400 patients required 1329 admissions for treatment of complications. Exactly 100 of these were for 'acute abdomen' but only five required an urgent operation, four for acute appendicitis and one for intestinal strangulation. Most had an extraperitoneal haematoma, which may lie in the anterior or the posterior abdominal wall. A haematoma in the anterior wall can produce a sharp localized tenderness but there will be little in the way of anorexia or vomiting. A posterior wall haemorrhage beneath the sheath of the iliacus or psoas muscle can, on the right side, produce a picture difficult to distinguish from acute appendicitis. There can be considerable tenderness and guarding over the right iliac fossa. However, the true diagnosis may be suggested by:

- marked hip flexion;
- paraesthesiae in the distribution of the femoral nerve, and perhaps quadriceps weakness;
- the absence of nausea and vomiting;
- an unexpectedly low haemoglobin.

In this situation, in which it is so undesirable to operate if it can be avoided, the next step is an urgent ultrasonic or CT scan that could demonstrate the presence of a haematoma. The chances of such a case being appendicitis are about 1 in 20, but close active observation will be needed to detect the few with appendicitis.

Haemophiliacs occasionally suffer from intussusception due to a local haematoma in the intestinal wall: this acts as the head of the intussusception. If in the colon this can be diagnosed, and perhaps treated, with the help of a barium enema. In the small intestine, diagnosis is more difficult. It should be possible to palpate a tender mobile mass which will be quite unlike any finding in extraperitoneal bleeding. Any strangulating obstruction is likely to be more serious because of the greater tendency to haemorrhage.

Alimentary bleeding is fairly common (in Anscombe's study there were 107 cases among 1329 patients' admissions). There are two complicating factors to be taken into account. Aspirin and NSAID may inadvertently have been used (perhaps to relieve haematoma pain) and alcohol is potentially dangerous also. Liver disease due to viral infection is common: although hepatitis B is now almost totally preventable, haemophiliacs who received factor concentrates up to the last few years are almost all positive for HCV and some have significant liver damage, even cirrhosis. Early endoscopy is especially important in these patients in order to deal expeditiously with any varices.

Once a haemophiliac develops a peptic ulcer the risk of recurrent haematemesis is high. Some 10–13% of adult haemophiliacs suffer from peptic ulceration and every effort must be made to achieve healing.

In a bleeding episode the aim is to obtain a level of the deficient factor to allow satisfactory haemostasis for the operation and the initial phase of wound healing. A variety of products are available to replace this deficient factor. The recommended product is recombinant factor VIII concentrate which is not derived from human plasma and avoids the risk of transmission of viral infection. If this is not available, a high-purity plasma-derived concentrate that is treated to kill virus particles should be used.

The aim of replacement therapy is to have the factor VIII coagulant level at approximately 100% at the time of surgery and to maintain it over 50% for 5–7 days postoperatively. This requires that factor VIII concentrate is given every 8–12 hours and requires close monitoring to ensure the adequacy of replacement. Close liaison with the haematology laboratory is essential.

15.6.2.2 Bleeding associated with anticoagulant therapy

The increasing use of warfarin in the treatment of patients with vascular disease means that inadvertent overdosage is a significant cause of bleeding episodes. The coincidental use of aspirin and NSAIDs is a factor in at least a quarter of alimentary haemorrhagic episodes. Most present with haematemesis or melaena, but some 10% of intramural haematomas of the duodenum (p. 435) are due to anticoagulant overdosage.

When a patient on anticoagulants requires an urgent operation, it is found that an INR of less than 2.5 allows adequate haemostasis. The first decision concerns the need for continued warfarin therapy after the operation. While this is essential in patients with an artificial heart valve, in most other cases the patient can be assessed individually for the balance of risks of bleeding versus further thrombosis.

If ongoing warfarin therapy is not indicated, the anticoagulant effect can be reversed with vitamin K and a coagulation factor product. Currently a combination of the vitamin-K-dependent factors (prothrombin, factors VIII, IX and X) is recommended if available, or fresh frozen plasma. The advantage of the coagulation factor complex is that it is treated to destroy viruses; thus the risk of transfusion-related viral infection is greatly reduced. If the patient is at ongoing risk of venous thrombosis postoperatively, warfarin should be stopped and coagulation corrected as above, aiming for an INR below 2.5 at the time of surgery and starting heparin prophylaxis postoperatively.

Patients with artificial heart valves present the greatest problems. A suggested approach is to have the INR below 2.5 at the time of surgery, then to fully anticoagulate the patient with heparin (APTT ratio 2) until warfarin can be restarted. The advantage of heparin is that it can be more rapidly reversed if significant bleeding occurs.

Plan of management:

1. Check INR and platelet count.
2. If INR <2.5 withhold warfarin and proceed with surgery.
3. If INR >2.5 withhold warfarin and give coagulation factor concentrate, e.g. HTDEFIX, dose 50 IU FIX/kg, or give fresh frozen plasma 10 ml/kg. If warfarin is not to be continued postoperatively give vitamin K 5–10 mg i.v. Check INR – if below 2.5 proceed with surgery.
4. Restart warfarin 24–48 hours postoperatively when satisfied with haemostasis. If concerned about haemostasis consider using i.v. heparin which can be rapidly reversed.

15.6.2.3 Acute haemolytic crisis

An acute haemolytic crisis, with rapidly increasing pallor, anaemia and icterus, may be associated with abdominal pain and tenderness. There is usually some fever, headache and pain in the back, which improve with blood transfusion.

15.6.3 OTHER CONDITIONS

Polycythemia vera is characteristically plethora, cyanosis and splenomegaly. Headache is troublesome. When the PCV rises above 55% infarcts are likely to occur as a result of spontaneous thrombosis. These may affect the spleen, or mesenteric vessels, with consequent acute abdominal complications.

Patients with neutropenia due, for instance, to chemotherapy may develop 'neutropenic typhlitis' (p. 544).

In all these situations, early and continuing cooperation with a haematologist is vital.

15.7 VASCULITIS

Vasculitis interferes with circulation in small vessels and the consequent complications of haemorrhage and visceral perforation can be the first sign of systemic lupus erythematosus (SLE) and polyarteritis nodosa (PAN). In PAN there is necrosis of the media of arterioles, with consequent formation of small aneurysms. In SLE there is vasculitis of small arteries and veins leading to thrombosis and focal ischaemia (Stoddard *et al.*, 1978).

These conditions are uncommon, and do not often cause acute abdominal disease. They appear in three forms:

- **Haemoperitoneum**. A ruptured aneurysm on a mesenteric arteriole can rupture and cause abdominal swelling and increasing signs of internal haemorrhage.

- **Intestinal perforation**. Thrombosis of mesenteric arterioles can lead to necrosis and perforation of bowel. Zizic *et al.* (1982) saw six perforations due to SLE and five due to PAN, affecting both large and small bowel. In our only experience of this, a man of 31 had been unwell for several weeks and then suddenly felt epigastric pain and showed signs of general peritonitis. He had a perforation of the stomach and microscopy of stomach and omentum showed arteritis with medial necrosis.
- **Intestinal haemorrhage**. The vasculitis may lead to necrosis of the mucosa and brisk haemorrhage into the lumen of the bowel.

When recovery follows closure or resection of affected bowel, these patients require long-term treatment with chemotherapy and corticosteroids.

Henoch–Schönlein purpura (p. 117) is due to vasculitis in small vessels, often secondary to streptococcal infection in young people.

15.8   THE IMMUNOCOMPROMISED PATIENT

This group now includes a considerable number of patients – those receiving **chemotherapy** (either for malignant disease, or as an element of organ and bone marrow transplantation), or on long-term **corticosteroids**, or patients with **HIV/AIDS**.

Opportunistic infections of the gastrointestinal tract, causing pain and diarrhoea, and the problems of Kaposi's sarcoma in AIDS patients have been referred to in Chapter 2.

Transplantation surgery is associated with some general surgical complications. Steed *et al.* (1985) reviewed 143 patients undergoing heart and heart–lung transplantation; 40 suffered surgical complications, including ten who needed a laparotomy, mostly for intestinal perforation and ulceration, and others had pancreatitis. These occurred as long as 21 months after the operation and were presumably due to the effects of immunosuppressive drugs.

The **ileocaecal syndrome**, or neutropenic enterocolitis or typhlitis, is particularly seen during chemotherapy for the leukaemias, and it has also been seen in HIV patients. Inflammation and ulceration of the ileocaecal angle and ascending colon presents with signs of RLQ tenderness, sometimes a mass, and sometimes peritonitis due to perforation. CT scanning and laparoscopy can be very helpful in diagnosis.

Initial management consists of intravenous fluids, and broad-spectrum antibiotics, which should be given in an intensive care unit. Careful active observation by the same surgeon is essential, because some of these patients resolve on watchful conservative management. Parenteral nutrition may be needed. In some patients signs of peritonitis due to perforation develop and then resection with ileostomy and a mucous fistula will probably be safest. The subject is well reviewed by Williams and Scott (1997).

15.9   DISEASES OF THE NERVOUS SYSTEM

Meningitis occasionally presents with acute abdominal pain and tenderness in the RLQ. There may be several hours delay before headache and neck stiffness appear.

Herpes zoster in the pre-eruption stage can be difficult to detect unless it is recognized that the pain is of nerve-root distribution. There may be erythema of overlying skin, but it may be several days before the eruption appears.

Anterior poliomyelitis can present with severe abdominal pain and vomiting in the preparalytic stage. There is often headache, and some neck stiffness can suggest a neurological disease.

Tabes dorsalis, with its attacks of epigastric pain and vomiting, is hardly ever seen. Absent knee jerks and pupils that react to accommodation but not to light will be found.

It must be remembered that patients who are **paraplegic** through spinal injury or nervous disease can become seriously constipated, and occasionally **stercoral ulceration** will occur.

15.10   TOXIC CAUSES

A wide variety of substances can cause severe abdominal pain, vomiting and collapse. Arsenic, copper, mercury and chromium are acutely toxic to the alimentary tract, as are organophosphates, poisonous fungi and the bites of some snakes and scorpions.

Lead intoxication is of more gradual onset. Mann (1962) found 61 patients in the West of Scotland in the 1950s; 12 were admitted to surgical wards with severe colic and abdominal tenderness and guarding, of whom six had a laparotomy. A good history can reveal the vital fact that the patient works with lead and this was true of five of the six operated upon. There may be signs of wrist- and foot-drop. The blue lead line on the gums is rarely seen but the blood film shows punctate basophilia.

For emergency treatment intravenous sodium/calcium edetate (75 mg/kg daily for 5 days) is helpful.

REFERENCES

Anscombe, A. R. (1970) Surgery in haemophilia and allied disorders. *Ann. R. Coll. Surg. Engl.*, **47**, 125–138.

Campbell, I. W., Duncan, L. J. P., Innes, J. A. *et al.* (1975) Abdominal pain in diabetic metabolic decompensation. *J.A.M.A.*, **233**, 166–168.

Clark, O. H., Hall, A. D. and Schambelan, M. (1974) Clinical manifestations of adrenal haemorrhage. *Am. J. Surg.*, **128**, 219–224.

Davies, S. C. and Oni, L. (1997) Management of patients with sickle cell disease. *BMJ.*, **315**, 656–660.

Fitz-Hugh, T. (1934) Acute gonoccic perihepatitis of the right upper quadrant in women. *J.A.M.A.*, **102**, 2094–2096.

Goldberg, A. (1959) Acute intermittent porphyria: a study of 50 cases. *Q. J. Med.*, NS **28**, 183–209.

Heller, H., Sohar, E. and Sherf, L. (1958) Familial Mediterranean Fever. *Arch. Intern. Med.*, **102**, 50–71.

Leahy, A. L., Fogarty, E. E., Fitzgerald, R. J. *et al.* (1984) Discitis as a cause of abdominal pain in children. *Surgery*, **95**, 412–414.

MacSween, R. N. (1960) Acute abdominal crisis, circulatory collapse and sudden death in haemochromatosis. *Q. J. Med.*, NS **35**, 589–598.

Mann, T. S. (1962) Lead intoxication in the surgical wards. *Scot. Med. J.*, **7**, 36–41.

Rizza, C. R. (1994) Haemophilia and related inherited coagulation defects, in *Haemostasis and Thrombosis*, (eds A. L. Bloom, C. D. Forbes, D. P. Thomas *et al.*), Churchill Livingstone, Edinburgh, pp 819–841.

Shanahan, D., Lord, P. H., Grogono, J. *et al.* (1988) Clinical acute cholecystitis and the Curtis–Fitz-Hugh syndrome. *Ann. R. Coll. Surg. Engl.*, **70**, 44–46.

Steed, D. L., Brown, B., Reilly, J. J. *et al.* (1985) General surgical complications in heart-lung transplantations. *Surgery*, **98**, 739–744.

Stoddard, C. J., Kay, P. H., Simms, J. M. *et al.* (1978) Acute abdominal complications of systemic lupus erythematosus. *Br. J. Surg.*, **65**, 625–628.

Valerio, D. (1976) Acute diabetic abdomen in childhood. *Lancet*, **i**, 66–68.

Williams, N. and Scott, A. D. N. (1997) Neutropenic colitis: a continuing surgical challenge. *Br. J. Surg.*, **84**, 1200–1205.

Wood, J. J., Bolton, J. P., Connon, S. R. *et al.* (1982) Biliary-type pain as a manifestation of genital tract infection: the Curtis–Fitz-Hugh syndrome. *Br. J. Surg.*, **69**, 251–253.

Zizic, T. M., Classen, J. N. and Stevens, M. B. (1982) Acute abdominal complications of systemic lupus erythematosus and polyarteritis nodosa. *Am. J. Med.*, **73**, 525–531.

Index